Handbook of Nutritional Disorders

Handbook of Nutritional Disorders is a comprehensive handbook covering topics in nutrition, malnutrition, and clinical disorders associated with nutrition, from deficiency to toxicity. It includes information on carbohydrate, lipid, and protein metabolism disorders and vitamin and mineral abnormalities. The book details various types of supplements, feeding methods, and therapies for many specific patients. It aims to educate readers on ways to prevent disorders resulting from all kinds of malnutrition and their potentially severe complications.

Features

- Strong focus on diabetes, featuring information on various forms of the disease and treatment methods.
- Detailed discussion of lipids and related disorders – cardiovascular disease being the most frequent cause of death – informing users on the prevention and treatment of hypertension, myocardial infarction, and stroke.
- Contains information on selective nutritional disorders, including obesity, dehydration, imbalances, malabsorption, alcoholism, neuropsychiatric disorders, eating disorders, cancer, and pollutant poisonings.

Written for researchers, academics, and students in healthcare and nutrition, this book educates individuals on the prevention of disorders resulting from all types of malnutrition and their potentially severe complications.

Handbook of
Nutritional Disorders

Jahangir Moini, MD, MPH
Former Professor of Science and Health (retired)
Eastern Florida State College

Katia Ferdowsi, MD, MPH
Lecturer, Department of Health Sciences
University of Central Florida

CRC Press
Taylor & Francis Group
Boca Raton London New York

CRC Press is an imprint of the
Taylor & Francis Group, an **informa** business

Designed cover image: Shutterstock

First edition published in 2025
by CRC Press
2385 NW Executive Center Drive, Suite 320, Boca Raton, FL 33431

and by CRC Press
4 Park Square, Milton Park, Abingdon, Oxon, OX14 4RN

CRC Press is an imprint of Taylor & Francis Group, LLC

© 2025 Taylor & Francis Group, LLC

ISBN: 9781032590806 (hbk)
ISBN: 9781032591810 (pbk)
ISBN: 9781003453376 (ebk)

DOI: 10.1201/9781003453376

Typeset in Times
by codeMantra

Dedication

I dedicate this book to my precious grandchildren: Artemis, Anastasia, Anabelle, and Laila. It is also to my wonderful wife, Hengameh, and beautiful daughters, Mahkameh and Morvarid.

– Jahangir Moini

I dedicate this book to my beloved parents, Pooran and Hassan; my sister Kamila; my brothers, Kambiz and Kamran; my husband, Reza; and my lovely daughter, Donya, who is the whole world to me!

– Katia Ferdowski

Contents

PART I *Introduction*

PART II *Disorders of Carbohydrate Metabolism*

PART III   Disorders of Lipid Metabolism

PART IV   *Disorders of Protein Metabolism*

PART VI   Mineral Deficiency and Toxicity Disorders

PART VII   Selective Nutritional Disorders

Preface

Handbook of Nutritional Disorders is a comprehensive and easy-to-read resource that addresses the importance of combating undernutrition and overnutrition, which affect more than 1 billion people worldwide. Malnutrition is responsible for more than 50% of all childhood deaths, and its effects also include many types of chronic diseases as well as decreased economic productivity. Overnutrition has become a serious global threat to overall health, with more than 35% of the world's population being overweight. In the United States, nearly 70% of the population is overweight. All types of people are affected by malnutrition worldwide, and when it involves children under age 5, it can result in poor growth, delayed development, and lifelong health problems. Pregnant women suffering from malnutrition are more likely to have premature births and severe health complications, and their babies have an incidence of congenital disabilities. Malnutrition is a worldwide health crisis that must be addressed seriously by all healthcare professionals.

This book addresses the widespread need to fill the gap in malnutrition resources. It contains detailed information about the prevalence of nutritional disorders and epidemics. It discusses dietary requirements and focuses on populations most affected by nutritional disorders and individual nutritional effects on various body systems. It also focuses on clinical treatments and costs. The issues of malnutrition are globally significant for people of all ages, from infants to older people. This book provides detailed information about how poor nutrition causes health problems worldwide, often severe and life-threatening.

Handbook of Nutritional Disorders is written in a highly engaging style, offering excellent material flow complemented with numerous figures and tables. Each chapter begins with an overview of the topics discussed. Each section ends with "Check Your Knowledge" questions about the most essential information. The text features practical applications for use in clinical practice.

Additionally, there are "You Should Remember" boxes about specific topics. The book covers significant diseases caused by poor diet and nutrition, offering suggestions for preventing malnutrition by improving diet. The text includes bulleted lists and critical terms. In addition, the book consists of actual clinical case studies, which feature essential questions of thinking. The answers to these questions are provided in Appendix A at the end of the book. In the final part of each chapter is a "Further Reading" section that lists additional sources of information on the topics discussed in this book.

Acknowledgments

The authors appreciate the contributions of everyone who assisted in creating this book, including T&F Senior Editor Randy Brehm, Editorial Assistant Tom Connelly, Production Editor Iris Fahrer, Project Manager Vinodhini Kumaran, and Greg Vadimsky.

About the Authors

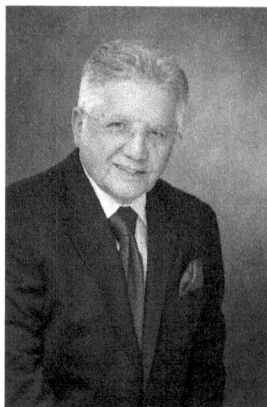

Dr. Jahangir Moini was an assistant professor at the Department of Epidemiology and Preventive Medicine, Tehran University Medical School, for 9 years. He worked as the Director of Epidemiology for the Brevard County Health Department for 18 years. In addition, he worked as the Director of Science and Health for Everest University in Melbourne, FL, for 15 years. Furthermore, he worked as a professor of science and health at Everest for 24 years and at Eastern Florida State College for 6 years, respectively, but he is now retired. Dr. Moini has been an international author for 25 years and has written 58 books. His *Anatomy & Physiology for Healthcare Professionals* was translated and released in Japan and South Korea in 2020. His *Complications of Diabetes Mellitus* was translated into Spanish in 2023.

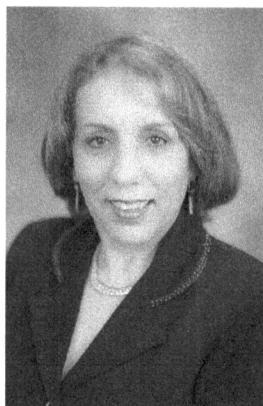

Dr. Katia Ferdowsi is a lecturer at the Department of Health Sciences, University of Central Florida. She holds a medical degree from Azad University, Tehran Medical Branch, and a Master of Public Health degree from Shiraz University of Medical Sciences in Iran, where she also completed her residency in community medicine. She is a coauthor of two books.

Part I

Introduction

1 Healthy Nutrition

OVERVIEW

Healthy eating refers to foods that give individuals the nutrients they need to maintain their health, feel good, and have energy. Proteins, carbohydrates, fats, water, vitamins, and minerals include these nutrients. Two areas we have the most control over are our diet and exercise. These can significantly affect the overall health and be some of the main factors in preventing disease and other complications later in life. A proper diet and regular exercise are helpful for preventive measures. Nutrition is consuming, absorbing, and using nutrients the body needs to grow, develop, and maintain life. To receive adequate nutrition, people must consume a healthy diet consisting of various nutrients – the substances in foods that nourish the body. A healthy diet protects against chronic noncommunicable diseases like heart disease, diabetes, and cancer. Staying healthy is at the top of nearly everyone's priority list, and our daily choices can determine how healthy we are. Not everything is in our control, but our habits and approaches to health can often make a difference between being healthy and unhealthy. Nutrition is a critical part of health and development. Better nutrition is related to improved infant, child, and maternal health; robust immune systems; safer pregnancy and childbirth; lower risk of noncommunicable diseases (such as diabetes and cardiovascular disease); and longevity.

THE ROLE OF NUTRITION

The role of nutrition is to support the everyday health and development of the human body. When food is adequate, people of all ages have better muscular health. The immune system is strengthened, pregnancy and childbirth are safer, fewer noncommunicable diseases, and longevity is improved. Better health from good nutrition also means that learning is enhanced, along with productivity. In most developed nations, federal agencies provide detailed dietary and nutritional recommendations and guidelines. In the United States, the Department of Health and Human Services (HHS) and the Department of Agriculture (USDA) publish an annual report about the latest nutritional guidelines every 5 years. Nutrition requires basic dietary guidelines. These include the following:

- *A variety of vegetables* – including those that are dark green, orange, and red, as well as legumes and starchy vegetables
- *Fat-free or low-fat dairy products* – milk, yogurt, cheese, and fortified soy products
- *Fruits* – especially whole fruits
- *Grains* – especially whole grains
- *Healthy oils*
- *Protein foods* – lean meats, poultry, seafood, legumes, nuts, seeds, and soy products

Additional guidelines focus on the limitations of certain foods. Those recommended to be limited include saturated fats, trans fats, sodium, and added sugars. Various nutrient-dense foods are recommended to be consumed in specific daily amounts across all the guided food groups. The goal is to ensure sufficient carbohydrates, fats, proteins, vitamins, minerals, and water. Therefore, these nutrients can support all body cells and tissues.

Nutrition studies food nutrients, how the body uses them, and the relationships between diet, health, and disease. It also focuses on how humans use dietary choices to reduce disease risks, excessive or deficient nutrients, and allergies. When nutrients are imbalanced in the diet, the risks of certain health conditions increase.

DOI: 10.1201/9781003453376-2

TABLE 1.1

The Roles of Various Nutritional Components

Nutrient	Role
Carbohydrates	Provide a good energy source, plus structural constituents for the formation of cells
Proteins	Required for tissue formation, cell repair, and production of hormones and enzymes; essential for building strong muscles and a healthy immune system
Fats	Provide stored energy; function as structural cellular components and signaling molecules for proper cellular communication; also provide insulation to vital organs and help maintain body temperature
Water	Transports essential nutrients throughout the body as well as waste products for disposal; also aids in body temperature maintenance
Minerals	Regulate body processes; required for normal cell function; also make up body tissues
Vitamins	Regulate body processes while promoting normal body system functions

Macronutrients are nutrients needed in relatively large quantities. They include carbohydrates (sugars, starches, and fibers), proteins (amino acids), fats (lipids), and water. **Micronutrients** are nutrients needed in smaller amounts, which include minerals. The minerals most required by the human body include potassium, sodium, calcium, phosphorus, magnesium, zinc, iron, manganese, copper, and selenium. Vitamins are also needed in small quantities, including water-soluble vitamins (B vitamins and vitamin C) and fat-soluble vitamins (A, D, E, and K) – some nutrients function as *antioxidants*, including vitamins, minerals, proteins, and other molecules. Antioxidants function to remove toxic substances (free radicals, which are also called reactive oxygen species). **Table 1.1** summarizes the roles of various nutritional components.

Registered dietitian nutritionists study food, nutrition, and dietetics. Dietitians work in private and public healthcare, education institutes, corporations, research facilities, and the food industry. Nutritionists can study nutrition independently or through formal education and have fewer qualifications than registered dietitian nutritionists. They often work in the food industry and food science and technology sectors. These professionals work to provide optimal nutrition for their patients to ensure the best possible health, functioning, growth, development, and quality of life.

Check Your Knowledge

1. What are the primary dietary guidelines for good nutrition?
2. What types of foods must be limited to achieve good nutrition?
3. What are macronutrients and micronutrients?

HEALTH PROMOTION

Health promotion is the process of enabling humans to increase control over and improve their health. The World Health Organization (WHO) has established health promotion conferences to increase power and improve global health. Therefore, health promotion focuses on individual behaviors and a more comprehensive range of social and environmental interventions. It includes concentrating on quitting smoking, increasing access to healthy foods, increasing physical activity, preventing excessive alcohol use, promoting lifestyle changes and disease management, promoting reproductive health, promoting clinical preventive services, and promoting community water fluoridation. The following three basic health promotion strategies are widely used:

- *Health communication helps us better understand health needs and make crucial individual health decisions.* It encourages healthy activities and improves health literacy while understanding cultural considerations about health. Examples include influenza (flu) vaccination posters, health screening brochures, and heart disease discussions with patients.

- *Health education* teaches about various health conditions to improve preventive methods and early treatments. It is often focused on target populations, such as poorer neighborhoods that lack sufficient ways to learn about nutrition, physical activities, and conditions such as type 2 diabetes mellitus.
- *Policy, systems, and environmental changes* – It focuses on creating smoke-free areas and safety equipment in the workplace, using innovations, technologies, or certifications to change how health problems are managed, and improving living environments with more availability of nutritious food and more recreational areas such as parks.

Health promotion and disease prevention programs focus on keeping people healthy by teaching them about healthy choices and behaviors. Changes that reduce the risks of developing chronic diseases and other **morbidities** can be taught. Disease prevention differs from health promotion because it focuses on specific efforts that help reduce the development and severity of chronic diseases and other morbidities.

In the United States, health promotion is widely encouraged and supported by the Centers for Disease Control and Prevention (CDC), with its Coordinating Center for Health Promotion; the National Institute for Occupational Safety and Health, with its Total Worker Health program; and the United States Army Center for Health Promotion and Preventive Medicine. Nongovernmental organizations involved in health promotion include the Public Health Education and Health Promotion Section (part of the American Public Health Association), the National Commission for Health Education Credentialing, the Wellness Council of America, and the Utilization Review Accreditation Commission. The program known as Healthy People 2030 sets data-driven national objectives to improve health and well-being. It includes 358 objectives as well as developmental and research objectives. These objectives are classified as health conditions, behaviors, populations, settings/systems, and social determinants. The health conditions section includes:

- Addiction
- Arthritis
- Blood disorders
- Cancer
- Chronic kidney disease
- Chronic pain
- Dementias
- Diabetes
- Foodborne illness
- Healthcare-associated infections
- Heart disease and stroke
- Infectious disease
- Mental health and mental disorders
- Oral conditions
- Osteoporosis
- Overweight and obesity
- Pregnancy and childbirth
- Respiratory disease
- Sensory or communication disorders
- Sexually transmitted infections

Health behaviors include child and adolescent development, drug and alcohol use, emergency preparedness, family planning, health communication, injury prevention, nutrition and healthy eating, physical activity, preventive care, safe food handling, sleep, tobacco use, vaccination, and violence prevention. Populations include adolescents, children, infants, LGBT individuals, men, older adults, parents or caregivers, people with disabilities, women, and the workforce.

Settings and systems include the community, environmental health, global health, healthcare, health insurance, health information technology (IT), health policy, hospital and emergency services, housing and homes, public health infrastructure, schools, transportation, and the workplace. Social determinants of health include the following:

- Economic stability
- Education access and quality
- Healthcare access and quality
- Neighborhood and built environment
- Social and community context

Healthy People 2030 includes a vision and mission, foundational principles, overarching goals, and a plan of action. Its framework was based on recommendations from the Secretary's Advisory Committee on National Health Promotion and Disease Prevention Objectives for 2030. Healthy People 2030 addresses personal health literacy and organizational health literacy and defines each of them as follows:

- *Personal health literacy* – the degree to which individuals can find, understand, and use information and services to inform health-related decisions and actions for themselves and others
- *Organizational health literacy* – the degree to which organizations fairly (equitably) enable individuals to find, understand, and use information and services to inform health-related decisions and actions for themselves and others

These new definitions emphasize individuals' abilities to use health information instead of just understanding it. They focus on the ability to make well-informed decisions instead of just appropriate choices and incorporate a public health perspective. These definitions also acknowledge that organizations have a responsibility to address health literacy.

YOU SHOULD REMEMBER

The term "wellness" is related to health promotion and disease prevention. It is defined as attitudes and actively formed decisions that contribute to an individual's positive health behaviors and outcomes. Typical activities for health promotion, disease prevention, and wellness programs include communication (raising awareness), education, and changes in policy, systems, and living and working environments.

Check Your Knowledge

1. What are examples of health promotion?
2. What are the three primary health promotion strategies?
3. What do the social determinants of health include?

FOOD, ENERGY, AND NUTRIENTS

A healthy and balanced diet provides nutrients that the body uses for fuel. The energy produced helps the heartbeat. Usually, the brain remains active, the muscles function precisely, and the bones and other body tissues are built and strengthened. The body needs three significant nutrients for energy: carbohydrates, lipids (fats), and proteins.

ENERGY

Carbohydrates provide energy for the brain, muscles, heart, and lungs. Lipids provide energy, help manufacture the coverings around nerves, and produce some hormones. Proteins provide power and help build and repair cells and tissues. The body needs them to be healthy. A good balance also helps regulate body weight. Carbohydrates, lipids, and proteins are organic, meaning they comprise hydrogen, oxygen, and carbon structures. When **oxidized**, energy is released and becomes available for cells. Although vitamins are also organic, they do not provide power.

The energy released from food is measured in calories or kilocalories (kcal). One calorie is the amount of heat necessary to raise the temperature of 1 g of water by 1°C (0.8°F). Though calories are commonly used, the correct clinical term is *kilocalories*. While carbohydrates and proteins contain 4 kcal/g, lipids provide more than twice the energy at 9 kcal/g. The kcal of any specific food is based on the amount of carbohydrate, lipid, and protein energy it contains. When energy-yielding foods are consumed, other nutrients (vitamins, minerals, and water) are also usually ingested. Though alcohol provides 7 kcal/g, it is not a nutrient since the body does not require it. Moderate consumption of alcohol may be protective against heart disease.

Check Your Knowledge

1. What are the three major nutrients needed for energy?
2. Which major nutrient provides the most kilocalories?

CARBOHYDRATES

Carbohydrates, or carbs, are sugar molecules. Along with proteins and fats, carbohydrates are the primary nutrients in foods and drinks. They are a primary fuel source for the body, consisting of simple and complex carbohydrates, including starches and fibers. Carbohydrates comprise carbon, hydrogen, and oxygen at their chemical level. Food containing carbohydrates is converted into glucose or blood sugar by the digestive system during digestion. **Simple carbohydrates** are found in fruits, milk, and sweeteners such as sugar, honey, and high-fructose corn syrup. **Complex carbohydrates** are found in cereals, fruits, grains, pasta, and vegetables. Except for fiber, all carbohydrates are broken down into glucose units, a simple carbohydrate. Glucose provides the best, most efficient type of energy – especially for the brain and muscles.

Carbohydrates can be *monosaccharides, disaccharides,* or *polysaccharides* (see **Figure 1.1**). These carbohydrates are explained in greater detail below:

- *Monosaccharides* – single units of sugar with examples including glucose, galactose (primarily available in milk and dairy products), and fructose (mostly in fruits and vegetables)
- *Disaccharides* – two joined sugar molecules with examples including lactose (glucose+galactose) found in milk and sucrose (glucose+fructose), which is also known as *table sugar 3*
- *Polysaccharides* – chains of many sugars consisting of hundreds or thousands of monosaccharides; they act as food stores, with examples including **glycogen, starches**, and **cellulose**

Monosaccharides and disaccharides are simple carbohydrates, while polysaccharides are complex carbohydrates. Simple carbohydrates are sugars consisting of one or two molecules. They provide quick energy, but hunger soon returns. Complex carbohydrates have long chains of sugar molecules, maintain fullness for longer, and contain more vitamins, minerals, and fibers.

Types of Carbohydrates

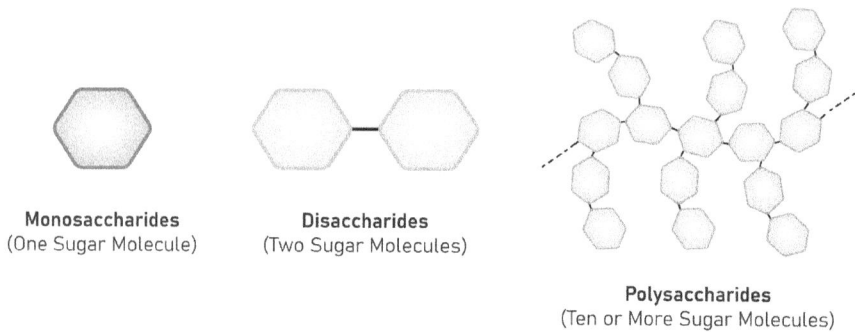

Monosaccharides
(One Sugar Molecule)

Disaccharides
(Two Sugar Molecules)

Polysaccharides
(Ten or More Sugar Molecules)

FIGURE 1.1   Types of carbohydrates.

Fiber is also a type of carbohydrate that the body cannot digest. Though most carbohydrates are broken down into glucose molecules, fiber cannot be broken down into sugar molecules. Instead, it passes through the body undigested, providing no energy. Even so, fiber is required for good health. Dietary fiber benefits the digestive system and the absorption of foods. It helps prevent constipation and may reduce colon cancer and heart disease risks. Fiber is a complex carbohydrate that helps the body to feel full, making overeating less likely. Another benefit is that fiber can help lower cholesterol and blood glucose. It is found in many plant foods, including beans, fruits, nuts, seeds, vegetables, and whole grains.

The most crucial fact about carbohydrates is the *type*, not the quantity. Healthy whole grains such as whole wheat bread, rye, barley, and quinoa are better than highly refined white bread or the fast food favorite item known as French fries. Carbohydrates are widely present in healthy and unhealthy foods, including beans, milk, popcorn, cookies, soft drinks, spaghetti, corn, and fruit pies. The most abundant forms of carbohydrates are sugars, fibers, and starches. Carbohydrates provide the body with glucose needed to support functions and physical activity.

Sugars are simple carbohydrates because they are in the most basic form. They include types that are found naturally in fruits, milk, and vegetables. However, they can also be added to candy, desserts, processed foods, and sodas. Starches are complex carbohydrates made of a large amount of connected simple sugars. The body must break starches down into sugars to use them to generate energy. Examples of starches include bread, cereals, and pasta. Also, some vegetables contain starches, including corn, peas, and potatoes.

The healthiest sources of carbohydrates are unprocessed or slightly processed beans, fruits, vegetables, and whole grains. They promote good health by delivering fiber, **phytonutrients**, minerals, and vitamins. Poorer and less healthy sources of carbohydrates include pastries, sodas, white bread, and other highly processed or refined foods. They contain easily digested carbohydrates, contributing to weight gain, slowing weight loss, and promoting heart disease and diabetes mellitus.

YOU SHOULD REMEMBER

The Healthy Eating Plate should be used to balance the diet, and half of the plate should be filled with healthy carbohydrates such as vegetables (but not potatoes) and fruits. Whole grains should fill up about one-fourth of the scale, and the final fourth should be healthy proteins. Each day should start with whole grains; lunch or snacks should utilize whole-grain bread. Instead of bread, brown rice or quinoa should be included. Whole fruits are much better than fruit juices, usually highly sweetened. Beans and other legumes are excellent sources of slowly digested carbohydrates.

Generally, the amount of carbohydrates that should be consumed varies based on age, gender, health, and whether an individual wants to lose or gain weight. On average, 45%–65% of daily calories should come from carbohydrates. On the *Nutrition Facts* labels, based on a 2,000-calorie diet per day, the daily value is 275 grams of carbohydrates (containing 900 to 1,300 calories). Some people use low-carbohydrate diets to lose weight, consuming between 25 g and 150 g of carbs daily. While this may be safe, a healthcare provider should always be consulted before starting the diet since it can limit the amount of fiber consumed and may be hard to follow over the long term.

The **glycemic index** classifies carbohydrate-containing foods according to their ability to increase blood glucose. Weight-loss diets based on the glycemic index usually suggest limiting foods that are higher on the index. These foods include potatoes, white bread, and snacks or desserts containing refined flour. Many healthy foods, such as whole grains, legumes, fruits, vegetables, and low-fat dairy products, are lower on the glycemic index.

Carbohydrates are the body's primary fuel sources; during digestion, starches and sugars are broken down into simple sugars and absorbed into the bloodstream. From the blood, glucose enters cells with the help of insulin. Extra glucose is stored in the liver and muscles or converted to fat. Excessive consumption of carbohydrates can increase blood glucose so much that **hyperglycemia** develops, which is a risk factor for diabetes. If insufficient carbs are consumed, *hypoglycemia* may result.

YOU SHOULD REMEMBER

The American Heart Association recommends the following rules concerning carbohydrates: limit foods that are high in processed, refined simple sugars that provide calories but very little nutrition; get more complex carbohydrates and healthy nutrients by eating more fruits and vegetables; and focus on whole-grain rice, bread, and cereals while consuming beans, lentils, and dried peas.

The brain is the only carbohydrate-dependent organ in the body. It exclusively uses glucose to function, and brain cells need twice the energy of any other cells in the body. Only some animal products contain carbs, such as the lactose in milk and other dairy products, a disaccharide (sugar). The term *carbohydrate* means "carbon" plus "hydrate" (hydrogen plus oxygen). Carbohydrates are the only fuel source metabolized quickly enough to support extreme exercise. When an individual begins a low-carb diet, there is dramatic weight loss initially, but this is usually water weight. The body calls on its reserves when low amounts of carbs are provided. Glycogen is released and bound up significantly in water. As the body burns through the glycogen, the water is also removed. Overall, carbohydrates are the most critical energy source for the body. It stores carbs in reserves so that the body must use them, even if they are reduced in the diet.

Check Your Knowledge

1. What provides the most efficient type of energy for the body?
2. What are the healthiest sources of carbohydrates?
3. What are the brief descriptions of monosaccharides, disaccharides, and polysaccharides?

LIPIDS

Lipids are fatty compounds that perform a variety of functions in the body. They are the most source form of energy in foods and as stored energy in the body. Lipids also play roles in forming cell membranes and help control what goes in and out of the cells. They help move and store energy, absorb vitamins, and produce hormones. Having too much lipids is harmful. Dietary lipids contain

essential fatty acids and fat-soluble vitamins. Lipids help improve the tastes of foods in which they are present and are divided into the following categories:

- *Triglycerides* are esters formed from glycerol and three fatty acid groups. They are the main constituents of natural fats and oils, and their high concentrations in the blood indicate an increased risk of stroke.
- *Phospholipids* are a type of lipid molecule that is the main component of the cell membrane. Lipids include fats, waxes, and some vitamins, among others. Each phospholipid comprises two fatty acids, a phosphate group, and a glycerol molecule. When many phospholipids line up, they form a double layer characteristic of all cell membranes.
- *Sterols* are isoprenoid-derived lipids with essential roles in cell structure, function, and physiology. As crucial components of biological membranes, sterols interact with phospholipids and proteins within the membrane, thereby regulating membrane fluidity, permeability, and membrane protein functions.

Lipids are essential components of cell membranes, and the fundamental structure of the membrane is the **phospholipid bilayer**, which forms a stable barrier between two aqueous compartments. In the case of the plasma membrane, these compartments are the inside and the outside of the cell: the two fatty acid tails (**hydrophobic**) and a phosphate group (**hydrophilic**). Phospholipids are **amphipathic (see Figure 1.2)**. There are two types of fatty acids. **Saturated fatty acids** are hydrocarbon chains that are linear and unbranched. This indicates the number of hydrogen molecules bonded to each carbon. Saturated fats are found as solids at average room temperature and pressure. They are also called "bad fats" because they can cause health hazards such as arterial blockage and cancer when consumed.

At the same time, **unsaturated fatty acids** have one or multiple carbon-carbon double bonds. This suggests that a few hydrogen molecules are bonded to each carbon. Unsaturated fats are liquid at average room temperature and pressure. They are extracted from natural, healthy sources, such as nuts. They are called "good fats."

Both **lecithin** and **cholesterol** are consumed in food and manufactured by the body. Fatty acids are carbon chains with different lengths and amounts of hydrogen saturation. Saturated fats are

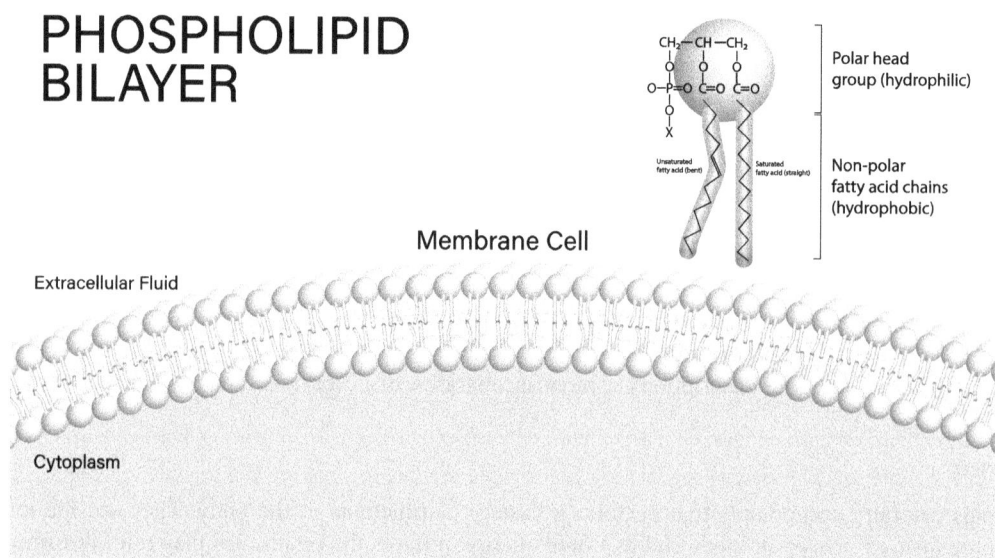

FIGURE 1.2   The cell membrane structure showing the phospholipid bilayer.

found in various fat-containing foods, and **trans fats** come from processed fats. These types of fats, along with dietary cholesterol, are linked to increased blood lipid levels. Increased blood lipids from any source result in risk factors for coronary artery disease. Since cancer and coronary artery disease are among the illnesses that claim the highest number of lives, it is essential to consume better types of fats and only moderate amounts of cholesterol. The six functions of lipids are as follows:

- Energy storage and production
- Chemical messengers
- Cholesterol formation
- Body temperature regulation
- Formation of **prostaglandin**
- Membrane lipid layer formation

Fatty acids, triglycerides, **glycerophospholipids**, **sphingolipids**, and steroids are divided into simple and complex lipids. Fats may be esters or oils. Esters are made up of glycerol and fatty acids, while oils are fats that are in a liquid form. Waxes are esters of fatty acids with monohydric alcohols and higher molecular weight. They have more than just alcohol and fatty acid inside them. Waxes are usually produced as a source of protection, such as ear wax, which protects against dust and germs. Glycolipids (glycosphingolipids) are lipids with fatty acids, sphingosine, and carbohydrates. Other complex lipids include **sulfolipids** and amino lipids. **Lipoproteins** also belong to this group. Steroids have cholesterol, various hormones, and the plant pigment **chlorophyll**. The body produces hormones such as testosterone and estrogen via cholesterol.

There are several different types of cholesterol based on various types of lipoproteins: **very low-density lipoproteins** (VLDLs), **low-density lipoproteins** (LDLs), and **high-density lipoproteins** (HDLs). Those with the lowest density are **chylomicrons**, which transport absorbed lipids from the gastrointestinal (GI) tract. The primary source of VLDLs is the liver. They transport triglycerides from the liver to the peripheral tissues – primarily the fatty tissues. Once the triglycerides are "unloaded," the remaining lipoproteins are called LDLs and are rich in cholesterol. LDLs also transport cholesterol to peripheral tissues so that cells can synthesize membranes or hormones or store them to be used later.

Most cells (besides hepatic and intestinal cells) obtain most of the cholesterol they require for membrane synthesis from the blood. A cell that needs cholesterol makes membrane receptor proteins for LDLs. LDLs bind to the receptors and are engulfed by endocytosis. Endocytotic vesicles fuse with lysosomes, where cholesterol is freed up to be used. When excessive cholesterol gathers in a cell, it reduces the cell's cholesterol synthesis plus the synthesis of LDL receptors.

HDLs are rich in phospholipids and proteins. Their primary function is to gather and transport excess cholesterol from the peripheral tissues back to the liver, which can be broken down and sent to bile. The liver manufactures protein envelopes of HDL particles, ejecting them into the bloodstream in collapsed form. Once in the blood, the incomplete HDL particles fill up cholesterol from tissue cells and arterial walls. HDLs also provide steroid-producing organs, such as the adrenal glands and ovaries, with their needed cholesterol.

In adults, a good total cholesterol level is below 200 mg/deciliter of blood. Levels above this are associated with atherosclerosis, clogging arteries and causing strokes and heart attacks. Clinically, it is more important to determine the various subtypes of cholesterol rather than total cholesterol. High levels of HDLs are considered to be good because the cholesterol is soon degraded. HDL levels above 60 mg/dL protect against heart disease, while below 40 mg/dL are undesirable. Generally, average HDL levels are 40–50 mg/dL in men and 50–60 mg/dL in women. For LDL, 160 mg/dL levels are considered undesirable. When LDLs are excessive, cholesterol deposits in arterial walls can lead to death. Cholesterol and hypercholesterolemia are discussed in greater detail in **Chapter 5**.

Check Your Knowledge

1. What are the descriptions of triglycerides, phospholipids, and sterols?
2. What are the differences between saturated fatty acids and unsaturated fatty acids?
3. What are the impacts of saturated fats and trans fats on health?

PROTEINS

Proteins are highly complex substances present in all living organisms. They are of great nutritional value and are directly involved in the chemical processes essential for life. They perform a wide range of functions involved in the structure of bones, enzymes, muscles, blood, hormones, cell membranes, and the immune system. A protein molecule is enormous compared with molecules of sugar or salt and consists of many amino acids joined together to form long chains, much like beads arranged on a string. To create all of the proteins required for life, 20 amino acids are needed. The body forms some amino acids but does not produce the essential amino acids that must be consumed in the diet. There are nine essential amino acids: histidine, isoleucine, leucine, lysine, methionine, phenylalanine, threonine, tryptophan, and valine. The **nonessential amino acids** are alanine, asparagine, aspartic acid, glutamic acid, and serine. There are also conditional amino acids, which include arginine, cysteine, glutamine, glycine, proline, and tyrosine. Some experts recognize a 21st amino acid called selenocysteine, derived from **serine,** when protein biosynthesis occurs.

Animal sources of amino acids and proteins include meats (fish and poultry) and dairy products such as milk and cheese. Plant sources include grains, legumes, nuts, seeds, and numerous vegetables (though vegetable protein is in lesser amounts). Though required for nutrition, excessive dietary proteins may be harmful as they can lead to overworking physical systems. Excessive proteins are broken down into amino acids, used for energy, or broken down further as part of metabolic processes and then stored as body fat or excreted via the kidneys in the urine.

Proteins exist in every cell of the body. They are the most satiating macronutrients, which explains why high-protein diets help promote weight loss and maintenance. The body is unable to store proteins, unlike carbohydrates and lipids. A protein's lifespan is only two days in the body, yet about one-fifth of body weight is proteins. Regarding protein content in fish, yellowfin tuna contains the most (about 30 g per 100 g serving), followed by anchovies (29 g), salmon (27 g), halibut (27 g), snapper (26 g), and tilapia (26 g). Low-sodium parmesan cheese has the highest sodium content (41.6 g per 100 g serving). Pumpkin seeds have the highest sodium content (33 g per 100 g serving).

Check Your Knowledge

1. What are essential amino acids?
2. What are some animal and plant sources of proteins?
3. Which foods have the highest sources of protein?

VITAMINS

Vitamins help other nutrients during digestion, absorption, metabolism, and excretion. The human body requires 13 different vitamins, each with a specific function. These include water-soluble and fat-soluble vitamins. Water-soluble vitamins dissolve in water, while fat-soluble vitamins dissolve in fats. The following are the 13 required vitamins:

- Water-soluble vitamins:
  - Vitamin B1 – thiamine – plays a vital role in the growth and function of various cells.
  - Vitamin B2 – riboflavin – helps reduce oxidative stress and inflammation of nerves.
  - Vitamin B3 – niacin – helps the body use food energy and keeps the nervous, digestive, and integumentary systems healthy.

- Vitamin B5 – pantothenic acid – is required to make coenzyme A (CoA), which helps enzymes build and break down fatty acids.
- Vitamin B6 – pyridoxine – is required for the body to utilize energy and produce red blood cells and for proper nerve function.
- Vitamin B7 – biotin – is needed to metabolize carbohydrates, fats, and amino acids.
- Vitamin B9 – folate or folic acid – helps form DNA and RNA and is involved in protein metabolism.
- Vitamin B12 – cobalamin – is needed to form red blood cells and DNA, function, and develop brain and nerve cells.
- Vitamin C – ascorbic acid – is required to form blood vessels, cartilage, muscle, and collagen and is vital for healing.
- Fat-soluble vitamins:
  - Vitamin A – retinol or retinoic acid – increases skin cell production, exfoliates the skin, and increases collagen production.
  - Vitamin D – calciferol – helps the body absorb calcium and phosphorus.
  - Vitamin E – tocopherol or alpha-tocopherol – boosts the immune system, helps prevent blood clots, and prevents cell damage caused by free radicals.
  - Vitamin K – phylloquinone or menaquinones – helps make proteins for blood clotting and building bones.

Vitamins are found in many foods, with fruits and vegetables being among the best sources. Since certain foods contain more quantities of specific vitamins, a variety of foods should be consumed regularly to get the best and most complete vitamin content. **Table 1.2** summarizes the best food sources for each vitamin.

TABLE 1.2
The Best Food Sources of Each Vitamin

Vitamin	Best Food Sources
B1	Organ meats, eggs, nuts, seeds, whole grains, enriched grains, legumes, peas
B2	Eggs, dairy products, organ meats, leafy greens, lean meats, legumes, nuts
B3	Eggs, saltwater fish, poultry, enriched and whole grains, legumes, avocados, potatoes
B5	Cabbage-family vegetables (broccoli, cabbage, brussels sprouts, kale), eggs, organ meats, poultry, milk, mushrooms, legumes, lentils, white and sweet potatoes, whole grains
B6	Meat and poultry, nuts, whole grains, avocados, bananas, legumes
B7	Chocolate, egg yolks, legumes, nuts, dairy milk, organ meats, pork, yeast
B9	Asparagus, broccoli (and other cabbage-family greens), leafy greens, beets, yeast, fortified grains, lentils, oranges, wheat germ, peanuts
B12	Eggs, dairy products, poultry, beef, pork, shellfish, organ meats, fortified foods
C	Citrus fruits, mangos, papayas, kiwi, pineapple, cantaloupe, berries, broccoli, brussels sprouts, cabbage, lettuce, turnip greens, spinach, collard greens, cauliflower, sweet potatoes, winter squash, red and green peppers, tomatoes
A	Eggs, organ meats, fish, fortified milk and cereals, carrots, sweet potatoes, bell peppers, cantaloupe, squash, mangos (and other red, yellow, and orange plant foods), dark leafy greens (such as kale, spinach, arugula), broccoli
D[a]	Fatty fish, egg yolks, beef liver, mushrooms, fortified milk, cheese made with fortified milk, fortified foods (orange juice, cereal, soy milk, yogurt)
E	Peanuts, almonds, hazelnuts, pumpkin seeds, sunflower seeds, wheat germ oil, safflower oil, sunflower oil, soybean oil, leafy green vegetables, mangos, avocados, asparagus, red bell pepper, fortified foods
K	Eggs, poultry, pork, beef, organ meats, leafy green vegetables, broccoli, cabbage, brussels sprouts, cauliflower

[a]*Note:* Sunshine is the best source of vitamin D, and it is hard to get enough vitamin D from food sources alone.

MINERALS

Minerals are found in body fluids and have structural functions, such as in the bones and teeth. They affect fluids, influencing muscle function and the central nervous system. The 16 essential minerals are classified as either significant minerals *(macrominerals)* or **trace elements** *(microminerals)* based on the quantities that the body needs. However, it is essential to understand that all minerals are equally important regardless of the amount. The 17 essential minerals include:

- *Major minerals* – needed in amounts of 100 mg to 1 g
  - Calcium
  - Phosphorus
  - Magnesium
  - Sodium
  - Potassium
  - Chloride
  - Sulfur
- *Trace elements* – required in much smaller amounts
  - Iron
  - Iodine
  - Manganese
  - Zinc
  - Copper
  - Fluoride
  - Cobalt
  - Molybdenum
  - Selenium
  - Chromium

Minerals are found in many dairy products, fruits, legumes, meats, and vegetables. Though they are generally hard to degrade, some are lost during food processing. One good example is when whole wheat flour is processed or refined to white flour. This results in phosphorus and potassium, two essential minerals, being lost and not replaced.

Calcium is essential for bone and teeth formation. It also aids in blood clotting, maintaining normal muscle and heart rhythm, and keeps many enzymes in the body functioning normally. Like calcium, phosphorus is essential for the formation of bones and teeth. It is also vital to energy production and is used to form nucleic acids like DNA. Phosphorus, like calcium, is essential for bone and tooth health and metabolizing energy. Without phosphorous, the body cannot turn food into power and strength. Phosphorus is vital to kidney and liver function. Foods high in phosphorus are also usually high in protein. Dairy, beef, chicken, and even cola beverages have a high phosphorus content.

Like calcium and phosphorus, the body requires magnesium to form bones and teeth. Magnesium is also necessary to keep nerves and muscles functioning normally and to activate various enzymes. Magnesium is the seventh most abundant element in the body, following calcium, phosphorus, sulfur, potassium, sodium, and chlorine. About 70% of magnesium is present in the bones and teeth. The remainder is found in the soft tissues and extracellular fluids. Magnesium plays a significant role in maintaining the electrical potential across muscle and nerve membranes. The master molecule of the body is DNA, which is involved in protein synthesis and uses magnesium in protein formation. Magnesium is essential in storing and releasing chemicals in the adenosine diphosphate/triphosphate energy system. Consequently, magnesium is stored in large quantities in the mitochondria, the powerhouse of body cells.

The most significant electrolyte minerals in body fluids are sodium and potassium. Sodium is necessary for maintaining proper nerve and muscle function. Most human sodium requirements are obtained from sodium chloride (table salt). The Recommended Daily Amount (RDA) for table salt varies considerably based on climate conditions, body temperature, exercise, disease conditions, and renal function. The RDA for an adult in a **temperate climate** is about 500 mg.

Balancing electrolytes requires potassium, much like sodium. Potassium is also essential for proper nerve and muscle function. Potassium and sodium play significant roles in water metabolism. Sodium is the major component of the cations of extracellular fluids. Just as calcium and magnesium interact, sodium and potassium closely interact with macro minerals. Chlorine is an essential mineral, functioning as a crucial electrolyte. The chloride ion participates with sodium, potassium, bicarbonate, and carbonic acid, playing a significant role in water metabolism, osmosis, and acid-base balance.

YOU SHOULD REMEMBER

The role of nutrition begins when we are embryos because this is where cellular formation occurs. Therefore, physicians recommend that pregnant women consume many fresh fruits and vegetables rich in micronutrients. A lack of a nutritious diet can lead to fetal death or functional changes in neonatal organs. These babies also have higher risks of cardiovascular disease and poor organ function.

Check Your Knowledge

1. What are the water-soluble and fat-soluble vitamins?
2. What are the seven major minerals?
3. What are the most important electrolyte minerals in body fluids?

WATER

Water is a significant component of every body tissue; humans can only live for a few days without it. It is the most essential nutrient of all. Water breaks down substances so that they can be reformed for use by the body. In the blood, water provides the material in which nutrients are transported to and from cells. Most people need to drink more water daily. Generally, 9–13 cups of water should be consumed daily. This quantity comes from actual servings of water itself and water present in foods and other beverages.

Clinical Case Studies

CLINICAL CASE STUDY 1.1

A 53-year-old woman has a history of type 2 diabetes mellitus, arthritis, hypertension, and hyperlipidemia. She is currently taking a variety of medications for her condition. Examination reveals a 150/92 mm Hg blood pressure and higher-than-normal heart and respiration rates. Laboratory analysis shows high blood glucose, glycosylated hemoglobin, LDL cholesterol, and triglycerides. The patient admits to eating a lot of high-carbohydrate snacks and only walking occasionally due to arthritic pain in her knees. She gets no other form of exercise. At 5'2" tall, she weighs 150 pounds. The patient asks for help turning her life around to lose weight and feel better.

CRITICAL THINKING QUESTIONS

1. What is the description of health education that this patient needs?
2. What is the definition of triglycerides?
3. How do carbohydrates, lipids, and proteins provide energy to the body?

CLINICAL CASE STUDY 1.2

A 45-year-old obese man goes for his annual medical checkup. Though he has no history of coronary artery disease, he had deep vein thrombosis several months previously. His father has a lipid disorder, and his mother had a myocardial infarction at age 51. The patient drinks at least two cans of beer daily and smokes half a pack of cigarettes. His heart rate is elevated, his blood pressure is 145/101 mm Hg, his weight is 299 pounds, and his waist circumference is 43″. He is taking warfarin, hydrochlorothiazide, and a multivitamin with added minerals. Tests reveal he has severe hyperlipidemia, and he admits to enjoying fried and fatty foods much more than healthier alternatives.

CRITICAL THINKING QUESTIONS

1. What does health promotion concentrate on?
2. What are the primary dietary guidelines required for good nutrition?
3. Since this patient is consuming a poor diet, what are the two types of carbohydrates, and in which foods are they found?

CLINICAL CASE STUDY 1.3

A 57-year-old nearly obese woman has been diagnosed with colorectal cancer. No one in her family ever had the condition, and the patient admits to a lifelong preference for red meat. She has always "hated" vegetables and only consumes them in limited quantities. The patient states that she has eaten some red meat nearly every day of her life. While she likes fruits better than vegetables, she also seldom eats them, and many of her food choices are high in fat and low in fiber. She also enjoys processed meats such as smoked pork, deli meats, and bacon. The patient is counseled about the effects of her diet on her health.

CRITICAL THINKING QUESTIONS

1. What is fiber, and in which foods is it found?
2. What are the healthiest sources of carbohydrates?
3. What are the different types of cholesterol?

FURTHER READING

1. Anderson, J.J.B., Root, M.M., and Garner, S.C. (2014). *Human Nutrition: Healthy Options for Life*. Jones & Bartlett Learning.
2. Edelman, C.L., and Kudzma, E.C. (2017). *Health Promotion Throughout the Life Span*, 9th Edition. Mosby.
3. Fertman, C.I., and Grim, M.L. (2021). *Health Promotion Programs: From Theory to Practice*, 3rd Edition. Sophe / Jossey-Bass.
4. Frenn, M., and Whitehead, D.K. (2021). *Health Promotion: Translating Evidence to Practice*. F.A. Davis.
5. Geissler, C., and Powers, H. (2017). *Human Nutrition*, 13th Edition. Oxford University Press.
6. Gropper, S.S., and Smith, J.L. (2012). *Advanced Nutrition and Human Metabolism*, 6th Edition. Cengage Learning.
7. Lanham-New, S.A., Hill, T.R., Gallagher, A.M., and Vorster, H.H. (2019). *Introduction to Human Nutrition (The Nutrition Society Textbook Series)*, 3rd Edition. Wiley Blackwell.

8. Medeiros, D.M., and Wildman, R.E.C. (2018). *Advanced Human Nutrition*, 4th Edition. Jones & Bartlett Learning.
9. Noland, D., Drisko, J.A., and Wagner, L. (2020). *Integrative and Functional Medical Nutrition Therapy: Principles and Practices.* Humana Press.
10. Reeder, A., and Couey, R. (2014). *Nutrition Manual: Discover the Answer to All Your Health Questions.* (Treasures of Health) – Designed Publishing.
11. Rosenthal, J. (2021). *Integrative Nutrition: A Whole-Life Approach to Health and Happiness*, 5th Edition. Integrative Nutrition LLC.
12. Ross, A.C., Caballero, B., Cousins, R.J., Tucker, K.L., and Ziegler, T.R. (2013). *Modern Nutrition in Health and Disease*, 11th Edition. Wolters Kluwer/Lippincott, Williams, and Wilkins.
13. Schiff, W.J., and Keck, T.L. (2021). *Nutrition for Healthy Living*, 6th Edition. McGraw Hill.
14. Spano, M.A., Kruskall, L.J., and Thomas, D.T. (2017). *Nutrition for Sport, Exercise, and Health.* Human Kinetics.
15. Stephenson, T.J., Sanctuary, M.R., and Passerrello, C.W. (2021). *Human Nutrition:* Science for Healthy Living, 3rd Edition. McGraw Hill.
16. Stipanuk, M.H., and Caudill, M.A. (2018). *Biochemical, Physiological, and Molecular Aspects of Human Nutrition*, 4th Edition. Saunders.
17. Sutherland, M. (2023). *The Science of Nutrition and Health.* Sutherland.
18. Willett, W.C., and Skerrett, P.J. (2017). *Eat, Drink, and Be Healthy: The Harvard Medical School Guide to Healthy Eating.* Free Press.

2 Digestion, Absorption, and Metabolism

OVERVIEW

The digestive system, which extends from the mouth to the anus, is responsible for receiving food, breaking it down into nutrients (digestion), absorbing the nutrients into the bloodstream, and eliminating the indigestible parts of food from the body. Digestion is essential because the body needs nutrients from food and drinks to work correctly and stay healthy. A series of steps break down foods into their parts. Various mechanical, electrical, and chemical bonds unite foods. Digestion breaks these bonds and separates the constituents into individual components. Therefore, digestion takes care of the body's various needs for absorption. Absorption is the process of moving nutrients from the intestines into the bloodstream. Most nutrients are absorbed through the small intestine's lining, but water-soluble nutrients are absorbed differently than fats or fat-soluble compounds. Metabolism converts nutrients into forms that can be used or stored and shapes that will be excreted from the body. The sequence of absorption and metabolism is different for different foods. Metabolism is often a multistep process, with one phase occurring in the small intestine and the final step in the liver and other tissues.

THE DIGESTIVE SYSTEM

The digestive system is primarily organized into the *alimentary canal* and the *accessory digestive organs*. It extends from the mouth to the anus. It is responsible for receiving food, breaking it down into nutrients, absorbing the nutrients into the bloodstream, and eliminating the indigestible parts of food from the body.

GASTROINTESTINAL TRACT

The *gastrointestinal tract* (GI tract) is also called the **alimentary canal**. The organs of the GI tract are the mouth, pharynx, esophagus, stomach, small intestine, large intestine, rectum, and anus (see **Figure 2.1**). While alive, the GI tract is about 25 feet (7.62 m) in length because of smooth muscle tone. After death, the loss of muscle tone causes it to lengthen to 30 feet (9 m). The digestive system also includes organs outside the digestive tract, such as the salivary glands, pancreas, liver, and gallbladder.

As food is broken down in the GI tract, nutrients become available to the body. There are six essential activities involved, which include the following (also shown in **Figure 2.2**):

- *Ingestion* – eating; taking of food into the mouth and digestive tract.
- *Propulsion* – voluntary swallowing and involuntary **peristalsis**, with alternating powerful waves of contraction and relaxation of the muscles of the organ walls; food is squeezed through the GI tract and mixed; peristalsis is shown in **Figure 2.3**.
- *Mechanical breakdown (mechanical digestion)* physically prepares food for digestion via **enzymes** and also increases the surface area of food that has been ingested. Automated processes include chewing, mixing food with saliva via the tongue, churning food in the stomach, and **segmentation**, which combines food and digestive juices. This improves absorption by repeatedly moving various portions of food masses over the intestinal wall.

DOI: 10.1201/9781003453376-3

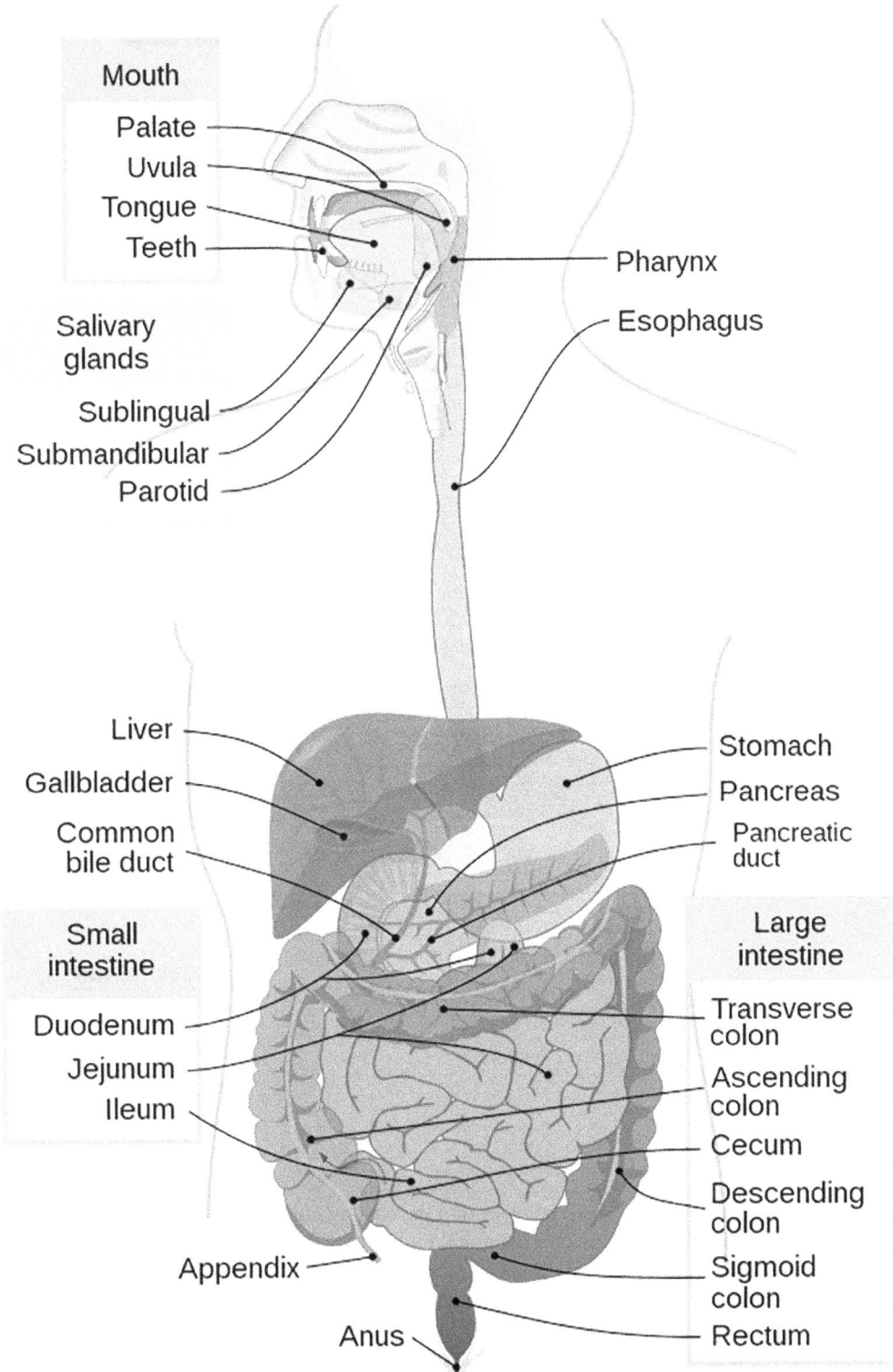

FIGURE 2.1   The alimentary canal (GI tract) and accessory digestive organs.

DIGESTION PROCESSES

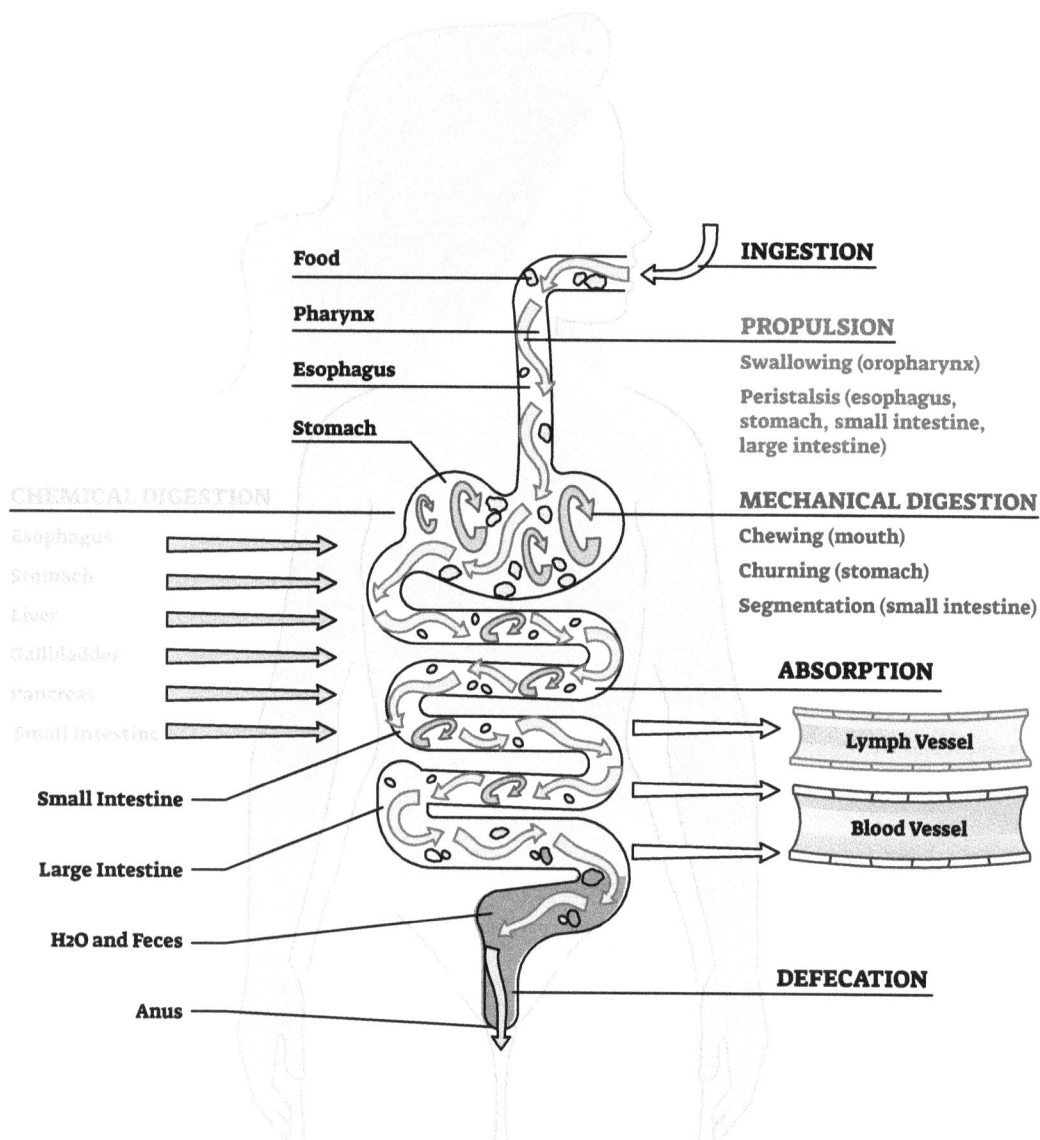

FIGURE 2.2 The six activities of the digestive tract.

- *Chemical digestion* – enzymes secreted into the cavity (lumen) of the GI tract break down complex food molecules into their chemical building blocks, a catabolic process.
- *Absorption* – the passage of digested end products, vitamins, minerals, and water from the GI tract's lumen through **mucosal cells** via active or passive transport into the bloodstream or lymph fluid.
- *Excretion (defecation)* – eliminates substances that cannot be digested from the body, through the anus, such as feces.

PERISTALSIS

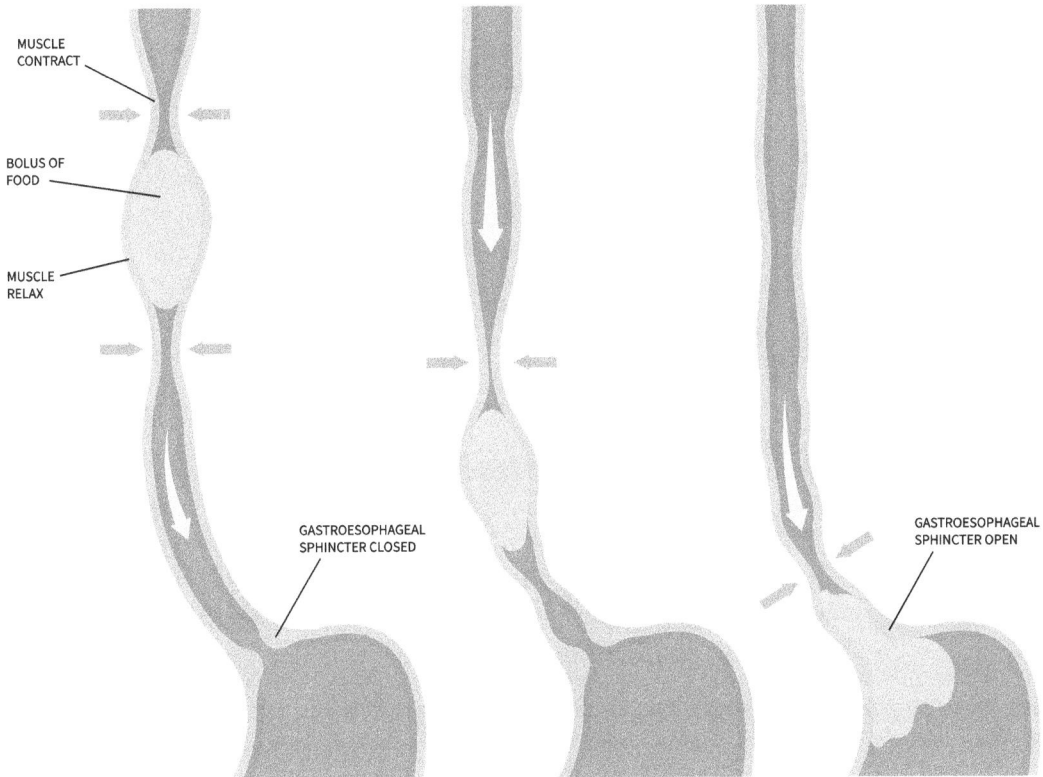

MUSCLE
CONTRACT

BOLUS OF
FOOD

MUSCLE
RELAX

GASTROESOPHAGEAL
SPHINCTER CLOSED

GASTROESOPHAGEAL
SPHINCTER OPEN

FIGURE 2.3   Peristalsis.

While some organs, such as the mouth and anus, have singular functions, most digestive system activities require several organs to work together as the food slowly moves along the tract. Food passes into the **oropharynx** and **laryngopharynx**. Contraction of the pharyngeal constrictor muscles propels food into the esophagus.

Esophagus

A muscular tube of about 10 inches (25 cm) in length: while food moves through the laryngopharynx, the **epiglottis** closes off the larynx so that food will be routed posteriorly into the esophagus. The esophagus pierces the diaphragm at the **esophageal hiatus** and enters the abdomen. It joins the stomach at the **cardiac orifice** in the abdominal cavity. The gastroesophageal sphincter also called the cardiac sphincter, surrounds this orifice. It functions as a sphincter, yet is only evidenced by a slight thickening of the circular smooth muscle nearby. The diaphragm surrounds this sphincter and helps keep it closed when food is not swallowed. The esophagus is protected from stomach acid reflux by mucous cells on both sides of the sphincter.

Deglutition (swallowing) occurs after the tongue has compacted food into a *bolus*. More than 22 muscle groups are implicated. After a food bolus is in the mouth, the phases of deglutition include the *buccal and pharyngeal-esophageal stages*. A bolus or small amount of saliva leaves the mouth, stimulating tactile receptors of the posterior pharynx. The next phase then begins. The pharyngeal-esophageal stage is involuntary and controlled by the brain's medulla and pons (swallowing center). The **vagus nerves** play the most significant role, transmitting motor impulses from the swallowing center to the pharyngeal and esophageal muscles. After entering the pharynx, food causes the respirator to be briefly inhibited. All routes except the one needed into the digestive tract are blocked.

Swallowing

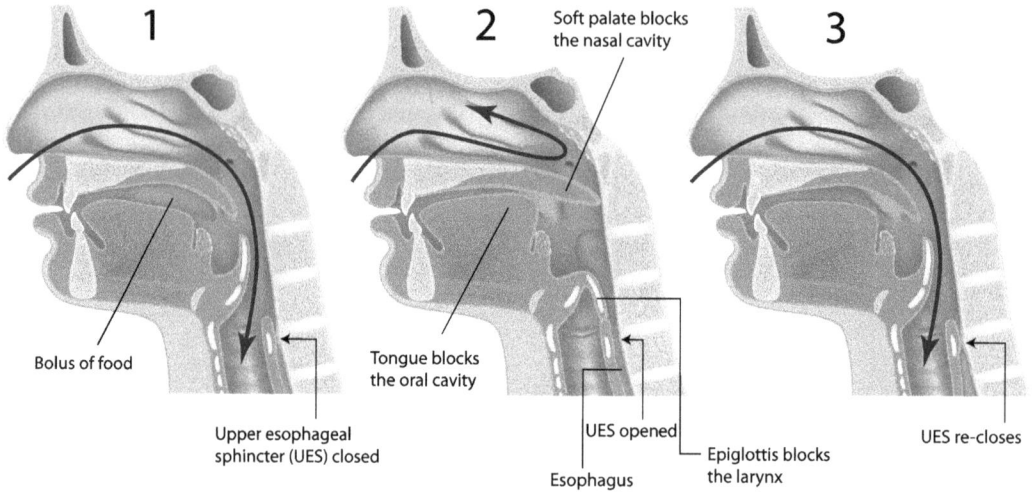

FIGURE 2.4 The processes of deglutition (swallowing).

Solid foods take about 8 seconds to pass from the oropharynx into the stomach. Fluids pass in 1–2 seconds due to the effects of gravity the deglutition (swallowing) processes are shown in (**Figure 2.4**).

Stomach

Below the esophagus, the GI tract expands, forming the stomach. It holds food temporarily and further degrades food with physical and chemical actions. The stomach is the widest part of the digestive system, and it not only digests food but also stores it. It can hold just over 1 L of food at once. It can take 4–6 hours or longer to digest a meal; the higher the fat content, the longer it takes. The food is converted into a thick juice called **chyme**, which is then moved into the small intestine. The stomach lies in the upper left quadrant of the peritoneal cavity, beneath the diaphragm. In adults, the stomach is between 6 and 10 inches long (15–25 cm), with diameter and volume depending on the contained food. When empty, the stomach has a volume of approximately 50 mL. Its cross-sectional diameter is only slightly larger than the large intestine. It can hold up to one gallon (4 L) of food and extend almost to the pelvis when extremely distended. While empty, the stomach collapses inward. The mucosa and submucosa create ample longitudinal folds known as **rugae**.

The small cardia surrounds the cardiac orifice, where food enters the stomach from the esophagus. The fundus is dome-shaped, below the diaphragm, and bulges superolateral toward the cardia. The midportion is called the *body*. It is continuous and inferior to the *pyloric part*, shaped like a funnel. The wider, superior **pyloric antrum** becomes narrowed, forming the **pyloric canal**, which ends at the **pylorus**, a structure continuous with the duodenum via the *pyloric sphincter* or *valve*. This sphincter controls stomach emptying.

The stomach has a convex lateral surface (greater curvature) and a concave medial surface (lesser curvature). Extending from the curvatures are the omenta (two mesenteries) that help bind the stomach to the body wall and other digestive organs. The **lesser omentum** continues from the liver to the lesser curvature, becoming continuous with the visceral peritoneum that covers the stomach. The **greater omentum** is draped inferiorly from the greater curvature, protecting the coiled small intestine. Fibroelastic capsules superiorly and dorsally wrap the spleen and transverse large intestine before blending into the **mesocolon**. This is a dorsal mesentery, securing the large intestine to the parietal peritoneum of the posterior abdominal wall. The greater omentum has many fat deposits and extensive collections of lymph nodes. Immune cells and macrophages inside the nodes monitor the peritoneal cavity and intraperitoneal organs.

STOMACH

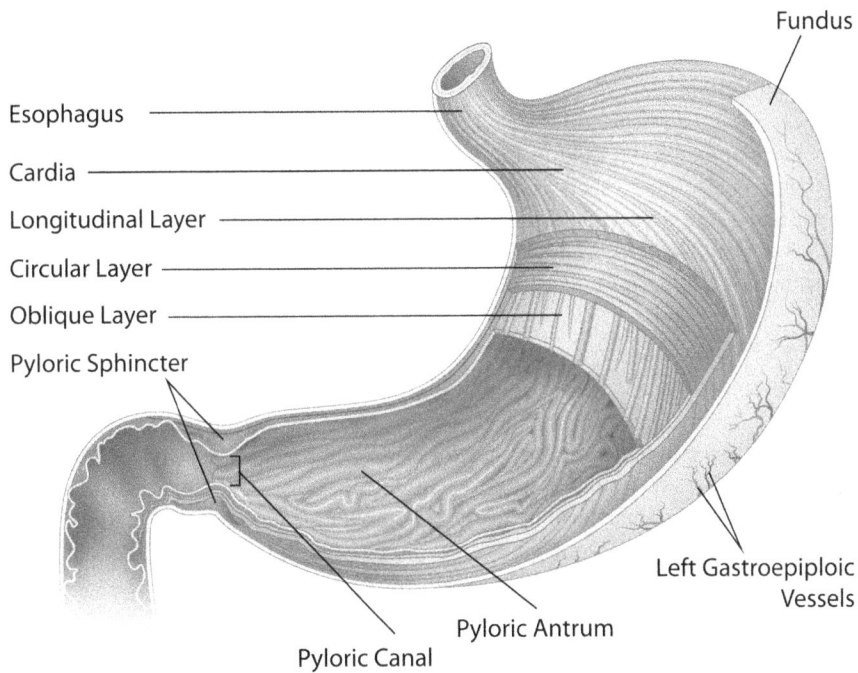

FIGURE 2.5   Anatomy of the stomach.

The autonomic nervous system serves the stomach. From the thoracic splanchnic nerves, sympathetic fibers relay through the celiac ganglion. The vagus nerve supplies the parasympathetic fibers. The gastric and splenic branches of the celiac trunk provide the stomach's arterial supply. Related veins form part of the **hepatic portal system**, eventually draining into the hepatic portal vein. The major areas of the stomach are shown in **Figure 2.5**.

Gland Cells

The stomach contains large cells that produce most of the stomach's secretions. They are as follows:

- *Mucous neck cells* – are mainly found within the neck of the stomach and scattered more deeply within the glands. These cells produce a thin and soluble mucus that is highly different from the mucus secreted by the mucous cells of the surface epithelium. The function of this acidic mucus needs to be understood.
- *Chief cells* – are found mainly in the basal regions of the gastric glands; these cuboidal cells produce **pepsinogen**, the inactive form of **pepsin**. When stimulated, the initial pepsinogen molecules they release are activated by hydrochloric acid in the apical portion of the gland. Once pepsin is present, it catalyzes the conversion of pepsinogen to pepsin. A small peptide fragment must be removed from the pepsinogen to do this. This causes it to change its shape and expose its active site. It is a positive feedback process limited by the amount of pepsinogen present. Chief cells secrete lipases that comprise approximately 15% of total GI lipolysis.
- *Parietal cells* – are scattered throughout the chief cells and are primarily closer to the lumen portions of the glands. These cells secrete hydrochloric acid as well as intrinsic factors. Appearing oval under a light microscope, the cells have three pitchfork-shaped

protuberances with dense microvilli, providing a large surface area for the secretions into the stomach lumen. Hydrochloric acid causes the stomach contents to be highly acidic, with a pH between 1.5 and 3.5 – this is required for the activation and the highest activity of pepsin, which digests proteins. Acidity aids digestion by denaturing proteins while breaking down the cell walls of plant foods. It is strong enough to destroy many of the ingested bacteria and foods. Intrinsic factor, a glycoprotein, is needed for the small intestine to absorb vitamin B12.

- *Enteroendocrine cells* – usually located deep in the gastric glands – release chemical messengers into the interstitial fluid of the lamina propria. Some, such as **histamine** and **serotonin**, have local effects, such as **paracrine**. Others, such as **somatostatin**, act as local paracrine and as hormones that diffuse into blood capillaries, influencing some digestive system target organs. **Gastrin** is a hormone that is essential for the regulation of stomach secretion and motility. **Table 2.1** presents the hormones and paracrine that function in digestion.

YOU SHOULD REMEMBER

Heartburn is a burning, radiating substernal pain caused by stomach acid regurgitating into the esophagus. It is the first symptom of gastroesophageal reflux disease (GERD). It resembles the feelings of a heart attack and is usually caused by excessive eating or drinking, obesity, pregnancy, and running. Heartburn is also common when a person has a hiatal hernia, causing gastric juice to enter the esophagus—especially when lying down. Frequent, prolonged episodes can lead to esophagitis, esophageal ulcers, and esophageal cancer.

TABLE 2.1
Hormones and Paracrine That Function as Part of Digestion

Substance	Site of Production	Stimulus for Production	Target Organ and Activity
Gastrin	Stomach mucosa G cells	Food (especially partly digested proteins) in the stomach (via chemical stimulation); acetylcholine from nerve fibers	*Stomach parietal cells* – increases HCl secretion, stimulates gastric emptying *Small intestine* – stimulates contraction of muscle *Ileocecal valve* – relaxes it *Large intestine* – stimulates mass movements
Histamine	Stomach mucosa	Food in the stomach	*Stomach* – activates parietal cells to release HCl
Serotonin	Stomach mucosa	Food in the stomach	*Stomach* – causes contraction of muscle
Somatostatin	Stomach mucosa; duodenal mucosa	Food in the stomach; stimulation by sympathetic nerve fibers	*Stomach* – inhibits gastric secretions *Pancreas* – inhibits secretion *Small intestine* – inhibits GI blood flow, reducing intestinal absorption *Gallbladder/liver* – inhibits contraction, bile release

(Continued)

TABLE 2.1 (*Continued*)
Hormones and Paracrine That Function as Part of Digestion

Substance	Site of Production	Stimulus for Production	Target Organ and Activity
Cholecystokinin (CCK)	Duodenal mucosa	Fatty chyme and partially digested proteins	*Stomach* – inhibits secretory activity *Liver/pancreas* – potentiates actions of secretin on these organs *Pancreas* – increases output of pancreatic juice, which is rich in enzymes *Gallbladder* – stimulates it to contract and expel bile *Hepatopancreatic sphincter* – relaxes it, allowing entry of bile and pancreatic juice into the duodenum
Glucose-dependent insulinotropic peptide (GIP, or gastric inhibitory peptide)	Duodenal mucosa	Fatty chyme	*Stomach* – inhibits hydrochloric acid (HCl) production *Pancreatic beta cells* – stimulates release of insulin
Intestinal gastrin	Duodenal mucosa	Acidic and partly digested foods in duodenum	*Stomach* – stimulates gastric glands and motility
Motilin	Duodenal mucosa	Fasting; periodic release every 1½–2 hours by neural stimuli	*Proximal duodenum* – stimulates the migrating motor complex
Secretin	Duodenal mucosa	Acidic chyme and partly digested proteins and fats	*Stomach* – inhibits gastric gland secretion, gastric motility *Pancreas* – increases output of pancreatic juice that is rich in bicarbonate ions; potentiates action of cholecystokinin *Liver* – increases bile output
Vasoactive intestinal peptide (VIP)	Enteric neurons	Chyme containing partly digested foods	*Small intestine* – stimulates buffer secretion, increases blood flow through intestinal capillaries, relaxes intestinal smooth muscle *Pancreas* – increases secretion *Stomach* – inhibits acid secretion

Check Your Knowledge

1. What are the organs of the GI tract?
2. What is the pharyngeal-esophageal phase of deglutition?
3. What are the various cells of the stomach?

Small Intestine

The small intestine extends from the pyloric sphincter to the ileocecal valve, emptying into the large intestine. The small intestine finishes the process of digestion, absorbs nutrients, and passes the remaining residue to the large intestine. The small intestine has three parts: the **duodenum**, **jejunum**, and **ileum**. It helps continue to digest food coming from the stomach. The small intestine absorbs vitamins, minerals, carbohydrates, fats, proteins, and water from food so that the body can use these nutrients. The plicae circulares, villi, and microvilli increase the absorptive surface area of the small intestine. Exocrine cells in the mucosa secrete mucus, peptidase, sucrase, maltase, lactase, lipase, and enterokinase. Endocrine cells secrete **cholecystokinin** (CCK) and **secretin**.

The most crucial factor for regulating secretions in the small intestine is the presence of chyme. This is primarily a local reflex action in response to chemical and mechanical irritation from the chyme and a response to enlargement of the intestinal wall. This is a direct reflex action and means that more secretion will occur with a more significant amount of chyme. Concerning absorption, carbohydrates are absorbed in the duodenum, while proteins are found in the jejunum. The jejunum also functions to absorb most fats. The ileum involves the absorption of vitamin B12.

Large Intestine

The large intestine includes the colon, rectum, and anus. It is a long tube that continues from the small intestine as food nears the end of its journey through the digestive system. The large intestine turns food waste into stool and excretes it from the body. The large intestine consists of eight parts: the cecum, appendix, ascending colon, transverse colon, descending colon, sigmoid colon, rectum, and anal canal (see **Figure 2.6**). The large intestine absorbs water and salts from the material that has not been digested as food, removing any remaining waste products.

ANATOMY OF THE LARGE INTESTINE

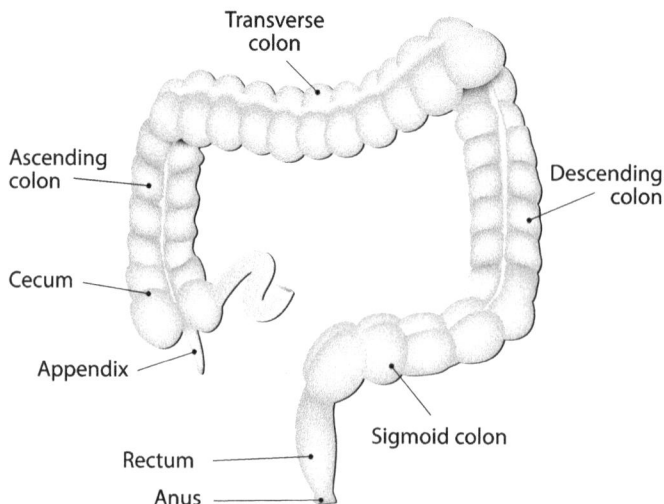

FIGURE 2.6   Anatomy of the large intestine.

The **bacterial flora**, also known as the *bacterial microbiota* of the large intestine, contains thousands of bacterial types. Some colonize the colon via the anus, while others enter from the small intestine, avoiding antimicrobial defenses. The gut bacteria help recover energy from indigestible foods and synthesize vitamins. The bacteria ferment some indigestible carbohydrates and **mucin** within the gut's mucus, resulting in short-chain fatty acids, which can be absorbed and used as fuel for the body. **Fermentation** also produces various gases, such as dimethyl sulfide, which smells nasty. Approximately 500 mL of **flatus** is made daily, especially when foods containing indigestible carbohydrates (such as beans) are consumed. Also, the gut bacteria synthesize B complex vitamins and some of the vitamin K required by the liver to produce clotting proteins.

The immune system destroys any bacteria that could pass through the mucosal barrier. However, the gut bacteria also instruct the immune system not to respond excessively to their presence. Beneficial bacteria suppress harmful bacteria and are present in much higher numbers. The immune system prevents bacteria from entering the body via the gut epithelium. Dendritic cells evaluate microbial **antigens** in the lumen and then migrate to lymphoid follicles in the gut mucosa, triggering an IgA antibody-mediated response occurring only within the lumen. Therefore, the bacteria cannot enter tissues deep into the mucosa, where they could cause a widespread systemic reaction. The types of bacteria present influence the balance between various T cell subtypes. This affects the balance between pro-inflammatory and anti-inflammatory responses. When the ratio of bacterial microbiota fails, inflammatory bowel disease may develop.

In the large intestine, most movements are **haustral contractions**, which are slow and segmented, lasting approximately 60 seconds and occurring about every 30 minutes. They are most common in the ascending and transverse colon, mixing food residue and aiding in water absorption. Mass peristalsis consists of long, slow, powerful contractile waves. It occurs three or four times daily, forcing residue toward the rectum, mostly during or after eating. Food in the stomach activates the small intestine's gastroileal reflex and the colon's propulsive gastrocolic reflex. Dietary fiber strengthens colonic contractions and softens the feces. It contains undigested food residue, mucus, epithelial cells sloughed off, bacteria, and water. Out of every 500 mL of food residue that enters the cecum per day, about 150 mL becomes feces.

The defecation reflex is initiated once mass peristalsis forces feces into the rectum and stretches its walls. It is a parasympathetic spinal reflex, causing the sigmoid colon and rectum to contract as the internal anal sphincter relaxes. As feces moves toward the anal canal, the brain receives messages that allow us to decide whether the voluntary, external anal sphincter should open or temporarily remain constricted. If defecation is delayed, the reflex contractions stop in a few seconds, and the rectal walls relax. The process continues until elimination occurs.

During defecation, the rectal muscles contract to expel feces. The glottis closes, and the diaphragm and abdominal wall muscles voluntarily tighten, increasing intra-abdominal pressure. This is also known as the **Valsalva maneuver**. The levator ani muscle is also contracted, lifting the anal canal superiorly. This leaves feces below the anus, outside of the body. Infants do not have the control of the external anal sphincter, so involuntary or automatic defecation occurs. It also happens in people who have experienced a spinal cord transection.

YOU SHOULD REMEMBER

The large intestine makes up about one-fifth of the entire GI tract. It is responsible for processing indigestible food material after most nutrients are absorbed in the small intestine.

Peritoneum

Most digestive organs are within the abdominopelvic cavity. The **peritoneum** is a slippery **serous membrane** (see **Figure 2.7**). The *visceral peritoneum* covers the outer surfaces of most digestive organs. It is continuous with the *parietal peritoneum*, which lines the walls of the body. In between is the *peritoneal cavity*, a thin potential space containing slippery serous fluid. This fluid allows digestive organs to move quickly across each other and along the body walls while aiding digestion. A **mesentery** extends to the digestive organs out from the body walls. Each mesentery provides paths for blood vessels, lymphatics, and nerves that reach the viscera, hold organs in place, and store fat. Most areas of the mesentery are dorsal, attached to the posterior abdominal wall. There are also ventral mesenteries, such as the one extending from the liver to the anterior abdominal wall. Some

PERITONEUM

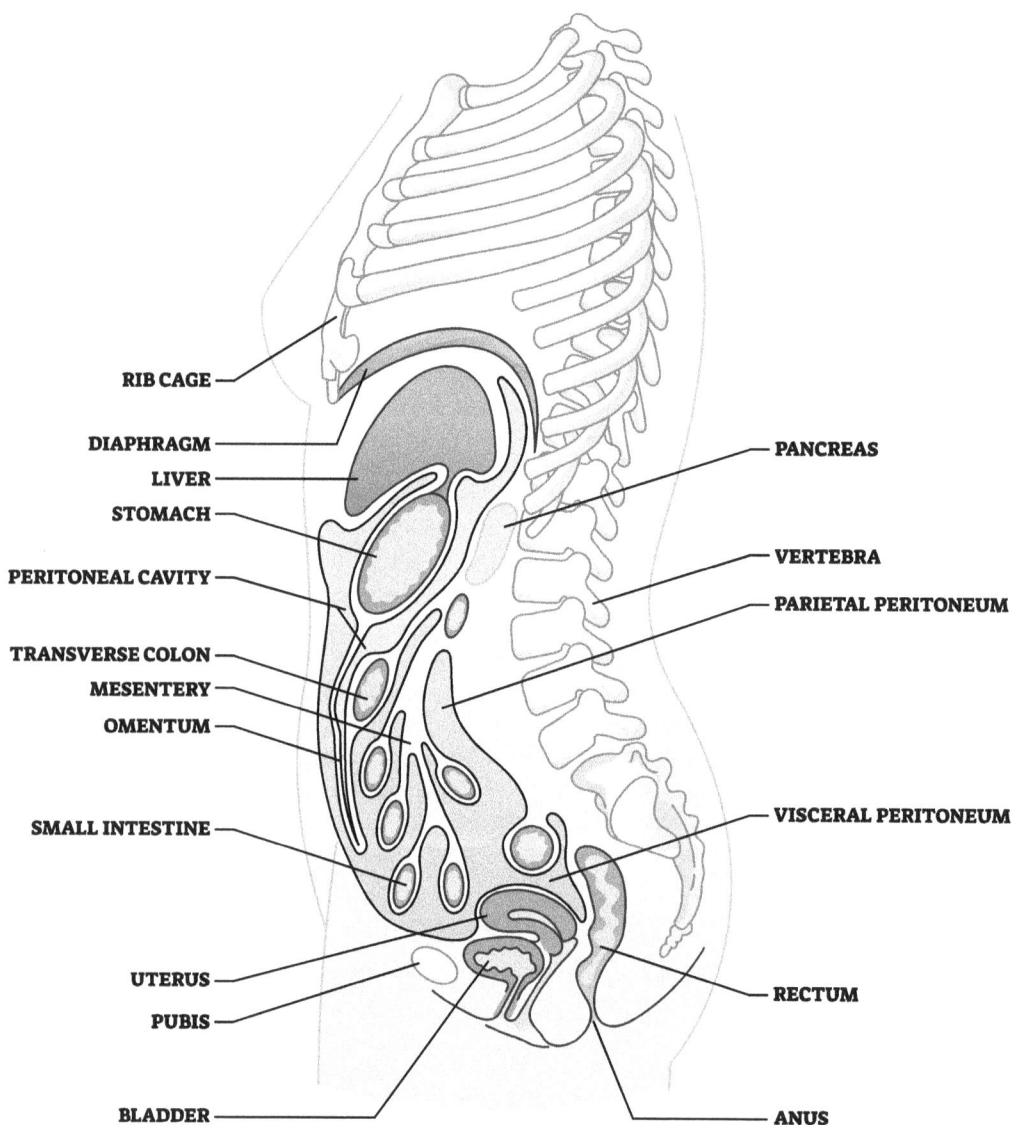

FIGURE 2.7   The peritoneum.

digestive organ mesenteries have identifying names, such as the **omenta**. Others are referred to as *ligaments*, though they are not the same fibrous ligaments that connect bones.

A mesentery does not suspend some digestive organs. During development, some portions of the small intestine adhere to the dorsal abdominal wall, losing their mesentery and then lying posterior to the peritoneum. These organs (most of the pancreas, duodenum, and parts of the large intestine) are retroperitoneal. In contrast, digestive organs like the stomach retain their mesentery and stay within the peritoneal cavity.

If the peritoneum becomes inflamed, it is called **peritonitis.** It is caused by piercing wounds to the abdomen, perforating ulcers that cause stomach juices to leak into the peritoneal cavity, or inadequate sterile technique during abdominal surgery. Most cases of peritonitis are caused by a **burst appendix**, which causes feces (and its bacteria) to spread over the peritoneum. The peritoneal coverings usually stick together around the area of infection, which localizes it and allows **macrophages** to stop it from spreading. However, it can be fatal when peritonitis spreads throughout the peritoneal cavity. The infectious debris must be removed to the greatest extent possible, and massive doses of antibiotics are required.

Check Your Knowledge

1. What are the functions of the small intestine?
2. What are the movements of the large intestine?
3. What are the descriptions of the peritoneum and mesentery?

ACCESSORY DIGESTIVE ORGANS

The accessory digestive organs include the teeth, tongue, salivary glands, pancreas, liver, and gallbladder. The accessory digestive glands produce many secretions that help break down food. The primary function of the teeth is rumination, which involves cutting, mixing, and grinding food to allow the tongue and oropharynx to shape into a bolus that can be swallowed. The salivary glands lubricate the mouth, aid in swallowing and digestion, and protect the teeth against harmful bacteria. There are three major types of salivary glands: sublingual, submandibular, and parotid. Human salivary glands produce 0.5–1.5 L of saliva daily while participating in the digestion of triglycerides and starches by secreting lipases and amylases.

Pancreas

The pancreas is an elongated, tapered organ across the back of the abdomen, behind the stomach. The right side of the organ is called the head and is the most comprehensive portion, lying in the curve of the duodenum (see **Figure 2.8**). The exocrine cells secrete digestive enzymes. These enzymes are secreted into a network of ducts that join the central pancreatic duct, which runs the entire length of the pancreas. The enzymes secreted by the exocrine cells of the pancreas help break down carbohydrates, fats, proteins, and nucleic acids in the duodenum. In an inactive form, these enzymes travel down the pancreatic duct into the bile duct. When they enter the duodenum, they become activated. The exocrine tissues also secrete bicarbonate to neutralize stomach acid in the duodenum, the first section of the small intestine. The endocrine portion of the pancreas, which consists of the islets of Langerhans, secretes hormones into the bloodstream. The main hormones secreted by the endocrine amount are insulin and **glucagon**, which regulate the glucose level in the blood, and somatostatin, which prevents insulin and glucagon release.

About 1,200–1,500 mL of clear pancreatic juice is produced daily, mainly in water. It also contains enzymes and electrolytes, most of which are bicarbonate ions. Therefore, pancreatic fluid has a high pH that helps neutralize acidic chyme that enters the duodenum, providing the best environment for intestinal and pancreatic enzymes. These enzymes include the following:

PANCREAS

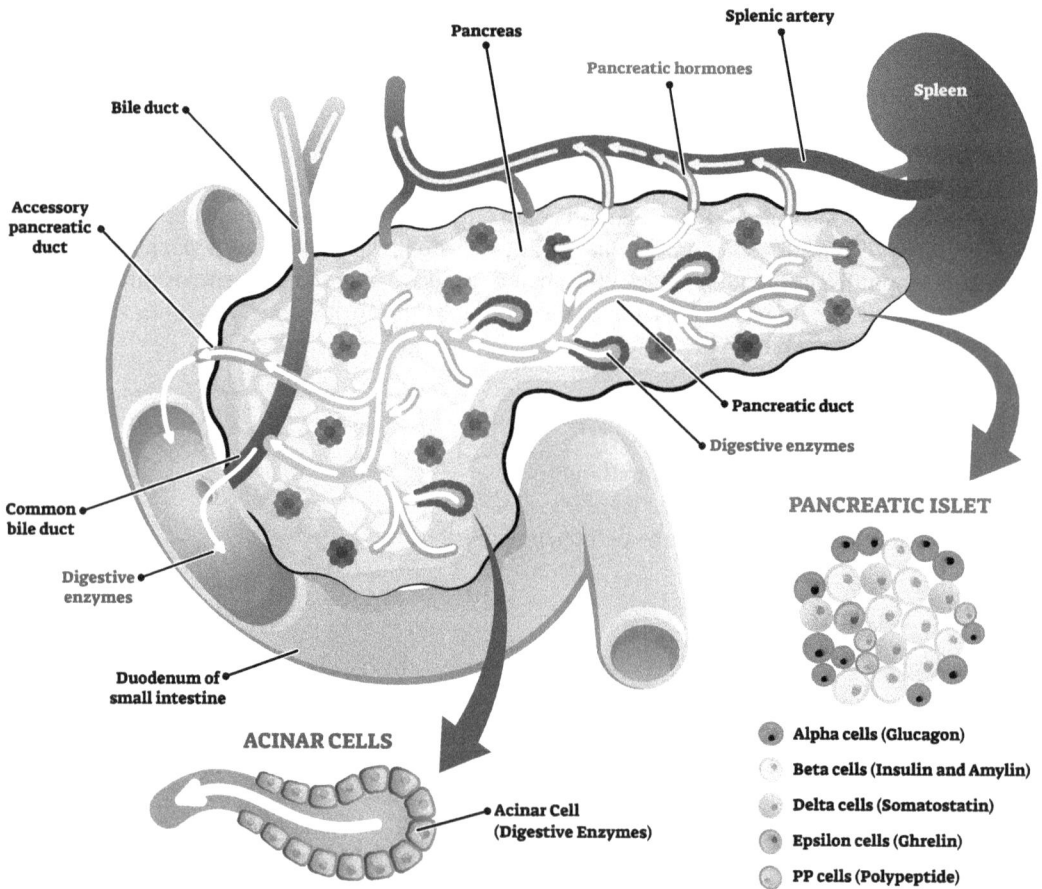

FIGURE 2.8   The pancreas.

- *Amylase* – for starch
- *Lipases* – for lipids
- *Nucleases* – for nucleic acids
- *Proteases* – for proteins

Like the pepsin in the stomach, pancreatic proteases are produced and released in inactive forms. They are activated within the duodenum, where they function, protecting the pancreas from self-digestion. In the duodenum, **enteropeptidase** activates *trypsinogen* to **trypsin**, activating more trypsinogen. It also starts *procarboxypeptidase in its active form, carboxypeptidase, and chymotrypsinogen in* its active form, **chymotrypsin**.

Liver

The liver is located in the upper right portion of the abdominal cavity, beneath the diaphragm, on top of the stomach, right kidney, and intestines. It consists of four lobes: the more extensive right and left lobes and the smaller caudate and quadrate lobes (see **Figure 2.9**). The **falciform ligament** divides the left and right lobes, which connect the liver to the abdominal wall. The right lobe is separated from the left lobe by a deep fissure. The falciform ligament is also known as the *round*

YOU SHOULD REMEMBER

The pancreas produces essential enzymes and hormones, while the liver is vital for metabolism, detoxification, digestion, and many other functions. Together, they work to maintain healthy blood glucose levels and other activities. The pancreas has exocrine functions, including enzymes to help break down food, and endocrine functions that manufacture and release insulin, glucagon, and other hormones.

LIVER

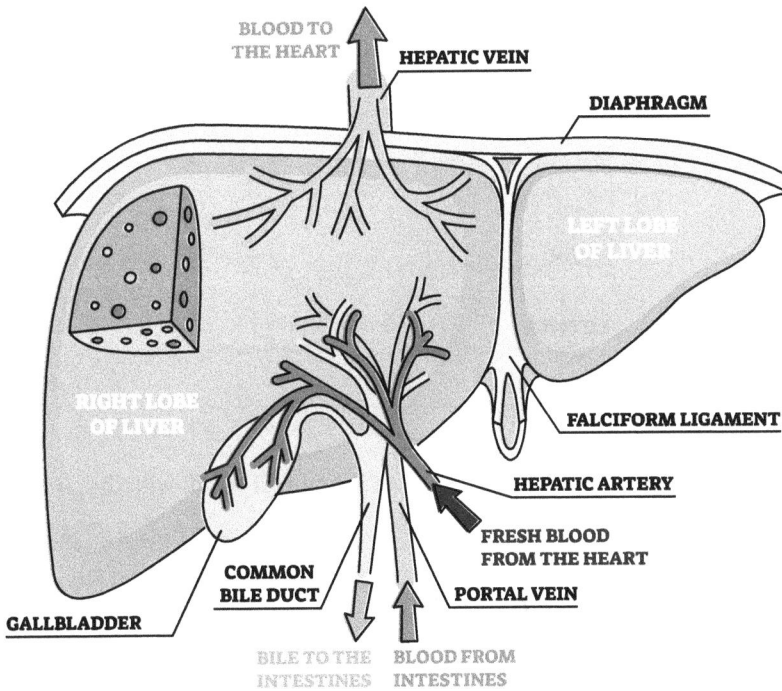

FIGURE 2.9   The liver.

ligament or the **ligamentum teres** and is a fibrous remnant of the umbilical vein that was present in the fetal period. The visceral peritoneum encloses the rest of the liver except for the top area, which contacts the diaphragm.

The liver is anchored to the lesser curvature of the stomach by the *lesser omentum*. The proper hepatic artery, portal vein, and everyday hepatic duct travel through the lesser omentum. The hepatic artery is good, and the hepatic portal vein enters the liver at the **porta hepatis**. Bile exits the liver lobes through the right and left hepatic ducts. They fuse, forming the large common hepatic duct, which continues downward toward the duodenum. Along the way, the duct fuses with the **cystic duct** that drains the gallbladder to form the **bile duct**.

Liver lobules are about the size of sesame seeds and comprise the liver's structural and functional units. Each is six-sided (hexagonal), consisting of plates of **hepatocytes** stacked like bricks. The hepatocyte plates radiate outward from a central vein that runs within the longitudinal axis of the lobule (see **Figure 2.10**). The liver's primary function is to process the nutrient-rich blood it

HEPATIC LOBULE

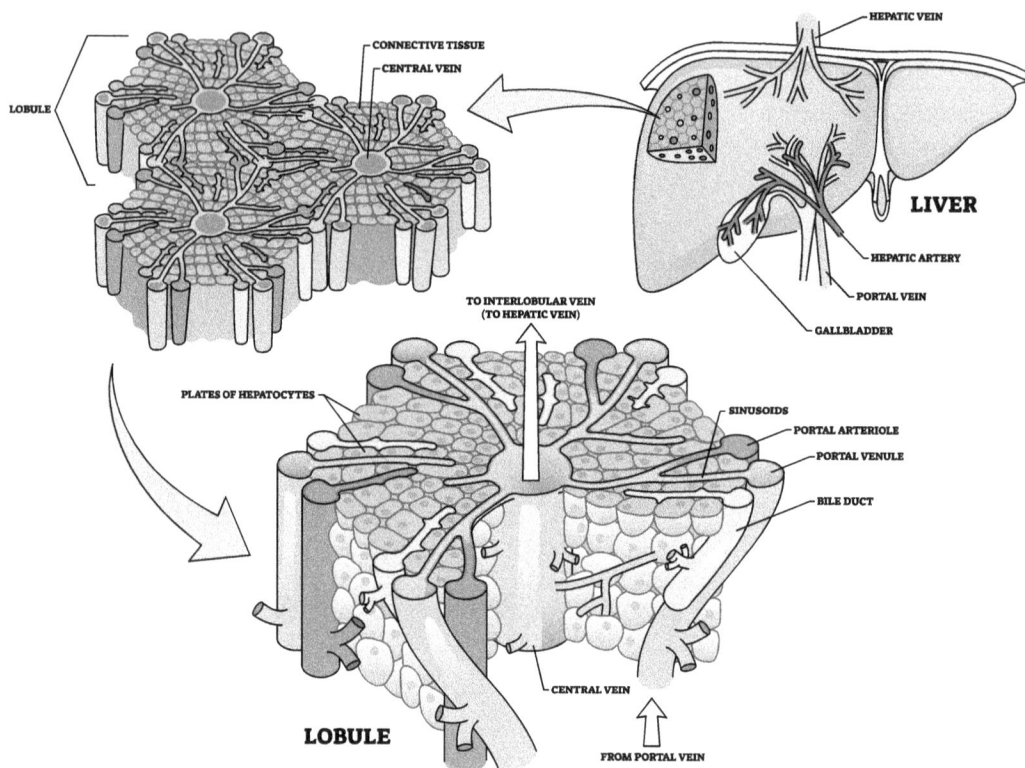

FIGURE 2.10   The liver lobules.

receives. At each of the six corners of a liver lobule is a **portal triad**, with the *portal tract region*, which is named because it contains the following:

- One branch of the *hepatic artery* – which supplies oxygen-rich arterial blood to the liver
- One branch of the *hepatic portal vein* – which carries venous blood containing nutrients from the digestive viscera
- One *bile duct*

Between the hepatocyte plates are enlarged **liver sinusoids** that are extremely fenestrated (perforated). Blood from the hepatic portal vein and hepatic artery proper moves from the triad regions through the sinusoids, emptying into the central vein. Eventually, the blood enters the hepatic veins that drain the liver, emptying into the inferior vena cava. Star-shaped *stellate macrophages* form part of the sinusoid walls, removing debris, including bacteria and worn-out blood cells.

The hepatocytes have significant amounts of rough and **smooth endoplasmic reticulum**, peroxisomes, **Golgi apparatus**, and mitochondria. They can secret about 900 mL of bile daily, process bloodborne nutrients, store fat-soluble vitamins, and play roles in detoxification (including removing ammonia from the blood and converting it to urea). Secreted bile flows through tiny **bile canaliculi**, running between hepatocytes toward the bile duct branches of the portal triads. Apical membranes of nearby hepatocytes form the walls of the canaliculi. Blood and bile flow in opposite directions in the liver lobules. Bile that enters the ducts eventually leaves the liver through the common hepatic duct and moves toward the duodenum.

The liver is the largest solid organ in the body, weighing about three pounds in adults. It is an essential organ that performs over 500 vital functions. These include removing waste products and foreign substances from the bloodstream, regulating blood sugar levels, and creating essential nutrients. Some of the most critical functions of the liver include the following:

- *Albumin production* – albumin is a protein that keeps fluids in the bloodstream from leaking into surrounding tissues. It also carries hormones, vitamins, and enzymes through the body.
- *Bile production* – bile is a fluid critical to the digestion and absorption of fats in the small intestine.
- *Blood filtration* – all the blood leaving the stomach and intestines passes through the liver, which removes toxins, byproducts, and other harmful substances.
- *Regulation of amino acids*—The production of proteins depends on amino acids. The liver ensures that amino acid levels in the bloodstream remain healthy.
- *Regulation of blood clotting* – blood clotting coagulants are created using vitamin K, which can only be absorbed with the help of bile, a fluid the liver produces.
- *Infection resistance* – as part of the filtering process, the liver removes bacteria from the bloodstream.
- *Storage of vitamins and minerals* – the liver stores significant amounts of vitamins A, D, E, K, and B12, as well as iron and copper.
- *Processing of glucose* – the liver removes excess glucose (sugar) from the bloodstream and stores it as glycogen. As needed, it can convert glycogen back into glucose.

Check Your Knowledge

1. What do the exocrine enzymes of the pancreas do?
2. What does the portal tract region of the liver contain?
3. What are the most critical functions of the liver?

Gallbladder

The gallbladder lies in the right upper quadrant of the abdomen, affixed to the undersurface of the liver, at the **fossa** (see **Figure 2.11**). It is attached to the rest of the extrahepatic biliary system via the cystic duct. The liver produces bile, which is drained into the gallbladder and stored until needed for digestion. The gallbladder's primary function is to store bile. This muscular organ also concentrates and releases bile into the digestive system. When bile is needed, the gallbladder contracts, forcing the fluid through a tube called the cystic duct.

YOU SHOULD REMEMBER

Gallstones are lumps of solid material formed in the gallbladder. They usually appear similar to small stones or gravel yet can be as small as grains of sand or as large as pebbles. Gallstones sometimes fill the gallbladder. About one in four women and one in eight men develop them; the leading cause is cholesterol. Cholesterol stones form when cholesterol levels in the bile are much higher than the bile acid levels, causing the cholesterol to solidify.

DIGESTION

Digestion is a catabolic process. It breaks down large food molecules into chemical building blocks, known as *monomers*, via enzymes secreted in the lumen of the alimentary canal. The mouth and its accessory digestive organs are involved in the ingestion, chewing (which starts mechanical

Gallbladder and Extrahepatic Bile Ducts

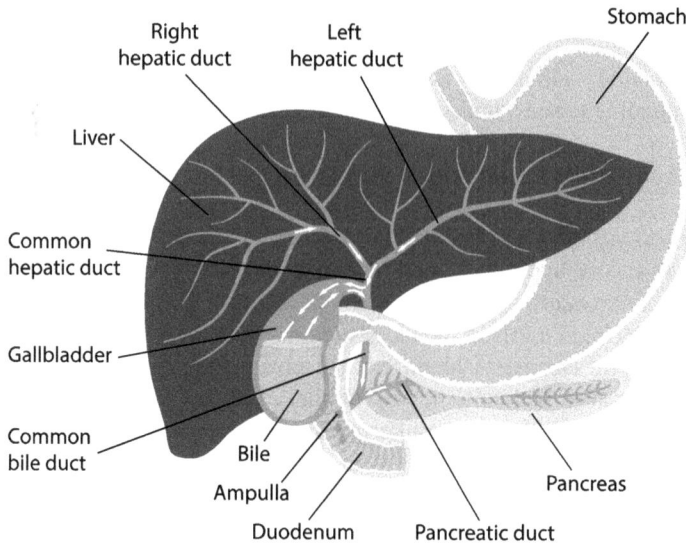

FIGURE 2.11   The gallbladder.

breakdown), swallowing (which creates propulsion), and initiation of the digestion of polysaccharides. As food enters the mouth, **mastication** initiates mechanical breakdown. The food is held between the teeth by the cheeks and lips. The tongue mixes food with saliva to soften it. The teeth reduce solid foods into smaller pieces. Mastication is partially voluntary as well as reflexive. While we voluntarily put food into the mouth and contract the jaw muscles, patterns and rhythm of jaw movements are controlled mainly by stretch reflexes, also in response to pressure input from receptors of the cheeks, gums, and tongue. They can also be voluntary. Carbohydrate digestion begins in the mouth via the amylase of the salivary glands.

The stomach is involved in propulsion, mechanical breakdown, digestion, and absorption. Protein digestion begins in the stomach. It is the primary type of enzymatic breakdown occurring in the organ. Hydrochloric acid produced by stomach glands denatures dietary proteins, preparing for enzymatic digestion. *Pepsin* is the most critical protein-digesting enzyme produced by the gastric mucosa. The stomach glands of infants also secrete *rennin,* an enzyme that acts upon *casein* (milk protein), converting it to a thick substance that resembles sour milk. Fat digestion mainly occurs in the small intestine, though gastric and lingual lipases affecting the acidic pH of the stomach also play a role. Though the stomach does not handle much absorption, alcohol, and aspirin, which are lipid soluble, easily pass from the stomach mucosa into the bloodstream.

The only function of the stomach essential to life is the secretion of intrinsic factors. These factors are needed for the intestinal absorption of vitamin B12 to produce mature erythrocytes. The gastric mucosa usually releases up to 3 L of gastric juice daily. Hormonal control of gastric secretion is generally regulated by **gastrin**, which stimulates the stomach's secretion of hydrochloric acid by **parietal cells**.

The cephalic (reflex) phase occurs before food enters the stomach and is a few minutes long, triggered by smells, tastes, sights, or thoughts of food. The vagus nerve stimulates the gastric glands to prepare for digestive actions. The gastric phase occurs as food reaches the stomach, lasting 3–4 hours, providing 66% of the released gastric juice. Stomach distension activates stretch receptors, initiating short and long reflexes. With long reflexes, impulses travel to the **medulla oblongata** and back to the stomach through vagal fibers. Chemical stimuli, from partially digested proteins, caffeine, and increasing pH, activate gastrin-secreting enteroendocrine cells (G cells) in the antrum of the stomach. Gastrin stimulates the parietal cells to secrete HCl by acting directly on cell receptors and producing G cells to release histamine.

When protein-rich foods are in the stomach, the gastric content pH usually increases since proteins become buffers, tying up hydrogen ions. The increase in pH stimulates gastric secretion and HCl release. This provides the amount of acid needed to digest protein. The higher the protein content in foods, the more gastric secretion and HCl will be released. With protein digestion, the gastric contents slowly become more acidic, further inhibiting gastrin-secreting cells. This is a negative feedback mechanism. It helps maintain the best pH and condition needed for gastric enzyme functionality.

Gastric secretion is inhibited when gastric contents are highly acidic, with a pH below 2. This often occurs between meals. Anything that triggers the fight-or-flight response inhibits gastric secretion since the sympathetic division dominates the parasympathetic (vagal) controls related to digestion. Triggers include anxiety, fear, and stress.

For gastric secretion, the intestinal phase begins with a short stimulatory component followed by inhibition. The first stimulatory portion begins when partially digested food fills the duodenum of the small intestine. Intestinal mucosal cells are then stimulated to release intestinal gastrin. This hormone encourages gastric glands to continue secreting a brief stimulatory effect since inhibitory stimuli will override it as the intestine fills up.

The actions of the duodenum that slow down gastric secretion are influenced by four primary factors: distention of the duodenum or the presence of either acidic, fatty, or hypertonic chyme. The same factors also decrease gastric emptying. They protect the small intestine from being excessively acidic. Additionally, they avoid a large influx of chyme from overwhelming the duodenum's absorptive and digestive abilities. They do this by matching the amount of chyme entering the small intestine's processing ability. There are two ways in which inhibition is achieved, as follows:

- *Enterogastric reflex* – the duodenum inhibits acid secretion within the stomach via brief reflexes throughout the enteric nervous system and more prolonged reflexes involving the vagus and sympathetic nerves.
- *Enterogastrones* – related hormones are released by scattered enteroendocrine cells in the duodenal mucosal epithelium. The two most critical enterogastrones are secretin and CCK. Collectively, enterogastrones inhibit gastric secretion and have other activities.

The small intestine is where most lipid digestion occurs since the pancreas is the primary source of the **lipases**, which digest fat. In the small intestine, digestion and absorption of lipids require the following processes:

- *Emulsification* – since triglycerides and their breakdown products are insoluble in water, they require bile salts to be digested in the small intestine's watery environment. Bile salts significantly increase the surface area exposed to pancreatic lipases, breaking large globules of fat into many smaller droplets. Bile salts have nonpolar (hydrophobic) and polar (ionized hydrophilic) regions. Fatty droplets are removed from large fat globules to form a stable **emulsion**. No chemical bonds are broken, but emulsification reduces attraction between fat molecules, allowing them to be more widely dispersed.
- *Digestion* – the breakdown of triglycerides is catalyzed by pancreatic lipases. Two fatty acid chains are slipped off to yield free fatty acids and monoglycerides.
- *Formation of micelles* – liberated monoglycerides and free fatty acids are quickly associated with bile salts and **lecithin** to form **micelles**. They are similar to emulsion droplets but about 500 times smaller. Micelles diffuse between microvilli to contact the apical cell surface closely.
- *Diffusion* – after reaching the enterocytes, various lipid substances leave the micelles and move through the apical plasma membrane via simple diffusion.

- *Formation of chylomicrons* – the smooth endoplasmic reticulum converts free fatty acids and monoglycerides back into triglycerides, combined with lecithin and other phospholipids plus cholesterol. These are then coated with proteins, forming **chylomicrons**.
- *Transport of chylomicrons* – milky white and too large to pass through enterocyte plasma membranes or basement membranes of blood capillaries. Instead, vesicles containing chylomicrons move to the basolateral membrane. They are extruded by exocytosis and enter the more permeable lacteals. Therefore, most fat enters the lymphatic stream to be distributed, and eventually, chylomicrons empty into the venous blood through the thoracic duct.

The triglycerides of chylomicrons are then hydrolyzed to free fatty acids and glycerol by lipoprotein lipase. The fatty acids and glycerol pass through the capillary walls to be used for energy by tissue cells or stored as fats in the adipose tissue. Liver cells endocytose and process any residual chylomicron materials. Passage of short-chain fatty acids does not require bile salts or micelles; they diffuse into the portal blood for distribution. Fat absorption is mainly completed in the ileum, but when bile is absent, this is a prolonged process, and most fat passes into the large intestine to be lost in the feces.

Pancreatic nucleases hydrolyze nucleic acids to **nucleotide** monomers. *Nucleosidases* and *phosphatases* break the nucleotides apart, releasing their nitrogenous bases, pentose sugars, and phosphate ions. Breakdown products of nucleic acid digestion are transported across the epithelium and then enter the blood. The small intestine absorbs dietary vitamins, while the large intestine absorbs some B and K vitamins manufactured by GI bacteria. Most water-soluble (B and C) vitamins are absorbed through specific active or passive transporters. *Intrinsic factors* in the stomach bind to vitamin B12. The vitamin B12–intrinsic factor complex binds to specific mucosal receptor sites in the terminal ileum, triggering active uptake via endocytosis.

Absorbed electrolytes come from ingested foods as well as GI secretions. While most ions are actively absorbed along the small intestine, iron and calcium are mostly absorbed only in the duodenum. Sodium ions are actively pumped out of enterocytes by a sodium-potassium pump after entering the cells. Bicarbonate is secreted into the lumen in the small intestine's terminus in exchange for chloride. Potassium ions move passively across the intestinal mucosa via facilitated diffusion. When water is absorbed from the lumen, increasing potassium levels in the chyme creates a concentration gradient. Anything interfering with water absorption reduces potassium absorption and pulls potassium ions from the interstitial space into the intestinal lumen.

Iron is actively transported into mucosal cells to bind to **ferritin**. Intracellular iron–ferritin complexes act as storehouses for iron. When iron reserves are depleted, iron uptake from the intestine and its release to the bloodstream speed up. In the blood, iron binds to **transferrin**. Calcium absorption is highly related to the blood levels of ionic calcium. Active vitamin D promotes the active absorption of calcium. Decreased blood levels of ionic calcium encourage the release of parathyroid hormone (PTH) from the parathyroid glands. Then, PTH stimulates the kidneys' activation of vitamin D to calcitriol, speeding up calcium ion absorption in the small intestine.

About 9 L of water, mainly from GI tract secretions, enters the small intestine daily. About 95% of water is absorbed in the small intestine by osmosis. Most of the remainder is interested in the large intestine, with only about 0.1 L left behind to soften the feces. Water is usually absorbed at 300–400 mL/hour. *Net osmosis* occurs when a concentration gradient is established via the active transport of solutes (mainly sodium) into mucosal cells.

YOU SHOULD REMEMBER

There are five basic steps related to how humans absorb nutrients. They include chewing and introducing enzymes in the mouth, churning and mixing with gastric juice in the stomach, contact and absorption in the small intestine, entering the bloodstream, and using carrier proteins that bring nutrients into cells. The small intestine pulls glucose, amino acids, fatty acids, vitamins, and minerals out of food so that cells can use them.

Check Your Knowledge

1. What is the gallbladder's primary function?
2. What is the only function of the stomach that is essential to life?
3. In the small intestine, what do digestion and absorption of lipids require?

ABSORPTION

Absorption is how substances move from the lumen of the GI tract into the body. Since tight junctions join enterocytes (epithelial cells) of the intestinal mucosa at their apical surfaces, substances, in most cases, cannot move between cells. Materials must instead pass through enterocytes. They enter an enterocyte via its apical membrane from the lumen of the tract, then exit through the basolateral membrane into the interstitial fluid on the opposite side of the cell. Upon reaching the interstitial fluid, substances diffuse into blood capillaries. From the capillary blood in the **villus**, they move in the hepatic portal vein to get to the liver. However, some lipid digestion products do not. Instead, they enter the **lacteal** in the villus and are carried in the lymphatic fluid to the blood.

Because of the structure of the plasma membrane, nonpolar substances can be absorbed passively. These substances can dissolve in the lipid cord of the membrane, while all others must have a carrier mechanism. Most nutrients are absorbed by active transport directly or indirectly driven by the metabolic energy of **adenosine triphosphate** (ATP). Up to 10 L of food, liquids, and GI secretions enter the alimentary canal daily. However, 1 L or less will reach the large intestine. Nearly all foods, 80% of electrolytes, and most water will be absorbed in the small intestine. Though absorption occurs through the small intestine, most are completed when the chyme reaches the ileum. The primary role of the ileum is to reclaim bile salts so that they can be recycled back to the liver for resection. Carbohydrates are digested and absorbed via the following processes:

- *Pancreatic amylase* – breaks down starch and glycogen into **oligosaccharides** and disaccharides. It acts upon starchy foods and other digestible carbohydrates that are not broken down by salivary amylase. About 10 minutes after they enter the small intestine, starches are entirely converted to oligosaccharides, the most common resulting substance being *maltose.*
- *Brush border enzymes* – break oligosaccharides and disaccharides into monosaccharides. The most important of these enzymes are *dextrinase* and *glucoamylase.* They act on oligosaccharides of more than three simple sugars and on maltase, sucrase, and lactase, which hydrolyze *maltose, sucrose,* and *lactose* into their constituent monosaccharides.
- *Monosaccharides* – are transported across the apical membrane of the **enterocyte**. Glucose and galactose, freed by the breakdown of starch and disaccharides, are moved into enterocytes via secondary active transport with sodium. However, fructose enters the cells via facilitated diffusion. Proteins that transport monosaccharides into cells are located near disaccharidase enzymes on the brush border. They combine with monosaccharides as disaccharides are broken down.
- *Facilitated diffusion* – allows all monosaccharides to exit across the basolateral membrane and pass into the capillaries via intercellular clefts.

Some polysaccharides, such as *cellulose,* cannot be broken down, so they function to provide fiber and move food through the GI tract.

Inside the GI tract, digested proteins include about 125 g of dietary proteins per day, 15–25 g of enzyme proteins secreted by various glands, and protein from sloughed and disintegrating mucosal cells. A healthy person digests much of this protein to its amino acid monomers. Protein digestion starts in the stomach as pepsinogen, secreted by chief cells, is activated to become pepsin, which has the most vital functions in the stomach's 1.5–2.5 acidic pH range. Pepsin hydrolyzes 10%–15%

of ingested protein. The high pH of the duodenum inactivates it. The digestion and absorption of proteins in the small intestine is summarized as follows:

- *Pancreatic proteases break down proteins and their fragments* – they become smaller pieces and some actual amino acids. Protein fragments that enter the small intestine are affected by many proteolytic enzymes. The proteins are cleaved into smaller particles by trypsin and chemotrypsin. Carboxypeptidases split off an amino acid, one at a time, from the end of a polypeptide chain with a carboxyl group.
- *Brush border enzymes break down oligopeptides and dipeptides into amino acids* – individual amino acids are liberated from the ends of peptide chains as carboxypeptidases and aminopeptidases. Dipeptidases break pairs of amino acids apart. Interactions between the enzymes, trypsin, and chymotrypsin speed up the process by attacking internal parts of proteins.
- *Amino acids are transported across enterocytes' apical membranes* – most carriers, such as those for glucose and galactose, are coupled to active sodium transport. Short chains of two or three dipeptides and tripeptides are actively absorbed via hydrogen ion-dependent cotransport. Inside enterocytes, they are digested to their amino acids.
- *Amino acids exit the basolateral membrane through facilitated diffusion* – they enter capillaries through intercellular clefts.

METABOLISM

Metabolism is a collective term. Substances are continually built up and torn down. **Anabolism** describes all reactions building larger molecules or structures from smaller ones. **Catabolism** describes all processes breaking down complex systems into simpler ones. There are three primary stages involved, as follows:

- *Stage 1* – digestion and absorption, with absorbed nutrients transported in the bloodstream to tissue cells.
- *Stage 2* – in tissue cells' cytoplasm, newly arriving nutrients are built into lipids, proteins, and glycogen, an essential metabolic intermediate.
- *Stage 3* – in the mitochondria, oxygen is used to complete the breakdown of remaining products; most are converted to *acetyl CoA*, producing carbon dioxide and water, requiring large amounts of ATP.

Catabolic reactions known as **cellular respiration** include glycolysis, the citric acid cycle, and oxidative phosphorylation. Some released energy is captured to form ATP. As ATP is hydrolyzed, enzymes shift phosphate groups to other molecules, known as *phosphorylated*. The body also stores energy in fuels, such as glycogen and fats, mobilizing the stores later to produce ATP for the cells to use.

Regarding carbohydrate metabolism, glucose enters tissue cells via diffusion, which insulin enhances. Glucose is phosphorylated to *glucose-6-phosphate* via the transfer of one phosphate group to its sixth carbon during a coupled reaction with ATP. Phosphorylation traps glucose inside cells. Most cells cannot reverse the reaction because they lack the enzymes needed. The response keeps intracellular glucose levels low. The only cells that can change this reaction are intestinal epithelial cells, kidney tubule cells, and liver cells. Catabolic and anabolic pathways for carbohydrates all start with glucose-6-phosphate. There are three significant phases of glycolysis, as follows:

- *Sugar activation* – glucose is phosphorylated twice and converted to fructose-1,6-bisphosphate.
- *Sugar cleavage* – fructose-1,6-bisphosphate is split into two 3-carbon fragments (either glyceraldehyde 3-phosphate or dihydroxyacetone phosphate).

- *Sugar oxidation + ATP formation* – The removal of hydrogen oxidizes two 3-carbon fragments, and some glucose energy is transferred to nicotinamide adenine dinucleotide (NAD) ions. Inorganic phosphate groups with high-energy bonds are attached to each oxidized piece. Once these terminal phosphates are split, the captured energy forms four ATP molecules.

The final products of glycolysis are two **pyruvic acid** molecules, two molecules of reduced NAD ions, and two hydrogen ions. Glycolysis can continue only if the reduced coenzymes formed are relieved of their extra hydrogens. When oxygen is not present sufficiently, hydrogen atoms are unloaded back onto the pyruvic acid, reducing it and yielding lactic acid. When oxygen becomes available, lactic acid is oxidized to pyruvic acid, entering aerobic pathways and completely rusting to water and carbon dioxide. The next stage of glucose oxidation is the **citric acid cycle**, which occurs in the mitochondrial matrix. There are three processes:

- *Decarboxylation* – one carbon is removed from pyruvic acid and released as carbon dioxide gas. CO_2 diffuses out of cells into the blood and is expelled by the lungs.
- *Oxidation* – the remaining 2-carbon fragment is oxidized to acetic acid by removing hydrogen atoms, which are picked up by NAD ions.
- *Formation of acetyl CoA* – acetic acid is combined with coenzyme A to produce **acetyl coenzyme A** (acetyl CoA), which is now ready to enter the citric acid cycle and be broken down into mitochondrial enzymes.

As the cycle continues, citric acid atoms are rearranged to produce intermediate molecules, most of which are **keto acids**. Finally, acetic acid is absent, and a pickup molecule called *oxaloacetic acid* is regenerated. Though glycolysis is exclusive to carbohydrate oxidation, breakdown products of carbohydrates, fats, and proteins feed into the citric acid cycle. They are oxidized for energy.

YOU SHOULD REMEMBER

The term "metabolism" refers to chemical reactions in the body. Every cell continually experiences metabolic reactions. Problems with metabolism can result in illness, and one of the most common metabolic diseases is diabetes mellitus. It occurs when the body cannot process glucose and other sugars properly. Metabolic processes are also linked to diseases such as cancer.

Check Your Knowledge

1. How are most nutrients absorbed?
2. How are carbohydrates digested and absorbed?
3. What are the three primary stages involved in catabolism?

GLYCOGENESIS

While most glucose is used to generate ATP molecules, this does not mean that unlimited amounts of glucose result in infinite ATP synthesis. This is because the cells cannot store large amounts of ATP. Along with cellular respiration, carbohydrate metabolism ensures the right amount of glucose in the bloodstream. When more glucose is available, it can quickly be oxidized, increasing intracellular ATP concentration and eventually inhibiting glucose catabolism, causing glucose to be stored as glycogen or fat. Since the body can store much more fat than glycogen, fats comprise 80%–8%

of stored energy. The first of the three processes is **glycogenesis**. When high levels of ATP begin to shut down glycolysis, glucose molecules are combined in long chains, forming glycogen. This is the animal carbohydrate storage product. Glycogenesis starts as glucose enters cells and is phosphorylated to glucose-6-phosphate. It is then converted to its isomer, which is called *glucose-1-phosphate*. The last phosphate group is split off, and *glycogen synthase*, an enzyme, catalyzes the attachment of glucose to the enlarging glycogen chain. Liver and skeletal muscle cells are the most active in glycogen synthesis and storage.

Glycogenolysis

When blood glucose levels decrease, splitting occurs in the process known as **glycogenolysis**. An enzyme, *glycogen phosphorylase*, regulates phosphorylation and splitting of glycogen. Glucose-1-phosphate is released and then converted to glucose-6-phosphate. This form can enter the glycolysis pathway so that it can be oxidized for energy. In most cells, especially muscle cells, glucose-6-phosphate from glycogenolysis is trapped since it cannot cross cell membranes. Hepatocytes and some cells of the kidneys and intestine contain glucose-6-phosphatase; the enzyme then removes the terminal phosphate, producing free glucose. Since glucose can quickly diffuse from cells into the blood, the liver can use glycogen stores to provide blood glucose for other organs when its levels drop. Liver glycogen is an essential energy source for skeletal muscles that have run out of glycogen reserves.

Gluconeogenesis

When insufficient glucose is metabolized, glycerol and amino acids are converted to glucose. **Gluconeogenesis** is the process of forming new glucose from non-carbohydrate molecules. It occurs in the liver. Gluconeogenesis happens when dietary sources and glucose reserves are used up, and blood glucose levels decrease. The process protects the body – primarily the nervous system – from the harmful effects of hypoglycemia by ensuring that ATP synthesis continues.

ELIMINATION

Food molecules that cannot be digested or absorbed must be eliminated from the body. The removal of indigestible wastes through the anus, in the form of feces, is called elimination (defecation). The process occurs via contraction of the rectal muscles, relaxation of the internal anal sphincter, and an initial contraction of the skeletal muscle of the external anal sphincter. The defecation reflex is primarily involuntary. The autonomic nervous system controls it, though the somatic nervous system plays a role in maintaining the timing of elimination.

Common problems with elimination include constipation and diarrhea. Constipation is a condition in which the feces are hardened because excess water is removed from the colon. Oppositely, diarrhea occurs if not enough water is removed from the waste. Many bacteria, such as those that cause cholera, affect the proteins needed for water reabsorption in the colon and result in excessive diarrhea.

CLINICAL CASE STUDY 1

A 59-year-old man went to his physician because of being woken up in the middle of the night with abdominal pain. This happened several nights per week. The man also complained of occasional discomfort during the afternoons. The pain affected the man's appetite since he felt that perhaps certain foods were causing the pain. The patient was referred to a specialist in internal medicine, and an endoscopy was performed. The result was a diagnosis of a peptic ulcer. Analysis of a tissue sample taken from the ulcer site also showed an infection with *Helicobacter pylori* bacteria. The patient was prescribed two antibiotics and a medication to decrease stomach acid secretion.

CRITICAL THINKING QUESTIONS

1. What causes the environment of the stomach to be highly acidic?
2. What helps to neutralize acidic chyme as it exits the stomach?
3. When the gastric contents have a pH below 2, what is inhibited?

CLINICAL CASE STUDY 2

A 16-year-old girl was taken by her parents to a pediatrician because of anemia, anorexia, and minor abdominal pain. Family history is negative for malabsorption or inflammatory bowel disease. Examination revealed the girl's abdomen to be slightly protruded and hyperresonant, with hyperactive bowel sounds. Tests revealed mild anemia, iron deficiency, and steatorrhea, suggesting some malabsorption condition. Biopsies from the duodenal and proximal jejunal area revealed severe villus atrophy, consisting of flat mucosa with deep crypts. Further testing resulted in a diagnosis of celiac disease. The girl was started on a strict gluten-free diet, and her symptoms resolved.

CRITICAL THINKING QUESTIONS

1. What is the process of absorption in the GI tract?
2. What are the absorptive functions of the duodenum and jejunum?
3. What increases the absorptive area of the small intestine?

CLINICAL CASE STUDY 3

A 32-year-old man is evaluated for hypertension whose father also has hypertension. Both his mother and grandmother have diabetes mellitus. The patient has gained 15 pounds over the last year and seldom exercises. Examination and testing have revealed moderate central obesity, elevated LDL cholesterol, low HDL cholesterol, elevated triglycerides, and elevated fasting blood glucose. The patient has met the diagnostic criteria for metabolic syndrome and prediabetes. He is at high risk of developing type 2 diabetes. Therefore, he has started an exercise and weight loss program and enrolled with a nutritional counselor.

CRITICAL THINKING QUESTIONS

1. When does diabetes mellitus occur?
2. What are the three stages of normal metabolism?
3. What are the three processes involved in the regulation of blood glucose?

FURTHER READING

1. Bagchi, D., and Ohio, S.E. (2021). *Nutrition and Functional Foods in Boosting Digestion, Metabolism and Immune Health.* Academic Press.
2. Bender, D.A. (2014). *Introduction to Nutrition and Metabolism,* 5th Edition. CRC Press.
3. Da Poian, A.T., and Castanho, M.A.R.B. (2021). *Integrative Human Biochemistry: A Textbook for Medical Biochemistry,* 2nd Edition. Springer.
4. De Oliveira, M.R. (2022). *The Amazing Universe of Human Metabolism.* De Oliveira.
5. Frayn, K., and Evans, R. (2019). *Human Metabolism: A Regulatory Perspective.* Wiley Blackwell.
6. Frayn, K.N. (2022). *Understanding Human Metabolism.* Cambridge University Press.
7. Gropper, S.S., Smith, J.L., and Carr, T.P. (2021). *Advanced Nutrition and Human Metabolism,* 8th Edition. Cengage Learning.
8. Kang, J. (2018). *Nutrition and Metabolism in Sports, Exercise, and Health,* 2nd Edition. Routledge.
9. Katz, D.L., Essel, K.D., Friedman, R.S.C., Joshi, S., Levitt, J., and Yeh, M.C. (2022). *Nutrition in Clinical Practice,* 4th Edition. Wolters Kluwer.
10. Kohlmeier, M. (2015). *Nutrient Metabolism: Structures, Functions, and Genes,* 2nd Edition. Academic Press.

11. Lanham-New, S.A., Macdonald, I.A., and Roche, H.M. (2010). *Nutrition and Metabolism*, 2nd Edition. Wiley Blackwell.

12. Miller, S. (2022). *Metabolism Made Simple: Making Sense of Nutrition to Transform Metabolic Health.* Lioncrest Publishing.

13. Mitchell, T. (2018). *Digestive System & Metabolism*, Volume 4. Master Books.

14. Nelson, D.L., and Cox, M.M. (2021). *Lehninger: Principles of Biochemistry*, 8th Edition. W.H. Freeman.

15. Pontes, S., Boaventura, J., and Santana, N. (2022). *Introduction to Human Metabolism: Health in Brief.* Our Knowledge Publishing.

16. Prasad, A. (2013). *Trace Elements and Iron in Human Metabolism (Topics in Hematology).* Springer.

17. Rosenthal, M.D., and Glew, R.H. (2011). *Medical Biochemistry: Human Metabolism in Health and Disease.* Wiley.

18. Sutherland, M. (2023). *The Science of Nutrition and Health.* Sutherland.

19. Vanderkooi, J.M. (2012). *Your Inner Engine: An Introductory Course on Human Metabolism (The Human Body).* Vanderkooi.

Part II

Disorders of Carbohydrate Metabolism

3 Diabetes Mellitus

OVERVIEW

Diabetes mellitus, as one of the different types of glucose intolerance disorders, is a chronic metabolic disease involving inappropriately elevated blood glucose levels. It has several categories, including type 1, type 2, gestational diabetes, neonatal diabetes, and secondary causes due to endocrinopathies. Diabetes mellitus, especially type 2 diabetes, is an epidemic requiring global attention as cardiovascular disease (CVD) risk, in addition to neuropathy, nephropathy, retinopathy, and mortality through macrovascular complications, even in early or pre-stages. Because of its asymptomatic onset and progression, population-based screening is essential for the early detection of diabetes mellitus before developing vascular complications. Many modifiable risk factors, such as dyslipidemia, hyperglycemia, and hypertension, must be controlled to prevent CVD in people with established diabetes mellitus. Diabetes is the most common metabolic disease in humans. Type 1, insulin-dependent, or juvenile-onset diabetes mellitus is characterized by onset in childhood or early adolescence. Gestational diabetes mellitus is a condition characterized by glucose intolerance during pregnancy. Neonatal diabetes mellitus is rare within the first 6 months of life. Our bodies need insulin to help our cells make energy. Infants with this condition do not produce enough insulin, which increases blood glucose levels.

STRUCTURE OF THE PANCREAS

The pancreas is below and behind the stomach, in front of the spine. It is a spongy gland that is 12–15 cm (6–10 inches) long and is primarily retroperitoneal. The head of the pancreas is on the right side of the abdomen. The gland is connected to the first section of the small intestine, the *duodenum*, via the small *pancreatic duct*. The narrow *tail* of the pancreas extends to the left side of the body (see **Figure 3.1**).

The pancreatic tissues contain approximately 1–2 million clusters of cells called the pancreatic islets or **islets of Langerhans.** The pancreatic islets comprise less than 2% of the total pancreatic tissues. They are essential because they secrete hormones to regulate **glycemia and** blood glucose concentration. Each islet is about 75 by 175 micrometers and contains between just a few cells and approximately 3,000 cells. There are three primary types of these cells: the alpha cells, which comprise 20% of the total cells; the beta cells (70%); and the delta cells (5%). All the islet cells directly respond to nutrient levels related to eating and fasting in the blood. About 5% of pancreatic cells are pancreatic polypeptide cells (PP cells). There are four types of hormone-secreting cells, which include the following:

- *Alpha cells* – which secrete glucagon
- *Beta cells* – which secrete insulin and amylin
- *Delta cells* – which secrete gastrin and somatostatin
- *F (PP) cells* – which secrete PP

The pancreas is essential in converting food into fuel for the body's cells. Its exocrine glands produce digestive enzymes, including trypsin and chymotrypsin, to digest proteins. The pancreas also produces amylase to digest carbohydrates and lipase to break down fatty acids and cholesterol. The pancreas's endocrine functions occur via the pancreatic islets, mainly via the hormones **insulin** and **glucagon**.

DOI: 10.1201/9781003453376-5

PANCREAS

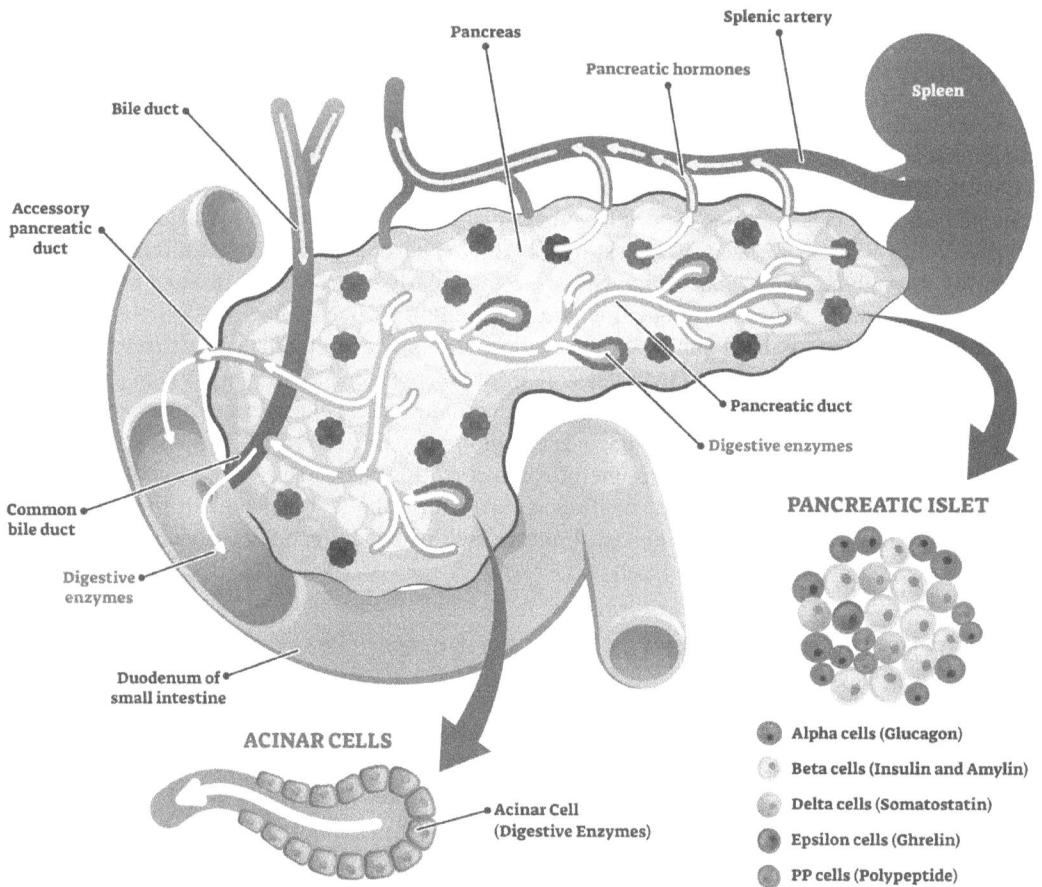

Splenic artery

Pancreas

Pancreatic hormones

Spleen

Bile duct

Accessory
pancreatic
duct

Pancreatic duct

Digestive enzymes

Common
bile duct

PANCREATIC ISLET

Digestive
enzymes

Duodenum of
small intestine

ACINAR CELLS

Acinar Cell
(Digestive Enzymes)

- Alpha cells (Glucagon)
- Beta cells (Insulin and Amylin)
- Delta cells (Somatostatin)
- Epsilon cells (Ghrelin)
- PP cells (Polypeptide)

FIGURE 3.1   The pancreas.

Alpha Cells

The alpha (α) cells secrete glucagon between meals, increasing blood glucose. Glucagon is essential in the liver for **glycogenolysis** and **gluconeogenesis.** Glycogenolysis occurs when glycogen is degraded into glucose. Gluconeogenesis is the synthesis of glucose from proteins and fats. Both processes release glucose into the blood circulation, raising blood glucose levels. Glucagon, in the adipose tissue, stimulates the release of free fatty acids and the **catabolism** of fats. Glucagon is secreted in response to increasing amino acid levels in the blood after high-protein meals. Amino acid absorption is promoted by glucagon, providing cells with raw materials required for gluconeogenesis.

Beta Cells

The beta (β) cells secrete the hormones insulin and **amylin**. Insulin is concerned with the abundance of nutrients and is secreted during and after meals as blood nutrient levels increase. Beta cells quickly respond to spikes in blood glucose concentrations by secreting stored insulin while producing more insulin. It regulates the rate of glucose uptake into many different cells. The main component of glucose in maintaining normal cell function is the sensitivity of insulin receptors. Insulin resistance is linked to diabetes, hypertension, and CVDs. The adipocytes release altered hormones in obese patients, significantly affecting insulin sensitivity.

A hormone from bone **osteoblasts**, known as *osteocalcin*, helps stimulate the multiplication of beta cells, secretion of insulin, and tissue sensitivity to insulin. The liver, adipose tissue, and skeletal muscles are directly targeted by insulin. When nutrients are sufficient, insulin stimulates the cells to absorb, store, and metabolize amino acids, fatty acids, and glucose. As a result, insulin lowers blood glucose levels and nutrients while encouraging fat, glycogen, and protein synthesis. This action promotes the storage of excessive nutrients to be used later. Insulin also enhances the growth and differentiation of cells. Insulin antagonizes glucagon to suppress the use of stored fuels. Muscles and adipose cells need insulin to use glucose, but glucose is absorbed and used by the brain, kidneys, liver, and red blood cells without any requirement for insulin. However, insulin still promotes the synthesis of glycogen in the liver. When there is an insulin insufficiency or inactive, diabetes mellitus develops.

Amylin is another beta-cell hormone that helps reduce **postprandial** spikes in blood glucose. It is also called *islet amyloid polypeptide*. Amylin slows stomach emptying, regulates the secretion of acids, bile, and gastric enzymes, restricts glucagon secretion, and stimulates the sense of fullness or *satiety* so that overeating will not occur. Therefore, it acts with antihyperglycemic effects. Aggregation of amylin has cytotoxic effects, encouraging a loss of beta cells in type 2 diabetes or when islet cells are transplanted. *Amylomimetics* are new drugs to treat type 1 and type 2 diabetes.

Check Your Knowledge

1. What do the alpha and beta cells of the pancreas secrete?
2. What processes are essential for glucagon in the liver to carry out?
3. How do beta cells respond to spikes in blood glucose?

DELTA CELLS

The delta (δ) cells secrete **somatostatin**, also known as *growth hormone-inhibiting hormone*. These cells are located in the pancreatic islets, stomach, and intestines. The secretion of somatostatin occurs while the beta cells release insulin – somatostatin, along with amylin, limits stomach acid secretion. The secretion of somatostatin is influenced mainly by the peptide hormones **urocortin** and **ghrelin**. Under an electron microscope, delta cells have smaller, slightly more compacted granules than beta cells.

Delta cells in the stomach contain cholecystokinin B receptors (CCKBRs), which respond to **gastrin**. The delta cells also have *muscarinic acetylcholine (M_3) receptors*, which react to acetylcholine (ACh). The CCKBRs increase somatostatin output, while the M_3 receptors decrease it. Vasoactive intestinal peptide acts upon delta cells, causing more somatostatin to be released. Inside the stomach, somatostatin directly affects the acid-producing parietal cells. It does this via a G-protein-coupled receptor that inhibits adenylate cyclase, antagonizing the stimulatory effect of histamine and reducing acid secretion. Somatostatin directly decreases stomach acid by preventing the release of hormones such as gastrin and secretin. This slows down the digestive process.

F (PP) CELLS

PP cells, formerly known as gamma cells (γ-cells) or F cells, are cells in the pancreatic islets (islets of Langerhans) of the pancreas. Their primary role is to help synthesize and regulate the release of PP, after which they have been named. PP cells are more concentrated in the head of the pancreas. PP cells secrete PPs, which inhibit GI movement, pancreatic secretion, and gallbladder contraction. The nervous system also regulates islet endocrine function, which has sympathetic and parasympathetic nerve endings.

YOU SHOULD REMEMBER

Amylin is a centrally acting, neuroendocrine hormone synthesized with insulin in the beta cells of pancreatic islets. Co-secretion is provoked by nutrient influx to the gastrointestinal tract, signaling the need to restore blood glucose homeostasis.

Check Your Knowledge

1. What is the general role of the pancreas?
2. What are the four types of hormone-secreting cells in the pancreas?
3. What are the functions of amylin, osteocalcin, glucagon, and somatostatin?

The Role of Insulin in Metabolism

Insulin is a critical regulator of glucose, lipid, and protein metabolism. It suppresses hepatic glucose and triglyceride production. Insulin inhibits adipose tissue lipolysis and whole-body and muscle proteolysis while stimulating glucose uptake. Women are more sensitive to insulin regarding glucose metabolism in the liver and muscles, while there are no differences between men and women in insulin action on lipolysis. Differences exist in regulating plasma triglyceride concentration and protein metabolism by insulin and in changes in insulin action in response to stimuli such as weight loss and exercise, which alter insulin sensitivity.

Insulin is an *anabolic hormone*. It elicits metabolic effects throughout the body. By monitoring glucose levels, amino acids, **keto acids**, and fatty acids circulating in the plasma, the β cells regulate insulin production as needed. The overall role of insulin is to control energy conservation and utilization during fasting and feeding. The role of insulin in cellular and molecular metabolism is explained as follows:

- *Cellular metabolism* – the insulin-dependent cascade is carried out by muscles, vascular endothelium, heart, and liver cells. In these cells, the response generated by the effects of insulin is tissue-specific. In adipose tissue, skeletal muscles, and the heart, glucose is metabolized via glucose uptake into cells. In the vascular endothelium and nature, the result is vasodilation through **nitric oxide** production. In the liver, there is a decrease in gluconeogenesis and increased glycogenesis. Insulin also affects lipid and protein metabolism, stimulating **lipogenesis** and protein synthesis while inhibiting lipolysis and degradation.
- *Molecular metabolism* – preproinsulin is the original insulin precursor, consisting of proinsulin and signal peptide sequences. Once it is translocated into the endoplasmic reticulum, preproinsulin cleaves at its signal peptide. This releases proinsulin, later cleaved by a trypsin-like enzyme, releasing insulin and a C-peptide. Until metabolically required, insulin is stored in glucose-regulated secretory vesicles as *zinc insulin hexamers*.

Insulin also affects lipid and protein metabolism, inflammation, and vasodilation. It increases the expression of certain lipogenic enzymes so that an increase in fatty acid generation increases glucose uptake by the cells. Ultimately, insulin decreases serum-free heavy acid levels. The regulation of protein breakdown is influenced by insulin's downregulation of hepatic and muscle cell enzymes responsible for protein degradation. The actions of insulin within endothelial cells and macrophages have anti-inflammatory effects. It stimulates the endothelial nitric oxide synthetase expression, releasing nitric oxide and resulting vasodilation. Insulin also suppresses nuclear factor-kappa-B in the endothelial cells. Additionally, insulin suppresses the generation of oxygen radicals and reactive oxygen species.

YOU SHOULD REMEMBER

Insulin plays a role in glucose and glycogen metabolism. Two signaling cascades carry out the homeostasis of glucose metabolism: insulin-mediated glucose uptake and glucose-stimulated insulin secretion. In the liver, insulin affects glycogen metabolism by stimulating glycogen synthesis.

Check Your Knowledge

1. What is the role of insulin in overall metabolism?
2. What are the differences between cellular and molecular metabolism?
3. What are the actions of insulin within endothelial cells and macrophages?

INSULIN RESISTANCE

Insulin resistance is described as an impaired biological response to exogenously administered insulin or to endogenously secreted insulin. The condition mainly causes decreased insulin-stimulated glucose transport and metabolism in the adipocytes and skeletal muscles. Insulin resistance is also signified by impaired insulin suppression of adipocyte lipolysis and glucose output from the liver. There are disorders of multiple metabolic pathways that involve the metabolism of amino acids, glucose, and lipids.

- *Many factors influence insulin sensitivity* – including age, ethnicity, weight, body fat (primarily abdominal), medications, and the amount of physical activity. Insulin resistance is most likely very influential in developing impaired glucose tolerance and diabetes. The condition is regularly found in patients with type 2 diabetes and is present years before the disease manifests. Insulin resistance predicts the development of diabetes.
- *However, diabetes is not commonly seen in insulin-resistant persons without a certain amount of beta-cell dysfunction* – it occurs in first-degree relatives of type 2 diabetes patients, even when they are not obese. This means that there is a vital genetic component. Environmental factors also strongly influence genetic predisposition to insulin resistance and diabetes.

Beta-cell dysfunction is partially caused by decreased beta-cell mass. There is a progressive decrease in the weight and number of these cells. They are susceptible to high levels of glucose and free fatty acids. The function of their **endoplasmic reticulum** is interrupted, and apoptosis occurs. Inflammation and changes in adipokines also cause dysfunction. Many inflammatory **cytokines** are toxic to the beta cells. The **endoplasmic reticulum** decreases insulin synthesis, so many obesity-related causes of insulin resistance also cause programmed beta-cell death (apoptosis). Abnormally high levels of glucagon aid in increased hepatic glucose production, resulting in hyperglycemia. Amylin suppresses **glucagon** release from the alpha cells and aids in pancreatic islet-cell destruction via abnormal amyloid polypeptide deposition. **Incretins** are released in response to food intake that increases beta-cell sensitivity to circulating glucose levels, improving insulin responsiveness to meals. Decreased levels of **ghrelin** are linked to hyperinsulinemia and hyperleptinemia. Reduced amounts of circulating ghrelin are related to altered insulin secretion, resistance, and obesity.

The development of type 2 diabetes is complicated and not well understood. When insulin secretion cannot compensate for insulin resistance, hyperglycemia develops. While insulin resistance is characteristic of type 2 diabetes, there is often beta-cell dysfunction and impaired insulin secretion. This includes inadequate initial-phase insulin secretion due to intravenous glucose infusion, lack of pulsatile insulin secretion, increased proinsulin secretion that signals deficient insulin processing, and accumulation of islet amyloid polypeptide, a protein usually secreted with insulin. Hyperglycemia may impair insulin secretion because high glucose levels desensitize beta cells, cause glucose toxicity with beta-cell dysfunction, or both. Usually, it takes years for these changes to develop along with insulin resistance.

Some genetic determinants exist, but diet, exercise, and lifestyle are involved. Adipose tissues increase plasma levels of free fatty acids that can impair insulin-stimulated glucose transport and muscle glycogen synthase activity. The fatty tissues appear to have endocrine functions. They release *adipocytokines* that may be metabolically needed, such as adiponectin, or harmful, such as IL-6, **leptin**, resistin, and tumor necrosis factor-alpha. Insulin resistance in older people is also related to previous intrauterine growth restriction and low birth weight. This may be related to prenatal environmental influences on glucose metabolism. In type 2 diabetes, obesity and weight gain are important factors for insulin resistance.

Check Your Knowledge

1. What is insulin resistance?
2. What factors influence insulin sensitivity?
3. How is insulin resistance implicated in the development of type 2 diabetes?

HYPERGLYCEMIA

Hyperglycemia means high blood glucose. It occurs when the body has too little insulin or cannot use it properly. A *hyperglycemic hormone* can raise blood glucose concentrations. Counter-regulatory hormones include glucagon, catecholamines, growth hormone, and glucocorticoid hormones. Insulin is classified as a *hypoglycemic hormone* because it decreases blood glucose levels. Hyperglycemia may result when a person with type 1 diabetes has not taken enough insulin. If a person has type 2 diabetes, the body may have enough insulin, but it is not as effective as needed. Hyperglycemia can also be caused by overeating or exercising insufficiently, illness or emotional stress, or due to the *dawn phenomenon*, in which a surge of hormones is naturally produced between 4:00 a.m. and 5:00 a.m.

Hyperglycemia also causes high levels of glucose in the urine, frequent urination, and increased thirst. Blood glucose must be monitored regularly, and patients must understand the range for average blood glucose. Often, exercise can lower blood glucose levels, but if the stores are 240 mg/dL or higher, the urine needs to be checked for ketones. If ketones are present, exercise must be avoided since it can cause blood glucose levels to go even higher. Meal sizes can also be reduced; for some patients, medications may need to be changed in quantity and schedule. Types of diabetes that are caused by hyperglycemia are discussed in detail later.

HYPOGLYCEMIA

Hypoglycemia occurs when blood glucose levels are lower than the standard range. It requires immediate treatment and is generally signified by a fasting blood sugar of 70 mg/dL or 3.9 mmol/L. High-sugar foods, drinks, or medications are essential to get blood glucose back into the standard range. Over the long term, treatment requires identifying and treating the actual cause of hypoglycemia.

Epidemiology

The prevalence of hypoglycemia is generally 5%–10% of people who have the suggestive symptoms. The global incidence of severe hypoglycemia events is 4,800 per 100,000 patients annually.

The global incidence of moderate hypoglycemia events is 13,100 per 100,000 patients annually. Rates of hypoglycemia are increasing in children under 6 years of age. Patients with type 1 diabetes have an increased frequency of symptomatic hypoglycemia of about one severe episode per year. The proportion of patients with diabetes mellitus with an observed extreme hypoglycemia event in insulin-treated type 2 diabetes is about 30% of the rate seen with type 1 diabetes. The event rate for severe hypoglycemia ranges from 40% to 100% of patients with type 1 diabetes. There is no gender or racial predilection for hypoglycemia.

Etiology and Risk Factors

Hypoglycemia is often related to diabetes treatment, though other drugs and various conditions can also cause low blood sugar in people who do not have diabetes. Drinking alcoholic beverages heavily without eating can keep the liver from releasing glucose from its glycogen stores into the bloodstream and can lead to hypoglycemia. Other medications can cause hypoglycemia, especially in children or people with kidney failure, such as quinine (Qualaquin), used to treat malaria. Other hypoglycemia causes include severe liver illnesses such as hepatitis or cirrhosis, severe infections, kidney disease, and advanced heart disease. Kidney disorders can also keep the body from properly excreting medications. This can affect glucose levels due to a buildup of drugs that lower blood sugar levels.

Hypoglycemia can occur with malnutrition and starvation when insufficient amounts of food and the glycogen stores the body needs to create glucose are used up. The eating disorder called *anorexia nervosa* is one example of a condition that can cause hypoglycemia and result in long-term starvation. A rare tumor of the pancreas (insulinoma) can cause too much insulin to be produced, resulting in hypoglycemia. Other tumors also can result in excessive production of insulin-like substances. Unusual cells of the pancreas that produce insulin can result in excessive insulin release, resulting in hypoglycemia. Specific adrenal gland and pituitary tumor disorders can produce inadequate hormones that regulate glucose production or metabolism. Children can have hypoglycemia if they have insufficient growth hormone. In general, hypoglycemia is much more dangerous than hyperglycemia. Extremely low blood sugar can do permanent damage and cause severe brain injury relatively quickly. Severe hypoglycemia lasting 90 minutes or more results in brain cell death within 1 week. Hyperglycemia also has adverse effects but usually causes harm over a more extended period, including complications of diabetes such as neuropathy.

Risk factors for developing hypoglycemia include hepatic insufficiency, sepsis, paraneoplastic syndromes, glycogen storage diseases, counter-regulatory hormone deficiencies, hypoadrenocorticism, pregnancy, and iatrogenic insulin overdose. Erythrocytosis and leukocytosis may also be implicated.

Clinical Manifestations

The signs and symptoms of hypoglycemia include shaking, sweating, headache, dizziness or light-headedness, numb lips, tongue, or cheek, difficulty concentrating, fatigue, hunger, nausea, tachycardia, nervousness, irritability, and anxiety. In severe cases of hypoglycemia, signs and symptoms include loss of coordination, blurry vision or **tunnel vision**, slurred speech, confusion, seizures, and loss of consciousness.

Diagnosis

Diagnosis is via a blood glucose meter test that reveals blood glucose to be 70 mg/dL or less.

Treatment

The mainstay of therapy for hypoglycemia is glucose. Pure glucose is available in tablets, gels, and other forms. Commonly, four glucose tablets (usually available OTC) can be taken, or one serving of *glucose gel*, five to six pieces of hard candy or jelly beans, four ounces of fruit juice or regular (not diet) soda, or one tablespoon of sugar, corn syrup, or honey. Generally, food or drinks with

15–20 g of carbohydrates can return blood glucose levels to the safe range. Other medications may be administered based on the underlying cause or the accompanying symptoms. In the case of severe hypoglycemia, a glucagon injection or intravenous glucose may be needed.

Blood glucose levels should be checked 15 minutes after eating or drinking something. If they are still low, another 15–20 g of carbohydrates should be consumed. This is repeated until the blood glucose is above 70 mg/dL. A snack or meal should be consumed to keep it from dropping again. If a patient usually takes insulin with food, additional insulin is generally unnecessary when consumed with a snack or meal. Some people can take a reduced insulin dose to ensure blood glucose does not increase too quickly. For emergency treatment, glucagon is available in a syringe kit or as a premixed, ready-to-use injection and a powdered nasal spray.

Prevention

Blood glucose must be monitored to prevent hypoglycemia. This may need to be done several times daily or weekly. Careful monitoring is the only preventive method to ensure blood glucose remains within the target range.

YOU SHOULD REMEMBER

Hyperglycemia occurs when blood sugar levels are too high. People develop hyperglycemia if their diabetes is not treated correctly. Hypoglycemia sets in when blood sugar levels are too low. This is usually a side effect of treatment with blood-sugar-lowering medication.

Check Your Knowledge

1. What are the causes of hyperglycemia?
2. How prevalent is hypoglycemia?
3. What are the clinical manifestations of hypoglycemia?

TYPES OF DIABETES MELLITUS

The three primary types of diabetes mellitus are type 1, 2, and gestational diabetes. However, five subgroups of diabetes are explained as follows:

- *Severe autoimmune diabetes (SAID)* – also classified as type 1 diabetes, the immune system produces antibodies that destroy the insulin-producing beta cells as an autoimmune response. Close blood glucose and insulin replacement must be monitored with daily injections or an insulin pump.
- *Severe insulin-deficient diabetes (SIDD)* – similar to SAID, the body does not produce enough insulin, but no antibodies are present. Instead, damage to the insulin-producing cells causes insufficient production of insulin. This subgroup has the highest risk of vision loss. Management is similar to SAID's, but oral medications may also be needed.
- *Severe insulin-resistant diabetes (SIRD)* –occurs when the body does not respond to insulin. Patients in this subgroup are usually overweight and have a higher risk of kidney disease. Management plans for this subgroup are the least effective. Patients with this subgroup may benefit the most from new diagnostics and more intensive treatments.
- *Mild obesity-related diabetes (MOD)* – patients are very overweight and have some amount of insulin resistance, which is not as severe as in SIRD; however, this subgroup is related to obesity.

- *Mild age-related diabetes (MARD)* – patients are elderly, with a milder form of diabetes than those that developed it in middle age; this is the most common subgroup.
- *Mature-onset diabetes of the young (MODY)* is a mutation in a single gene (monogenic) of beta cells that causes a defect in insulin synthesis. This is an autosomal dominant genetic disorder, and patients show manifestations of diabetes before the age of 25.

Type 1 Diabetes Mellitus

Type 1 diabetes mellitus was previously called *insulin-dependent* or *juvenile-onset* diabetes mellitus. It is a chronic disease caused by pancreatic insufficiency of insulin production. There are two forms of type 1 diabetes. Type 1A is the most common form and immune-mediated, and type 1B is rare and idiopathic. Type 1A has three subgroups: polygenic, monogenic, and latent autoimmune diabetes in adults (LADA). Type 1 diabetes is the primary disease in children and adolescents, making up 5%–10% of all cases. It is rare during the first 9 months of life and is at its highest incidence at 12 years of age. Lacking insulin, glucose cannot enter the cells that require insulin-mediated glucose uptake. This can cause extremely high levels of blood glucose and potentially life-threatening *diabetic ketoacidosis*. This suggests that a more vigorous autoimmune response occurs with type 1 diabetes in young children. Type 1 diabetes is an autoimmune disease in which cytotoxic CD8-T lymphocytes attack and destroy the pancreatic islets.

Epidemiology

The incidence of type 1 diabetes is increasing by 2%–5% globally. Prevalence is about one in every 300 people by the age of 18. In 2021, approximately 8.4 million people have type 1 diabetes globally. Of these, 1.5 million were younger than 20, 5.4 million were between ages 20 and 59, and 1.6 million were 60 or older. In the United States, Caucasians develop type 1 diabetes more often than African Americans, Hispanics, or Latinos.

Etiology and Risk Factors

Type 1 diabetes is caused by an autoimmune reaction that destroys the pancreatic essential cells, resulting in insulin becoming unable to be manufactured. This can go on for months to years before symptoms manifest. An imbalance between available insulin and the amount required will cause elevated blood glucose. Target tissue insulin resistance, relative insulin insufficiency, or both conditions cause the imbalance. Insulin resistance fails to inhibit endogenous glucose production in the liver. It also causes a failure of glucose uptake and glycogen synthesis in the skeletal muscles after meals. Additionally, it causes a loss and inhibits the activation of hormone-sensitive lipase in the fatty tissues. This leads to excess triglyceride breakdown in the adipocytes and excessive circulation of free fatty acids.

Clinical Manifestations

The development of type 1 diabetes occurs in three stages, as follows:

- *Stage 1* – asymptomatic; characterized by average fasting glucose, standard glucose tolerance, and presence of two or more pancreatic autoantibodies
- *Stage 2* – a presence of two or more pancreatic autoantibodies plus **dysglycemia**, with impaired fasting glucose of 100–125 mg/dL or impaired glucose tolerance (2-hour plasma glucose of 140–199 mg/dL, or a hemoglobin A1c between 5.7% and 6.4%); individuals remain asymptomatic
- *Stage 3* – diabetes or hyperglycemia with clinical symptoms and two or more pancreatic autoantibodies

The signs and symptoms of type 1 diabetes sometimes appear suddenly. **Polydipsia**, **polyuria**, **polyphagia**, loss of weight without trying to do so, irritability, other mood changes, tiredness, weakness, blurry vision, and, in children, bed-wetting after never previously having had the problem.

Diagnosis

The diagnosis of type 1 diabetes mellitus is based on a **glycated hemoglobin** (A1C) test, a random blood sugar test, and a fasting blood sugar test. The glycated hemoglobin test shows the average blood glucose level for the past 2–3 months, measuring the amount of blood glucose attached to the oxygen-carrying protein in red blood cells, known as *hemoglobin*. The higher the levels, the more hemoglobin will be present with glucose attached. An A1C level of 6.5% or more on two tests indicates diabetes. If the A1C test is unavailable, or some conditions can make it inaccurate (pregnancy or an uncommon hemoglobin variant), the other two tests may be chosen.

A blood sample is taken after fasting overnight in the fasting blood sugar test. A fasting blood sugar level of less than 100 mg/dL (5.6 mmol/L) is healthy. However, a story from 100 to 125 mg/dL (5.6–6.9 mmol/L) is considered "prediabetes." If the group is 126 md/dL (7 mmol/L) or more on two separate tests or a random blood sugar of 200 mg/dL or more with hyperglycemia symptoms confirms the diagnosis of type 1 diabetes. The presence of ketones in the urine also suggests type 1 diabetes.

Treatment

Treatments for type 1 diabetes include insulin, counting carbohydrates, fats, and protein, regular blood glucose monitoring, a healthy diet, exercising regularly, and maintaining a healthy weight. The goal is to keep daytime blood glucose levels before meals between 80 and 130 mg/dL (4.44–7.2 mmol/L). After-meal numbers should be at most 180 mg/dL (10 mmol/L) 2 hours after eating. Insulin options include short-acting, rapid-acting, intermediate-acting, long-acting, and ultra-long-acting insulins. They may be delivered by injections or with an insulin pump. Some patients also require antihypertensive medications, aspirin, and cholesterol-lowering drugs. Life activities that may need to be modified include driving, working, pregnancy, and managing concurrent health conditions. Potential future treatments include pancreas transplantation and islet-cell transplantation.

Prevention

No one knows how to prevent type 1 diabetes, but it can be treated successfully by physician follow-up recommendations for a healthy lifestyle and managing blood sugar.

YOU SHOULD REMEMBER

Experts think type 1 diabetes is caused by genes and factors in the environment, such as viruses, that might trigger the disease. Researchers are working to pinpoint the causes of type 1 diabetes through studies.

Check Your Knowledge

1. What are the three primary types of diabetes mellitus?
2. What is type 1 diabetes caused by?
3. What are the three stages of development of type 1 diabetes?

Type 2 Diabetes Mellitus

Type 2 diabetes mellitus, also called non-insulin-dependent diabetes or adult-onset diabetes, is one of the most common health conditions today. It is a heterogeneous disorder believed to represent many different primary environmental and genetic abnormalities that lead to relative insulin deficiency. Type 2 diabetes is more common in males than females and usually occurs after the age of 40. However, when diagnosed before age 40, the average reduction in lifespan is 12 years in males but 19 years in females.

Type 2 diabetes is about 90%–95% of all disease cases. The most common cause of insulin resistance is weight gain or obesity. As body mass index (BMI) increases, so does the risk of developing diabetes. Genetic syndromes may also cause insulin resistance, autoantibodies to insulin, primary target cell defects, increased insulin degradation when there is excessive energy (more than the body can store), and insulin-mediated cellular glucose uptake changes.

Adipokines are hormones released by adipocytes or macrophages infiltrating adipose tissue in response to the increase in fat mass. They induce low-grade chronic inflammation, insulin resistance, and obesity-associated diseases. There are increased serum levels of leptin, known as *leptin resistance*, and increased serum levels of **resistin**, with decreased **adiponectin** levels. The altered adipokines affect body tissues and the functions of the hypothalamus and pancreas.

Epidemiology

Type 2 diabetes accounts for approximately 90% of global cases of diabetes. It is a current epidemic in developed and developing countries but is most common in non-European countries. For example, on the island of Nauru in the Pacific, nearly 40% of adults have diabetes. The disease was almost nonexistent in this location 50 years ago. Current diabetes statistics show that 77% of global diabetes patients live in lower- or middle-income countries, with about 179 million people believed to be undiagnosed. The epidemic is growing since current estimates are much higher than predictions made 10 years ago.

Since 1940, type 2 diabetes has been increasing in the United States. It has doubled in all adult age groups in just the past 25 years. Type 2 diabetes varies between ethnic groups but is most common in African-American women. It affects 34% of people between the ages of 65 and 74. A **metabolic syndrome** increases the likelihood of developing type 2 diabetes and related cardiovascular complications. It is common in overweight children and adolescents and affects about 55 million Americans. According to the American Diabetes Association, approximately 25% of Americans aged 65 or older have type 2 diabetes. Metabolic syndrome will be discussed in more detail in **Chapter 24**.

In 2017, the Centers for Disease Control and Prevention (CDC) estimated that 30.3 million people in the United States (9.4% of the population) had diabetes. They also believed that 8.1 million (27.8%) were undiagnosed. In 2017, the CDC estimated that 84.1 million people (37% of adults older than 20) had prediabetes and were at a high-risk level for developing diabetes. In 2017, approximately 462 million individuals were affected by type 2 diabetes, corresponding to 6.28% of the world's population (4.4% of those aged 15–49 years, 15% of those aged 50–69, and 22% of those aged 70+), or a prevalence rate of 6,059 cases per 100,000. Over 1 million deaths per year can be attributed to diabetes alone, making it the ninth leading cause of mortality. The burden of diabetes mellitus is rising globally and much faster in developed regions, such as Western Europe. The gender distribution is equal, and the incidence peaks at around 55. The global prevalence of type 2 diabetes is projected to increase to 7,079 individuals per 100,000 by 2030, reflecting a continued rise across all regions. There are concerning trends of rising prevalence in lower-income countries. Urgent public health and clinical preventive measures are warranted. By 2,045, this number is expected to reach 693 million.

Etiology and Risk Factors

The etiology of type 2 diabetes mellitus includes a family history of diabetes, unhealthy diet, overweight, increasing age, physical inactivity, ethnicity, and hypertension. Extra abdominal fat is linked to insulin resistance, CVD, and type 2 diabetes. With insulin resistance, the body requires more insulin to help glucose enter the cells. Specific genes also make individuals more likely to develop type 2 diabetes. The disease tends to run in families and is more common in African Americans, Alaska natives, Native Americans, Asian Americans, Hispanics/Latinos, native Hawaiians, and Pacific Islanders. Genes also increase risks for type 2 diabetes by increasing the tendency to become overweight or obese.

Risks are doubled if a parent or sibling has diabetes and increased by four times if two or more first-degree relatives have the condition. Unknown environmental factors are believed to play a role, but this is still being studied. The most important environmental risk factor is central (abdominal) or visceral obesity. Medical conditions that may increase the risks for type 2 diabetes include the following:

- *Acanthosis nigricans* – a skin condition in which the skin appears darker than usual. There are soft brown to black patches of skin on the back of the neck, armpit, elbows, and, sometimes, the knees (see **Figure 3.2**). The condition is most common in obese people when their bodies are overproducing insulin. Patients with this condition are twice as likely to have type 2 diabetes mellitus as those without it.
- *Hypertension* – greater than 130/80 mm Hg. According to the American Diabetes Association, hypertension plus type 2 diabetes is much more likely to be fatal because it dramatically increases the risks of heart attack or stroke. Chronic hypertension can also cause faster development of Alzheimer's disease and dementia.
- *Hypercholesterolemia* – high insulin levels in the blood have a terrible effect on the number of cholesterol particles in the bloodstream. They raise the amount of "bad" LDL cholesterol, which is the type that usually forms plaques in the arteries while lowering the number of "good" high-density lipoprotein (HDL) cholesterol, which helps clear out plaques before they can break off and cause a heart attack or stroke. Diabetes also usually causes higher levels of triglycerides in the blood. Increased LDL cholesterol is often seen when insulin resistance is present, even during prediabetes. With type 2 diabetes, the plaques in the arteries usually have more fat content and are less fibrous than in type 1 diabetes. This is a much more dangerous condition than a heart attack or stroke. The American Diabetes

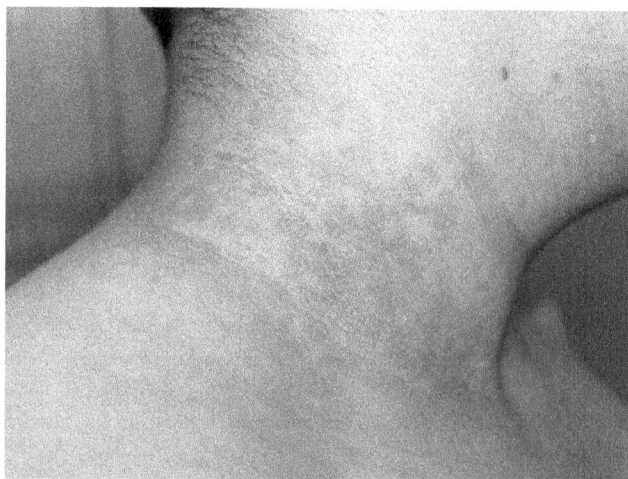

FIGURE 3.2   Acanthosis nigricans.

Association recommends checking cholesterol levels at least once yearly and more often when they are high and not controlled by medication. For those with diabetes and known coronary heart disease, LDL levels should be below 70 mg per deciliter (mg/dL).

- *Triglyceride levels* – (250 or higher). Normal triglyceride levels are below 150 mg/dL. Leftover calories are stored in body cells as triglycerides. Aside from a poor diet, triglyceride levels can increase because of renal failure, genetics, low thyroid hormone levels, and certain medications. A good diet is low in carbohydrates, sugars, saturated fat, and trans fats. A significant amount of fatty fish, nuts, seeds, avocados, and olive oil should be consumed. Smoking also increases triglyceride levels, as does excessive alcohol intake. Additional risk factors for type 2 diabetes include low HDL or "good" cholesterol, a history of gestational diabetes or giving birth to a baby weighing nine pounds or more, a history of heart disease or stroke, and depression.
- *Polycystic ovary syndrome (PCOS)* – affects between 5% and 20% of women and is the most common reproductive hormone disorder of women of childbearing age. It is also the number one cause of female infertility. This condition is diagnosed when there are irregular or absent periods, elevated male sex hormones, ovaries with large amounts of cysts, and other symptoms (skin discolorations, painful menstruation, depression, mood disorders, lack of sex drive, and excess abdominal fat). Between 50% and 90% of women with PCOS have insulin resistance, and women with this condition are three to five times more likely to develop type 2 diabetes.
- *Prediabetes* – higher-than-normal blood sugar levels, but not yet at diabetes levels. The progression from prediabetes to type 2 diabetes is slower when the diet consists of many plant-based, non-processed foods and overall lower body fat. Physical exercise, including strength training, is very effective in keeping type 2 diabetes from developing.

Clinical Manifestations

Patients with type 2 diabetes usually have less severe insulin deficiency than those with type 1. There is often an insidious onset of hyperglycemia, and many patients have no initial symptoms. If the disease progresses without treatment, there may be symptoms of coronary artery, cerebrovascular, or peripheral artery disease. Many patients have chronic skin infections. The clinical manifestations of type 2 diabetes are summarized in **Table 3.1**.

Type 2 diabetes may present with symptomatic hyperglycemia but is often asymptomatic. The condition is usually detected because of routine tests. Initial symptoms may be those of diabetic

---

TABLE 3.1
Type 2 Diabetes Clinical Manifestations

Clinical Manifestation	Examples
Fatigue, lethargy	Changes in metabolism cause poor use of food products
General pruritus	Since glycosuria and hyperglycemia encourage fungal growth, women often develop candidal infections that result in pruritus
Paresthesias	Commonly develop due to diabetic neuropathies
Recurrent infections (boils, carbuncles, skin infections); prolonged wound healing	Increased glucose levels stimulate growth of microorganisms; healing is slowed due to impaired blood supply
Visual changes	Water balance fluctuates in the eyes due to elevated blood glucose, and blurred vision occurs; another cause of visual loss is diabetic retinopathy

complications. The disease may have been developing for quite some time. A hyperosmotic coma sometimes occurs first, often due to stressors or impaired glucose metabolism caused by corticosteroids and other drugs.

Diagnosis

Diagnosis of type 2 diabetes uses the same criteria as for type 1. For prediabetes, annual monitoring is required. The classic signs and symptoms of type 1 diabetes mellitus (polyuria, polydipsia, and polyphagia) are not as common in type 2. Vision changes, headache, increased fatigue, and lethargy may lead to a diagnosis of type 2 diabetes. Diagnostic tests include the oral glucose tolerance test (OGTT), hemoglobin A1c level, C-peptide insulin level, and islet-cell antibody level. Diagnosis is only made after laboratory tests reveal glycosuria or hyperglycemia. Usually, diagnosis is made after routine blood testing in asymptomatic people. Today, regular glucose testing is recommended for everyone older than age 45. Diagnosis may also occur after the patient seeks medical attention for fatigue, dizziness, or blurred vision.

Treatment

Treatment of type 2 diabetes begins with dietary changes. Carbohydrates, fats, and proteins are individualized based on the patient's goals, preferences, and eating patterns. Most patients with diabetes consume approximately 45% of their calories as carbohydrates, followed by 25%–35% as fats. Only 10%–35% are consumed as proteins.

In 2018, the Food and Drug Administration (FDA) reported that a severe genital infection was linked to type 2 diabetes patients who took *sodium-glucose cotransporter-2 (SGLT2) inhibitors.* One person died, and 11 people were hospitalized. These agents had been approved in 2013 to lower blood sugar in adults with type 2 diabetes. The FDA now requires drug labeling for SGLT2 inhibitors to describe this risk. These agents include canagliflozin (Invokana®) and empagliflozin (Jardiance®). Patients are at risk of the infection known as Fournier's gangrene, a sporadic yet life-threatening bacterial infection of the tissue under the skin surrounding the genital area. The bacteria usually enter via a wound and spread quickly. Diabetes is a risk factor for developing this type of gangrene. Of the 12 cases, seven were males and five were females. Some survivors required multiple disfiguring surgeries and developed complications. The infections developed within several months of the patients using the medications. In managing patients who have type 2 diabetes, the following must be considered before prescribing medications.

People with type 2 diabetes with slightly elevated plasma glucose are placed on a healthy diet and exercise regimen, followed by a single oral antihyperglycemic medication, if indicated. Oral additional medicines (combination therapy) may be added. When two or more drugs are ineffective, insulin is administered. With more significant glucose elevations upon diagnosis, lifestyle changes and oral antihyperglycemics are usually started simultaneously.

Dietary Considerations

Limiting carbohydrate intake and substituting some fat calories with monounsaturated fats will lower triglycerides, and "good" HDL cholesterol will increase. Monounsaturated fats include olive oil, canola oil, and oils from avocados and nuts. In high doses, omega-3 fatty acids lower plasma triglycerides and VLDL cholesterol and reduce platelet aggregation. A high intake of alpha-linolenic acid is beneficial in the secondary prevention of coronary heart disease. Good diets are rich in fruits and vegetables, supplying extensive information on natural **antioxidants**.

For sweetening foods, options include **saccharin** (Sweet and Low), a nonnutritive sweetener. Aspartame (NutraSweet) comprises two primary amino acids, aspartic acid, and phenylalanine, creating a nutritive sweetener 180 times sweeter than sucrose. Aspartame cannot be used in cooking or baking because high temperatures destroy it. Other products that assist in dietary treatment include sucralose (*Splenda*) and acesulfame potassium (*DiabetiSweet, Sunett, Sweet One*). These nonnutritive sweeteners are heat-stable.

A highly effective natural sugar substance, *fructose*, causes only slightly increased plasma glucose levels and does not require insulin for utilization. However, large amounts of fructose (up to 20% of total calories) cause potential adverse effects, raising serum cholesterol, LDL cholesterol, and triglycerides. Therefore, it is not advantageous to be used as a sweetener for people with diabetes. An option is to eat fruits and vegetables (containing natural fructose) or moderate intake of foods sweetened with fructose.

Sugar alcohols are also known as polyalcohols or **polyols**. They are commonly used sweeteners and *bulking agents*. Naturally present in many fruits and vegetables, they can also be made from glucose, sucrose, and starch. Examples of sugar alcohols include *sorbitol, mannitol, xylitol, isomalt, lactitol, hydrogenated starch hydrolysates, and maltitol*. These are not as easily absorbed as sugar, so they do not raise blood glucose levels as much as conventional types of sugar. However, they increase blood glucose and may cause bloating and diarrhea if consumed in large amounts. Sugar alcohols are often used in food products sold as "sugar-free": chewing gum, hard candies, lozenges, and sugar-free ice cream.

Exercise

Exercise is essential and is very effective in increasing insulin sensitivity in humans. Adequate training reduces postprandial blood glucose levels, insulin requirements, and cholesterol and triglyceride levels. Exercise also increases HDL cholesterol and is a valuable adjunct to weight loss. It should be noted that hypoglycemia can occur while exercising if the patient is receiving insulin or sulfonylurea therapy.

Surgery

For the morbidly obese who are unresponsive to diet and exercise, bariatric surgery may be required. Gastric bypass surgery achieves significant improvements in glycemic control for diabetic patients. Medications are used for most people with type 2 diabetes, with oral hypoglycemic agents being the treatment of choice. However, some older patients continue to self-inject insulin. In the later stages of type 2 diabetes, insulin may be needed due to loss of beta-cell function. The risks of hypoglycemia must always be taken into account. There are several categories of medications used to treat type 2 diabetes. These include the following:

- *Medications that act on the sulfonylurea receptor complex of beta cells* – sulfonylureas are the most widely prescribed drugs for hyperglycemia. They include *acetohexamide, chlorpropamide, glimepiride, glipizide, glyburide, Glynase, tolazamide*, and *tolbutamide*. The meglitinide analog *repaglinide* and the delta-phenylalanine derivative *nateglinide* bind the sulfonylurea receptor, stimulating insulin secretion.
- *Medications that mostly lower glucose levels by affecting the liver, skeletal muscles, or fatty tissues* – while metformin (a *biguanide* also available in an extended-release form) works mainly in the liver, other drugs primarily affect the skeletal muscles and adipose tissues. These include the peroxisome proliferator-activated receptor agonists (PPARs) called *rosiglitazone* and *pioglitazone*. These drugs are also classified as *thiazolidinediones*.
- Medications mainly affecting glucose absorption are classified as alpha-glucosidase inhibitors, including two drugs (*acarbose* and *miglitol*).
- Medications that mimic the effects of incretin or lengthen its actions are GLP-1 receptor agonists and DPP-4 inhibitors. The GLP-1 receptor agonists include *albiglutide, dulaglutide, exenatide, long-acting-release-exenatide, liraglutide,* and *lixisenatide*. The DPP-4 inhibitors include *alogliptin, linagliptin, saxagliptin,* and *sitagliptin*.
- *Medications inhibiting the reabsorption of filtered glucose in the kidneys are SGLT2 inhibitors, including canagliflozin, dapagliflozin,* and *empagliflozin*.

- *Other medications include pramlintide, which lowers glucose by suppressing glucagon and slowing* gastric emptying. Other drugs called *bromocriptine* and *colesevelam* have unknown mechanisms for reducing blood glucose.

Prevention

As the global population has become less and less active over decades, reduced exercise has resulted in a massive increase in type 2 diabetes. Advanced technology allows us to interact with others quickly and easily without physically traveling as often. Recreation involving computers, television, and video games can be done inside the home and nearly anywhere else. Fast food and vending machines supply drinks and foods with low nutrition, high calories, and large amounts of fat and carbohydrates.

The American Diabetes Association recommends preventing type 2 diabetes by restricting caloric intake and getting regular physical exercise. Saturated fat must be reduced to less than 7% of daily calories. Trans fats must be avoided entirely. Alcohol consumption must be limited to no more than two servings per day. Whole grains and monounsaturated fats are encouraged frequently. At least 14 g of dietary fiber must be consumed per day. Carbohydrate intake must be restricted. Foods with a high glycemic index must be limited, including sweetened beverages and desserts. The total average daily calories should be monitored. A physician should regularly check vital signs such as blood lipids, pressure, and glucose.

According to the CDC, more than one out of every three adults have prediabetes, and 90% do not know it. The National Diabetes Prevention Program can help people make lifestyle changes to prevent or delay type 2 diabetes and its related health problems. Blood sugar testing can reveal the condition quickly. Losing 5%–7% of body weight can significantly lower the risk of developing type 2 diabetes. Regular physical activity means at least 150 minutes per week of brisk walking or a similar activity – only 30 minutes a day for 5 days per week.

YOU SHOULD REMEMBER

In the United States, 96 million adults have prediabetes. More than eight in ten of them do not know they have it. With prediabetes, blood sugar levels are higher than usual but not high enough for a type 2 diabetes diagnosis. Prediabetes raises the risk of type 2 diabetes, heart disease, and stroke.

Check Your Knowledge

1. How common is type 2 diabetes?
2. What medical conditions may increase the risks for type 2 diabetes?
3. What are the general treatment options for type 2 diabetes?

GESTATIONAL DIABETES

Gestational diabetes can develop during pregnancy in women who do not have diabetes. Every year, 2%–10% of pregnancies in the United States are affected by gestational diabetes. Managing gestational diabetes will help ensure healthy pregnancies and infants. Affected babies are more likely to develop obesity and type 2 diabetes later in life. Untreated, gestational diabetes can result in a baby's death before or shortly after birth. Also, women with diabetes are about five times more likely to have a stillbirth.

Gestational diabetes is a condition in which a hormone made by the placenta typically prevents the body from using insulin. Glucose builds up in the bloodstream instead of being absorbed by the cells. Unlike type 1 diabetes, gestational diabetes is not caused by a lack of insulin but by other hormones produced during pregnancy that can result in insulin resistance. Gestational diabetic symptoms disappear following delivery. Although the cause is unknown, some theories exist on why the condition occurs. Although any woman can develop gestational diabetes during pregnancy, some of the factors that may increase the risk include the following:

- Being overweight or obese
- Family history of diabetes
- Having given birth previously to an infant weighing greater than 9 pounds
- Age (women who are older than 25 are at a greater risk for developing gestational diabetes than younger women)
- Race (women who are African-American, American Indian, Asian American, Hispanic or Latino, or Pacific Islander have a higher risk)
- Prediabetes, also known as impaired glucose tolerance

Although increased glucose in the urine is often included in the list of risk factors, it is not believed to be a reliable indicator for gestational diabetes.

The placenta supplies a growing fetus with nutrients and water and produces a variety of hormones to maintain the pregnancy. Some hormones (estrogen, cortisol, and human placental lactogen) can block insulin. This is called the *contra-insulin effect* and usually begins about 20–24 weeks into the pregnancy. As the placenta grows, more hormones are produced, and the risk of insulin resistance becomes more significant. Usually, the pancreas can make additional insulin to overcome insulin resistance, but when insulin production is not enough to overcome the effect of the placental hormones, gestational diabetes results.

Gestational diabetes often has no symptoms or may be mild, such as having a stronger thirst than usual or urinating more frequently. Gestational diabetes is sometimes related to the hormonal changes of pregnancy that make the body less able to use insulin. Genes and extra weight may also play a role. The most common period for gestational diabetes is between 24 and 28 weeks of pregnancy. Diagnostic tests include the glucose challenge and OGTTs. If the glucose challenge test results show high blood glucose, the woman will return for an OGTT test to confirm the diagnosis of gestational diabetes. Managing gestational diabetes includes following a healthy eating plan and being physically active. Insulin may be required if the patient's eating plan and physical activity are insufficient to keep blood glucose in your target range.

Prevention

The chance of developing gestational diabetes can be lowered by losing extra weight (if a woman is overweight) before becoming pregnant. Being physically active before and during pregnancy also may help prevent gestational diabetes.

Check Your Knowledge

1. What percentage of pregnancies are affected by gestational diabetes?
2. Which factors increase risks for gestational diabetes?
3. In which period does gestational diabetes most commonly occur?

NEONATAL DIABETES

Neonatal diabetes is a rare form that occurs in the first 6 months of life. Affected infants do not produce enough insulin, so blood glucose levels increase. Neonatal diabetes is often mistaken for the much more common type 1 diabetes, but that condition usually occurs in children older than

6 months. Fetuses with neonatal diabetes do not grow normally in the uterus, and newborns may be tiny for their gestational age, known as *intrauterine growth restriction.*

Epidemiology

Half of infants with neonatal diabetes will have a lifelong condition known as *permanent neonatal diabetes mellitus.* This occurs in one of every 260,000 infants globally. The other half of infants with neonatal diabetes will have the state disappear within the first 12 weeks of life, though it can recur. This is called *transient neonatal diabetes mellitus.*

Etiology and Risk Factors

Neonatal diabetes is a monogenetic disease caused by single-gene mutations. In most cases, the gene mutation is inherited. The only risk factor is having a causative gene mutation.

Clinical Manifestations

As glucose leaves the body through the urine, the signs and symptoms of neonatal diabetes may include increased wet diapers, appetite, and dehydration. Parents should immediately alert their child's pediatrician if these signs or symptoms occur.

Diagnosis

Neonatal diabetes is diagnosed when a physician finds elevated glucose levels in an infant's blood or urine. Genetic testing can also help properly diagnose it.

Treatment

Neonatal diabetes is often treated with insulin. Sometimes, when a specific gene mutation is known, oral medications may be used.

Prevention

There is no current way to prevent neonatal diabetes.

YOU SHOULD REMEMBER

Macrosomia is the predominant adverse outcome and the main factor linked to neonatal complications. Poor maternal glycemic control, especially in the context of maternal type 2 diabetes and obesity, increases the risk of all adverse neonatal outcomes, most strikingly, the risk of perinatal mortality and congenital disabilities.

Check Your Knowledge

1. When does neonatal diabetes occur?
2. What are the signs and symptoms of neonatal diabetes?
3. What are the diagnostic requirements and treatments for neonatal diabetes?

OBESITY AND DIABETES

Obesity is defined as *excessive adipose tissue mass.* This does not always mean it is equivalent to increased body weight. By numerical standards, lean but extremely muscular people can be overweight without increased adiposity. Obesity is also defined by considering how it relates to morbidity or mortality. The most common method of gauging obesity is the BMI. This equals body weight in kilograms (kg) divided by square meters (m^2) of height. Obesity can also be assessed with *anthropometry*, which measures the thickness of skinfolds, *densitometry* (underwater weighing), computed tomography (CT), magnetic resonance imaging (MRI), and *electrical impedance*. According to the *Metropolitan Life Tables*, the BMI "midpoint" for men and women of all heights and body frames ranges from 19 to 26 kg/m^2. However, women have a higher body fat percentage at a similar BMI. Based on substantial morbidity information, a BMI of 30 is usually the obesity threshold for both men and women.

BMIs of 25 or higher are linked to slowly worsening risks for morbidity from all causes (including metabolic, cancer-related, and cardiovascular-related causes). The term *overweight* is used by most healthcare practitioners for individuals with BMIs between 25 and 30. These BMIs are medically significant, and therapeutic intervention should occur when there are adiposity-influenced risk factors such as glucose intolerance and hypertension.

Intra-abdominal and abdominal subcutaneous fat are of more clinical concern than subcutaneous fat in the buttocks and lower extremities. The most important complications of obesity in men and women include insulin resistance, diabetes, hyperlipidemia, hypertension, and, only in women, **hyperandrogenism**. The systemic complications of obesity may be related to adipokines secreted by stored adipocytes.

Obesity is a pandemic condition that increases risks for type 2 diabetes. Approximately 2.1 billion people globally are *overweight* or *obese*. In America, an estimated 160 million people are either obese or overweight. Of these, 78 million are obese, a higher figure than in any other country. Adults are not the only people affected since nearly 30% of younger people under 20 are either obese or overweight. Of children under 18 years, about 13% are obese. Risk factors for obesity include interactions of **genotypes** and environmental factors such as diet and physical activity.

Obesity has different effects on various ethnic groups. It is much more likely to develop in African-Americans, Hispanics, American Indians, and Pacific Islanders than Caucasians. For unknown reasons, Asians have a higher risk for type 2 diabetes than Caucasians; it occurs at a lower BMI and fat mass than in other groups. This may be linked to the fact that Asians have a mean lower fat mass at every decade of life compared to Caucasians, African-Americans, and Puerto Rican Hispanics. There are also higher rates of hypertension, diabetes, and hyperuricemia in people from Taiwan compared to African-Americans or Caucasians, based on the level of BMI. According to the CDC, the number of overweight and obese individuals of both genders has risen since 1960. In the last decades, the percentage of adults aged 20 or older who are overweight or obese has increased to 54.9%.

Check Your Knowledge

1. What is the most common method of gauging obesity?
2. What are the most critical complications of obesity?
3. In which groups of people is obesity most likely to develop?

DIETARY COMPONENTS

Dietary fiber has been shown to help decrease risks. Increased risks for type 2 diabetes also result in increased risks for coronary heart disease and gallbladder disease. Whole grains are protective against type 2 diabetes, along with cereal fiber and dietary magnesium. Soluble fiber inhibits the absorption of macronutrients, reduces postprandial glucose responses, and helps to balance blood lipids. However, reduced risks for diabetes are more significantly linked to insoluble fiber, also known as *cereal fiber*. High magnesium intake has an overall risk reduction for type 2 diabetes of 23%. Magnesium has significant chemopreventive activity against the condition. Food sources with large amounts of magnesium include green leafy vegetables, nuts, and whole grains. Intracellular magnesium is an essential cofactor for several enzymes required for carbohydrate metabolism. When deficient, insulin resistance can be triggered by reduced intracellular insulin signaling.

Trans fatty acids increase the risks for type 2 diabetes. Polyunsaturated fatty acids protect against the disease, and other types of fat are neutral in their effects. Consumption of processed meats also increases risks, while a high intake of linoleic acid reduces chances. For diabetic patients, a diet rich in monounsaturated fat improves both glycemic and lipoprotein levels and dramatically improves health. High-fructose corn syrup has become a standard component of many popular food products. It is a mixture of about 55% fructose and 42% sucrose, with the remaining percentage comprising other ingredients, and is the only sweetening agent in soft drinks. Overconsumption of this agent harms glucose metabolism. There are significant increases in blood concentrations of fasting glucose, postprandial triacylglycerol, and apolipoprotein-B, the main protein of the low-density lipoprotein that carries cholesterol to the tissues while decreasing insulin response. High-fructose corn syrup increases lipogenesis, promotes dyslipidemia, reduces sensitivity to insulin, and increases visceral adiposity in overweight or obese adults. Fructose does not stimulate insulin secretion or the release of leptin. Since insulin and leptin are critical to regulating food intake and body weight, high fructose levels may increase energy uptake and weight gain.

DIABETIC KETOACIDOSIS

Diabetic ketoacidosis is a severe complication of diabetes mellitus that may be life-threatening. It develops when the body does not have enough insulin to allow blood glucose into the cells to be used for energy. Instead, the liver breaks down fat for fuel, producing ketones. When too many ketones are made too quickly, they can accumulate to dangerous levels. Diabetic ketoacidosis is a true medical emergency that requires immediate treatment.

EPIDEMIOLOGY

Diabetic ketoacidosis is most common among people with type 1 diabetes, though it can also develop in those with type 2 diabetes.

Etiology and Risk Factors

The most common causes of diabetic ketoacidosis are illness and problems with insulin. Eating and drinking may be significantly reduced when sick, making blood glucose levels difficult to manage. Insulin-related causes include missing insulin shots, a clogged insulin pump, or taking the wrong insulin dose. Other causes of diabetic ketoacidosis include heart attack, stroke, physical injuries, alcohol or drug use, and medications such as certain diuretics or corticosteroids. The most significant risk factors for diabetic ketoacidosis are type 1 diabetes and regularly missing needed insulin doses.

Clinical Manifestations

Insulin deficiency and increased counter-regulatory hormones (glucagon, catecholamines, and cortisol) cause the body to metabolize triglycerides and amino acids for energy. Serum levels of glycerol and free fatty acids increased due to uncontrolled lipolysis. Alanine levels rise due to muscle catabolism. Glycerol and alanine provide a substrate for gluconeogenesis in the liver, stimulated by excessive glucagon accompanying insulin deficiency. Glucagon stimulates the mitochondrial conversion of free fatty acids into ketones. Ketogenesis proceeds in the absence of insulin. Acetoacetic acid and beta-hydroxybutyric acid create metabolic acidosis. Acetone from metabolized acetoacetic acid accumulates in the serum and is slowly removed via respiration.

Hyperglycemia from insulin deficiency causes osmotic diuresis, leading to significant losses of water and electrolytes in the urine. Urinary excretion of ketones results in losses of excessive sodium and potassium. Even with a large total body potassium deficit, initial serum potassium is usually normal or elevated due to the extracellular migration of potassium caused by acidosis. Potassium levels generally decrease even more during treatment as insulin therapy drives potassium into the cells. If the serum potassium is not monitored and adequately replaced, life-threatening hypokalemia may develop.

Diabetic ketoacidosis usually develops slowly. Initial symptoms include extreme thirst and significantly increased urination. If untreated, more severe symptoms can appear quickly. They have fast and deep breathing, dry mouth and skin, facial flushing, a "fruity" smell of the breath, headache, muscle aches or stiffness, extreme tiredness, nausea, vomiting, and stomach pain. Sometimes, diabetic ketoacidosis is the initial sign of undiagnosed diabetes mellitus.

Diagnosis

Blood tests for diabetic ketoacidosis include blood glucose ketone levels and acidity. Other tests include blood electrolyte tests, urinalysis, chest X-rays, and an electrocardiogram.

Treatment

Treatment for diabetic ketoacidosis usually occurs in the hospital's emergency department or after admission. Treatments include fluid replacement, electrolyte replacement, insulin, and medications for any underlying illnesses.

Prevention

Methods to prevent diabetic ketoacidosis include checking blood glucose regularly, incredibly when sick, keeping blood glucose levels within the target range as much as possible, taking all prescribed medications as instructed, and discussing with a physician how to adjust insulin based on foods that are eaten, physical activity levels, and during an illness.

Check Your Knowledge

1. What dietary components increase the risks for type 2 diabetes?
2. How does diabetic ketoacidosis develop?
3. How do the symptoms of diabetic ketoacidosis develop over time?

HYPEROSMOLAR COMA

Hyperosmolar coma is also known as *hyperosmolar hyperglycemic syndrome (HHS)* and *nonketotic hyperglycemic syndrome*. It is a true hyperglycemic crisis characterized by severe hyperglycemia, hyperosmolality, and dehydration without significant ketoacidosis.

EPIDEMIOLOGY

Hyperosmolar coma is most common in people older than 65 and causes ten times more deaths than diabetic **ketoacidosis**. As many as 20% of patients with hyperosmolar coma die. Overall mortality rates vary between 5,000 and 20,000 of every 100,000 affected individuals. Hyperosmolar coma is more common in African-American males than in any other group.

Etiology and Risk Factors

Hyperosmolar coma is caused by type 2 diabetes mellitus due to a combination of absolute or relative insulin deficiency in the setting of increased **counter-regulatory hormones**. Other causes include dehydration, infections, heart attack, stroke, medications that decrease the effects of insulin, medications or conditions that increase fluid loss, and incorrect use of prescribed diabetes medications. Risk factors include infections, heart attack, stroke, recent surgery, **heart failure**, impaired thirst, older age, poor kidney function, poor diabetes management, and incurred use of diabetes medications.

Clinical Manifestations

Elevated counter-regulatory hormones initiate hyperosmolar coma by stimulating hepatic glucose production through glycogenolysis and gluconeogenesis, leading to hyperglycemia, intracellular water depletion, and osmotic diuresis. The signs and symptoms of hyperosmolar coma include polyuria, polydipsia, weight loss, dehydration, weakness, mental status changes, lethargy, focal neurologic deficits, seizures, and low body temperature.

Diagnosis

Diagnosing hyperosmolar coma includes plasma glucose, blood urea nitrogen, serum creatinine, serum osmolality, serum and urine ketones, arterial pH, bicarbonate level, urinalysis, and complete blood count with differential. Electrolyte testing is also required. Identifying any precipitating illness via EKG, blood, urine, sputum cultures, and chest X-rays is essential. Consideration should be made for testing drug and alcohol levels, salicylate levels, tricyclic antidepressant levels, cardiac biomarkers, lactate, and serum lipase. For severe neurologic signs or no improvement in consciousness, urgent brain imaging is required, such as CT scans.

Treatment

Treatment for hyperosmolar coma includes management of the underlying illness, fluid resuscitation, improving mental status, re-establishing euglycemia, replenishing electrolytes and minerals, and preventing complications. The initial evaluation should focus on airway, breathing, and circulation status, and the mental and volume quality should be assessed. Serum glucose should be measured every hour. Electrolytes should be supplied every few hours, and close attention should be paid to cardiopulmonary status during volume resuscitation.

Prevention

Methods of preventing hyperosmolar coma include regular physician visits, emphasizing the importance of insulin during illnesses, emphasizing the correct use of insulin as prescribed, reviewing blood glucose goals, having medications available to manage fevers and treat infections, using an easily digestible liquid diet containing carbohydrates and sodium when nauseated, and educating family members about the patient's management.

Check Your Knowledge

1. In which individuals are hyperosmolar coma most common?
2. What are the risk factors for hyperosmolar coma?
3. What are the treatments for hyperosmolar coma?

CLINICAL CASE STUDY 1

A 53-year-old man is being assessed because of altered mental status. He knows his name but needs clarification about the current time, location, and what is happening around him. His pulse is regular, but his skin is pale and clammy, and he is sweating. Respirations are normal. The patient's wife informs the physician that he is a type 1 diabetic, had a typical breakfast in the morning, and took his usual insulin dose. There are no signs of a stroke. He has an ulcer on his right foot that has been infected for a few days. The patient's blood glucose is low, and it is determined that he is in a state of hypoglycemia. Once oral glucose is administered, the patient returns to normalcy within a few minutes. The physician explains what happened.

CRITICAL THINKING QUESTIONS

1. What blood levels generally indicate hypoglycemia?
2. How common is hypoglycemia in type 1 diabetics?
3. What is the mainstay of treatment for hypoglycemia?

CLINICAL CASE STUDY 2

A 70-year-old woman has had type 2 diabetes for 15 years. She has gained 11 pounds over the past 6 months, admits to not adhering to her medications well, and has also developed foot pain. She takes glyburide (DiaBeta) and atorvastatin (Lipitor) daily. When she misses a dose of the glyburide, it is usually due to feelings of dizziness and sweating, which are adverse effects of the drug. The patient states she does not test her blood glucose levels at home. History evaluation reveals that both of the patient's parents had type 2 diabetes as well. The patient has never seen a dietitian whose diet history shows excessive bread and pasta consumption. She is a former smoker and consumes two glasses of red wine at each dinner. When questioned about her elevated blood pressure, she is unaware that it needs to be maintained at 130/80 mm Hg or less for both heart and kidney health. The patient has never had a foot exam and has not been instructed in preventive foot care.

CRITICAL THINKING QUESTIONS

1. In which individuals are type 2 diabetes more common and more severe?
2. What are the epidemiological statistics about type 2 diabetes in the United States?
3. What are the dangers of having hypertension with type 2 diabetes?

FURTHER READING

1. Castro, M.R. (2022). *Mayo Clinic: The Essential Diabetes Book: A Complete Guide to Prevent, Manage, and Live With Diabetes*, 3rd Edition. Mayo Clinic Press.
2. Cohn, R.M. (2022). *Diagnosis and Treatment of Diabetes and its Complications*. American Medical Publishers.
3. Effiong, K. (2023). *Complications of Type 2 Diabetes: How to Prevent Them: Medical Review*. Effiong.
4. Fleming, S. (2023) *Gestational Diabetes: Nutrition, Complications and Treatment*. American Medical Publishers.
5. Franz, M.J., Evert, A.B., and Franz, M.J. (2017). *Guide to Nutrition Therapy for Diabetes*. American Diabetes Association.
6. Fried, R., and Carlton, R.M. (2018). *Type 2 Diabetes: Cardiovascular and Related Complications and Evience-Based Complementary Treatments*. CRC Press.
7. Grace, R.C. (2021). *Diabetes Mellitus: Practical Guide to the Causes, Symptoms, Prevention and How to Avoid Complications of Diabetes Mellitus*. Grace.
8. Graham, K., and Shomali, M. (2020). *Complete Diabetes Guide: Advice for Managing Type 2 Diabetes (Health and Wellness)*, 2nd Edition. Robert Rose.
9. Hale, G. (2023). *The Ultimate Guide to Manage Latent Autoimmune Diabetes in Adults*. Hale.
10. Kirkman, M.S. (2022). *Medical Management of Type 1 Diabetes*, 8th Edition. American Diabetes Association.
11. Lyons, M.D., McDonnell, P.J., and Schmidt, J.M. (2022). *The Washington Manual of Outpatient Internal Medicine*, 3rd Edition. Wolters Kluwer.
12. Mauricio, D., and Alonso, N. (2023). *Chronic Complications of Diabetes Mellitus: Current Outlook and Novel Pathophysiological Insights*. Academic Press.
13. Maurya, R.C. (2023). *Diabetes, Complications, and Remedies: A Comprehensive View*. Lap Lambert Academic Publishing.
14. Meneghini, L.F. (2020). *Medical Management of Type 2 Diabetes*, 8th Edition. American Diabetes Association.

15. Moini, J., Adams, M., and LoGalbo, A. (2022). *Complications of Diabetes Mellitus: A Global Perspective*. CRC Press.

16. Morgan, W. (2021). *Diabetes Mellitus: History, Chemistry, Anatomy, Pathology, Physiology, and Treatment*. Legare Street Press.

17. Rodriguez-Saldana, J. (2019). *Diabetes Textbook: Clinical Principles, Patient Management, and Public Health Issues*. Springer.

18. Ryan, J. (2023). *Diabetes Complications, Comorbidities, and Related Disorders*. American Medical Publishers.

19. Umpierrez, G.E. (2014). *Therapy for Diabetes Mellitus and Related Disorders*, 6th Edition. American Diabetes Association.

20. White, Jr., J.R. (2020). *Guide to Medications for the Therapy of Diabetes Mellitus*. American Diabetes Association.

4 Hereditary Carbohydrate Disorders

OVERVIEW

Hereditary disorders occur when parents pass the defective genes that cause these disorders on to their children. Inherited metabolic disorders are rare genetic conditions that cause a person's metabolism not to work correctly. Metabolism is the essential chemical process that converts food into energy and removes toxins from the body. Defects in genes passed down from parents can result in abnormal chemical reactions that interfere with metabolism. Many of the clinical features of the inherited disorders of carbohydrate metabolism are caused by the following: Lack of glucose for the metabolism of the brain, muscle, liver, or kidney (in circumstances in which ketone bodies cannot be used), Inability to break down glucose to pyruvate. Disorders of carbohydrate metabolism occur in many forms. The most common disorders are acquired. Acquired or secondary derangements in carbohydrate metabolism, such as diabetic ketoacidosis, hyperosmolar coma, and hypoglycemia, affect the central nervous system. Symptoms include severe hypoglycemia, intolerance to fasting, and liver enlargement.

GALACTOSEMIA

Galactosemia is a disorder of carbohydrate metabolism due to inherited deficiencies in enzymes that convert galactose to glucose. It results in hepatic and renal dysfunction, cataracts, cognitive deficits, and premature failure of the ovaries. Galactose is present in dairy products, fruits, and vegetables. **Autosomal recessive** enzyme deficiencies cause three clinical syndromes: *galactose-1-phosphate uridyl transferase deficiency, galactokinase deficiency,* and *uridine diphosphate galactose 4-epimerase deficiency.*

EPIDEMIOLOGY

The incidence of classic galactosemia, caused by galactose-1-phosphate uridyl transferase deficiency, is 1 in every 62,000 births, and the carrier frequency is 1 in 125. The incidence of galactokinase deficiency is 1 in every 40,000 births. The incidence of the benign form of uridine diphosphate galactose 4-epimerase deficiency is 1 in every 23,000 births (in Japan). The estimated incidence in the United States is 1 in 53,000. There is no incidence data available for the severe form. Galactosemia occurs in all races; however, its variants are based on the exact gene defect. The variants are most notable among African Americans.

Etiology and Risk Factors

Galactose-1-phosphate uridyl transferase (GALT) deficiency causes *classic galactosemia*. In some cases, the enzyme is missing entirely. **Mutations** of this gene, as well as the genes called GALK1 and GALE, are implicated. These genes provide instructions for making enzymes essential for processing dietary galactose. They break down galactose into glucose and other molecules the body can store or use for energy. The primary risk factor for galactosemia is having both parents who are carriers of the gene for galactosemia.

DOI: 10.1201/9781003453376-6

Clinical Manifestations

Galactose-1-phosphate uridyl transferase deficiency causes infants to become anorectic and jaundiced within days or weeks after consuming breast milk or lactose-containing formula. Manifestations include **hepatomegaly**, vomiting, **lethargy**, poor growth, diarrhea, septicemia (usually with *Escherichia coli*), and renal dysfunction (signified by aminoaciduria, **Fanconi syndrome**, and proteinuria). The renal dysfunction leads to **metabolic acidosis** and edema. In some cases, hemolytic anemia also occurs. Without treatment, children are shorter than usual. They develop balance, cognitive, gait, and speech deficits during adolescence. Many develop cataracts, **osteomalacia** (due to hypercalciuria), and premature ovarian failure. With the *Duarte variant*, the phenotype is much milder.

With galactokinase deficiency, patients develop cataracts due to the production of **galactitol,** which osmotically damages lens fibers. Idiopathic intracranial hypertension, also known as *pseudotumor cerebri*, only occurs rarely. There are benign and severe **phenotypes** with galactosemia called uridine diphosphate galactose 4-epimerase deficiency. The benign condition only affects the red and white blood cells, causing no clinical abnormalities. The severe form causes a syndrome identical to classic galactosemia, though some patients develop hearing loss.

Diagnosis

The diagnosis of galactosemia is clinically based and supported by elevated levels of galactose, plus the presence of reducing substances such as galactose or galactose 1-phosphate in the urine. Diagnosis is confirmed via DNA or enzyme analysis of red blood cells, liver tissue, or both. Routine neonatal screening is performed in the United States for galactose-1-phosphate uridyl transferase deficiency. In diagnostic laboratories, gas-chromatographic determination of urinary sugars and sugar alcohols demonstrates elevated galactose and galactitol concentrations, which are used to detect galactosemia.

Treatment

The treatment of galactosemia eliminates all sources of dietary galactose – mainly lactose, which is a source of galactose. Lactose is present in all dairy products, breast milk, milk-based infant formulas, and as a food sweetener. Many patients require vitamins and supplemental calcium. For patients with **epimerase deficiency**, some galactose intake is needed to ensure enough uridine-5′-d iphosphate-galactose (UDP-galactose) for specific metabolic processes.

Prevention

There is no known way to prevent galactosemia. Genetic counseling may be undertaken if the condition is present or there is a family history. Genetic counselors can help determine the risk of passing the infection to offspring.

YOU SHOULD REMEMBER

Adults with galactosemia can live relatively everyday lives, but those who experience symptoms as children may continue to experience lifelong symptoms. Some signs may come and go depending on how well adults maintain their restricted diet. Others, such as hormone deficiencies, are common despite treatment.

YOU SHOULD REMEMBER

Sucrose intolerance is a type of carbohydrate malabsorption that is more common than previously believed. The affected individual cannot digest sucrose (table sugar), the primary sugar in many fruits, maple syrup, and some vegetables. The sucrase-isomaltase enzyme is expressed on the surface of the small intestine's cells. It digests sucrose molecules, which are then absorbed into the bloodstream. The sucrose is not absorbed when the enzyme is present in insufficient amounts. Instead, it passes into the colon, where intestinal bacteria digest it, producing the condition's symptoms.

SUCROSE INTOLERANCE

Sucrose intolerance is a type of carbohydrate malabsorption that is caused by sucrase-isomaltase deficiency. It causes postprandial cramping, bloating, gas, and diarrhea – all symptoms that mimic those of irritable bowel syndrome. Accurate diagnosis of sucrose intolerance requires a sucrase enzyme assay of duodenal biopsies obtained via endoscopy.

EPIDEMIOLOGY

Sucrose intolerance was previously believed to be a rare condition that was always discovered in early childhood. Today, we understand that it may affect a much more significant percentage of the population, even into adulthood. The highest prevalence rates are in the **Inuit populations** of Greenland (5%–10%), Alaska (3%–7%), and Canada (approximately 3%). In Europe, the prevalence of descent is between 0.05% and 0.2%. There is a lower incidence in African Americans and Hispanics compared to Caucasians.

Etiology and Risk Factors

Sucrose intolerance is caused by sucrase-isomaltase deficiency. The inability to digest sucrose normally is usually due to genetics. It can also be caused by **irritable bowel syndrome** and aging. If this is the situation, treatment of the underlying illness is required.

Clinical Manifestations

The symptoms of sucrose intolerance include abdominal cramps, bloating, diarrhea, vomiting, hypoglycemia, headaches, poor weight gain and growth, and excess gas production. These are difficult to distinguish from **irritable bowel syndrome**. Sucrose intolerance associated with IBS refers to the unwanted fermentation in the large intestine due to sucrose not being broken down generally in the small intestine, leading to uncomfortable IBS symptoms.

Diagnosis

The best method of diagnosing sucrose intolerance is a sucrase enzyme assay of duodenal biopsies obtained via **endoscopy**. Also, hydrogen-methane or 13-C sucrose breath tests are noninvasive screening methods. In the 13-C sucrose breath test, the patient consumes a solution containing a modified form of sucrose, then breaths into a bag 30, 60, and 90 minutes afterward. The air chemistry is assessed, quantifying the amount of sucrase-isomaltase enzyme activity in the patient's body.

When an intestinal biopsy is performed, it is advantageous because sucrase-isomaltase enzyme activity, plus other digestive enzymes produced in the same region, can be measured. These include lactase and maltase. If more than one food intolerance is suspected or the diagnosis is not specific, this diagnostic method may be preferred.

Treatment

Sucrose intolerance is treatable when there is an underlying nongenetic cause. Unfortunately, there is no way for most patients to restore normal levels of the sucrase-isomaltase enzyme. Once diagnosed, treatment is with various combinations of supplemental enzymes and changes in the diet. A prescription enzyme supplement is available and helps patients tolerate sucrose foods. It is given before meals. The enzyme must be refrigerated, which is challenging to use during travel. Patients learn to adapt their diet to avoid all sucrose foods in those situations.

Prevention

The only way to prevent sucrose intolerance is to avoid all sucrose foods. These foods include table sugar, cane sugar, beet sugar, date sugar, coconut sugar, granulated sugar, powdered or confectioner's sugar, brown sugar, raw sugar, turbinado sugar, demerara icing, molasses, sucanat, caramel, maple syrup, cane juice, apricots, apples, bananas, grapefruit, cantaloupe, peaches, pineapple, oranges, honeydew, mangos, raisins, dates, canned fruit in syrups, any fruits that are sweetened with added sugar, fruit juices, all dried beans, baked beans, lentils, green peas, soybeans, sweet pickles, store-bought spaghetti sauce, flavored or sweetened milk, flavored or sweetened yogurt, sweetened condensed milk, ice cream, certain processed cheese spreads, carbonated sweetened drinks and sodas, vegetable juices, milk shakes, malts, sweetened tea, sweetened coffee, powdered beverages, milk flavorings and syrups, milk substitutes, chocolate, desserts made with sugar, jams, jellies, sauces, chutneys, ketchup, sweet relish, barbecue sauce, mayonnaise, high-sugar salad dressings, sausages, ham, hot dogs, deli meats, liverwurst, pates that are cured with sucrose, coconut, coconut milk, creams used in cooking, breads and cereals that list sugar in the first four ingredients, nuts, and nut butters.

YOU SHOULD REMEMBER

Congenital sucrase-isomaltase deficiency is inherited in an autosomal recessive pattern, with variants in both gene copies in each cell. Parents of individuals with such an **autosomal recessive** condition carry one copy of the altered gene but may not have any signs or symptoms.

Check Your Knowledge

1. What does galactosemia cause?
2. What are the symptoms of sucrose intolerance?
3. What is the only way to prevent sucrose intolerance?

GLYCOGEN STORAGE DISORDERS

Glycogen storage disorders are another form of carbohydrate metabolism disorder. There are various types, all caused by deficiencies of enzymes involved in glycogen synthesis or breakdown. The defects may occur in the liver or muscles, causing hypoglycemia or deposition of abnormal types of glycogen or its intermediate metabolites in tissues.

EPIDEMIOLOGY

The incidence of glycogen storage disorders is estimated at 1 in 25,000 births. This may be underestimated since milder subclinical forms may be undiagnosed. Type I glycogen storage disease occurs in about 1 of every 100,000 births, though its prevalence in Ashkenazi Jews is about 1 in 20,000. These disorders affect males and females in nearly equal numbers in any given population group.

Etiology and Risk Factors

Glycogen storage disorders are hereditary, occurring when both parents have a gene mutation that affects how glycogen is stored or used. Most appear because parents pass on the same abnormal gene to their children. The age of onset, clinical manifestations, and severity vary by type. Risk factors are increased if a family member has a glycogen storage disorder.

Clinical Manifestations

The signs and symptoms of glycogen storage disorders include jaundice, malaise, weight loss, chronic abdominal pain, inability to concentrate, and bruises. In some cases, hypoglycemia, hepatomegaly, exercise intolerance, muscle cramps, weakness, cirrhosis with dysplastic nodules, and splenomegaly are present. These disorders sometimes affect the myocardial tissue, leading to cardiomyopathy and cardiac conduction defects.

Diagnosis

Diagnosis of glycogen storage disorders is based on history, examination, and detection of glycogen plus intermediate metabolites in tissues via Ultrasound, MRI, CT, or biopsy. Confirmation is by DNA analysis, or less often, by detecting a significant decrease of enzyme activity in the liver, muscles, skin fibroblasts, or red blood cells. Another diagnostic method is to see a lack of increased venous lactate with forearm activity or ischemia. GSD II (Pompe disease) is part of the newborn screening panel in many areas of the United States.

Treatment

Treatments vary by the type of glycogen storage disorder present but usually include dietary supplementation with cornstarch. This provides a sustained source of glucose for the hepatic subtypes, while exercise avoidance is needed for the muscle subtypes.

Prevention

There is no way to prevent glycogen storage disorders, but early treatment can help control them once they have manifested.

YOU SHOULD REMEMBER

Because they affect many organ systems, type II glycogen storage disorder (Pompe's disease) and GSD type IV (Andersen's disease) are challenging to treat and can be fatal. Research into enzyme replacement therapy and gene therapy is promising, which may improve the outlook for the future.

Check Your Knowledge

1. Where may the defects of glycogen storage disorders occur?
2. What are the signs and symptoms of glycogen storage disorders?
3. Which glycogen storage disorders can be fatal?

HEREDITARY FRUCTOSE INTOLERANCE

Hereditary fructose intolerance is a metabolic disorder caused by a deficiency of enzymes. The condition can be asymptomatic or cause hypoglycemia. Fructose is a monosaccharide present in significant concentrations in fruit and honey. It is a constituent of sucrose and sorbitol. Hereditary fructose intolerance includes fructose 1-phosphate aldolase B deficiency, fructokinase deficiency, and *fructose-1,6-biphosphatase.*

EPIDEMIOLOGY

The incidence of fructose 1-phosphate aldolase B deficiency is estimated at 1 in every 20,000 births. Fructokinase deficiency is about 1 in every 130,000 births. The incidence of fructose-1,6-biphosphatase poverty is unknown.

Etiology and Risk Factors

Inheritance of fructose 1-phosphate aldolase B deficiency is autosomal recessive. Inheritance of fructokinase deficiency is also autosomal recessive, as is the legacy of lack of fructose-1,6-biphosphate.

Clinical Manifestations

Fructose 1-phosphate aldolase B deficiency causes the clinical syndrome of hereditary fructose intolerance. Infants are healthy until they ingest fructose. Then, fructose 1-phosphate accumulates. This causes hypoglycemia, nausea, vomiting, abdominal pain, sweating, confusion, excessive sleepiness, **tremors**, lethargy, failure to thrive, mental deterioration, and coma. Repeated ingestion of fructose-containing foods can lead to liver and kidney damage. Liver damage can result in jaundice, hepatomegaly, and cirrhosis. Continued exposure to fructose may result in seizures, coma, and, ultimately, death from liver and kidney failure. Due to the severity of symptoms experienced when fructose is ingested, most people with hereditary fructose intolerance develop a dislike for fruits, juices, and other foods containing fructose.

Fructokinase deficiency causes benign elevation of blood and urine fructose levels, known as *benign fructosuria*. Otherwise, this condition is asymptomatic, diagnosed incidentally when a non-glucose-reducing substance is found in the urine. A deficiency of fructose-1,6-biphosphatase involves gluconeogenesis. This results in fasting hypoglycemia, ketosis, and metabolic acidosis. The flaw can be fatal in neonates. Febrile illnesses can trigger episodes of this type of fructose intolerance.

Diagnosis

Diagnosis of fructose 1-phosphate aldolase B deficiency is based on the signs and symptoms related to recent fructose intake. It is confirmed by DNA analysis. Earlier, confirmatory testing used liver biopsy or induction of hypoglycemia by fructose infusion (200 mg/kg, intravenously). Diagnosis and identification of **heterozygous** carriers of the gene mutation can also be made by direct DNA analysis.

Treatment

The short-term treatment of fructose 1-phosphate aldolase B deficiency is glucose. The long-term treatment requires the exclusion of dietary fructose, sucrose, and sorbitol. Often, patients develop a natural aversion to foods that contain fructose. Treatment usually provides an excellent prognosis. The acute treatment of fructose-1,6-biphosphatase deficiency is oral or IV glucose. Tolerance to fasting usually increases with age.

Prevention

Only the primary manifestations of hereditary fructose intolerance can be prevented with dietary restrictions of fructose, sucrose, **sucralose**, and sorbitol. During hospitalizations, fructose-containing IV fluids, infant formulas, and medications must be avoided.

YOU SHOULD REMEMBER

Hereditary fructose intolerance is an autosomal recessive disease characterized by a lack of the enzyme called aldolase B. This essential enzyme is responsible for breaking fructose-1-phosphate into glyceraldehyde and dihydroxyacetone phosphate.

Check Your Knowledge

1. In hereditary fructose intolerance, what happens once fructose is ingested?
2. Can hereditary fructose intolerance be fatal?
3. What are the short-term and long-term treatments?

PYRUVATE METABOLISM DISORDERS

Pyruvate is an essential substrate in carbohydrate metabolism. Pyruvate metabolism disorders are other types of carbohydrate metabolism disorders. An inability to metabolize pyruvate causes **lactic acidosis**, plus various central nervous system (CNS) abnormalities. The two examples of these disorders are *pyruvate dehydrogenase deficiency* and *carboxylase deficiency*. Pyruvate dehydrogenase is a multi-enzyme complex needed to generate acetyl CoA from pyruvate for the Krebs cycle (see **Figure 4.1**). PC deficiency may be primary or secondary to holocarboxylase synthetase, biotin, or biotinidase deficiencies.

EPIDEMIOLOGY

The incidence of pyruvate dehydrogenase deficiency is unknown but is estimated to be less than 1 in every 50,000 births. The incidence of primary PC deficiency is about 1 in every 250,000 births, but it is higher in some Native American populations.

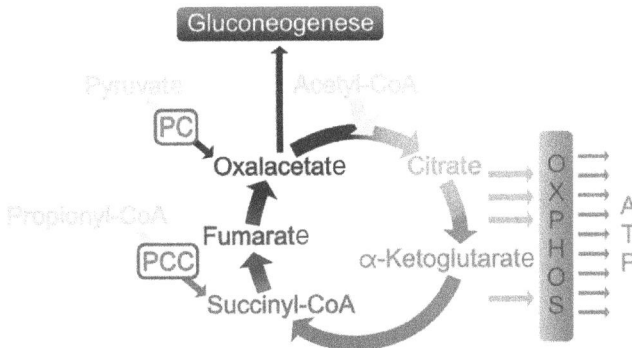

FIGURE 4.1   Generation of acetyl CoA during the Krebs cycle.

Etiology and Risk Factors

Mutations in the gene that provides instructions for making E1 alpha, the PDHA1 gene, are the most common cause of pyruvate dehydrogenase deficiency, involved in about 80% of cases. There are no specific risk factors. PC deficiency is caused by PC gene mutations, which provide instructions for making the PC enzyme.

Clinical Manifestations

Clinical manifestations are varied but include lactic acidosis and CNS malformations. Other post-natal changes include cystic lesions of the brainstem, cerebral cortex, and **basal ganglia**, as well as **ataxia** and psychomotor retardation. Pyruvate carboxylase is an enzyme needed for gluconeogenesis from pyruvate and alanine generated in muscles. Both primary or secondary forms of PC deficiency cause lactic acidosis. Psychomotor retardation with seizures and spasticity are significant manifestations. Secondary PC deficiency is similar, with failure to thrive, infantile spasms, tonic-clonic seizures, and other signs of organic aciduria.

Diagnosis

Diagnosis of pyruvate dehydrogenase deficiency is confirmed with enzyme analysis of skin fibroblasts, DNA testing, and sometimes both. Pyruvate carboxylase deficiency is suspected in patients with non-specific clinical signs. Diagnosis requires identifying test abnormalities in amino acid, organic acid, glucose, and ammonia serum concentrations. A pyruvate carboxylase enzyme activity assay that shows a deficiency of the enzyme in fibroblasts is also diagnostic, along with mutations in the PC gene via molecular genetic testing. Laboratory abnormalities include hyperammonemia, ketoacidosis, elevated plasma lysins, citrulline, alanine, and proline, and increased alpha-ketoglutarate excretion.

Treatment

There is no effective treatment for pyruvate dehydrogenase deficiency. However, a low-carbohydrate or ketogenic diet plus dietary thiamin (vitamin B1) supplementation can be beneficial. There is also no effective treatment for PC deficiency. Some patients with the primary form and those with the secondary structure require biotin supplementation, 5–20 mg orally once daily.

Prevention

There are no specific methods of prevention of pyruvate metabolism disorders.

HUNTER SYNDROME

Hunter syndrome, also known as *serotonin syndrome*, is a potentially life-threatening condition that results from increased CNS serotonergic activity. It is usually drug-related. The syndrome can occur with therapeutic drug use, self-poisoning, or usually, unintended drug interactions between two serotonergic drugs. When the syndrome is severe, complications include metabolic acidosis, **rhabdomyolysis**, seizures, acute kidney injury, and disseminated intravascular coagulation. These complications are likely caused by severe hyperthermia and excessive muscle activity.

Epidemiology

Hunter syndrome can occur in all age groups. However, the incidence is still being determined since mild cases are often overlooked or dismissed. The syndrome is estimated to occur in 1 out of every 100,000–170,000 males. Females can be carriers of the genetic mutation that causes mucopolysaccharidosis type II (MPS II).

Etiology and Risk Factors

Hunter syndrome can result from agonism, antagonism, or both of varying combinations of serotonergic agents. Some illicit drugs and dietary supplements are also associated. Risk factors only include the use of two or more serotonergic drugs.

Clinical Manifestations

In most cases, Hunter syndrome manifests within 6–24 hours of a change in dose or initiation of a drug, with widely varying signs and symptoms. These manifestations are grouped as the following:

- *Mental status alterations* – **agitation**, anxiety, delirium, easy startling, restlessness
- *Autonomic hyperactivity* – diarrhea, vomiting, hypertension, hyperthermia, tachycardia, **diaphoresis**, shivering
- *Neuromuscular hyperactivity* – extensor plantar responses, hyperreflexia, muscle hypertonia or rigidity, **myoclonus**, tremor (these manifestations may be more extreme in the legs compared to the arms)

Symptoms usually resolve within 1 day but can last longer after using drugs with a long half-life or active metabolites (such as monoamine oxidase or selective serotonin reuptake inhibitors).

Diagnosis

The diagnosis of Hunter syndrome is clinical. The *Hunter criteria* are preferred because they are easy to use and offer perfect accuracy. They have nearly 85% sensitivity and more than 95% specificity compared to a toxicology diagnosis. The criteria require that a serotonergic drug has been taken and that the patient has one of the following:

- Muscle hypertonia
- Ocular or inducible clonus (plus either agitation, diaphoresis, or a body)
- Temperature higher than 100.4°F (38°C)
- Spontaneous clonus
- Tremor with hyperreflexia

Systemic infections, drug or alcohol withdrawal, and toxicities must be ruled out. It can be challenging to differentiate Hunter syndrome from **neuroleptic malignant syndrome** because of similar symptoms. Testing to exclude other disorders, such as CSF analysis for CNS infections and urine testing for abused drugs, should be done. Some tests may be needed to identify complications if the syndrome is severe. These include platelet count, serum electrolytes, **creatine kinase**, renal function tests, prothrombin time, and testing for urine myoglobin.

Treatment

The prognosis is usually good once Hunter syndrome is detected and treated quickly. All serotonergic drugs must be stopped. Mild symptoms can be relieved with a benzodiazepine for sedation, with resolution occurring in 1–3 days. The patient must be observed for several hours or more when symptoms resolve quickly. Most patients will require hospitalization for additional tests, treatments, and monitoring. For severe cases, an intensive care unit is needed. Hyperthermia is treated with cooling. Some patients require neuromuscular blockage with appropriate sedation, muscle paralysis, or other measures. Treatment of autonomic abnormalities with medications must be with shorter-acting drugs such as esmolol or nitroprusside. This is because abnormalities such as hypertension or tachycardia can change rapidly. If symptoms continue, cyproheptadine, a serotonin antagonist, can be given orally or crushed and given via nasogastric tube (12 mg, then 2 mg every 2 hours until effective).

Prevention

Preventing Hunter syndrome requires awareness of the toxic potential of serotonergic agents.

Check Your Knowledge

1. Can pyruvate metabolism disorders affect the central nervous system?
2. How can drugs influence the development of Hunter syndrome?
3. What are the different groups of manifestations of Hunter syndrome?

HURLER SYNDROME

Hurler syndrome is the most severe form of *mucopolysaccharidosis type 1(MPS1)*, a rare hereditary lysosomal storage condition. In this condition, the cells cannot break down long chains of sugar molecules called glycosaminoglycans (formerly called mucopolysaccharides). As a result, the molecules build up in different body parts and cause various health problems.

Epidemiology

Life expectancy for children diagnosed with Hurler syndrome is short due to the life-threatening symptoms. Hurler syndrome affects an estimated 1 of every 100,000 newborns. Males and females are equally affected. Less severe forms of MPS I affect almost 1 of every 500,000 newborns.

Etiology and Risk Factors

Hurler syndrome can affect any child because of a random genetic mutation. If there is a history of MPS I in the family, there is an increased risk of having a child with Hurler syndrome. If both parents carry a nonworking copy of the gene related to this condition, their children have a 25% (1 in 4) chance of developing the disease. People with MPS I do not make an enzyme called lysosomal alpha-L-iduronidase; glycosaminoglycans build up and damage organs, including the heart.

Clinical Manifestations

Hurler syndrome often appears between ages 3 and 8. Children with severe MPS I develop symptoms earlier than those with the less severe form. It causes skeletal and joint abnormalities, specific facial characteristics (large head, excessive hair growth, cloudy eyes, a low nasal bridge, and full cheeks and lips), issues with cognitive development, heart and lung problems, and enlargement of the liver and spleen (see **Figure 4.2**). Many affected children are of shorter than average stature. There may be recurrent ear, sinus, and pulmonary infections or an eventual need for breathing assistance or surgery to repair symptomatic organ damage. Symptoms begin in early childhood and continue through adolescence. There are developmental delays and a progressive decline in how the child learns and retains information. Symptoms may include cardiomyopathy, hearing loss, hydrocephalus, enlarged organs, glaucoma, tight muscles, carpal tunnel syndrome, joint disease, respiratory infections, sleep apnea, difficulty breathing, and hernias. During the first year of life, characteristics include short stature **dysostosis**, thoracic-lumbar kyphosis, and excessive hair growth.

Diagnosis

Amniocentesis or chorionic villus sampling can diagnose a child with Hurler syndrome before birth. After birth, the syndrome can be diagnosed via physical examination and an enzyme activity assay for confirmation. Sometimes, X-rays, echocardiograms, and blood or urine tests are also needed.

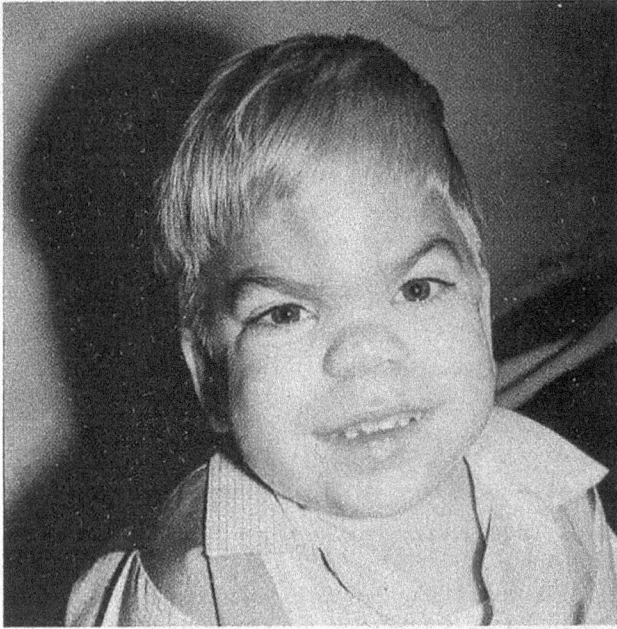

FIGURE 4.2   Facial characteristics of Hurler syndrome.

Treatment

Hurler syndrome treatment focuses on preventing and managing symptoms with enzyme replacement therapy or hematopoietic stem cell transplant (HSCT). Replacing damaged enzymes can stop signs from worsening and potentially reverse complications. After diagnosis, regular injections of alpha L-iduronidase (Aldurazyme) will be given. The frequency of injections is based on how severe the condition is and will continue throughout life. For children under age two and some over age 2, HSCT can prolong life expectancy in extreme cases, prevent disease progression, preserve cognitive function, and reduce somatic symptoms. Stem cells from donors with functional enzymes in the bone marrow's hematopoietic cells replace damaged cells in the patient via chemotherapy. Other options include surgery (to repair or replace heart valves, replace the corneas, repair bone growth abnormalities, or repair hernias), hearing aids, and pain-relieving medications.

Prevention

Hurler syndrome is not preventable, so anyone planning on becoming pregnant should discuss genetic counseling and testing to understand the risks of having a child with the condition. It is unfortunately common for diagnosed children to have a short life expectancy of about 10 years due to the severe symptoms of the syndrome affecting the heart and lungs.

Check Your Knowledge

1. How does Hurler syndrome affect life expectancy?
2. When does Hurler syndrome often appear?
3. What are the treatment options for Hurler syndrome?

MORQUIO SYNDROME

Morquio syndrome is a rare genetic condition affecting a child's bones, spine, organs, and physical abilities. It is also known as *mucopolysaccharidosis type IV (MPS IV)*, in which the body cannot process specific sugar molecules called glycosaminoglycans (GAGs). In Morquio syndrome, the particular GAG that builds up in the body is called keratan sulfate. The buildup of GAGs in different body parts causes symptoms in many organs. The sugar chains accumulate in the cells, blood, tendons, and ligaments, resulting in damage over time. Morquio syndrome is another example of mucopolysaccharidosis.

EPIDEMIOLOGY

Morquio syndrome is a rare inherited condition, estimated to occur in 1 of every 200,000 births. There must be sufficient epidemiological information on whether the syndrome affects particular groups more than others.

Etiology and Risk Factors

Morquio syndrome is an autosomal recessive genetic condition, so both parents must carry the gene and pass it to the child. Each person has two copies of the genes needed to break down **keratan sulfate**, but only one healthy copy is required. Both parents pass down one defective copy to their child, resulting in a child with no functional copies of the gene. As such, the body cannot break down keratan sulfate for disposal. The incompletely broken down GAGs remain stored in cells in the body, causing progressive damage. Babies may show little sign of the disease, but as more and more cells become damaged, symptoms start to appear.

Clinical Manifestations

Signs and symptoms of Morquio syndrome usually appear between ages 1 and 3. Types A and B have similar presentations, but Type B generally has milder symptoms. Morquio syndrome causes progressive changes to the skeleton of the ribs and chest, which may lead to neurological complications such as nerve compression. Patients may also have hearing loss and clouded corneas. Intelligence is usually average unless a patient has untreated hydrocephalus. Physical growth slows and often stops around age 8. Skeletal abnormalities include a bell-shaped chest, scoliosis, kyphosis, shortened long bones, and **hip dysplasia** (see **Figure 4.3**). The bones that stabilize the connection between the head and neck can be malformed (odontoid hypoplasia). Restricted breathing, joint stiffness, and heart disease are also common. Children with the more severe form of MPS IV may not live beyond their twenties or thirties.

Diagnosis

Many children with Morquio syndrome are diagnosed with orthopedic conditions, including scoliosis, **kyphosis**, narrow chest, **skeletal dysplasia**, joint diseases, and leg deformities. In some cases, these conditions are present at birth and can be treated when the child is very young. Diagnosis of Morquio syndrome begins with a thorough medical history and physical examination. Diagnostic methods may include genetic testing, X-ray images of the bones, MRI scans of the organs and other structures, echocardiograms, and laboratory testing.

Treatment

Treatment for Morquio syndrome often requires a multidisciplinary team, including specialists from clinical genetics, orthopedics, pulmonology, and cardiology. The condition is progressive, so the patient's medical needs may change. Actual treatments are based on symptoms, and monitoring is required for all patients. Surgical intervention may be needed for scoliosis, kyphosis, and leg deformities. Enzyme replacement therapy can supply the body with the enzymes it cannot manufacture. It is infused intravenously and can improve many of the symptoms.

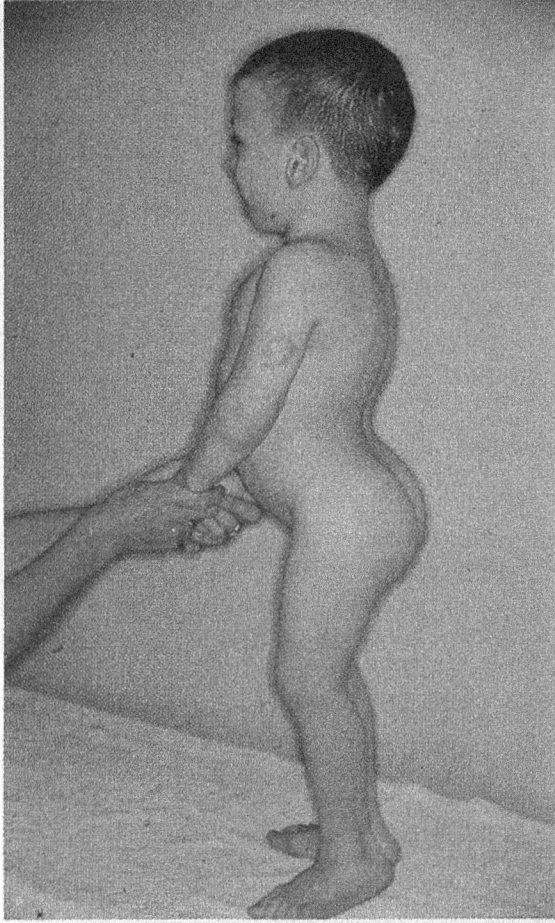

FIGURE 4.3   Skeletal abnormalities of Morquio syndrome.

Prevention

Though not preventable, Morquio syndrome can be improved by enzyme replacement therapy.

YOU SHOULD REMEMBER

The life expectancy of individuals with Morquio syndrome depends on the severity of symptoms. Severely affected individuals may survive only until late childhood or adolescence. Those with milder forms of the disorder usually live into adulthood, although their life expectancy may be reduced. Spinal cord compression and airway obstruction are significant causes of death in people with this condition.

MCARDLE SYNDROME

McArdle syndrome, also known as glycogen storage disease type 5 (GSD V), is a rare inherited condition in which the body cannot break down glycogen. The syndrome is autosomal recessive, so the child must receive a copy of the nonworking gene from both parents.

EPIDEMIOLOGY

McArdle syndrome is one of the most common glycogen storage disorders, but its exact prevalence is unknown. It is estimated to be 1 in every 100,000 patients in the United States. There is also some data from other countries: 1 in 170,000 in Spain and 1 in 350,000 in the Netherlands.

Etiology and Risk Factors

McArdle syndrome is caused by an error in the gene that makes the enzyme known as muscle glycogen phosphorylase. Therefore, the body cannot break down glycogen in the muscles. A family history of the syndrome increases the risk of developing it.

Pathophysiology

McArdle syndrome develops from a myophosphorylase deficiency (alpha-1,4-glucan orthophosphate glycosyl transferase). In normal individuals, myophosphorylase initiates glycogen breakdown by removing 1,4-glucosyl groups from glycogen by releasing glucose-1-phosphate.

Clinical Manifestations

Symptoms of McArdle syndrome usually start in childhood. However, it can be challenging to separate the symptoms from those of normal childhood, potentially delaying diagnosis until age 20 or 30. Symptoms may include burgundy (purple) colored urine, known as **myoglobinuria**, fatigue, exercise intolerance, poor stamina, muscle cramps or pain, and muscle stiffness or weakness.

Diagnosis

Tests to diagnose McArdle syndrome include **electromyography**, genetic testing, testing for lactic acid in the blood, MRI, muscle biopsy, testing for myoglobin in the urine, testing for ammonia in the plasma, and serum creatine kinase testing.

Treatment

There is no specific treatment for McArdle syndrome. Patients are advised to monitor physical limitations, warm up gently before exercising, avoid exercising too hard or too long, and eat enough protein. Some providers recommend eating sweet food before exercising to help prevent muscle symptoms. It is essential to check with a provider about receiving general anesthesia if surgery is needed.

Prevention

While McArdle syndrome is incurable, dietary changes and exercise strategies can help control it. A well-designed low or moderate-exercise routine can help the body maximize its ability to use glucose.

Check Your Knowledge

1. How is Morquio syndrome inherited?
2. What are the symptoms of McArdle syndrome?
3. What orthopedic conditions are involved in Morquio syndrome?

POMPE DISEASE

Pompe disease, also known as acid-maltase disease and glycogen storage disease II, is a rare genetic disorder that causes progressive weakness of the heart and skeletal muscles. The disease is linked to the buildup of glycogen in body cells. There are variable rates of disease progression and different ages of onset.

EPIDEMIOLOGY

The highest genetic prevalence for Pompe disease appears to be 1 in 12,125 in Eastern Asia. In Taiwan, the incidence is lower, estimated to be 1 in 34,348. In Finland, there have only been three cases ever reported. Incidence in the Netherlands is 1 in 40,000. In the United States, the incidence is 1 in 21,979– 27,800. In Mexico, the incidence is 1 in 20,018. There is no explanation for Pompe disease's varying prevalence and incidence in different countries.

Etiology and Risk Factors

Pompe disease is caused by mutations in a gene that makes the enzyme called *acid alpha-glucosidase (GAA)*, which the body uses to break down glycogen. The enzyme functions in the lysosomes.

Pathophysiology

Mutations of the GAA gene reduce or eliminate alpha-glucosidase, causing a buildup that seriously damages the skeletal and cardiac muscles. The severity of the disease and age of onset (which vary widely) are related to the level of enzyme deficiency. There are two forms, as follows:

- *Early-onset (infantile)* – due to complete or almost complete depletion of GAA
- *Late-onset (juvenile or adult)* – due to partial lack of GAA, which can begin in the first decade of childhood or well into adulthood

Clinical Manifestations

Signs and symptoms of early-onset Pompe disease include feeding problems, poor weight gain, difficulty breathing, muscle weakness, enlarged heart, **floppiness**, head lag, and often, an enlarged tongue. Without enzyme replacement therapy, most infants die from cardiac or respiratory complications before reaching 1 year of age. Signs and symptoms of late-onset Pompe disease mostly feature muscle weakness. This progresses to death from respiratory failure after several years. The heart is not usually involved.

Diagnosis

The diagnosis of Pompe disease begins with blood tests, which are confirmed through DNA testing. Other tests include sleep studies, breathing tests (pulmonary function tests), and electromyography. A complete patient and family history should be taken. Heart studies, including X-rays, electrocardiograms, and echocardiograms, may also be needed. For pregnant women at risk, a prenatal diagnosis may be made.

Treatment

Enzyme replacement therapy can help improve muscle tone and reduce glycogen storage in patients with Pompe disease. The following agents have been approved: alglucosidase alfa (Myozyme, for early-onset disease), a different formulation of alglucosidase alfa (Lumizyme, for patients of all ages), and aval glucosidase alfa-night (Nexviazyme) for patients age 1 year or older with late-onset Pompe disease.

Prevention

There is no prevention for Pompe disease, but supportive treatment and care are available. Without treatment, the condition will be fatal.

Check Your Knowledge

1. Where is Pompe disease most common?
2. What are the two forms of Pompe disease?
3. What factors of Pompe disease are fatal for infants?

CLINICAL CASE STUDY 1

A 26-year-old man had a 3-month history of jaundice, malaise, weight loss, chronic abdominal pain, and inability to concentrate. There were many bruises and purple striae on his skin. A complete blood count showed pancytopenia and raised lactate dehydrogenase. Blood film showed left-shifted neutropenia with thrombocytopenia with some target cells. Ultrasound revealed splenomegaly with a small low-attenuation liver lesion. MRI and CT revealed cirrhosis with dysplastic nodules and splenomegaly. A liver biopsy revealed a significant glycogen load in the hepatocytes. The patient was diagnosed with glycogen storage disorder III and referred to a liver specialist team for further monitoring and management.

CRITICAL THINKING QUESTIONS

1. What are the causes of glycogen storage disorders?
2. What are the clinical manifestations of glycogen storage disorders?
3. What are the treatments for glycogen storage disorders?

CLINICAL CASE STUDY 2

A 42-year-old woman was assessed for repeated nausea and vomiting after ingesting fruits, sucrose, or fructose-containing foods. Because of her lifelong history of these problems, hereditary fructose intolerance was suspected. Genomic DNA was extracted, and very detailed testing was undertaken. The patient had a known heterozygous pathogenic nonsense variant and a known pathogenic frame-shift variant. She was started on a fructose-restricted diet after counseling with a dietician.

CRITICAL THINKING QUESTIONS

1. What is fructose?
2. What can happen when an infant with hereditary fructose intolerance consumes fructose?
3. Which manifestations of hereditary fructose intolerance can be prevented?

CLINICAL CASE STUDY 3

A 22-month-old boy was brought to the emergency department by his mother because he had experienced abnormal movements for about 1 month. He tilted his head to the left side, had a left gaze deviation, and fencer posturing toward the left side for a few seconds within clusters that lasted up to 3 minutes. The child also had sudden, jerky, and purposeless movements in his arms. A video electroencephalogram revealed epileptic spasms, tonic-clonic seizures, and multifocal epileptiform discharges that were consistent with epileptic encephalopathy and infantile spasms. Previously, the boy had been diagnosed with pyruvate carboxylase deficiency as a neonate. Additional testing resulted in a diagnosis of new-onset infantile spasms and tonic-clonic seizures, expected to be due to the metabolic disorder known as PCD type A.

CRITICAL THINKING QUESTIONS

1. What are the two examples of pyruvate metabolism disorders?
2. What is pyruvate carboxylase?
3. What does the diagnosis of pyruvate carboxylase deficiency require?

FURTHER READING

1. Dickens, F., Randle, P.J., and Whelan, W.J. (2014). *Carbohydrate Metabolism and its Disorders.* Academic Press.
2. Ekvall, S.W., and Ekvall, V.K. (2017). *Pediatric and Adult Nutrition in Chronic Diseases, Developmental Disabilities, and Hereditary Metabolic Disorders*, 3rd Edition. Oxford University Press.
3. Fraites, Jr., T. (2019). *Muscle-directed Gene and Enzyme Replacement Therapies for Glycogen Storage Disorder Type II Pompe Disease.* Dissertation Discovery Company.
4. Garg, U., and Smith, L.D. (2017). *Biomarkers in Inborn Errors of Metabolism: Clinical Aspects and Laboratory Determination.* Elsevier.
5. Monch, E., and Moses, S.W. (2014). *Inherited Disorders of Carbohydrate Metabolism: Glycogen Storage Diseases and Deficiencies of Monosaccharide Metabolism.* Uni-Med Verlag AG.
6. Nyhan, W.L. and Hoffmann, G.F. (2020). *Atlas of Inherited Metabolic Diseases*, 4th Edition. CRC Press.
7. Reiser, S. (2019). *Metabolic Effects of Dietary Fructose (Revivals).* CRC Press.
8. Reuser, A.J.J., and Schoser, B. (2022). *Pompe Disease*, 3rd Edition. Uni-Med Verlag AG.
9. Roche, H.M., MacDonald, I.A., Schol, A., and Lanham-New, S.A. (2024). *Nutrition and Metabolism (The Nutrition Society Textbook)*, 3rd Edition. Wiley-Blackwell.
10. Saboowala, H. (2023). *Hurler Syndrome (Mucopolysaccharidosis Type I MPH I): Aetiology, History, Symptoms, and Treatment – An Overview.* Saboowala.
11. Salway, J.G. (2017). *Metabolism at a Glance*, 4th Edition. Wiley-Blackwell.
12. Sutherland, H.W., Stowers, J.M., and Pearson, D.W.M. (2012). *Carbohydrate Metabolism in Pregnancy and the Newborn IV.* Springer-Verlag.

Part III

Disorders of Lipid Metabolism

5 Hypercholesterolemia

OVERVIEW

Hypercholesterolemia is defined as a high blood cholesterol level. Cholesterol is a waxy substance produced by the liver and is a component of all cells found in the body.

All the cholesterol a person needs is produced in the liver, but another source is dietary cholesterol, which comes from animal food products such as meat, poultry, dairy, egg yolk, and fish. Such foods are rich in saturated and *trans* fats, which can trigger the liver to produce excess cholesterol. In some cases, this can lead to hypercholesterolemia. Cholesterol is required for various bodily functions, including synthesizing cell membranes and certain hormones and producing substances needed for fat digestion. However, a cholesterol level that is too high can increase the risk of coronary artery disease. There is a rise in levels of cholesterol and apolipoprotein B (apoB), a rich lipoprotein called low-density lipoprotein cholesterol (LDL-C). It is also known as dyslipidemia, encompassing elevated triglycerides, low high-density lipoprotein cholesterol (HDL-C), and qualitative lipid abnormalities. Hypercholesterolemia is a significant risk factor for atherosclerotic cardiovascular disease. This includes stroke, coronary heart disease, and peripheral arterial disease. It is usually asymptomatic until considerable atherosclerosis has developed.

LIPOPROTEINS

Cholesterol and triglycerides travel freely in the blood because they are insoluble. Therefore, they must be cut by specific proteins to be transported. These proteins are called **lipoproteins.** They are complex particles with a central core that contains cholesterol esters. They are surrounded by free cholesterol, phospholipids, and **apolipoproteins**, which facilitate the formation and function of lipoproteins (see **Figure 5.1**). Plasma lipoproteins can be divided into seven classes based on size, lipid composition, and apolipoproteins. The seven types of lipoproteins include the following:

- *Chylomicrons* – they are large triglyceride-rich lipoproteins produced in enterocytes from dietary lipids (fatty acids and cholesterol); they are composed of a primary central lipid core that mainly consists of triglycerides, but, like other lipoproteins, carry esterified cholesterol and phospholipids.
- *Chylomicron remnants* – they deliver dietary cholesterol to the liver to be incorporated into very LDLs, which are secreted in plasma.
- *Very low–density lipoproteins* (VLDLs) – contain the highest amount of triglycerides, which are considered "bad cholesterol" because they help build cholesterol on the walls of arteries. *They are* measured by laboratory testing.
- *Intermediate-density lipoproteins* – they are formed by the removal of triglycerides from VLDL by muscle and adipose tissue; these particles are enriched in cholesterol, contain apoB-100 and E, and are proatherogenic.
- *LDLs* – they are another type of "bad cholesterol"; it makes up most of the cholesterol in the body; the high levels of LDL-C increase the risks of heart disease and stroke.
- *HDLs* – they are "good cholesterol"; they absorb cholesterol in the blood and carry it back to the liver, which flushes it from the body. High levels of HDL-C can lower the risks of heart disease and stroke.
- *Lipoprotein A* – it is a type of LDL-C that is stickier than other types of LDL particles, so it may be more likely to cause blockages and blood clots in the arteries, resulting in very high risks of heart disease, stroke, and other severe conditions.

DOI: 10.1201/9781003453376-8

STRUCTURE OF DIFFERENT CLASSES OF LIPOPROTEINS

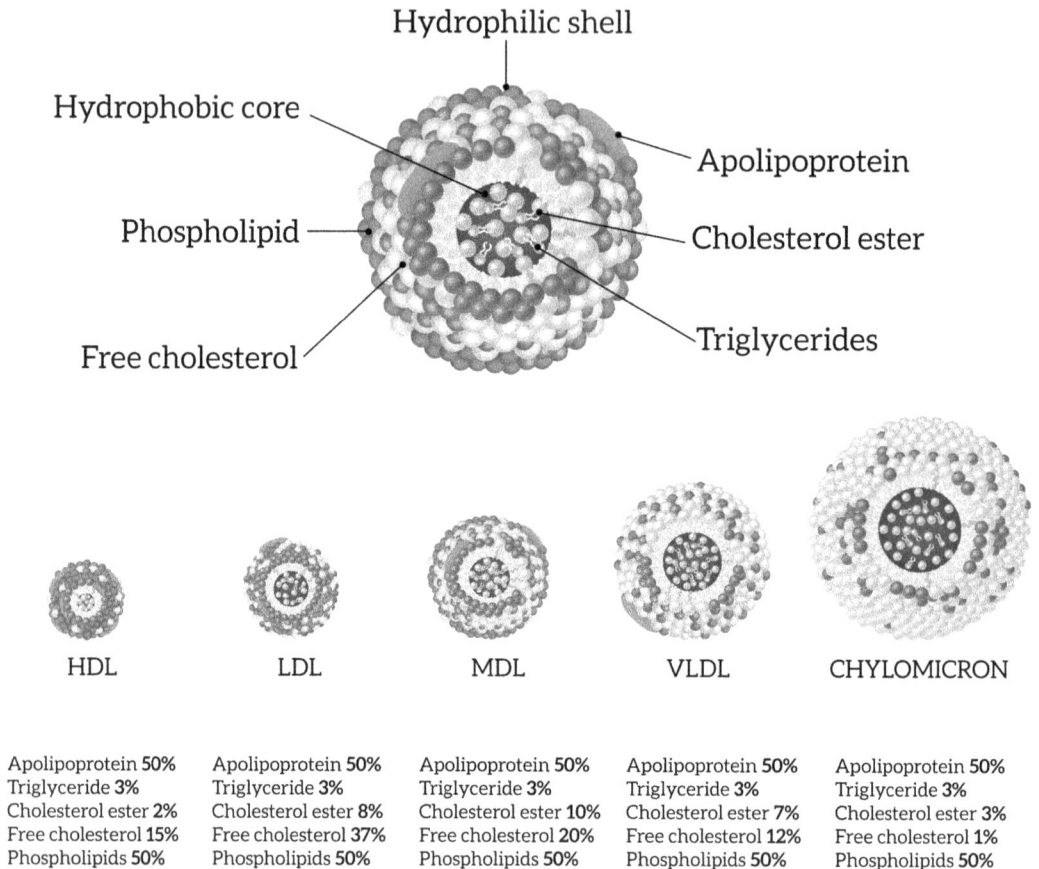

Apolipoprotein 50%	Apolipoprotein 50%	Apolipoprotein 50%	Apolipoprotein 50%	Apolipoprotein 50%
Triglyceride 3%	Triglyceride 3%	Triglyceride 3%	Triglyceride 3%	Triglyceride 3%
Cholesterol ester 2%	Cholesterol ester 8%	Cholesterol ester 10%	Cholesterol ester 7%	Cholesterol ester 3%
Free cholesterol 15%	Free cholesterol 37%	Free cholesterol 20%	Free cholesterol 12%	Free cholesterol 1%
Phospholipids 50%	Phospholipids 50%	Phospholipids 50%	Phospholipids 50%	Phospholipids 50%

FIGURE 5.1 The structure of lipoproteins.

Apolipoproteins have four primary functions in the body. They serve a structural role, act as ligands for lipoprotein receptors, guide the formation of lipoproteins, and activate or inhibit enzymes involved in lipoprotein metabolism.

The exogenous lipoprotein pathway begins with incorporating dietary lipids into **chylomicrons** in the intestine. In the circulation, the triglycerides carried in chylomicrons are metabolized in muscle and adipose tissue by lipoprotein lipase, releasing free fatty acids. These are then metabolized by muscle and adipose tissue, and **chylomicron remnants** are formed to be taken up by the liver.

The endogenous lipoprotein pathway begins in the liver by forming VLDL. The triglycerides carried in VLDL are metabolized in muscle and adipose tissue by lipoprotein lipase, which releases free fatty acids. Reverse cholesterol transport begins with the formation of new HDL by the liver and intestine. These small HDL particles acquire cholesterol and phospholipids from cells. The HDL then transports cholesterol to the liver, directly interacting with hepatic genes or indirectly transferring cholesterol to VLDL or LDL. Cholesterol **efflux** from macrophages to HDL is vital in protecting against atherosclerosis.

YOU SHOULD REMEMBER

The six lipoprotein particles are atherogenic, which causes cardiovascular disease.
   HDLs are anti-atherogenic and prevent cardiovascular disease.

Check Your Knowledge

1. What are lipoproteins?
2. Which lipoproteins are considered "good" and "bad" cholesterol?
3. How does the exogenous lipoprotein pathway begin?

CLASSIFICATIONS OF HYPERCHOLESTEROLEMIA

There is no definitive diagnostic definition of **hypercholesterolemia**. Plasma concentrations of atherogenic cholesterol are mainly determined by circulating cholesterol levels transported in the lipoproteins. These fractions of circulating cholesterol are the causal factor for atherosclerotic cardiovascular disease. To reduce the onset or occurrence of this condition, precise blood lipid measurements and reduction of circulating atherogenic lipoproteins are vital. The classifications of hypercholesterolemia include primary hypercholesterolemia, which is genetic, and secondary hypercholesterolemia, which is acquired. There can also be a multifactorial form of the condition that combines both etiologies.

PRIMARY HYPERCHOLESTEROLEMIA

Primary hypercholesterolemia, also known as *familial hypercholesterolemia*, affects the way the body processes cholesterol. People with this form have a higher risk of heart disease and early myocardial infarction. The genetic changes that cause primary hypercholesterolemia are inherited. The condition is present from birth, though symptoms often do not appear until adulthood. If an individual inherits the situation from both parents, symptoms usually appear during childhood. This is a rare and more severe subtype, and if untreated, it usually causes death before the age of 20.

Epidemiology

Primary hypercholesterolemia may be more common in populations such as Ashkenazi Jews, some groups of Lebanese people, French Canadians, South Africans, and Tunisians. In most countries, the condition affects an estimated one in every 200–300 people. It is believed to be the most common inherited condition that results in cardiovascular disease. Worldwide, about 30 million people are believed to be affected. The estimated FH prevalence displays a variation across ethnicity, ranging from 0.25% (1:400) to 0.52% (1:192), with the highest prevalence among black and brown and the lowest among Asian individuals. The differences observed suggest that targeted screening among subpopulations may increase the identification of cases and, thus, the opportunity for prevention.

Etiology and Risk Factors

Primary hypercholesterolemia is caused by a genetic alteration passed down from one or both parents. It is an autosomal dominant genetic disorder. Affected individuals are, therefore, born with the condition. It prevents the body from removing LDL, "bad cholesterol," resulting in a buildup in the arteries that leads to heart disease. Risk factors include having one or both parents with the causative gene alteration. Most people with the condition receive one affected gene, but rarely can a child receive the affected gene from both parents, leading to a more severe subtype.

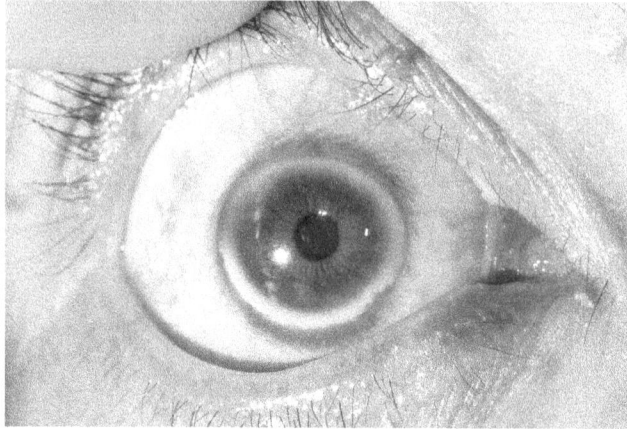

FIGURE 5.2 Arcus senilis.

Clinical Manifestations

Primary hypercholesterolemia means that there are very high levels of LDL-C in the blood, which can build up in the walls of arteries, narrowing and hardening them. This excess cholesterol is sometimes deposited in some skin regions called *xanthelasmas*. The most common areas for xanthelasmas in the skin are on the hands, elbows, and knees, but they can also occur around the eyes. Cholesterol deposits may thicken the Achilles tendon and some of the tendons in the hands. Corneal arcus may develop in the eyes, and a white or gray ring may form around the iris (see **Figure 5.2**). This is most common in older adults but can also occur in younger people. Primary hypercholesterolemia causes a higher risk of heart disease and death at a younger age. Heart attacks may occur before age 50 in men and before age 60 in women. Without diagnosis or treatment, the rarer, more severe subtype may be fatal before age 20.

Diagnosis

Primary hypercholesterolemia requires a detailed family history of any relatives with high cholesterol levels or heart disease, especially during childhood. Physical examination focuses on checking for cholesterol deposits in the skin around the hands, knees, elbows, and eyes. The tendons of the heel and writing may be thickened, and a gray or white ring may develop around the irises of the eyes. A person's first cholesterol screening test should occur between ages 9 and 11 and be repeated every 5 years. Cholesterol levels are measured in milligrams per deciliter of blood or millimoles per liter of blood. Adults with primary hypercholesterolemia usually have LDL levels over 190 mg/dL (4.9 mmol/L). Children often have LDL levels over 160 mg/dL (4.1 mmol/L). In severe cases, the LDL levels can be higher than 500 mg/dL (13 mmol/L).

A genetic test can confirm primary hypercholesterolemia but is not always required. It can also help determine whether other family members may be at risk. If one parent has primary hypercholesterolemia, each child has a 50% chance of inheriting the condition. Inheriting the altered gene from both parents can result in the rare, more severe subtype. Once the disease is diagnosed, all first-degree relatives (siblings, parents, and children) should also be tested. This allows for early treatment to begin if it is needed.

Treatment

Treatment of primary hypercholesterolemia focuses on reducing high LDL-C levels to lower the risks of heart attack and death. Medications are often required in various combinations for treatment. Medication options include statins, ezetimibe (Zetia), and the proprotein convertase subtilisin/kexin type 9 (PCSK9) inhibitors. Statins block the liver's ability to manufacture cholesterol and include drugs such as atorvastatin (Lipitor), fluvastatin (Lescol XL), lovastatin (Altoprev), pitavas-tatin (Livalo), pravastatin (Pravachol), rosuvastatin (Crestor), and simvastatin (Zocor). The drug known as ezetimibe limits the absorption of cholesterol contained in foods. This drug is often added when the statins do not reduce cholesterol sufficiently. The PCSK9 inhibitors are newer drugs, including alirocumab (Praluent) and evolocumab (Repatha). They help the liver absorb more LDL-C, lowering circulating cholesterol in the bloodstream. They are expensive drugs that are injected under the skin every few weeks. For severe cases of primary hypercholesterolemia, some patients must periodically undergo a procedure that filters excess cholesterol from the blood, and some require liver transplants.

Lifestyle changes can also help reduce heart disease risks and lower cholesterol. These include losing weight, eating a heart-healthy diet, exercising regularly, and avoiding smoking. The diet should focus on plant-based foods, including fruits, vegetables, and whole grains. Saturated fats and trans fats must be limited. Exercise should be gradually increased to at least 30 minutes of moderate-intensity activities five times weekly.

Prevention
Primary hypercholesterolemia cannot be prevented since it is an inherited condition. However, genetic testing can alert parents to the defective gene so that conceiving children can be evaluated.

YOU SHOULD REMEMBER

In the homozygous subtype, distinct functioning LDL receptors may be undetectable. Hereditary dyslipidemia involves a defect on chromosome 19, which prevents the body from removing LDL-C from the blood.

Check Your Knowledge

1. In which groups is primary hypercholesterolemia more common?
2. What is arcus senilis?
3. What are the medication options for primary hypercholesterolemia?

SECONDARY (ACQUIRED) HYPERCHOLESTEROLEMIA

Secondary (acquired) hypercholesterolemia is an abnormal increase in blood lipids, which include cholesterol and triglycerides. It does not cause noticeable symptoms but may increase the risks of heart attack and stroke. The condition develops due to lifestyle, underlying health conditions, or medications.

Epidemiology
Secondary hypercholesterolemia accounts for the majority of cases of hypercholesterolemia. Nearly 94 million adults aged 20 or older in the United States have total cholesterol levels of about 200 mg/dL, and 28% have levels above 240 mg/dL.

Etiology and Risk Factors
Secondary hypercholesterolemia results from lifestyle and other factors. An unhealthy lifestyle or acquired medical conditions, including underlying diseases and applied drugs, can be caus-ative. Unlike primary hypercholesterolemia, the causes of secondary hypercholesterolemia are usually modifiable. It may begin with endocrine disorders, renal disorders, liver diseases, stor-age diseases, and medications. Endocrine disorders include diabetes mellitus and **hypothyroidism**.

Renal conditions include **nephrotic syndrome** and **renal failure**. Foods that should be eliminated as much as possible include red, processed meats, commercial baked goods, and fried foods. Acquired metabolic disorders include metabolic syndrome and insulin resistance, while a congenital metabolic disease is type 1 diabetes mellitus. Overall, the metabolic disorders associated with secondary hypercholesterolemia include the following:

- *Diabetes mellitus* – type 1, type 2, and prediabetes – is associated with abnormal increases in triglycerides and VLDL-C.
- *Kidney diseases* – kidney failure, cirrhosis, chronic hepatitis C, nephrotic syndrome – are associated with high triglycerides and VLDL.
- *Hypothyroidism* – it is associated with high LDL.
- *Cholestatic liver disease* – it involves bile duct damage linked to elevated LDL.

Autoimmune diseases linked to secondary hypercholesterolemia include **Cushing's syndrome** and lupus. Also, eating disorders such as anorexia nervosa can cause abnormal total cholesterol and LDL elevations.

Certain medications impair the hormone-producing glands, alter blood chemistry, or interfere with lipid clearance. The drugs that are associated with secondary hypercholesterolemia include the following:

- *Estrogen* – it usually increases levels of triglycerides and HDL.
- *Birth control pills* – it may increase cholesterol levels as well as the risk of atherosclerosis, based on the type and progestin/estrogen dosage.
- *Beta-blockers* – it usually elevate triglycerides while lowering HDL; they are commonly prescribed for hypertension, glaucoma, and migraines.
- *Retinoids* – it may increase LDL and triglycerides; they are used to manage psoriasis and certain skin cancers.
- *Diuretics* – they usually increase LDL and triglyceride levels; they are used to reduce the buildup of body fluids.

Risk factors for secondary hypercholesterolemia include smoking and heavy alcohol use.

Clinical Manifestations

Secondary hypercholesterolemia may begin with endocrine disorders, renal disorders, medications, liver disease, storage disease, and other causes. Endocrine disorders include diabetes mellitus and hypothyroidism. Renal disorders include nephrotic syndrome and renal failure. Secondary hypercholesterolemia does not cause specific symptoms, but its effects include atherosclerosis, hypertension, heart attack, stroke, and related conditions. **Atherosclerosis** or hypertension can cause shortness of breath and fatigue, especially with exertion. If the disease is advanced, the following may develop:

- *Xanthomas* – yellowish fatty nodules under the skin, especially around the eyes, knees, and elbows
- *Hepatomegaly* – pain or fullness in the right upper abdomen due to liver enlargement
- *Splenomegaly* – pain or fullness in the left upper abdomen due to spleen enlargement
- *Corneal arcus (arcus senilis)* – a light-colored ring around the corneas

Diagnosis

A lipid panel is required to diagnose secondary hypercholesterolemia and to measure lipids in the blood after fasting for 10–12 hours. The board is measured in mg/dL. The desirable values for cholesterol and triglycerides, according to the CDC, are as follows:

- *Total cholesterol* – 150 mg/dL
- *LDL-C* – 100 mg/dL
- *Triglycerides* – less than 150 mg/dL
- *HDL-C* – greater than or equal to 40 mg/dL (in men) and 50 mg/dL (in women)

Creatinine, fasting glucose, liver enzymes, thyroid-stimulating hormone, and urinary protein should be measured. Lipid measurement should occur along with assessment for other cardiovascular risk factors, including smoking cigarettes, diabetes mellitus, hypertension, and a family history of coronary artery disease in a male first-degree relative before the age of 55 or a female first-degree relative before the age of 65.

Treatment

Since secondary hypercholesterolemia is acquired, lifestyle modifications are essential for treatment, along with cholesterol-lowering medications. Most underlying metabolic causes, such as diabetes mellitus and hypothyroidism, are chronic and must be controlled. Other reasons, such as hepatitis C, can be cured, though there can still be resultant damage to the liver, leading to elevated lipid levels even after treatment. Medication-induced hypercholesterolemia can often be stopped by stopping or lowering doses of the causative drug. Patients are advised to reduce their intake of saturated fats to less than 6% of total daily calories. They should be replaced with healthier polyunsaturated or monosaturated fats. Fruits, vegetables, whole grains, low-fat dairy products, and oily fish rich in omega-3 fatty acids should be increased.

Weight loss is recommended for obese and overweight people. Smoking and excessive alcohol use must be stopped. According to the American Heart Association, alcohol intake must be limited to two servings per day for men and one serving per day for women. Medications used include the drugs used for primary hypercholesterolemia, plus a few more:

- *Statins*
- *Ezetimibe*
- *PCSK9 inhibitors*
- *Bile acid sequestrants* – which clear bile from the body, forcing the liver to produce more bile and less cholesterol
- *Adenosine triphosphate-citrate lyase (ACL) inhibitors* – which inhibit the biosynthesis of cholesterol in the liver
- *Fibrates* – which is mainly used to reduce triglyceride levels and increase HDL levels
- *Niacin (nicotinic acid)* – which is a prescription form of vitamin B3; it may help reduce LDL and increase HDL

Prevention

Secondary (acquired) hypercholesterolemia prevention requires avoiding the condition's causative agents and risk factors.

YOU SHOULD REMEMBER

Familial hypertriglyceridemia is an inherited disorder characterized by VLDL production in the liver. As a result, an excess number of VLDL and triglycerides are present in the affected individual's lipid profile. This genetic disorder usually follows an autosomal dominant pattern of inheritance. The condition presents clinically in patients with mild to moderately elevated triglyceride levels. Familial hypertriglyceridemia is generally accompanied by comorbidities such as hypertension, obesity, and hyperglycemia.

Check Your Knowledge

1. How familiar is secondary hypercholesterolemia?
2. Which metabolic disorders are associated with secondary hypercholesterolemia?
3. What are the clinical manifestations of secondary hypercholesterolemia?

COMPLICATIONS OF HYPERCHOLESTEROLEMIA

Hypercholesterolemia can lead to atherosclerosis and increased strain on the heart. These can result in an increased chance of stroke or heart attack. Complications include increased mortality, coronary artery disease, peripheral artery disease, cancer, infection, adrenal failure, mental disorders, and suicide. Hypocholesterolemia predisposes to cognitive deficits that include dementias of Alzheimer's type. Abnormal cholesterol metabolism is also linked to neurodegenerative diseases such as Parkinson's, Huntington's, and **amyotrophic lateral sclerosis**. Life expectancy can be reduced by approximately 15–30 years without treatment.

CLINICAL CASE STUDY 1

A 10-year-old boy who was very overweight was brought by his parents to assess multiple yellowish plaques that were consistent with xanthomas in various parts of his body. The lesions had been present at birth but gradually increased in size and number over time. Family history revealed that his maternal grandfather had undergone coronary artery bypass grafting at age 60, and his father and both grandfathers had accumulations of lipid deposits around their eyes. The patient was started on lifestyle modifications, and a decision as to the use of medications was discussed with his parents.

CLINICAL CASE STUDY 2

A 73-year-old man has had hypercholesterolemia for many years. He was first diagnosed when he was in college. A variety of medications had been tried without success. Genetic testing revealed that the patient was affected by a heterozygous, damaging gene mutation that was the cause of his familial hypercholesterolemia. For unknown reasons, testing reveals that he has deficient levels of factors that would signify any significant atherosclerotic disease. He showed an absence of atherosclerotic disease compared to healthy individuals, even though he has had a longstanding history of familial hypercholesterolemia and several cardiovascular risk factors. This may be because his body mass index is average, he does not have hypertension, he has never smoked cigarettes, and he eats a healthy, low-carbohydrate diet.

CLINICAL CASE STUDY 3

A 51-year-old woman was hospitalized because of the signs and symptoms of hypercholesterolemia. She had a long history of poor diet, including many sweetened beverages and foods and a craving for red and processed meats. The patient admitted to seldom eating fruits, vegetables, or whole grains. She had developed soft yellow nodular lesions all over her body. Tests revealed significant atherosclerosis, putting her at high risk for a heart attack or stroke. Her LDL-C was 191 mg/dL, and she had hypertension and prediabetes. The patient was started on a new, healthier diet and enrolled in a regular exercise program supervised by her managed healthcare plan. She was also started on cholesterol-lowering medications.

1. How may secondary (acquired) hypercholesterolemia begin and progress?
2. What can atherosclerosis or hypertension cause before it becomes advanced?
3. What are the medication options for secondary hypercholesterolemia?

FURTHER READING

1. Buck, C. (2023). *Coronary Heart Disease: A Comprehensive Guide to Understanding, Treating, and Preventing It*. Buck.
2. Captain, J. (2017). *How to Have Naturally Healthy Cholesterol Levels*. CreateSpace Independent Publishing Platform.
3. Dach, J.L. (2018). *Heart Book: How to Keep Your Heart Healthy*. Medical Muse Press.
4. Gardiner, C. (2015). *Lipoproteins: Current Concepts*. Callisto Reference.
5. Jiang, X.C. (2020). *Lipid Transfer in Lipoprotein Metabolism and Cardiovascular Disease (Advances in Experimental Medicine and Biology, Book 1276)*. Springer.
6. Kendrick, M. (2021). *The Clot Thickens the Enduring Mystery of Heart Disease*. Columbus Publishing Ltd.
7. Kontush, A., and Chapman, M.J. (2011). *High-Density Lipoproteins: Structure, Metabolism, Function, and Therapeutics*. Wiley.
8. Kostner, K., Kostner, G.M., and Toth, P.P. (2023). *Lipoprotein(a) (Contemporary Cardiology)*. Humana Press.
9. Kumar, S.A. (2015). *Hypercholesterolemia*. IntechOpen.
10. Libonati, J.P. (2011). *Good Cholesterol Bad Cholesterol*. AuthorHouse.
11. Marinetti, G.V. (2012). *Disorders of Lipid Metabolism*. Springer.
12. McAuley, M. (2023). *Cholesterol Metabolism in Aging and Disease*. Academic Press.
13. Papademetriou, V., Andreadis, E.A., and Geladari, C. (2019). *Management of Hypertension: Current Practice and the Application of Landmark Trials*. Springer.
14. Ridgway, N., and McLeod, R. (2015). *Biochemistry of Lipids, Lipoproteins, and Membranes*, 6th Edition. Academic Press.
15. RN Review. (2017). *High Yield Concepts on Treatment Hyperlipidemia: A Study Guide for Nursing Students*. RN Review.
16. Schaefer, E.J. (2010). *High-Density Lipoproteins, Dyslipidemia, and Coronary Heart Disease*. Springer.
17. Steinmetz, A., Schneider, J., and Kaffarnik, H. (2012). *Hormones in Lipoprotein Metabolism (Recent Developments in Lipid and Lipoprotein Research)*. Springer-Verlag.
18. Tada, H. (2022). *The Effect of Diet on Cardiovascular Disease, Heart Disease, and Blood Vessels*. MDPI.
19. Truswell, A.S. (2010). *Cholesterol and Beyond: The Research on Diet and Coronary Heart Disease 1900–2000*. Springer.
20. United States Congress/House Committee. (2015). *Cholesterol Measurement: Error and Variability: Hearing Before the Subcommittee on Technology of the Committee on Science, U.S. House of Representatives, One-Hundred Fourth Congress, First Session*. Palala Press.
21. Vissers, M.N., Kastelein, J.J.P., and Stroes, E.S. (2010). *Evidence-Based Management of Lipid Disorders*. TFM Publishing Ltd.

6 Dyslipidemia and Atherosclerosis

OVERVIEW

Dyslipidemia is the imbalance of plasma cholesterol, triglycerides, or both – or a low high-density lipoprotein cholesterol level, contributing to atherosclerosis development. It can be hereditary or secondary. Lipid measurements are continuous, but a linear relation may exist between lipid levels and cardiovascular risks, meaning many people with normal cholesterol levels benefit from achieving even lower levels. Therefore, there are no numeric definitions of dyslipidemia. The term is used for lipid levels for which treatment has been beneficial. The most decisive proof is for lowering elevated low-density lipoprotein levels. The general population has less evidence of the benefits of reducing high triglyceride levels and increasing high-density lipoprotein cholesterol levels. Dyslipidemias have been traditionally classified by patterns of elevation in lipids and lipoproteins. However, today, primary or secondary dyslipidemias are characterized by increases in cholesterol only, increases in triglycerides, or increases in both.

DYSLIPIDEMIA

Dyslipidemia is the imbalance of lipids such as cholesterol, triglycerides, low-density lipoprotein (LDL), and low-high-density lipoproteins (HDL). This condition can result from diet, tobacco exposure, or genetics and leads to cardiovascular disease (CVD) with severe complications. Dyslipidemia is divided up into primary and secondary types. Primary dyslipidemia is inherited. Secondary dyslipidemia is an acquired condition. That means it develops from other causes, such as obesity or diabetes and genetics. In the majority of cases, **autosomal recessive** inheritance. It is one of the most prevalent monogenic disorders, identified in approximately one of every 500 individuals in the general population. Dyslipidemia may be asymptomatic but may lead to symptomatic vascular disease, including coronary artery disease, peripheral arterial disease, and stroke. High levels of triglycerides (more than 500 mg/dL) can result in acute pancreatitis. High triglyceride levels can cause hepatosplenomegaly, confusion, dyspnea, and **paresthesias**.

The goal of treatment is to reduce the risk of **atherosclerosis**. Lifestyle, medications, and **statins** are often required. Patients may need to reduce or eliminate saturated and trans fats, exercise regularly, maintain a healthy weight, and quit smoking. In most patients with newly diagnosed dyslipidemia, and when a component of the lipid profile has worsened, tests for secondary causes should be done. Creatine, fasting glucose, liver enzymes, thyroid-stimulating hormone (TSH), and urinary protein should be measured.

Screening for dyslipidemia is done using a fasting lipid profile. Lipid measurement should occur along with assessment for other cardiovascular risk factors, including diabetes mellitus, hypertension, smoking, and family history of coronary artery disease in a male first-degree relative before age 55 or a female first-degree relative before age 65.

Children with risk factors such as diabetes, hypertension, and a family history of severe hyperlipidemia should have a fasting lipid profile once between ages 2 and 8. For children with no risk factors, the lipid profile is done once before puberty—usually between ages 9 and 11—and again between ages 17 and 21. Adults are screened at age 20 and every 5 years after that.

DOI: 10.1201/9781003453376-9

YOU SHOULD REMEMBER

Hyperlipidemia refers to high levels of LDL or triglycerides. Dyslipidemia can refer to groups that are either higher or lower than the normal range for those blood fats.

Check Your Knowledge

1. What is the definition of dyslipidemia?
2. What conditions may dyslipidemia lead to?
3. How is screening for dyslipidemia done?

ATHEROSCLEROSIS

Atherosclerosis is a common condition that develops when a sticky substance called plaque builds up inside the artery. The development of plaques collects in the lumens of routes such as the coronary, carotid, and cerebral arteries (see **Figure 6.1**). The patchy plaques comprise lipids,

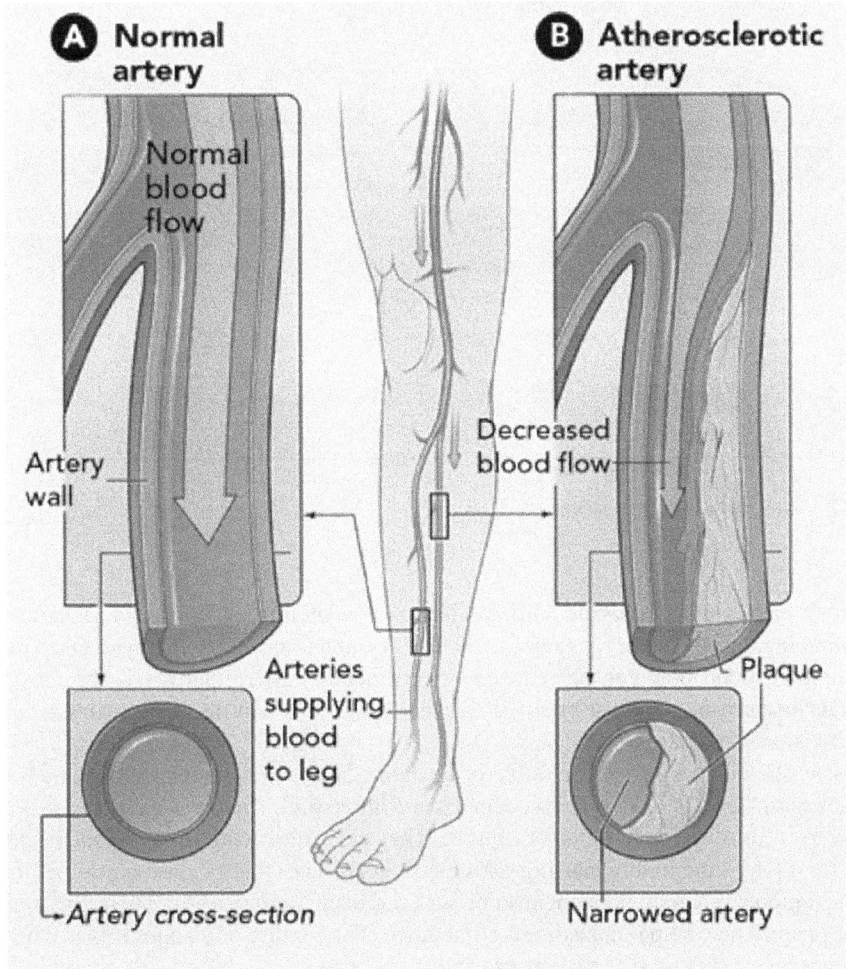

FIGURE 6.1   An artery with plaque buildup.

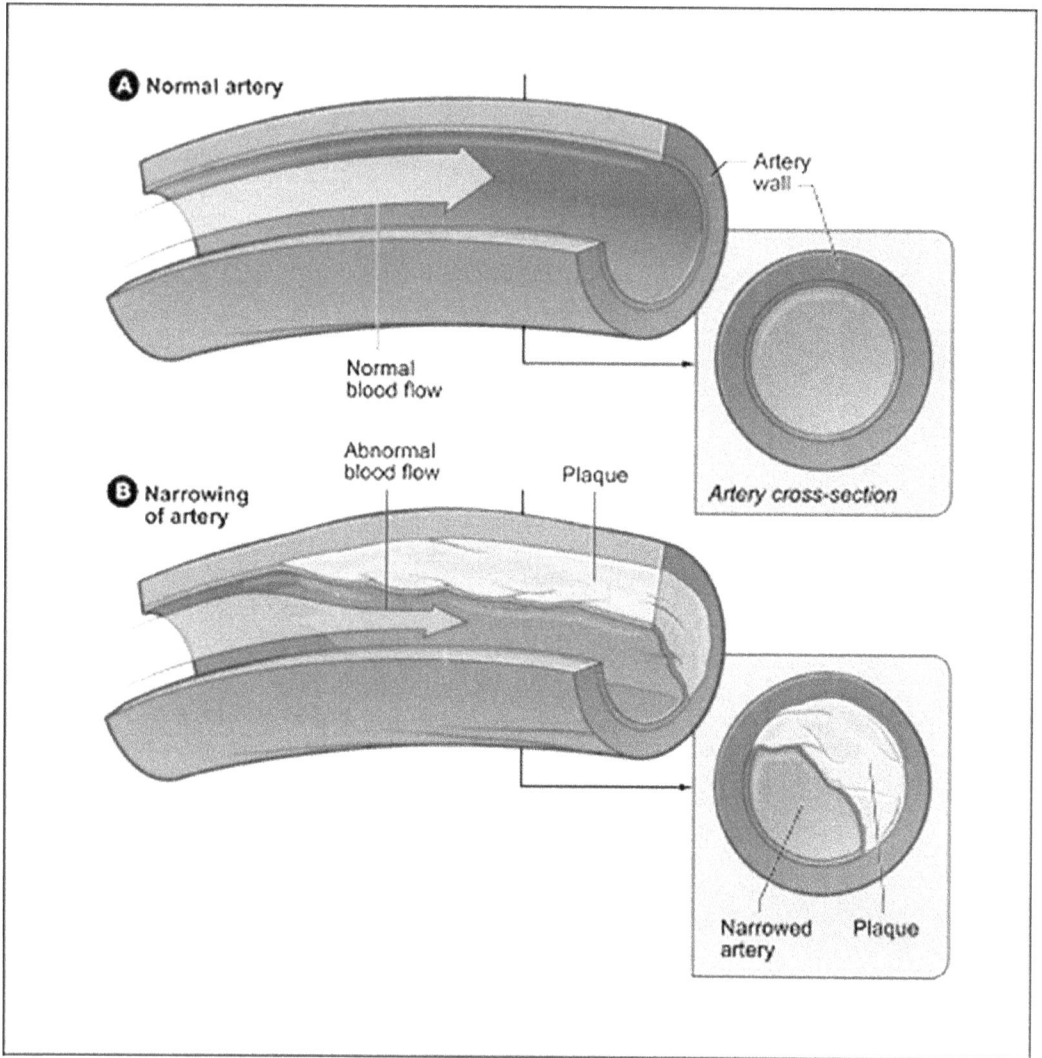

FIGURE 6.2   The course of atherosclerosis.

inflammatory, and connective tissue. Atherosclerosis is related to dyslipidemia, diabetes mellitus, cigarette smoking, family history, hypertension, obesity, and a sedentary lifestyle. Once the plaques grow or rupture, blood flow can be reduced or obstructed. Atherosclerosis is the most common form of **arteriosclerosis**. Atherosclerosis is a severe condition resulting in coronary artery disease (CAD), heart attack, and stroke.

Atherosclerotic plaques are either stable or unstable. *Stable plaques* can grow slowly over several decades until stenosis or occlusion occurs (see **Figure 6.2**). *Unstable plaques* are weaker and more likely to erode, develop fissures, or rupture. They can cause acute **thrombosis**, occlusion, and infarction for a long time before causing extreme stenosis. Unstable plaques cause the majority of signs and symptoms. They do not appear to be severe during **angiography**. Therefore, stabilization of unstable plaques may help reduce disease and death. The rupture of plaques is based on activated **macrophages** inside that secrete **cathepsins** and collagenases.

EPIDEMIOLOGY

Disease linked to atherosclerosis is the leading cause of death in the United States. About half of Americans between ages 45 and 84 have atherosclerosis and do not know it.

Atherosclerosis is the primary cause of disease and death in most developed countries worldwide. Recently, age-related deaths have been decreasing in developed countries. After age 45, men have significant plaque buildup, and women have this after age 55. According to the Multi-ethnic Study of Atherosclerosis, non-Hispanic Caucasian adults have higher levels of atherosclerosis and related CAD than non-Hispanic African, Hispanic, and Asian adults. The top 10 countries with the highest rates of atherosclerosis include Slovakia, Hungary, Ireland, Czech Republic, Finland, New Zealand, United Kingdom, Iceland, Norway, and Australia – updated statistics for each of these are not well documented.

Slightly different statistics are available for deaths from atherosclerosis-related CAD and CVD. Countries with the most deaths from these conditions include Turkmenistan, Kazakhstan, Mongolia, Uzbekistan, Kyrgyzstan, Guyana, Ukraine, Russia, Afghanistan, Tajikistan, and the Republic of Moldova. All of these have more than 500 deaths per 100,000 population annually. Atherosclerosis is increasing in prevalence in developing countries. Incidence is predicted to grow as people in developed countries live longer.

ETIOLOGY AND RISK FACTORS

Atherosclerosis progresses slowly and can begin as early as childhood. In some patients, it goes more rapidly. High blood cholesterol and triglyceride levels and genetic variants of hypertension may cause atherosclerosis. Risk factors include **metabolic syndrome**, insulin resistance, diabetes mellitus, hypertension, smoking, obesity, and stress.

CLINICAL MANIFESTATIONS

Atherosclerosis is often asymptomatic until blood flow begins to be affected. Transient ischemic symptoms may appear when stable plaques enlarge and reduce the arterial lumen by 70% or more. These include **intermittent claudication**, stable exertional angina, and transient ischemic attacks. A lesion that does not limit blood flow can be affected by vasoconstriction so that severe or total stenosis develops. When an unstable plaque ruptures and occludes a significant artery and a superimposition of **embolism** or thrombosis, symptoms may develop, including unstable angina, heart attack, and ischemic stroke. **Aneurysms**, absent pulses, and sudden death may occur due to atherosclerosis (see **Figure 6.3**).

DIAGNOSIS

Diagnosis of atherosclerosis is based on whether the patient is symptomatic or asymptomatic. There must be an evaluation for the location and amount of vascular occlusion when there are signs and symptoms of ischemia. The patient's history is taken, followed by physical examination. Blood tests must be done to determine atherosclerosis – for example, fasting lipid profile, plasma glucose, and glycosylated hemoglobin (HbA1C) levels. Noninvasive imaging can evaluate the morphology and characteristics of atherosclerotic plaques. These methods include **angioscopy**, CT, three-dimensional vascular ultrasonography, and MR angiography.

A new method is recommended for estimating atherosclerotic CVD's 10-year and lifetime risks. It is based on age, gender, race, total cholesterol and HDL levels, diabetes mellitus, smoking status, and systolic BP. The American Heart Association recommends this method. The European Cardiovascular Society and European Atherosclerosis Society use Systemic Coronary Risk Estimation.

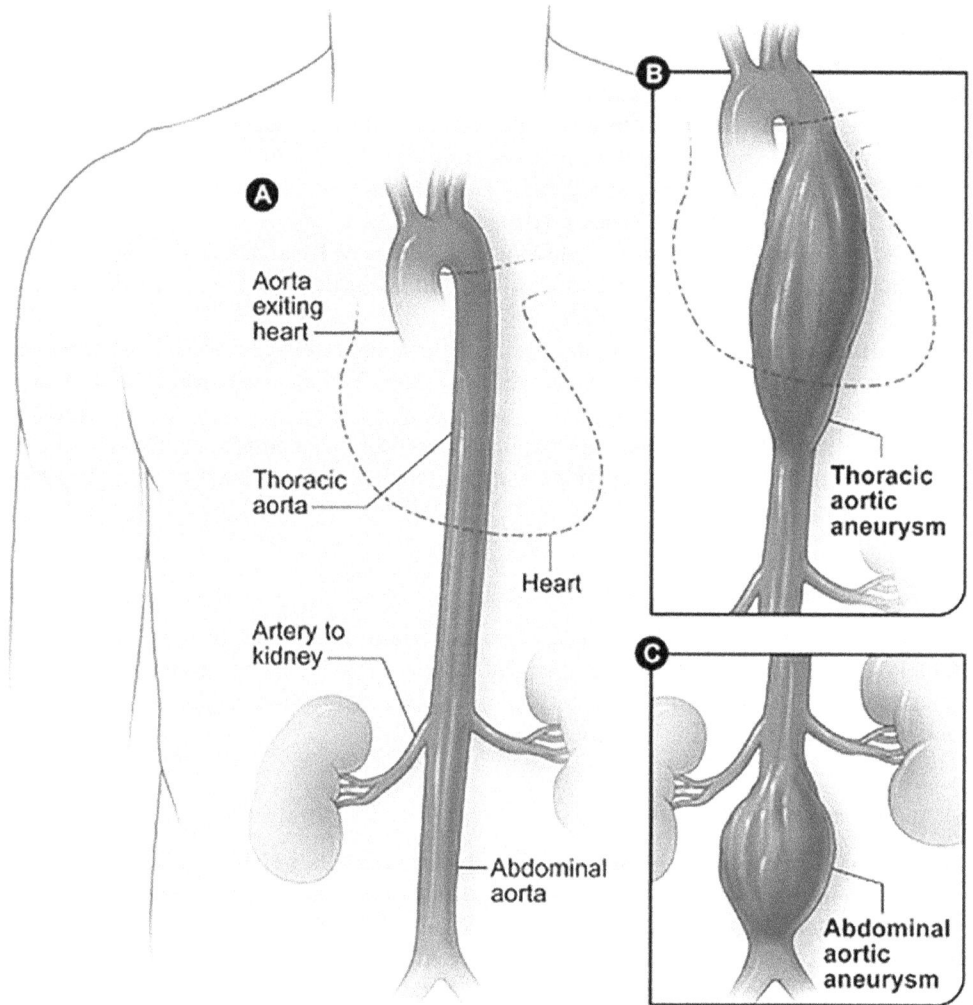

FIGURE 6.3   An aneurysm.

TREATMENT

Treatment of atherosclerosis includes changing lifestyle and medications to lower LDL in the blood. Patients must decrease their intake of saturated fat and refined carbohydrates and increase the types of carbohydrates that contain fiber. Caloric intake must be limited to keep weight gain in a normal range. Fat intake must be limited to no more than 20 g/day. This must consist of 6–10 g of polyunsaturated fat with equal omega-3 and omega-6 fatty acids. Trans fats also must be avoided.

Increased dietary fiber may affect glucose and insulin levels while decreasing total cholesterol. At least 5–10 g of soluble fiber, such as beans, oat bran, and soy products, should be consumed daily. The recommended daily amount of fiber decreases LDL by approximately 5%. Cellulose and lignin are forms of *insoluble fiber* that do not affect cholesterol but help reduce risks for colorectal cancer. Excessive fiber should be avoided because it interferes with some vitamins and minerals absorption.

PREVENTION

Preventing atherosclerosis involves quitting or avoiding smoking, managing hypertension and high cholesterol, becoming more physically active, eating a heart-healthy diet, and managing diabetes mellitus. Aerobic exercise is very beneficial for reducing atherosclerosis. At-risk patients should see their healthcare providers regularly for check-ups to check their BP and cholesterol levels.

YOU SHOULD REMEMBER

Though alcohol increases HDL and has anti-inflammatory, antioxidant, and antithrombotic properties, higher doses can cause severe health problems. The "good" effects of alcohol appear to be the same for moderate beer, wine, and problematic liquor consumption.

YOU SHOULD REMEMBER

Regular physical activity reduces the incidence of diabetes mellitus, dyslipidemia, hypertension, CAD, and atherosclerotic-related death. This is true whether there have been any previous ischemic events. It is recommended that patients engage in 30–45 minutes of walking, cycling, swimming, or running for 3–5 days per week. Aerobic exercise helps prevent atherosclerosis while promoting weight loss.

Check Your Knowledge

1. Which factors are related to atherosclerosis?
2. What are the descriptions of stable plaques and unstable plaques?
3. What are the clinical manifestations of atherosclerosis?

ATHEROMAS

Atheroma refers to the fatty material that clogs arteries. It builds up over time and can lead to complications. Atheroma (plaque) is the defining feature of a disease called atherosclerosis. When patients have atherosclerosis, meaning plaque buildup in their arteries. Atheromas encroach on the lumen of arteries that are medium to large. The plaques contain lipids, inflammatory cells, connective tissue, and smooth muscle cells. Atheromas may form because of various factors, including diabetes mellitus, dyslipidemia, cigarette smoking, family history, a sedentary lifestyle, hypertension, and obesity. Atherosclerosis is the most common form of arteriosclerosis, a general term for several disorders that result in thickening and loss of elasticity in the arterial wall. Atherosclerosis is the most severe and relevant form of arteriosclerosis because it causes stroke and CAD. The non-atheromatous forms of arteriosclerosis include arteriolosclerosis and **Mönckeberg arteriosclerosis**. Atheromas mainly develop through the continuous process of arterial wall lesions due to lipid retention by trapping in the intima by a matrix. This results in a modification that aggravates chronic inflammation of vulnerable sites in the arteries.

EPIDEMIOLOGY

Virtually everyone will develop some degree of atheromas as they age. For many people, they pose no risks. But when the atheromas become so large that they inhibit blood flow, serious problems can occur. This is more likely to happen if patients are overweight, have diabetes, smoke, or have hypertension. Atherosclerosis is quickly increasing in prevalence in low and middle-income countries. As people continue to live longer, the incidence will increase. It is the primary cause of morbidity and mortality in the United States and most developed countries. However, age-related deaths related to this condition are decreasing.

ETIOLOGY AND RISK FACTORS

Atheromas are caused by consuming high saturated fat, trans fat, cholesterol, and triglycerides, **rheumatoid arthritis**, hypertension, and diabetes mellitus. Risk factors for atheromas include aging, a family history of early heart disease, an unhealthy diet, diabetes mellitus, hypertension, high cholesterol, lack of exercise, obesity, **sleep apnea**, and smoking.

CLINICAL MANIFESTATIONS

The signs and symptoms of atheromas begin with an asymptomatic period that can last for decades. Once lesions impede blood flow, signs and symptoms develop. Symptoms vary depending on which arteries are affected and how much the atheroma blocks blood flow. When an artery supplying blood to the heart is affected by atheromas, the patient may experience heart attack or heart disease symptoms. When arteries in the neck that supply blood to the brain are restricted or blocked, you may experience a stroke or a transient ischemic attack (TIA). A TIA is a "mini" stroke with more fleeting neurological effects. Peripheral arteries that transport blood to the arms and legs may also be affected. However, the legs seem most prone to dangerous atheromas.

Transient ischemic symptoms can develop when stable plaques grow and reduce the arterial lumen by more than 70%. These include chest pain, cold sweats, dizziness, extreme tiredness, heart palpitations, dyspnea, nausea, and weakness. Symptoms of unstable atheromas cause acute occlusion of a major artery, with superimposition of thrombosis or embolism. This condition may cause stroke or *intermittent claudication*.

DIAGNOSIS

Diagnosing atheromas as part of atherosclerosis is based on the presence or absence of symptoms. Signs of ischemia are evaluated for the amount and location of vascular occlusion based on the organs involved. Noninvasive imaging techniques include 3-D vascular ultrasonography, CT scan, angiography, and magnetic resonance (MR) angiography.

A noninvasive alternative, **immunoscintigraphy**, uses radioactive tracers that localize in vulnerable plaques. Another newer approach is **positron emission tomography** (PET) of the vasculature to assess susceptible plaques. Some clinicians also measure serum markers of inflammation, which can be highly predictive of cardiovascular events.

TREATMENT

Treatment of atheromas and atherosclerosis requires aggressive modification of risk factors to slow progression and result in regression of existing plaques. Regarding cholesterol, "the lower, the better" is the approach that is favored. Lifestyle changes include diet modification, regular physical activity, and smoking cessation. Drugs to treat diabetes mellitus, dyslipidemia, and hypertension are often needed. These changes improve endothelial function, reduce inflammation, and improve clinical outcomes. Statins can decrease atherosclerosis-related illness and death even when serum cholesterol is normal or slightly high. Antiplatelet drugs are suitable for all patients with atherosclerosis. Patients with coronary artery disease may also benefit from ACE inhibitors and beta-blockers.

The diet must have less saturated fat, no trans fats, fewer refined carbohydrates, more fruits and vegetables, more fiber, and slight alcohol. Calorie intake must be limited to keep weight within the normal range. Fat intake is limited to 20 g/day, consisting of 6–10 g of polyunsaturated fat with omega-6 and omega-3 acids equal to 2 g or less of saturated fat and the remainder as monoun-saturated fat. Caloric deficiencies should comprise proteins and unsaturated fats instead of simple carbohydrates. Excessive fat and refined sugar must be avoided, especially when there is a risk of diabetes. Consumption of complex carbohydrates (whole grains and vegetables) is encouraged. In fruits and vegetables, phytochemicals called flavonoids are highly protective. Daily intake of at least 5–10 g of soluble fiber is recommended (via oat bran, beans, soy products, and psyllium), enough to decrease LDL by approximately 5%. Generally, foods rich in phytochemicals and vitamins are also rich in fiber.

Alcohol increases HDL and has undefined antithrombotic, antioxidant, and anti-inflammatory properties. About 30 mL of ethanol five to six times per week protects against coronary athero-sclerosis, but significant health problems may result in higher doses. Mortality rates are low-est for men who consume less than 14 drinks per week and women who consume less than nine drinks per week. The only dietary supplement proven to reduce risks for atherosclerosis is fish oil.

Regular physical activity, such as 30–45 minutes of walking, running, swimming, or cycling three to five times per week, reduces the incidence of hypertension, dyslipidemia, diabetes mellitus, myocardial infarction, and death that is attributable to atherosclerosis in patients that have or have not had any previous ischemia. There is an inverse linear relationship between aerobic physical activity and risk. Walking regularly increases the distance from which patients with peripheral vas-cular disease can walk without pain. Aerobic exercise helps prevent atherosclerosis and promotes weight loss. A physician should always direct it.

Antiplatelet drugs include aspirin, clopidogrel, prasugrel, and ticagrelor. Aspirin is the most widely used drug and may be considered the primary prevention of coronary atherosclerosis in high-risk patients. Each patient must be evaluated regarding the use of aspirin and the correct dos-age. Generally, 81–325 mg orally once per day is preferred. Clopidogrel (75 mg orally once per day) is substituted when ischemic events recur after taking aspirin or if the patient cannot tolerate aspirin. Prasugrel and ticagrelor are newer, more effective drugs for coronary disease prevention in certain patients.

Statins primarily lower LDL cholesterol. They are used as preventive therapy for clinical atherosclerotic cardiovascular disease when LDL cholesterol is at or higher than 190 mg/dL (4.92 mmol/L), the patient is 40–75 years of age (with LDL at 70–189 mg/dL [1.81–4.9 mmol/L]), or the patient is 40–75 years of age (with LDL 70–189 mg/dL and estimated 10-year risk of arte-riosclerotic cardiovascular disease of 7.5% or higher). Statins are also used for risk factors that include a family history of premature arteriosclerotic cardiovascular disease, high-sensitivity C-reactive protein levels, high coronary artery calcium scores, low ankle-brachial blood pressure indices, or chronic kidney disease not treated with dialysis or kidney transplantation. Statin treat-ment is classified as high, moderate, or down based on the treatment group and age. Response to therapy is determined by whether LDL levels decrease as expected based on the intensity of the treatment.

Other drugs used for atheromas and atherosclerosis include angiotensin-converting enzyme (ACE) inhibitors, angiotensin II receptor blockers, ezetimibe, and proprotein convertase subtilisin/ kexin type 9 (PCSK9) inhibitors. Rivaroxaban also decreases the risks of cardiovascular events via an unknown mechanism of action. When ezetimibe is added to standard statin therapy, it reduces cardiovascular events in those with a previous occasion and if the LDL is higher than 70 mg/dL. The PCSK9 inhibitors are most useful in patients with familial hypercholesterolemia, those with prior cardiovascular events with LDL not optimal even after statin therapy, and those who need lipid-lowering but have some amount of statin intolerance.

PREVENTION

Lifestyle factors can be taken to reduce the risks of atheromas and atherosclerosis. These include avoiding smoking, eating a healthy diet, having a low sodium intake, having regular physical activity, managing weight, drinking alcohol only in moderation, and controlling blood pressure and cholesterol levels.

YOU SHOULD REMEMBER

Atheroma plaques may be stable or unstable. Stable plaques regress, remain static or grow slowly over decades to eventually cause stenosis or occlusion. Unstable plaques may experience spontaneous erosion or ruptures, leading to acute thrombosis, occlusion, and infarction.

Check Your Knowledge

1. What do atheromas contain?
2. What are atheromas caused by?
3. What does the treatment of atheromas and atherosclerosis require?

FATTY STREAK

A **fatty streak** is simply the earliest visible lesion of atherosclerosis caused by an accumulation of lipid-laden foam cells in an artery's intimal layer. Over time, the heavy bar evolves into a fibrous plaque, the identifying factor of established atherosclerosis.

The matrix may have thrombi that are in different stages of organization. Calcium deposits may also be present (see **Figure 6.4**).

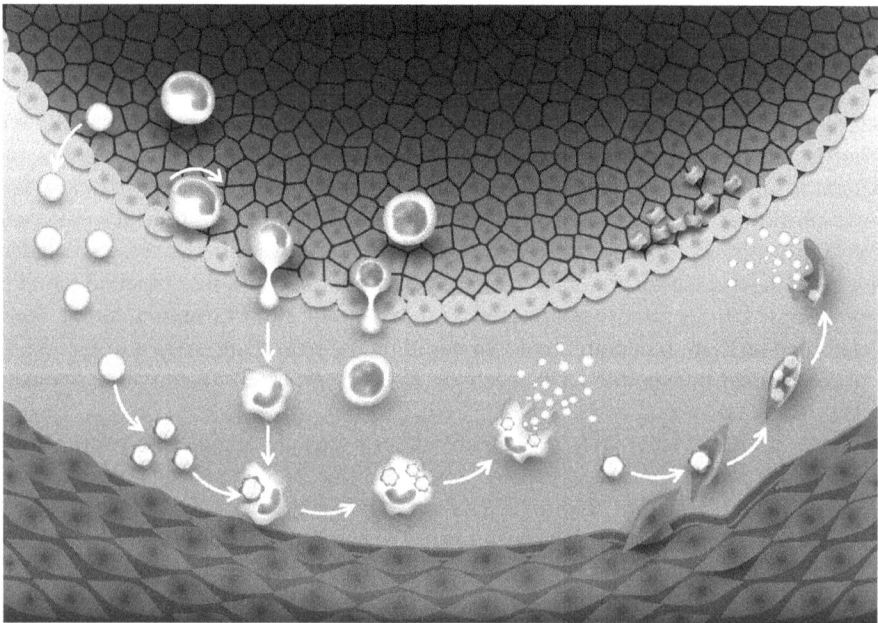

FIGURE 6.4   A fatty streak.

EPIDEMIOLOGY

The prevalence of fatty streaks in the coronary arteries increases with age, from about 50% at 2–15 to 85% at 21–39. The prevalence of raised fibrous-plaque lesions increases from 8% at 2–15 to 69% at 26–39.

ETIOLOGY AND RISK FACTORS

The cause of fatty streaks is the expansion of foam cells at the plaque site. By this stage, a lipid core has formed that will progress into a mature atherosclerotic plaque after an influx of different inflammatory cell types and extracellular lipids. Risk factors for fatty streaks include high cholesterol, hypertension, diabetes mellitus, tobacco use, obesity, lack of exercise, and a diet high in saturated fat.

CLINICAL MANIFESTATIONS

When a fatty streak develops, there are no signs or symptoms. Symptoms may begin later when the plaque becomes more prominent and the arterial lumens narrow.

DIAGNOSIS

A fatty streak is not generally diagnosed because it is an initial step in atherosclerosis. However, it is the first grossly visible lesion in this condition, appearing as an irregular yellow-white discoloration on the luminal surface of an artery.

TREATMENT

There is no treatment for fatty streaks. They are clinically harmless and potentially reversible, though progression to fibrous plaques and more advanced lesions often leads to a critical stage of atherosclerosis.

PREVENTION

Fatty streaks cannot be prevented, but they can be reversed with treatments for atherosclerosis.

Check Your Knowledge

1. What is a fatty streak?
2. What are the risk factors for fatty streaks?
3. How does a fatty streak appear in color?

GLYCEROL METABOLISM DISORDERS

Glycerol is a precursor for synthesizing triacylglycerols and phospholipids in the liver and adipose tissue. When the body uses stored fat as energy, glycerol and fatty acids are released into the bloodstream. Glycerol is metabolized predominantly in the liver, the first step presumably being **phosphorylation** to alpha-glycerophosphate. When ethanol is present in the blood, the rate of glycerol uptake by the splanchnic organs is reduced to about one-third of the control value. Glycerol is converted to glycerol-3-phosphate by the hepatic enzyme called *glycerol kinase*. The best example of these disorders is glycerol kinase deficiency (GKD).

EPIDEMIOLOGY

Glycerol metabolism disorders are rare, affecting fewer than 200,000 individuals in the United States. Due to their infrequency, these disorders have no significant epidemiological statistics.

ETIOLOGY AND RISK FACTORS

Glycerol metabolism disorders mainly result in glycerol kinase deficiency, which is an X-linked recessive enzyme defect that is heterozygous. Three clinically distinct forms of this deficiency have been proposed: infantile, juvenile, and adult. Many affected individuals also have a **chromosomal deletion** extending past the glycerol kinase gene into the contiguous gene region containing congenital adrenal hypoplasia and Duchenne muscular dystrophy genes. Therefore, a patient with glycerol kinase deficiency may have one more of these related diseases. The only risk factor is having this chromosomal deletion.

CLINICAL MANIFESTATIONS

Glycerol kinase deficiency causes the condition known as **hyperglycerolemia**, an accumulation of glycerol in the blood and urine. Excess glycerol in bodily fluids can lead to many potentially dangerous symptoms. Common symptoms include vomiting, hypotonia, and lethargy. These tend to be the only symptoms present in adult GKD, which have been found to present with fewer symptoms than infant or juvenile GKD. Symptoms visible at or shortly after birth include **strabismus**, seizures, metabolic acidosis, hypoglycemia, **cryptorchidism**, adrenal cortex insufficiency, and learning disabilities.

DIAGNOSIS

Diagnosing glycerol metabolism disorders involves detecting an elevated glycerol level in the serum and urine. It is confirmed by DNA analysis.

TREATMENT

Treatments for GKD are targeted to treat the symptoms because there are no permanent treatments for this disease. The primary way to treat these symptoms is through glucose infusion and corticosteroids. The steroid hormone regulates stress responses, carbohydrate metabolism, blood electrolyte levels, and other uses. Mineralocorticoids, such as aldosterone, control many electrolyte levels and allow the kidneys to retain sodium. Glucose infusion is coupled with insulin infusion to monitor blood glucose levels and keep them stable.

PREVENTION

There is no prevention for glycerol metabolism disorders because they are inherited.

YOU SHOULD REMEMBER

The best ways to lower triglycerides include losing weight, eating fewer calories, and exercising regularly (30 minutes daily). Diet changes may help avoid fats, sugar, and refined foods (simple carbohydrates such as sugar and foods made with white flour).

Check Your Knowledge

1. What is the best example of glycerol metabolism disorders?
2. What condition is caused by glycerol kinase deficiency?
3. What are the common symptoms of hyperglycerolemia?

KETONE METABOLISM DISORDERS

Episodes of metabolic decompensation characterize disorders of **ketone body** metabolism. **Diabetic ketoacidosis** is a condition that affects people with diabetes and people with undiagnosed diabetes. It happens when the blood turns acidic because it has too many ketones due to a lack of insulin. Diabetes-related ketoacidosis is life-threatening and requires immediate medical attention. Ketones are made in the liver from the breakdown of fats. They are formed when insufficient sugar or glucose supplies the body's fuel needs.

EPIDEMIOLOGY

The incidence is roughly two episodes per 100 patient-years of diabetes, with about 3% of patients with type 1 diabetes initially presenting with DKA.

ETIOLOGY AND RISK FACTORS

The disorders of ketogenesis cause hypoglycemia and encephalopathy. Diabetic ketoacidosis develops when ketone bodies build up during uncontrolled diabetes (usually type 1 diabetes).

CLINICAL MANIFESTATIONS

The signs and symptoms of diabetic ketoacidosis include nausea and vomiting, headache, dry skin and mouth, **tachypnea**, fruity-smelling breath, headache, polydipsia, polyuria, muscle aches, fatigue, and confusion.

DIAGNOSIS

A physical exam and blood tests can help diagnose diabetic ketoacidosis. In some cases, other tests may be needed to help determine the cause. Blood tests include blood sugar, ketone, pH, and urinalysis.

TREATMENT

Treatment for diabetic ketoacidosis usually involves replacing fluids by mouth or intravenously. IV electrolytes help the heart, muscles, and nerve cells function generally. In addition to juices and electrolytes, insulin is given via IV. A return to regular insulin therapy may be possible when the blood sugar level falls to about 200 mg/dL (11.1 mmol/L) and the blood is no longer acidic.

PREVENTION

The most important thing the patient can do to prevent DKA is to keep their diabetes well-managed. Monitoring blood sugar levels and taking insulin are the main factors for prevention.

Check Your Knowledge

1. What is diabetic ketoacidosis?
2. What do the disorders of ketogenesis cause?
3. What are the signs and symptoms of diabetic ketoacidosis?

COMPLICATIONS OF DYSLIPIDEMIA

Cholesterol is not bad because the body still needs cholesterol to synthesize hormones, vitamin D, and digestive fluids. Cholesterol also creates a metabolic environment for the organs to function smoothly. However, high cholesterol levels cause many dangerous diseases. Therefore, understanding dyslipidemia and its complications helps us take early measures to regulate blood fat levels, prevent diseases, ensure quality of life, and prolong life in the future. Severe or untreated dyslipidemia can lead to other conditions, including coronary artery disease (CAD) and peripheral artery disease (PAD). CAD and PAD can cause serious health complications, including heart attacks and strokes.

YOU SHOULD REMEMBER

The ketogenic diet typically consists of a high-fat, adequate-protein, and low-carbohydrate diet previously thought to be relatively safe for weight loss. However, when carbohydrates are entirely removed from the diet, an overproduction of ketone bodies results in ketoacidosis. Treatment should be aimed at halting the ketogenic process and patient education.

CLINICAL CASE STUDY 1

A 13-year-old obese boy is evaluated for dyslipidemia. His checkup at age 10 revealed highly elevated triglycerides and his parents were encouraged to improve the boy's diet. They find this hard to do because he consistently sneaks other foods out of the kitchen and eats them, preferring high-sugar and salty foods over more healthy choices. He seldom participates in any sports activities, and his only regular exercise is occasionally riding his bicycle. Physical examination revealed that the boy's body mass index was in the 98th percentile for his age. Blood tests showed all types of his cholesterol, except HDL, to be higher than usual.

CRITICAL THINKING QUESTIONS

1. What are the differences between primary and secondary dyslipidemia?
2. What tests are performed to assess dyslipidemia?
3. What testing is done for children with dyslipidemia?

CLINICAL CASE STUDY 2

A 52-year-old man has had dyslipidemia for several years without any cardiovascular complications. He has been treated with various lipid-lowering agents but is currently not on medication. His mother also had dyslipidemia with elevated triglycerides and LDL cholesterol, and she had a stroke at the age of 72 years. His maternal uncle has dyslipidemia and had a myocardial infarction at the age of 57 years. The patient does not follow any particular diet and does not exercise regularly. His blood pressure is 134/84 mm Hg, and he weighs 180 pounds, standing at 5 feet 9 inches in height.

1. What is the link between dyslipidemia, atherosclerosis, and other factors?
2. How is the screening for dyslipidemia done?
3. How could regular physical activity help this patient?

CLINICAL CASE STUDY 3

An 89-year-old woman was hospitalized due to chest pain and swelling in the left upper arm. She previously had angina that occurred after exertion. Physical examination revealed tachycardia and hypertension. Coronary angiography showed obstructions of 90% in the right coronary and 70% in the anterior interventricular artery. A successful coronary angioplasty with stent implantation in the coronary artery was completed, but the right coronary artery was occluded, and coronary angioplasty could not be done. About 2 weeks later, the patient underwent coronary angioplasty with stent implantation in the anterior interventricular coronary branch. She was given fenofibrate, followed by simvastatin. At 6 months of follow-up, the patient improved tremendously.

CRITICAL THINKING QUESTIONS

1. How is an unstable plaque related to angina?
2. How may atherosclerosis be prevented?
3. What is the result of the buildup of plaques in the arteries?

FURTHER READING

1. Baliga, R.R., and Cannon, C.P. (2011). *Dyslipidemia (American Cardiology Library)*. Oxford University Press.
2. Chopra, H.K., Nanda, N.C., Narula, J., Wander, G.S., Manjunaath, C.N., Chandra, P., Kumar, V., Ponde, C.K., and Pancholia, A.K. (2022). *Advances in Statin Therapy & Beyond in CVD (ASTC): A Textbook of Cardiology*. Jaypee Brothers Medical Publishers Ltd.
3. Covic, A., Kanbay, M., and Lerma, E.V. (2014). *Dyslipidemias in Kidney Disease*. Springer.
4. Davidson, M.H., Toth, P.P., and Maki, K.C. (2021). *Therapeutic Lipidology (Contemporary Cardiology)*, 2nd Edition. Humana Press.
5. Dureja, H., Narasimha Murth, S., Wich, P.R., and Dua, K. (2022). *Drug Delivery Systems for Metabolic Disorders*. Academic Press.
6. Garg, A. (2015). *Dyslipidemias: Pathophysiology, Evaluation, and Management (Contemporary Endocrinology)*. Humana Press.
7. Grundy, S.M. (2011). *Atlas of Atherosclerosis and Metabolic Syndrome*, 5th Edition. Springer.
8. Iacobellis, G. (2020). *Epicardial Adipose Tissue: From Cell to Clinic (Contemporary Cardiology)*. Humana Press.
9. Lee, S.H., and Kyoung Kang, M. (2021). *Stroke Revisited: Dyslipidemia in Stroke*. Springer.
10. Lipovetskiy, B. (2012). *Dyslipidemias and Atherosclerosis: Connections with Ischemic Disease of Heart and Brain*. Lap Lambert Academic Publishing.
11. Moini, J., Akinso, O., Ferdowski, K., and Moini, M. (2022). *Health Care Today in the United States*. Academic Press.
12. Myerson, M. (2018). *Dyslipidemia: A Clinical Approach*. Wolters Kluwer.
13. Patel, V.B. (2018). *The Molecular Nutrition of Fats*. Academic Press.
14. Ramji, D. (2022). *Atherosclerosis: Methods and Protocols (Methods in Molecular Biology, 2419)*. Humana Press.
15. Ridgeway, N., and McLeod, R. (2015). *Biochemistry of Lipids, Lipoproteins and Membranes*, 6th Edition. Academic Press.
16. Rippe, J.M. (2022). *Integrating Lifestyle Medicine in Cardiovascular Health and Disease Prevention*. CRC Press.

17. Schaefer, E.J. (2010). *High-Density Lipoproteins, Dyslipidemia, and Coronary Heart Disease*. Springer.
18. Thompson, D. (2015). *Dyslipidemia Essentials*. Foster Academics.
19. Von Eckardstein, A., and Binder, C.J. (2022). *Prevention and Treatment of Atherosclerosis: Improving State-of-the-Art Management and Search for Novel Targets (Handbook of Experimental Pharmacology, 270)*. Springer.
20. Young, R. (2016). *The Cause and Cure for Atherosclerosis and Coronary Artery Disease*. Hikari Omni Media.

7 Hypertension

OVERVIEW

Hypertension is a condition in which the blood vessels have persistently raised pressure. The blood pressure is made up of two numbers: systolic and diastolic. Most of the time, there are no apparent symptoms. Hypertension is a significant risk factor for cardiovascular disease. Lowering blood pressure has been shown to decrease complications. Globally, an estimated 26% of the world's population (972 million people) has hypertension, and the prevalence is expected to increase to 29% by 2025. Certain physical traits and lifestyle choices can increase the risk of hypertension. The pathophysiology of hypertension involves an impairment in renal pressure natriuresis. This is the feedback system in which hypertension causes an increase in sodium and water excretion by the kidney, which leads to a reduction in blood pressure. Hypertension can lead to a variety of complications, including heart attack, stroke, aneurysm, heart failure, kidney problems, eye problems, metabolic syndrome, changes in memory or understanding, and dementia.

PRIMARY HYPERTENSION

Hypertension is commonly referred to as *high blood pressure*. It is defined as a sustained elevation of resting systolic blood pressure of 130 mm Hg or higher, diastolic blood pressure of 80 mm Hg or higher, or both. Hypertension involves activation of the sympathetic nervous system and **renin-angiotensin system**, sodium retention, and various abnormalities. Obesity increases the risk for hypertension and is associated with increased blood flow, vasodilation, cardiac output, and glomerular filtration rate. As renal sodium retention increases, hypertension develops. Blood pressure (BP) levels are continuously related to stroke and coronary heart disease risks.

EPIDEMIOLOGY

Global uncontrolled hypertension affects more than 1.13 billion people. The prevalence of hypertension was highest in Africa (46%) for both genders. Generally, prevalence is higher in low- and middle-income countries than in high-income countries. Countries with the highest prevalence of hypertension are shown in **Figure 7.1**.

In the United States, about 116 million people have hypertension. While 81% are aware of their condition, only about 75% receive treatment, and only 24% have adequate blood pressure control. Adult hypertension is most common in African-Americans (56%) compared to Caucasians (48%) or Hispanics (39%)–see **Figure 7.2.** Morbidity and mortality are also more significant among African Americans. With age, blood pressure increases. About 70% of people over the age of 65 have hypertension. Higher BP increases morbidity and mortality risks. Globally, hypertension has an average incidence of 31.1% based on age, gender, and body type. The incidence of hypertension depends on age, gender, and body type. According to the WHO, hypertension accounts for 57 million disability-adjusted life years, or 3.7% of total DALYs. The CDC reports that total costs associated with hypertension in the United States exceed $131 billion annually. Globally, hypertension is estimated to cause about 7.5 million deaths annually.

DOI: 10.1201/9781003453376-10

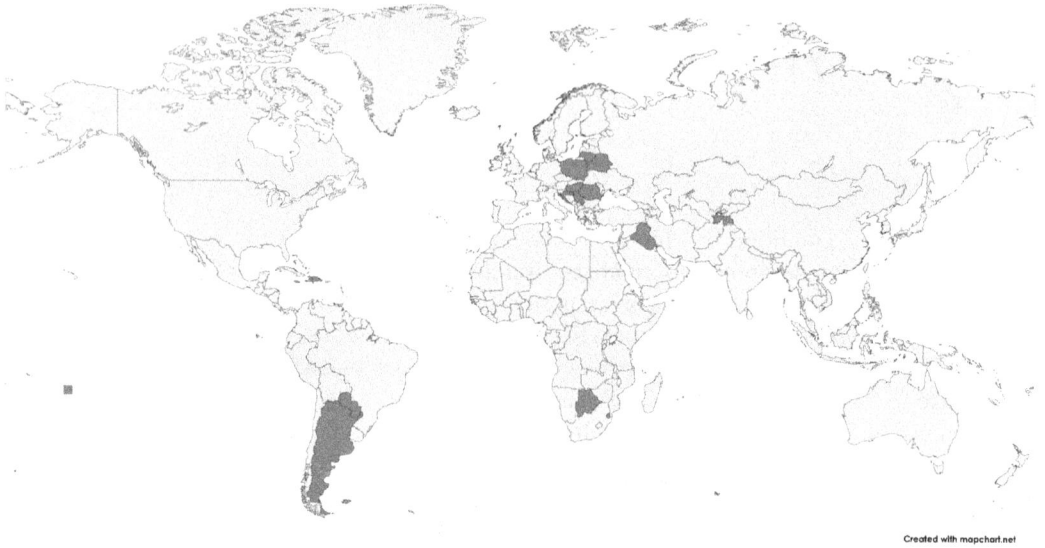

FIGURE 7.1   Countries with the highest prevalence of hypertension.

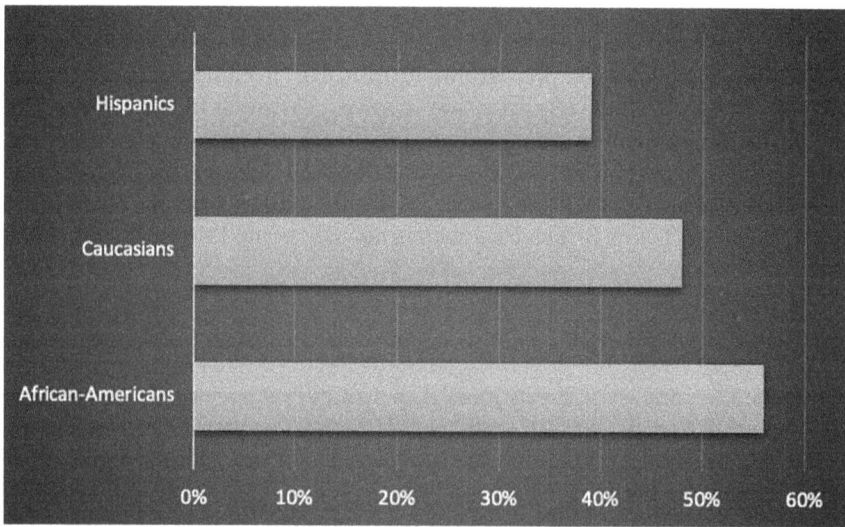

FIGURE 7.2   Percentages of adults with hypertension in various racial or ethnic groups.

ETIOLOGY AND RISK FACTORS

Hypertension is classified as *primary* (essential) in over 90% of cases and *secondary* in the remainder. Primary hypertension has multiple factors, and heredity is a predisposing factor. The exact causative mechanism needs to be more precise. Environmental factors include obesity, dietary sodium, and stress. These appear to affect only genetically susceptible individuals at younger ages. In patients over 65, high sodium intake is more likely to precede hypertension. Obesity, tobacco smoking, insulin resistance, and heavy alcohol consumption are additional risk factors.

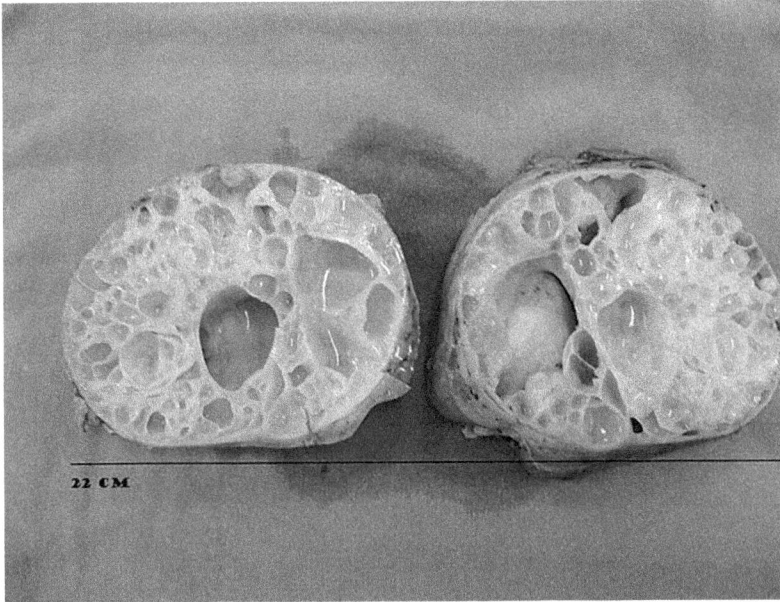

FIGURE 7.3   Polycystic renal disease.

CLINICAL MANIFESTATIONS

Early signs and symptoms of hypertension include dizziness, facial flushing, early morning headaches, **epistaxis**, vision changes, ear buzzing, and nervousness. Severe hypertension can cause fatigue, nausea, vomiting, confusion, anxiety, chest pain, and muscle tremors. Hypertensive emergencies can cause severe cardiovascular, neurologic, renal, and retinal symptoms. These include symptomatic coronary atherosclerosis, heart failure, hypertensive encephalopathy, heart attack, stroke, sexual dysfunction, and renal failure. Retinal changes include arteriolar narrowing, hemorrhages, exudates, and papilledema (see **Figure 7.3**).

The development of primary hypertension is highly complex and multifactorial. The kidneys are the contributing organs and the target organs of hypertension. Multiple organ systems interact with various mechanisms of independent or interdependent pathways. Factors include genetics, activation of the sympathetic nervous system and renin-angiotensin-aldosterone system, obesity, and high dietary sodium. Arterial hypertension is the condition of persistently elevated systemic blood pressure.

DIAGNOSIS

The diagnosis of primary hypertension is based on the presence of high blood pressure without any of the conditions that cause secondary hypertension. A medical history is reviewed to rule out these conditions. Suppose a patient has multiple elevated blood pressure readings; 24-hour ambulatory BP monitoring may be recommended. This measures the blood pressure over 1 day, even while the patient is asleep. Providers then take the average of these readings to confirm or rule out the diagnosis.

TREATMENT

Treatments for hypertension typically include lifestyle changes and medications. Various medications can lower blood pressure, including angiotensin-converting enzyme (ACE) inhibitors,

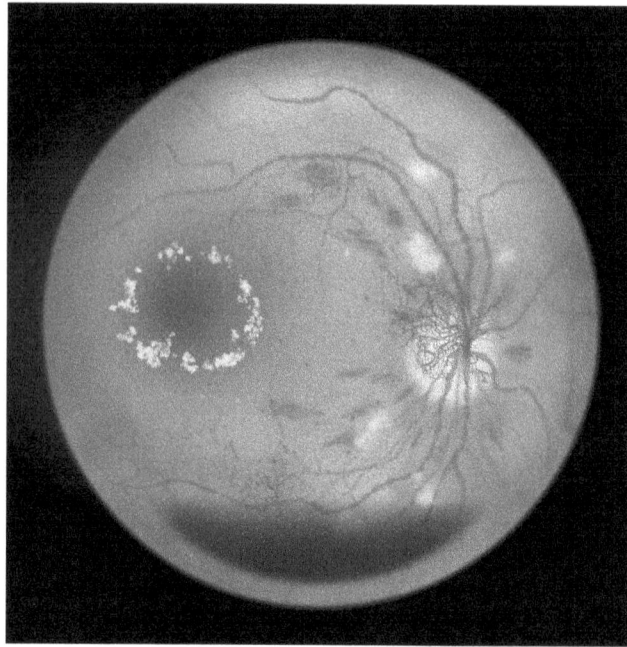

FIGURE 7.4 Retinal changes due to hypertension.

angiotensin II receptor blockers (ARBs), beta-blockers, calcium channel blockers, diuretics, and vasodilators. Control of BP can significantly reduce adverse consequences in both forms. Treatment targets are blood pressure lower than 120/80 mm Hg, regardless of age, up to 80. **Table 7.1** summarizes the categories of hypertension, showing target systolic and diastolic BP, according to the CDC and the American Heart Association (AHA). Generally, recommended lifestyle modifications include the following:

- Increased physical exercise
- Weight loss
- A diet rich in fruits, vegetables, whole grains, and low-fat dairy products with reduced saturated and total fat content
- Reduced dietary sodium
- Enhanced dietary potassium intake
- Moderate or no use of alcohol
- Smoking cessation

TABLE 7.1
Categories of Hypertension

Category	CDC Measurements	Category	AHA Measurements
Normal	Systolic: less than 120 mm Hg	Normal	Systolic: less than 120 mm Hg
	Diastolic: less than 80 mm Hg		Diastolic: less than 80 mm Hg
At risk (prehypertension)	Systolic: 120–139 mm Hg	Elevated	Systolic: 120–129 mm Hg
	Diastolic: 80–89 mm Hg		Diastolic: Less than 80 mm Hg
Hypertension	Systolic: 140 mm Hg or higher	Hypertension	Systolic: 130 mm Hg or higher
	Diastolic: 90 mm Hg or higher		Diastolic: 80 mm Hg or higher

PREVENTION

The only methods of preventing essential hypertension include weight loss, increased physical activity, moderation of alcohol intake, and a diet high in fruits, vegetables, and low-fat dairy products but lower in average sodium content.

YOU SHOULD REMEMBER

Low dietary calcium increases blood pressure, and supplemental calcium helps reduce blood pressure. Dietary calcium of 1,200–1,500 mg daily can reduce systolic and diastolic BP.

YOU SHOULD REMEMBER

Many people worldwide overuse table salt, and in some countries, such as the United States, individuals consume more than twice the recommended amount of salt daily. While most healthy adults should eat less than 2,300 mg of sodium daily, the average person consumes 2,900–4,300 mg daily. Other products used at the dinner table that contain high sodium levels include soy, fish, and sweet-and-sour sauces.

Check Your Knowledge

1. To which activated state is hypertension related?
2. How common is primary hypertension in comparison to secondary hypertension?
3. What is the diagnosis of primary hypertension based on?

SECONDARY HYPERTENSION

Secondary hypertension is caused by another medical condition, such as one that affects the kidneys, arteries, heart, or endocrine system. Secondary hypertension can also occur during pregnancy, along with thyroid problems and obstructive sleep apnea. Secondary hypertension differs from primary hypertension because the direct form has no definitive cause. Secondary hypertension is assessed using a blood pressure cuff, and multiple BP readings may be required.

EPIDEMIOLOGY

Secondary hypertension is present in approximately 10% of people diagnosed with hypertension and is common in younger individuals. It occurs in all groups, especially those with medical conditions that cause hypertension, such as kidney, artery, heart, or endocrine system problems.

ETIOLOGY AND RISK FACTORS

Common causes of secondary hypertension include primary aldosteronism, **parenchymal** diseases of the kidneys, renovascular disease, and sleep apnea. Renal parenchymal diseases include chronic **glomerulonephritis**, chronic **pyelonephritis**, and **polycystic renal disease** (see **Figure 7.3**). Other causes include Cushing syndrome**, pheochromocytoma**, hypothyroidism, hyperthyroidism, **acromegaly**, and **coarctation of the aorta**.

CLINICAL MANIFESTATIONS

The signs and symptoms of secondary hypertension are similar to those of primary hypertension. They include sweating, increased frequency or force of heartbeats, headaches, anxiety, weight gain or loss, weakness, abnormal growth of body hair, loss of menstrual periods, purple **striations** on the abdomen, fatigue or daytime sleepiness, intolerance to heat or cold, low potassium levels, snoring, and sleep apnea.

DIAGNOSIS

The diagnosis of secondary hypertension depends on the etiology and the risk factors. It is relatively rare. Not every patient with hypertension is tested for the secondary form. Factors that may require screening include patients under 30 years of age with no family history or other risk factors for hypertension, resistant hypertension (which does not improve despite optimal treatment with at least three BP medications), obesity, and indications of an underlying condition. Laboratory tests of blood or urine must be evaluated. Imaging such as a cross-sectional scan, computed tomography, and MRI are needed to diagnose secondary hypertension.

TREATMENT

Treatment of secondary hypertension is based on the underlying condition and includes a healthy, low-sodium diet, regular exercise, avoiding smoking, maintaining a healthy body weight, and limiting alcohol. If a tumor is found to be the cause of secondary hypertension, surgery may be required. For hormonal imbalances and other conditions, medications may be needed.

PREVENTION

The prevention of secondary hypertension requires a healthy lifestyle. A healthy diet is needed, with limited amounts of sodium and increased amounts of potassium. Foods should be lower in fat and include many fruits, vegetables, and whole grains. The *DASH eating plan* helps lower blood pressure. Regular exercise, including aerobic exercise, is essential. Maintaining a healthy weight helps control BP and reduces the risk of other health problems. Excessive use of alcohol raises blood pressure and adds extra calories, causing weight gain. Cigarette smoking should be avoided since it increases BP, heart attack, and stroke risks. Stress management is essential for improving emotional and physical health and lowering BP. Techniques include exercising, listening to music, meditating, and focusing on calm, peaceful thoughts.

YOU SHOULD REMEMBER

Blood pressure is linked to other medical issues. Lowering systolic BP may reduce health risks. It is essential not to ignore "white coat hypertension," which occurs in a medical office, because the patient may be at a much higher risk of developing sustained hypertension. It is essential to learn to cope with stress. Also, good sleep can prevent and manage hypertension. Additionally, excessive sodium (salt) raises BP.

Check Your Knowledge

1. What are the common causes of secondary hypertension?
2. What are the treatments for secondary hypertension?
3. Which dietary changes are advised for secondary hypertension?

ISOLATED SYSTOLIC HYPERTENSION

Isolated systolic hypertension occurs when the diastolic blood pressure is less than 80 mm of mercury (mm Hg) and the systolic blood pressure is 130 mm Hg or higher. It is the most common form of high blood pressure in people over 65.

EPIDEMIOLOGY

Isolated systolic hypertension is the predominant form of hypertension in older adults. It is estimated that 15% of people aged 60 and older have isolated systolic hypertension. About 30% of the same group have untreated isolated systolic hypertension, compared to 6% in adults aged 40–50 and 1.8% in adults between 18 and 39.

ETIOLOGY AND RISK FACTORS

Isolated systolic hypertension can be caused by atherosclerosis, hyperthyroidism, diabetes, obesity, and heart valve disease. High systolic blood pressure over time can increase the risk of strokes, heart disease, and chronic kidney disease. Risk factors include high cholesterol, diabetes, being inactive, being obese, using tobacco products, and eating foods that are processed or contain high levels of salt and fat.

CLINICAL MANIFESTATIONS

The symptoms of isolated systolic hypertension do not begin early on. Over time, without treatment, the condition harms the heart and causes chest pain, shortness of breath, headaches, and blurred vision.

DIAGNOSIS

Isolated systolic hypertension happens when the diastolic blood pressure is less than 80 mm Hg and the systolic blood pressure is 130 mm Hg or higher. The diagnosis begins with family history, dietary information, activity levels, and other medical conditions. The blood pressure will be checked at two or three different appointments. Other tests may include an electrocardiogram, a lipid panel, and other blood tests.

TREATMENT

The recommended goal for systolic pressure for adults younger than 65 with a 10% or higher risk of developing cardiovascular disease is less than 130 mm Hg. For healthy adults who are age 65 or older, the recommended treatment goal for systolic pressure is less than 130 mm Hg. Controlling isolated systolic hypertension to prevent health problems requires medication. However, the lower systolic blood pressure treatment mustn't cause the diastolic blood pressure to drop too low. That can cause other complications. In addition to medication, lifestyle changes can help improve the systolic blood pressure reading. Important changes include:

- Eating a healthy diet.
- Decreasing the amount of salt in the diet.
- Losing weight when indicated.
- Increasing moderate physical activity to at least 150 minutes a week.
- Drinking alcohol in moderation.

PREVENTION

The prevention of isolated systolic hypertension includes the management of diabetes and high cholesterol, exercising regularly, keeping BMI below 30, avoiding tobacco products, and avoiding processed foods or those containing high levels of salt and fat.

MALIGNANT HYPERTENSION

Malignant hypertension (MHT) occurs when a sudden rise in blood pressure occurs. It typically happens to people with hypertension. Other medical conditions, like a kidney injury or an endocrine disorder, can also cause it.

EPIDEMIOLOGY

The prevalence of MHT is relatively low in the general population, with an annual incidence rate of around 2 per 100,000 of the Caucasian population. Greater disease predisposition and worse prognosis are observed in the Afro-American population (7.3 new cases per 100,000 people/year).

ETIOLOGY AND RISK FACTORS

Uncontrolled hypertension is one of the leading causes of malignant hypertension. Other causes include adrenal disorders, **Conn's syndrome**, Cushing's syndrome, pheochromocytoma**,** a **renin-secreting tumor**, stroke, traumatic brain injury, medications, and substance and medication withdrawal.

CLINICAL MANIFESTATIONS

Signs and symptoms depend on which organs are affected. The patient may complain of headaches, pulmonary edema, chest pain, lower back pain, nausea and vomiting, dyspnea, blurred vision, delirium, and mood changes.

DIAGNOSIS

The clinical diagnosis of malignant hypertension is based on high blood pressure at or above 180/120 mm Hg and evidence of organ damage from a urinalysis, a chest X-ray, a fundoscopic eye exam, and blood tests. Other tests include a CT scan, an MRI, an EKG, and an echocardiogram.

TREATMENT

MHT requires emergency medical attention to limit organ damage and other severely high blood pressure complications. The first-line treatment is the administration of intravenous medications to lower blood pressure in a hospital setting. Antihypertensive drugs are administered via an intravenous (IV) line for quick onset of action.

IV beta-blockers (labetalol and esmolol) or calcium channel blockers (nicardipine and clevidipine) are administered to reduce systolic blood pressure levels by no more than 25% within 1 hour. They will aim to avoid low blood flow to the organs, which may worsen organ damage. If MHT is caused by a malignant tumor of the adrenal medulla, surgery is indicated.

PREVENTION

High blood pressure can often be prevented or reduced by eating healthily, maintaining a healthy weight, exercising regularly, drinking alcohol in moderation, and not smoking. Taking blood pressure medications and routine physical exams are essential for prevention.

RESISTANT HYPERTENSION

Resistant hypertension is defined as blood pressure that remains above normal despite concurrent use of three antihypertensive agents of different classes taken at maximally tolerated doses. One of these should be a diuretic selected based on kidney function. Resistant hypertension may be related to renal artery stenosis or sleep apnea.

EPIDEMIOLOGY

Resistant hypertension is the most common condition managed by primary care physicians. It accounts for 8.6% of all visits to a primary care physician. About 10% of hypertensive patients in Westernized countries have resistant hypertension. Primary care physicians can expect to encounter this condition in one of every 20 hypertensive patients.

ETIOLOGY AND RISK FACTORS

The etiology of resistant hypertension is uncertain. It is only related to secondary hypertension in a small minority of cases. The condition is probably multifactorial, linked to genetic factors, aberrant sympathetic nervous system activation, and altered renal sodium/water handling because of changes in the renin-angiotensin-aldosterone system. Risk factors for resistant hypertension include obesity, physical inactivity, foods high in salt, and heavy alcohol intake.

CLINICAL MANIFESTATIONS

The signs and symptoms may include headaches, dyspnea, chest pain, and epistaxis. In some cases, it may develop symptoms of heart failure, stroke, ischemic heart disease, and renal failure.

DIAGNOSIS

The diagnosis of resistant hypertension is based on ruling out non-adherence to BP medications, improper BP measurement, and the **white coat syndrome**.

TREATMENT

The treatment of resistant hypertension is based on underlying conditions and how well various medications are tolerated. Treatments include addressing causative needs, making lifestyle changes, and adjusting medications for the best type and dosage.

PREVENTION

The prevention of resistant hypertension is based on adequate medication treatments, sodium restriction, a diet similar to the Mediterranean diet, and physiologically individualized therapy based on renin-aldosterone phenotyping.

HYPERTENSION IN OLDER ADULTS

Hypertension is a significant health problem that is common in older adults. The vascular system changes with age. Arteries get stiffer, causing hypertension. This can be true even for people with heart-healthy habits who feel fine. Hypertension is a significant risk factor for cardiovascular events and mortality in older adults. Myocardial infarction, stroke, congestive heart failure, and peripheral arterial disease may be the consequences of hypertension in older adults. It is also a significant risk factor for sudden cardiac death, a dissecting aortic aneurysm, angina pectoris, left ventricular hypertrophy, thoracic and abdominal **aortic aneurysms**, chronic kidney disease, **atrial fibrillation**, diabetes mellitus, metabolic syndrome, vascular dementia, Alzheimer's disease, and ophthalmologic disease.

EPIDEMIOLOGY

About 60% of the population has hypertension by age 60. Approximately 65% of men and 75% of women develop hypertension by age 70. Hypertension is more common in older adults because the blood vessels of the vascular system become stiffer, which increases BP. This is true even for those with heart-healthy habits who feel fine.

ETIOLOGY AND RISK FACTORS

Hypertension increases in older people because the arteries lose flexibility, causing the heart to work harder to circulate oxygenated blood. This increases BP. Risk factors for hypertension in older adults include aging, genetics, being overweight or obese, not being physically active, consuming a high-sodium diet, and drinking too much alcohol.

CLINICAL MANIFESTATIONS

Hypertension characteristics in older adults include increasing systolic and **pulse pressure**, instability of BP, increased orthostatic and postprandial hypotension, increased "non-dipper-type nighttime BP," increased morning surge, increased white coat hypertension, the presence of auscultatory gaps (disappearance of Korotkoff sounds), and the presence of pseudohypertension.

DIAGNOSIS

The diagnosis of hypertension requires measurement of BP in the proper environment under optimum conditions. The patient must relax in a chair for at least 5 minutes with the arm resting. More than two readings of elevated BP on more than two occasions are needed to establish a diagnosis. White coat hypertension is more common among older patients, possibly related to increasing arterial stiffness; thus, ambulatory or out-of-office blood pressure readings are essential in the subgroup of patients with mildly elevated in-office BP readings. The 2017 ACC has set a blood pressure reading above 130/80 mm Hg to be considered hypertensive, while the European Society of Hypertension guidelines have maintained a blood pressure reading of ≥140/90 mm Hg to be considered hypertensive. Since high BP is primarily asymptomatic, structured community programs play an essential role in the diagnosis and have proven effective in diagnosing patients unaware they have hypertension.

TREATMENT

Antihypertensive therapy has been shown to reduce morbidity and mortality in older patients with elevated systolic or diastolic blood pressure. This benefit appears to persist in patients older than 80, but less than one-third of older patients have adequate blood pressure control. Systolic blood pressure is the most important predictor of cardiovascular disease. Blood pressure measurement in older persons should include an evaluation for orthostatic hypotension. Low-dose thiazide diuretics remain the first-line therapy for older patients. Beta-blockers, angiotensin-converting enzyme inhibitors, angiotensin-receptor blockers, and calcium channel blockers are second-line medications that should be selected based on comorbidities and risk factors.

PREVENTION

Preventive measures against hypertension in older adults include achieving a healthy weight, regular exercise, a heart-healthy diet, reducing sodium, drinking less alcohol, avoiding smoking, getting normal, healthy sleep, and managing stress.

HYPERTENSION DURING PREGNANCY

Hypertension during pregnancy can place extra stress on the heart and kidneys, leading to heart disease, kidney disease, and stroke. Hypertension also increases the risks of **preeclampsia**, preterm birth, **placental abruption**, and cesarean section.

EPIDEMIOLOGY

Hypertension during pregnancy is relatively standard. It affects one of every 12–17 pregnancies in women aged 20–44. Hypertension during pregnancy is more prevalent in African women.

ETIOLOGY AND RISK FACTORS

The most common causes of hypertension during pregnancy include obesity, diabetes mellitus, chronic hypertension before pregnancy, pre-existing medical conditions such as autoimmune diseases, maternal age of 35 or older, being pregnant for the first time, multiple gestations, and hypercholesteremia. Risk factors include a history of preeclampsia and kidney disease.

CLINICAL MANIFESTATIONS

Hypertension during pregnancy may be signified by protein in the urine, edema, weight gain, blurred or double vision, nausea, vomiting, and right-sided upper abdominal pain or pain around the stomach.

DIAGNOSIS

Gestational hypertension is defined as BP greater than or equal to 140 mm Hg (systolic) or 90 mm Hg (diastolic) on two separate occasions at least 4 hours apart after 20 weeks of pregnancy when the previous BP was normal. There is also an assessment for indications of poor cardiac function and impending heart failure.

TREATMENT

Intravenous labetalol and hydralazine have been first-line medications to manage acute-onset, severe hypertension in pregnant women. Oral nifedipine may also be considered a first-line therapy.

PREVENTION

Early and regular prenatal care is essential to prevent hypertension during pregnancy. Patients should discuss any medications taken and which are safe during pregnancy. It is necessary to keep track of BP at home with a blood pressure monitor. Patients should continue to choose healthy foods and maintain a healthy weight.

COMPLICATIONS OF HYPERTENSION

Excessive pressure on arterial walls from hypertension can damage blood vessels and organs. The higher the BP and the longer it is uncontrolled, the greater the damage. Complications include coronary artery disease, myocardial infarction, stroke, aneurysm, heart failure, kidney problems, eye problems, metabolic syndrome, changes in memory and cognition, and dementia.

CLINICAL CASE STUDY 1

A 46-year-old woman had a regular physical examination, during which her blood pressure was found to be highly elevated, at 170/98 mm Hg. She had no symptoms of hypertension, however. The patient acknowledged having a very stressful job but stated that she slept well at night and had no changes in mood, weight, or appetite. There was no history of cardiovascular disease in her family. The patient also stated that she has never drunk alcohol or smoked but has always drank two cups of coffee per day. She said that she tries to eat a healthy diet, but this is challenging with her job. She lacked sufficient exercise because she mostly sat at work or while driving. The patient was diagnosed with primary hypertension.

CRITICAL THINKING QUESTIONS

1. What are the early signs and symptoms of hypertension?
2. How may primary hypertension develop?
3. What are the generally recommended lifestyle modifications for hypertension?

CLINICAL CASE STUDY 2

A 27-year-old woman was hospitalized due to uncontrolled hypertension, a severe headache, and chest pain. The highest recorded BP for this patient was 200/120 mm Hg. The patient had no history of smoking or drinking and no family history of hypertension or cardiovascular disease. After a cross-sectional scan, computed tomography, MRI, and laboratory tests, she was diagnosed with pheochromocytoma. The epinephrine levels, norepinephrine, and metabolites in her urine and blood confirmed the diagnosis. The patient underwent surgery to remove the tumor from the left adrenal medulla, and then his BP remained successfully controlled.

CRITICAL THINKING QUESTIONS

1. What are the causes of malignant hypertension?
2. How is malignant hypertension diagnosed?
3. What are the treatments for malignant hypertension?

CLINICAL CASE STUDY 3

An 87-year-old man was assessed because of hypertension that had persisted for a few days. He regularly took his blood pressure at home as a precautionary measure. The man was overall in good health with no significant illnesses except for a chronic kidney disorder called renal artery stenosis. He regularly walked, exercised, and followed a strict Mediterranean diet plan. His sitting blood pressure was 160/94 mm Hg, and his pulse was 72 bpm. The patient was given an ACE inhibitor and metoprolol and then scheduled for regular checkups.

1. What does the pathophysiology of hypertension involve?
2. What are the common causes of secondary hypertension?
3. What does the prevention of secondary hypertension require?

FURTHER READING

1. Bakris, G.L., and Sorrentino, M.J. (2017). *Hypertension: A Companion to Braunwald's Heart Disease,* 3rd Edition. Elsevier.
2. Covic, A., Kanbay, M., and Lerma, E.V. (2017). *Resistant Hypertension in Chronic Kidney Disease.* Springer.
3. Earlstein, F. (2017). *Hypertension or High Blood Pressure Explained: The Ultimate Information Guide for Hypertension.* Pack & Post Plus, LLC.
4. Heazell, A., Norwitz, E.R., Knney, L.C., and Baker, P.N. (2010). *Hypertension in Pregnancy (Clinical Guides).* Cambridge University Press.
5. Jagdal, D. (2017). *Prevalence and Some Risk Factors of Isolated Systolic Hypertension.* Lap Lambert Academic Publishing.
6. Kaplan, N.M., and Victor, R.G. (2023). *Kaplan's Clinical Hypertension,* 11th Edition. Wolters Kluwer.
7. Leonetti, G., and Cuspidi, C. (2013). *Hypertension in the Elderly (Developments in Cardiovascular Medicine Book 157).* Springer.
8. Lerma, E., Berns, J.S., and Nissenson, A.R. (2012). *Current Essentials of Diagnosis and Treatment in Nephrology & Hypertension.* McGraw-Hill/Lange.
9. Malvasi, A., Tinelli, A., and Carlo Di Renzo, G. (2016). *Management and Therapy of Early Pregnancy Complications: First and Second Trimesters.* Springer.
10. Miller-Jones, E.R. (2012). *Complications of Hypertension: The Facts!* Facebook Publishing.
11. Morganti, A., Agabiti Rosei, E., and Mantero, F. (2020). *Secondary Hypertension: Updates in Hypertension and Cardiovascular Protection.* Springer.
12. Moulton, S.A. (2016). *Managing Hypertension: Tools to Improve Health and Prevent Complications (Health Topics).* McFarland.
13. Safar, M., and O'Rourke, M.F. (2010). *Arterial Stiffness in Hypertension: Handbook of Hypertension Series,* Volume 23. Elsevier.
14. Salvetti, M. (2016). *Resistant Hypertension: Practical Case Studies in Hypertension Management.* Springer.
15. Schwartz, G.D. (2023). *Mayo Clinic on High Blood Pressure: Your Guide to Managing Hypertension.* Mayo Clinic Press.
16. Weir, M.R., and Lerma, E.V. (2015). *Chronic Kidney Disease and Hypertension: Clinical Hypertension and Vascular Diseases.* Humana Press.
17. Zapata Gonzalez, Y., Collazo Nunez, D., and Messana Fulgueria, L. (2021). *Hypertension and Hemorrhage, Causes of Death in Pregnancy: Bleeding and Hypertension Complications During Pregnancy and Childbirth.* Our Knowledge Publishing.

8 Coronary Artery Disease

OVERVIEW

Coronary artery disease (CAD) is caused by plaque buildup in the walls of the arteries that supply blood to the heart. It occurs when coronary arteries supply the heart with enough blood, oxygen, and nutrients. Consuming a diet high in saturated fats, trans fats, and cholesterol has been linked to heart disease and atherosclerosis. Also, too much table salt in the diet can raise blood pressure. CAD is the most common type of heart disease, killing 375,476 people in 2021. About 1 in 20 adults age 20 and older have CAD. In 2021, about 2 in 10 deaths from CAD occurred in adults younger than 65 years old. Being overweight, smoking tobacco, being physically inactivity, and unhealthy eating are risk factors for CAD. A family history of heart disease also increases your risk for CAD, especially a family history of having heart disease at an early age (50 or younger). If a coronary artery becomes completely blocked, it can result in a heart attack. CAD can also lead to other health problems, like heart failure or dysrhythmia. Various treatments can reduce the symptoms and the risk of complications. Accurate, early diagnosis and treatment are imperative because of the extreme complications, socioeconomic factors, and deaths related to the disease.

STRUCTURE OF THE CORONARY ARTERIES

Coronary arteries supply blood to the **myocardium**. Like all other tissues in the body, the heart muscle needs oxygen-rich blood to function. Also, oxygen-depleted blood must be carried away. The coronary arteries wrap around the outside of the heart (see **Figure 8.1**). Small branches divide into the heart muscle to bring it blood. The right and left coronary arteries arise from the coronary sinuses in the root of the aorta, above the aortic valve orifice. The left main coronary artery supplies blood to the left ventricle and left atrium. The left anterior descending artery branches off the left coronary artery and supplies blood to the front of the left side of the heart. The circumflex artery branches off the left coronary artery and encircles the heart muscle. This artery supplies blood to

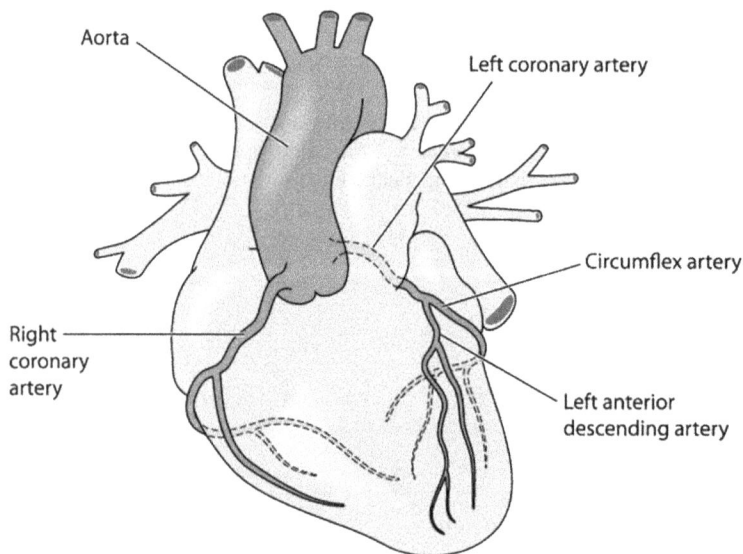

FIGURE 8.1 Structure of the coronary arteries.

DOI: 10.1201/9781003453376-11

the outer side and back of the heart. This artery supplies the anterior septum, which includes the proximal conduction system. It also provides the anterior free wall of the left ventricle (LV).

The circumflex artery is smaller than the LAD artery. It supplies the free wall of the lateral LV. The majority of people have the *right dominance* of the coronary arteries. The right coronary artery divides into smaller branches, including the right posterior and descending arteries. The left anterior descending artery and the right coronary artery help supply blood to the middle or septum of the heart. The right coronary artery continues along the atrioventricular (AV) groove and the right side of the heart. It supplies the right atrium, right ventricle, and often, the inferior myocardial wall.

CORONARY MICROVASCULAR DYSFUNCTION

Coronary microvascular dysfunction (CMD), also known as **microvascular angina** or *angina with no obstructive coronary artery disease,* is the constriction of coronary arteries that causes angina, even though the epicardial coronary arteries appear normal during angiography. Coronary microvascular dysfunction was previously called **syndrome X**. Patients experience typical angina relieved by rest or nitroglycerin, and coronary arteriograms show no atherosclerosis, embolism, or inducible arterial spasms. Some patients have ischemia that is found during stress testing.

The cause of the ischemia may be reflex intramyocardial coronary constriction plus reduced coronary flow reserve. Other patients have (CMD) which occurs within the myocardium. The abnormal vessels cannot dilate due to exercise or other cardiovascular stressors. There may also be increased sensitivity to cardiac pain. The outlook is better than for patients with proven coronary artery disease, but symptoms of ischemia can recur for years. Treatment focuses on controlling risk factors with lipid-lowering drugs and glycemic control. Many patients benefit from traditional anti-ischemic therapies such as beta-blockers and calcium channel blockers.

ANGINA PECTORIS AND ITS CLASSIFICATIONS

Angina pectoris results when oxygen supply and, occasionally, other nutrients are inadequate for the metabolic needs of the myocardium. It is a syndrome of precordial discomfort or pressure. It occurs because of transient myocardial ischemia without an infarction. Angina pectoris is usually brought on by exertion or psychologic stress and relieved by rest or sublingual nitroglycerin. It has several classifications, which include stable, unstable, and variant angina. Stable angina usually occurs with activity or emotional stress. Unstable angina often occurs while resting.

YOU SHOULD REMEMBER

Variant angina differs from stable angina in that it commonly occurs in individuals at rest or even asleep, whereas stable angina is generally triggered by exertion or intense exercise.

Check Your Knowledge

1. What are the coronary sinuses?
2. What is coronary microvascular dysfunction?
3. What is the classification of angina?

STABLE ANGINA

Stable angina pectoris is chest pain when the myocardium needs more oxygen than usual. Still, it is not getting oxygen at that moment because of heart disease. This can occur when it is cold outside or during exercise. In most cases, stable angina pectoris follows psychologic stress or physical exertion. It is often relieved by rest or by the use of nitroglycerin, administered sublingually. Angina is a common condition, especially in people over the age of 55. Type 2 diabetes is an additional and significant risk factor for angina pectoris.

Epidemiology

The prevalence of stable angina is challenging to determine since it is diagnosed based on patient history using clinical assessment. It is known to increase in prevalence with age for both men and women. In older adults between ages 65 and 84, stable angina affects 10%–12% of women yet is more prevalent in men, affecting 12%–14%. In the United States, almost 10 million people are diagnosed with stable angina yearly. There are slight variances in the percentage of people of various racial or ethnic groups affected by angina, as follows–this is also shown in **Figure 8.2**:

- *Non-Hispanic black women* – 6.7%
- *Hispanic women* – 4.5%
- *Non-Hispanic black men* – 4.4%
- *Non-Hispanic white women* – 4.1%
- *Non-Hispanic white men* – 4.1%
- *Hispanic men* – 3.5%

Etiology and Risk Factors

Stable angina pectoris is caused by a cardiac workload that requires more myocardial oxygen than the coronary arteries can supply via the oxygenated blood in the body. This occurs when the streets have narrowed, usually from coronary artery atherosclerosis and coronary artery spasms. Stable angina is less severe than unstable angina, but it can be painful or uncomfortable. Myocardial oxygen demand is determined by heart rate, systolic wall tension, and contractility. Therefore, the narrowing of a coronary artery usually causes angina during exertion. It is relieved by rest. Aortic stenosis, hypertension, aortic regurgitation, and hypertrophic cardiomyopathy can also increase the cardiac workload. If these are present, angina may occur with or without atherosclerosis. Angina can be precipitated or aggravated by a decreased oxygen supply due to severe hypoxia or anemia. Risk factors for stable angina include diabetes mellitus, being overweight or obese, a history of heart disease, high LDL, low HDL, hypertension, smoking, advancing age, male sex, and insufficient exercise. Cold weather, emotional stress, and large meals are also risk factors.

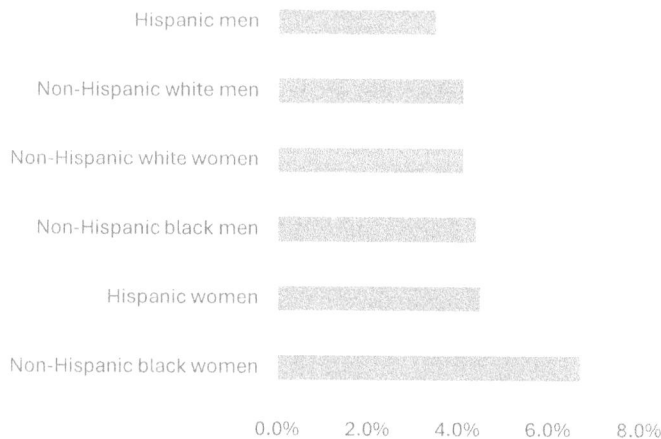

FIGURE 8.2 Percentages of various individuals with angina in the United States.

Clinical Manifestations

For some patients, angina pectoris is only a slight aching sensation. It can quickly become severe and intense, usually described as a crushing sensation but not usually described as pain. Chest pain from angina can radiate to the shoulders, arms, neck, or jaw (see **Figure 8.3**). Symptoms of **atypical angina** can be seen in some patients, particularly women and patients with diabetes. Angina symptoms can sometimes include shortness of breath, nausea, or upper abdominal pain. The patient often believes that indigestion is the cause. Ischemic symptoms usually require a minute or longer to resolve, so very brief sensations are generally not from angina. Pain from stable angina lasts an average of 1–15 minutes.

Nocturnal angina can occur if a dream or nightmare triggers significant changes in BP, pulse rate, and respiration. When lying down, venous return is increased, which stretches the myocardium and increases arterial wall stress. Oxygen demand is therefore increased. *Silent ischemia* may occur with CAD, especially in patients with diabetes mellitus. It may appear as a transient and asymptomatic ST-T heart abnormality. In radionuclide studies, there can be proof of asymptomatic myocardial ischemia during mental or physical stress. Silent ischemia and angina pectoris can exist together and occur at different times.

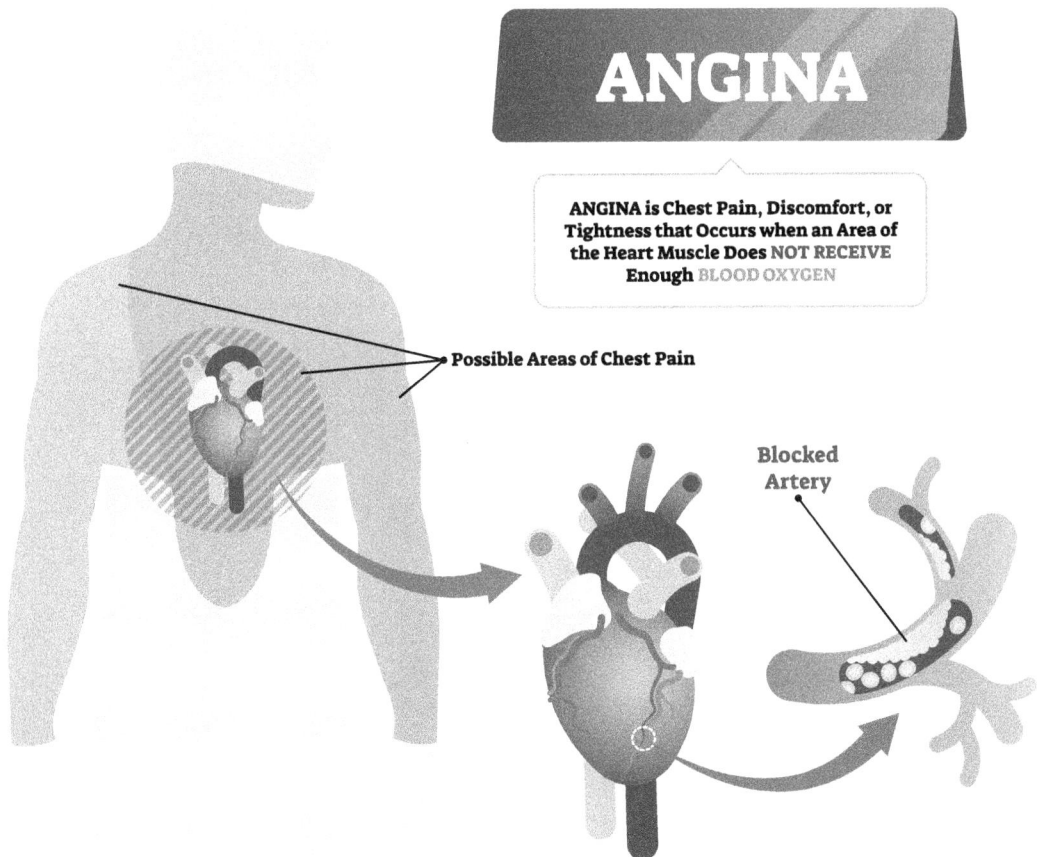

ANGINA

ANGINA is Chest Pain, Discomfort, or Tightness that Occurs when an Area of the Heart Muscle Does NOT RECEIVE Enough BLOOD OXYGEN

Possible Areas of Chest Pain

Blocked Artery

FIGURE 8.3   The radiation of chest pain from angina.

Diagnosis

A stable angina diagnosis is likely when a patient has chest discomfort caused by exertion and is relieved by rest. It is more accurate when significant risk factors for CAD are present. It is essential to understand that anxiety, panic attacks, costochondritis, G.I. disorders, and hyperventilation can also cause chest discomfort. A blood cholesterol profile is done. ECG is performed, and stress testing with ECG or myocardial imaging and coronary angiography may be ordered in some cases. Myocardial imaging methods include echocardiography, MRI, and radionuclide imaging.

Stress testing confirms the diagnosis and determines the extent of the disease. It helps identify exercise levels that the patient should tolerate and predicts the prognosis. Stress ECG testing is 70% specific and 90% sensitive for men with suspicious chest discomfort. In women, the specificity is lower, while the sensitivity is similar. This is especially true for women under 55, whose percentage is below 70%. Women with CAD are more likely than men to have an abnormal resting ECG. Coronary angiography is preferred to diagnose CAD but is not required to confirm the diagnosis in every case.

Cardiac MRI is an excellent method to evaluate a large number of abnormalities. It can determine CAD in several ways. There can be an assessment of blood flow in the coronary arteries, direct views of coronary stenosis, an examination of myocardial metabolism and perfusion, an evaluation of a myocardium that is either viable or infarcted, and an assessment of wall motion abnormalities. A cardiac MRI is indicated to evaluate cardiac structure and function and to assess myocardial viability. To diagnose and assess risks for patients with suspected or known CAD, specific forms of cardiac MRI include stress perfusion MRI and quantitative analysis of myocardial blood flow. A 24-hour **Holter monitoring device** is also helpful (see **Figure 8.4**).

Treatment

Sublingual nitroglycerin is the most effective drug for relieving symptoms during an acute angina attack. It is a solid smooth-muscle relaxant and also a vasodilator. Sublingual nitroglycerin can also be taken before exertion to prevent an attack. Effective relief occurs in 1.5–3 minutes in most cases,

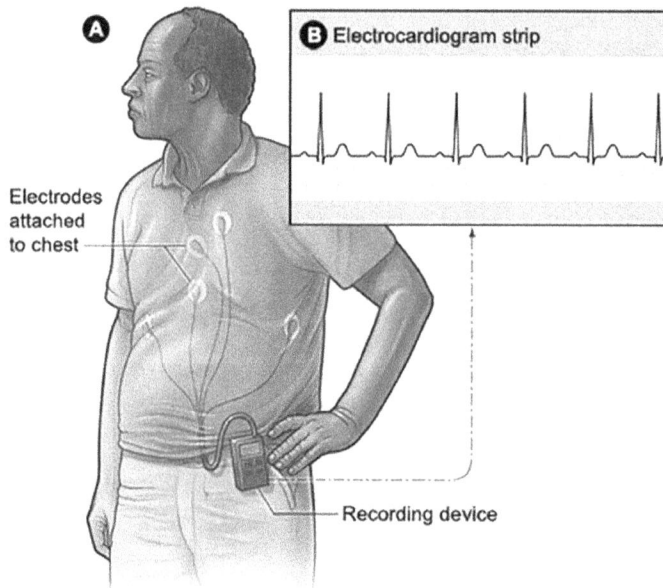

FIGURE 8.4   A Holter monitoring device showing (a) its components and (b) an electrocardiogram strip.

entirely in 5 minutes, lasting as long as 30 minutes. Doses can be repeated every 4–5 minutes, up to three times, if the effects are incomplete. The patient must always carry nitroglycerin, regardless of its dosage form, for prompt use when needed. If tablets are used, they must be stored in a light-resistant glass container that is tightly sealed to retain their potency. The drug deteriorates very quickly, so small amounts should be frequently purchased.

Antiplatelet drugs, beta-blockers, long-acting nitrates, and calcium channel blockers prevent ischemia. Antiplatelet drugs inhibit the aggregation of platelets. Aspirin binds to the platelets irreversibly, inhibiting platelet aggregation and cyclooxygenase. Other antiplatelet drugs include clopidogrel, prasugrel, and ticagrelor. These block platelet aggregations are induced by adenosine diphosphate. They can reduce the risk of MI or sudden death and are most effective when administered together. Patients who cannot tolerate one should receive one of the drugs that can be taken.

Calcium channel blockers are used for persistent symptoms after nitrates are used or if they cannot be tolerated. These blockers are best used if there is concurrent coronary spasm or hypertension. Dihydropyridines, including amlodipine, felodipine, and nifedipine, do not have chronotropic effects but have widely different adverse inotropic effects. The shorter-acting dihydropyridines can cause reflex tachycardia. They are linked to more deaths in patients with CAD and are not used alone to treat stable angina.

Sodium channel blockers and sinus node inhibitors can also stabilize angina. Ranolazine is a sodium channel blocker that treats chronic angina. Common adverse effects include constipation, dizziness, headaches, and nausea. Ivabradine, a sinus node inhibitor, inhibits the inward sodium/potassium current in the gated channel in sinus node cells. It slows down the heart rate without causing decreased contractility. Ivabradine is used for chronic stable angina pectoris when there is a normal sinus rhythm and the patient cannot tolerate beta-blockers. It is combined with beta-blockers when the patient's symptoms are not adequately controlled only by a beta-blocker, and the heart rate is more than 60 beats per minute.

Revascularization can be done if angina continues even with drug therapy and poor quality of life or if anatomic lesions found during angiography may cause death. This is done with percutaneous coronary intervention (PCI) such as angioplasty, stent placement, or coronary artery bypass graft (CABG). The choice is based on where the anatomic lesions are located, their severity, the surgical team's experience, and patient preference. The PCI procedure is often used for cases involving one or two vessels. It is also becoming more popular for three-vessel disease. However, long lesions, or those close to bifurcation points, are often not highly treatable with PCI. The process is being used for more complex cases today due to improvements in stent technology. It is usually used for unprotected left central coronary stenosis with no left anterior descending or circumflex graft.

For certain patients, CABG is highly effective. It is better than PCI for diabetic patients and those with multiple diseased vessels that will likely be responsive to grafting. Ideally, CABG is used for severe angina pectoris that is localized or for those with diabetes. Approximately 85% of patients have significant or total symptom relief. There is a positive relationship between graft patency and better exercise tolerance, as shown by exercise stress testing. However, exercise tolerance can remain better even with graft closure. Survival is improved with CABG for patients with the left central disease, a 3-vessel disease with poor LV function, and some patients with the 2-vessel disease.

Prevention

The best methods of preventing angina include a heart-healthy diet, avoiding smoking, limiting alcohol use, exercising regularly, maintaining a healthy weight, and keeping diabetes mellitus controlled.

YOU SHOULD REMEMBER

A coronary calcium scan is a unique CT scan of the heart. It looks for calcium deposits in the heart arteries. Calcium buildup can narrow the arteries and reduce blood flow to the heart. A coronary calcium scan may show coronary artery disease before patients have symptoms. Coronary calcium scan results can help determine the risk of heart attacks or strokes. Results from the scan may be used to plan or change treatment for coronary artery disease.

YOU SHOULD REMEMBER

There are "four E's" of stable angina. They include exercise, eating large meals, emotional stress, and exposure to cold temperatures. All of these increase the heart's workload. Stable angina is the most common type and has a regular, predictable pattern of pain and discomfort.

Check Your Knowledge

1. What is the cause of stable angina?
2. How does stress testing help confirm stable angina?
3. How does sublingual nitroglycerin work in the treatment of stable angina?

Unstable Angina

Unstable angina involves potentially dangerous and unpredictable changes, such as new-onset, resting, or increasing angina. These are serious if the chest discomfort is severe. It occurs from an acute coronary artery obstruction with no myocardial infarction. Rest angina usually lasts over 20 minutes; new-onset angina is at least class 3 in severity. Increasing angina is a previously diagnosed disease but has become more frequent, severe, of longer duration, or lower threshold.

An example is when a class 1 disease increases in severity to at least class 3. Therefore, unstable angina requires prompt diagnosis and treatment. Diabetic patients with unstable angina usually have more severe disease and poorer outcomes than nondiabetic patients.

Epidemiology

The most accurate global data on unstable angina is based on the Organization to Assess Strategies for Ischemic Syndromes Registry (OASIS-2). Aside from the United States, this registry contains data for Australia, Canada, Brazil, Poland, and Hungary. The mean age at diagnosis is between 62 and 65 years, with men diagnosed more than women in a ratio of slightly more than 1.5: 1. One exciting factor is that women diagnosed with unstable angina are approximately 5 years older than men when they are diagnosed. There is no specific racial or ethnic preference, except that black patients are often considered younger than other groups.

According to the American College of Cardiology and American Heart Association registry, every year in the United States, hospitalized patients have almost 1 million primary diagnoses of unstable angina. There may be as many cases that occur outside of hospitals that are unrecognized or managed on an outpatient basis. The average age of diagnosed patients is between 62 and 69, though 44% are 65 or older. Men are affected more than women, in a ratio of 1.5: 1. Most patients with unstable angina (60%–73%) are hypertensive, and hypercholesterolemia is present in 43%–50%. Unstable angina affects 66% of patients who previously had angina of any form. There are no specific racial or ethnic differences.

Etiology and Risk Factors

Unstable angina is caused by blood clots that block an artery wholly or partially. They can form, partially dissolve, and reform, with unstable angina occurring each time. The condition is related to coronary heart disease from the buildup of atherosclerotic plaques along arterial walls. Risk factors for unstable angina include diabetes mellitus, obesity, family history of heart disease, hypertension, high LDL, low HDL, male gender, tobacco use, and a sedentary lifestyle. Men are at the highest risk after age 45, and women are at the highest risk after age 55.

Clinical Manifestations

Chest pain or discomfort are the most common symptoms of unstable angina. However, these are usually more intense, longer in duration, precipitated by little exertion, or occur while resting. Unstable angina is classified by severity and the clinical situation as follows:

- *Class 1 severity*–the new onset of severe angina or increasing angina, but no angina at rest.
- *Class 2 severity*–there is angina at rest over the previous month but not within the preceding 48 hours; this is designated as subacute angina at rest.
- *Class 3 severity*–there is angina at rest over the preceding 48 hours; this is designated as acute angina at rest; the troponin status as negative or positive is evaluated, which affects the prognosis.
- *Clinical situation A*–the condition develops secondary to an extracardiac condition that worsens the myocardial ischemia, designated as secondary unstable angina.
- *Clinical situation B*–the condition develops without a contributing extracardiac need being present; the troponin status as negative or positive is evaluated, which affects prognosis; designated as primary unstable angina.
- *Clinical situation C*–the condition develops within 2 weeks of an acute MI, designated as post-myocardial infarction unstable angina.

The primary classification of the unstable angina level consists of a Roman numeral to assess the severity and a letter to assess the clinical situation; for example, the least severe would be class IA. There is a consideration of whether unstable angina occurs during treatment for chronic stable angina and if transient changes in the ST-T waves occur during the angina attack. If the discomfort has happened within 48 hours and no contributing extracardiac condition is present, the troponin levels may be measured to estimate the prognosis. Troponin-negative gives a better forecast than troponin-positive.

Diagnosis

For unstable angina, early stress testing cannot be performed. Diagnosis begins with an initial and serial ECG, plus serial measurements of **cardiac biomarkers**. This helps determine whether unstable angina is present or an acute MI is imminent. Non-ST-segment elevation MI (NSTEMI) or ST-segment elevation MI (STEMI) can be used for this determination. It is essential since fibrinolytics are helpful for patients with STEMI but can increase risks for patients with NSTEMI and unstable angina. For acute STEMI, urgent cardiac catheterization is required, but not usually for patients with NSTEMI or unstable angina. An ECG must be done within 10 minutes of the patient arriving at the chosen medical facility. During unstable angina, transient ECG changes may include ST-segment depression, elevation, or T-wave inversion. When unstable angina is suspected, a high-sensitivity assay of **cardiac troponin** must be done immediately and 3 hours later. When a standard troponin assay is used, it is performed at zero and 6 hours. The **creatinine kinase** will not be elevated. However, cardiac troponin may slightly increase, especially in the high-sensitivity troponin test. **Coronary cineangiography** can reveal coronary artery obstructions.

Treatment

Treatment of unstable angina begins with establishing an excellent intravenous route. Oxygen is usually given in 2 L via nasal cannula. Single-lead ECG monitoring is initiated. Before hospitalization, emergency medical personnel can lessen the risks of complications and death by monitoring the ECG, using nitrates to manage pain, and giving 325 mg of chewable aspirin. Once the diagnosis is confirmed within the emergency department, drug therapy and the scheduling of revascularization are confirmed. Urgent angiography with revascularization must occur if the patient is clinically unstable due to continuing symptoms, arrhythmias, or hypotensive. Morphine must be used carefully, such as when nitroglycerin is contraindicated, or the patient still has symptoms after nitroglycerin has been administered. Unstable angina can be complicated by recurring attacks, infarction, heart failure, or sustained and recurring ventricular arrhythmias.

Coronary artery bypass grafting is preferred over percutaneous coronary intervention (PCI) if the patient has *left central* or *left primary equivalent* angina, left ventricular dysfunction, or diabetes mellitus that is being treated. Lesions long or close to bifurcation points are often not successfully treated with PCI. All unstable angina patients are given anticoagulants, antiplatelet drugs, and antianginal drugs when chest pain is present. The drug regimen is based on a reperfusion strategy. Unless contraindicated, the medications for unstable angina include unfractionated or low-molecular-weight heparin (LMWH), aspirin, clopidogrel, or both, with alternatives to clopidogrel being prasugrel or ticagrelor, nitroglycerin or another antianginal drug; beta-blockers; ACE inhibitors; statins; and if PCI is done, a glycoprotein may be required. Aspirin is not of the enteric-coated type. Chewing the first dose before swallowing will speed up absorption and reduce short- and long-term risks of death.

Unless contraindicated, such as by active bleeding, low-molecular-weight heparin LMWH, unfractionated heparin, or bivalirudin are usually given. The LMWHs have lower risks for heparin-induced **thrombocytopenia**, better bioavailability, and are delivered via simple weight-based doses. Bivalirudin is preferred for patients with known or suspected occurrences of heparin-induced thrombocytopenia.

Nitroglycerin is usually used for chest pain, but sometimes morphine is needed. Nitroglycerin is preferred, but morphine is used if the patient is contraindicated to nitroglycerin, or maximal nitroglycerin therapy does not relieve pain. At first, nitroglycerin is given sublingually, which may be followed by a continuous IV drip if required. Morphine is given IV every 15 minutes as needed. Still, close monitoring is necessary due to the drug depressing respiration, being a solid venous vasodilator, and reducing myocardial contractility. Beta-blockers, ACE inhibitors, and statins are typically used as well. Beta-blockers are recommended, especially for high-risk patients, except if contraindicated because of asthma, **bradycardi**a, heart block, or hypotension. They reduce arterial pressure, contractility, and heart rate. This results in decreased oxygen demand and cardiac workload.

For patients who do not have angiography performed, options are based on whether there are high-risk features. These include recurring angina, heart failure, **ventricular fibrillation** or tachycardia after 24 hours, shock, or **murmurs**.

Prevention

Methods of preventing unstable angina include quitting smoking, avoiding secondhand smoke, exercising regularly, eating a heart-healthy diet to maintain a healthy weight, managing underlying conditions (diabetes mellitus, hypertension, and high cholesterol), and managing stress or depression.

YOU SHOULD REMEMBER

Unstable angina occurs with much less exertion than usual or when an individual undergoes no labor. With this type of angina, chest pain or pressure can lead to myocardial infarction. Physicians assess it with blood tests and electrocardiograms. Elevated cardiac troponin levels are expected in patients considered to have unstable angina.

Check Your Knowledge

1. In which age groups is unstable angina most common?
2. What are the three classes of unstable angina?
3. What is used to determine if an acute MI is imminent with unstable angina?

VARIANT ANGINA

Variant angina is also known as *Prinzmetal angina* and *angina inversa*. The condition is second-ary to epicardial coronary artery spasm, signified by angina symptoms occurring at rest but rarely after exertion. Many patients also have a significant obstruction of one or more major coronary arteries. If there is only mild obstruction or no *fixed obstruction*, the long-term outcome is better than when there are significant fixed obstructions. Having diabetes mellitus and variant angina affects the use of certain medications, such as bisoprolol, if there are large fluctuations in blood glucose levels. This is because the drug can mask the symptoms of hypoglycemia.

Epidemiology

Variant angina is rare, affecting between 2% and 10% of all angina patients. It usually occurs in younger-aged patients than the other forms of angina, mostly between ages 51 and 57. The condi-tion is not very well documented globally. About four out of every 100,000 Americans have variant angina in the United States. Men are slightly more affected than women. The disease is more com-mon in people of Japanese origin than in any other racial or ethnic group.

Etiology and Risk Factors

Variant angina is usually caused by smoking, hypertension, and high cholesterol. However, it can occur for unknown reasons in otherwise healthy people. While diabetes mellitus is not a direct cause of variant angina, it complicates cardiovascular disease, possibly resulting in variant angina. Risk factors include alcohol withdrawal, exposure to cold temperatures, various medications, stimu-lants such as cocaine, and stress.

Clinical Manifestations

Variant angina involves discomfort occurring mostly while resting, usually at night. The pain rarely occurs during exertion and is inconsistent unless there is a significant coronary artery obstruction. Variant angina often occurs regularly at specific times during each day. The pain can be extreme, lasting from several minutes to one-half hour. The pain can spread to the left arm, shoulder, neck, or head. Persistent spasms increase the risk of severe complications, including life-threatening arrhythmias or MI. Additional manifestations include chest tightness or pressure, heartburn, dizzi-ness, nausea, palpitations, and sweating.

Diagnosis

The diagnosis of variant angina is suspected because of an ST-segment elevation occurring during an attack. The ECG may have a stable yet abnormal pattern between episodes or even be expected. The diagnosis is confirmed by testing with ergonovine or acetylcholine. This may initiate a coro-nary artery spasm, identified by a significant ST-segment elevation on the ECG, or when a reversible spasm is seen during cardiac catheterization. Most diagnostic testing for variant angina is done in cardiac catheterization laboratories.

Treatment

Sublingual nitroglycerin is usually able to relieve variant angina quickly. Symptoms can be pre-vented by using calcium channel blockers. The most commonly used drugs in this class include sustained-release diltiazem, sustained-release verapamil (though doses must be reduced if there is kidney or liver dysfunction), and amlodipine (though amounts must be decreased with liver dysfunction or in elderly patients). These drugs do not appear to change the prognosis, however. Though not proven clinically, it is theorized that beta-blockers can worsen spasms by allowing alpha-adrenergic vasoconstriction to occur. For diabetic patients, bisoprolol must be used carefully since it can mask the symptoms of hypoglycemia. However, this is not an issue in nondiabetic patients with variant angina.

Prevention

The prevention of variant angina is based on lifestyle changes to remove the known causes and risk factors or to use medications to stop future attacks from occurring. It is essential to quit smoking, manage stress, exercise regularly but not to the point of causing hyperventilation, eat a heart-healthy diet, avoid frigid temperatures, engage in relaxation therapies, and monitor your body's circadian rhythms to prepare for the times of day in which the condition may occur regularly.

YOU SHOULD REMEMBER

Variant angina generally has an average survival of 5 years of 89%–97%. Mortality risks are more significant for patients with both variant angina and atherosclerotic coronary artery obstruction. Risks increase with more obstacles present. Usually, sublingual nitroglycerin can relieve variant angina quickly.

Check Your Knowledge

1. What are the primary causes of variant angina?
2. When is a diagnosis of variant angina suspected?
3. What are the most commonly used drugs for variant angina?

ACUTE CORONARY SYNDROMES

Acute coronary syndromes are outcomes of acute coronary artery obstruction. Severity is based on the location of the block and its degree. Uncontrolled angina and various types of MI, or sudden cardiac death, can occur. Diabetes mellitus is a significant risk factor. All acute coronary syndromes involve acute coronary ischemia: their symptoms, ECG results, and cardiac biomarkers. The uncontrolled angina subtype affects acute coronary insufficiency and pre-infarction angina, an *intermediate syndrome*. The cardiac biomarkers do not meet the criteria for MI. There is resting angina longer than 20 minutes, new-onset angina of at least class 3 severity, and increasing angina that becomes more regular, severe, and longer-lasting or rises quickly from class 1 to class 3 or higher. There may be ST-segment depression, T-wave inversion, or both.

Epidemiology

The global prevalence of acute coronary syndromes is as high as 13.5% of the population. The estimated incidence is 2,149 cases per 1 million population annually. Acute coronary syndromes represent about 1.8 million deaths per year. The ages at which acute coronary syndromes are most likely are over 30 (in men), over 40 (in women), and younger generations (in diabetic patients). Acute coronary syndromes occur much more often in men under age 60 than in women in the same age range, but most diagnosed patients over 75 are women. There are no significant differences in the preference for acute coronary syndromes between various racial or ethnic groups.

ETIOLOGY AND RISK FACTORS

An acute thrombus usually causes acute coronary syndrome in an atherosclerotic coronary artery. The plaque can become unstable or inflamed, then rupture or split. Thrombogenic material is exposed, activating platelets and the **coagulation cascade**, resulting in an acute thrombus. Cross-linking and aggregation of platelets occur. Even with a slight obstruction, atheromas can rupture and cause thrombosis. In more than half of all cases, pre-syndrome stenosis is less than 40%. While stenosis severity predicts the symptoms that will occur, it cannot always be predictive of acute thrombotic events. The thrombus quickly slows blood flow to areas of the myocardium. In most cases, spontaneous thrombolysis occurs. However, the obstruction does remain for long enough to cause tissue necrosis.

Rare causes of acute coronary syndromes include coronary artery **embolism** or dissection and coronary spasm. Embolism may be due to aortic, mitral valve stenosis, infective endocarditis, **atrial fibrillation**, or **marantic endocarditis**. Coronary artery dissection may occur in atherosclerotic or non-atherosclerotic coronary arteries. The non-atherosclerotic form is most common in women who are pregnant or have given birth, as well as in patients with connective tissue disorders such as fibromuscular dysplasia. Diabetic patients with acute coronary syndromes have increased mortality rates compared to nondiabetic patients. Diabetes mellitus is linked to a proinflammatory and prothrombotic state that can lead to plaque rupture. Risk factors for acute coronary syndromes, aside from diabetes, include increased age, hypercholesterolemia, hypertension, smoking, insufficient physical activity, an unhealthy diet, being overweight or obese, family history (of angina, heart disease, or stroke); personal history of hypertension, preeclampsia, or gestational diabetes, and the COVID-19 infection.

CLINICAL MANIFESTATIONS

Acute coronary syndromes cause a variety of symptoms. Stimuli from the heart and other thoracic organs cause discomfort. This is described as pressure, burning, indigestion, aching, sharp, or stabbing pain. It is difficult to assess the amount of ischemia present only by symptoms unless the infarction is extensive. The symptoms often mimic those of angina. Complications of acute coronary syndromes may involve electrical dysfunction, myocardial dysfunction, or valvular dysfunction. Electrical defects include arrhythmias and conduction defects. Myocardial effects include heart failure, interventricular septum rupture, **pseudoaneurysm**, ventricular aneurysm, cardiogenic shock, and mural thrombus formation. Valvular defects usually involve **mitral regurgitation**. Additional complications of acute coronary syndromes include recurring ischemia and pericarditis. If pericarditis occurs 2–10 weeks after an MI, it is called post-MI or **Dressler syndrome**.

DIAGNOSIS

Acute coronary syndromes are considered for patients with chest pain or discomfort over age 30 (male) or over age 40 (female)–except in diabetic patients, in which these syndromes occur in younger generations. The pain must be differentiated from pain caused by pneumonia, pericarditis, pulmonary embolism, costochondral separation, rib fracture, acute aortic dissection, esophageal spasm, renal calculi, splenic infarction, or abdominal disorders. It is important not to attribute any new symptoms to previous conditions such as hiatal hernia, gallbladder disease, or peptic ulcer.

An initial and serial electrocardiogram, plus a serial cardiac biomarker assessment, should be done to distinguish between the subtypes of acute coronary syndromes. Pulse **oximetry** is indicated. Chest X-rays are essential to assess any mediastinal widening, suggesting aortic dissection. An ECG is done within 10 minutes of the patient's arrival to evaluate treatments. Urgent cardiac catheterization may be needed. Careful reading of the ECG is required since there can be only slight ST-segment elevation. It is important not to focus on leads showing ST-segment depression. With the characteristic symptoms, ST-segment elevation on the ECG is 90% specific and 45% sensitive to diagnosing MI. Diagnosis is usually confirmed when serial tracings are taken every 8 hours for the first day, then daily if they show a slow evolution toward a more regular and stable pattern or the development of abnormal Q waves over several days. Cardiac biomarkers are the serum markers of myocardial cell injury released into the bloodstream following myocardial cell necrosis. Cardiac biomarkers appear at differing times, with levels decreasing at various rates. The newer testing allows for earlier MI identification and has become the primary cardiac biomarker assay in many locations.

Coronary angiography usually combines diagnosis with percutaneous coronary intervention. If possible, emergency coronary angiography is done stat after the onset of an acute MI. This has dramatically lowered complications and deaths and also improved outcomes in the long term. Angiography may be done if there is evidence of continuing ischemia based on ECG or symptoms, hemodynamic instability, recurring ventricular tachyarrhythmias, or anything else suggesting ischemia.

TREATMENT

Treatment of acute coronary syndromes is focused on interrupting thrombosis, relieving distress, limiting the size of infarctions, reversing ischemia, reducing cardiac workload, and preventing complications. Acute coronary syndromes are medical emergencies. Rapid diagnosis and treatment are essential. Aggression treatment for anemia, heart failure, or any other contributing conditions must exist. Any chest pain remaining after 12–24 hours must be assessed. It may indicate pericarditis, recurring ischemia, pneumonia, pulmonary embolism, gastritis, or an ulcer. A solid IV route is established, a nasal cannula usually gives oxygen, and continual single-lead ECG monitoring begins. Pre-hospital interventions include ECG, chewable aspirin, and nitrates for pain management. Morphine is only used cautiously.

Before or after discharge, patients often have stress testing based on individual features of their acute coronary syndrome. Physical activity slowly increases over the first 3–6 weeks after release. Moderate physical activities, including sexual intercourse, are encouraged. Most patients can return to complete activities after 6 weeks following an acute MI. Regular exercise programs are taught based on age, cardiac status, and lifestyle. After revascularization, supervised cardiac rehabilitation programs decrease mortality. The patient must be encouraged to modify risk factors and lifestyle and instructed that doing so can improve the prognosis.

Aspirin and other antiplatelet drugs reduce mortality and reinfarction following an MI. Long-term enteric-coated aspirin every day is recommended. Warfarin, with or without aspirin, also reduces mortality and reinfarction. Beta-blockers are commonly prescribed, including acebutolol, atenolol, metoprolol, propranolol, and timolol. They reduce deaths after MI by approximately 25% for 7 years or more. ACE inhibitors are also standard medications and are especially indicated after an MI if the ejection fraction is less than 40%. Statins are usually also prescribed and benefit nearly all post-MI patients. Statins generally continue throughout life, barring any extreme adverse effects, with doses increasing to a maximally tolerated level.

PREVENTION

Prevention of acute coronary syndromes requires the same lifestyle changes used to prevent coronary artery disease: quitting smoking, eating a heart-healthy diet, increasing physical activity, reducing stress, and taking medications that combat thrombocyte aggregation and facilitate the development of atherosclerotic plaques.

YOU SHOULD REMEMBER

Acute coronary syndromes are manifestations of coronary heart disease. They usually result from plaque disruption in the coronary arteries, known as atherosclerosis. Common risk factors include smoking, hypertension, diabetes mellitus, hyperlipidemia, the male gender, physical inactivity, family obesity, and poor nutrition.

Check Your Knowledge

1. How prevalent are acute coronary syndromes?
2. How does an acute thrombus cause an acute coronary syndrome?
3. What are the essential diagnostic procedures for acute coronary syndromes?

CLINICAL CASE STUDY 1

A 54-year-old man was hospitalized for symptoms of unstable angina. Three days before, he had awoken in the middle of the night with a solid precordial pain that lasted for 20 minutes. It radiated to his upper left arm and was accompanied by dyspnea. Tests showed no increase in myocardial injury markers, and an electrocardiogram did not suggest acute myocardial ischemia. The patient was given atenolol and aspirin and referred to the cardiology department for outpatient care. Two more episodes occurred while he was awaiting his appointment. The patient complained of dyspnea with exertion that had progressed over many years. He was a former smoker of 40 cigarettes daily and had hypertension controlled by medication. A stress test was positive for myocardial ischemia at the cardiology center, and the patient was admitted for coronary cineangiography. This procedure revealed a left main coronary artery free of obstructions, an anterior interventricular branch with an 80% obstructive lesion, and other lesions in various components. Coronary artery bypass graft surgery was scheduled.

CRITICAL THINKING QUESTIONS

1. What are the symptoms of unstable angina?
2. What is the cause of unstable angina?
3. What are the treatments for unstable angina?

CLINICAL CASE STUDY 2

A 66-year-old man arrived at the emergency department complaining of left-sided chest pain that radiated to his left arm. Past medical history included hypertension, uncontrolled diabetes mellitus, and hyperlipidemia. The patient stated that he could only walk about two city blocks before becoming fatigued. His chest pain was partially relieved by sublingual nitroglycerin. A 12-lead electrocardiogram revealed nonspecific T-wave inversions in the inferolateral leads, and aspirin was given, which fully resolved the chest pain. The patient was admitted to the telemetry floor for additional assessment. The presence of his risk factors for coronary artery disease and the ECG changes indicated that he was at an elevated risk for CAD. A cardiac troponin test was scheduled to exclude ongoing ischemic CAD before a stress test could be designed.

CRITICAL THINKING QUESTIONS

1. What are the symptoms of stable angina?
2. How could you diagnose stable angina?
3. What are the treatments for stable angina?

FURTHER READING

1. Aggarwal, N.R., and Wood, M.J. (2021). *Sex Differences in Cardiac Disease: Pathophysiology, Presentation, Diagnosis, and Management.* Elsevier.
2. Cooper, O. (2020). *Coronary Artery Disease: Causes, Diagnosis, and Management.* Hayle Medical.
3. De Lemos, J., Omland, T. (2017). *Chronic Coronary Artery Disease: A Companion to Braunwald's Heart Disease.* Elsevier.
4. Hanna, E.B. (2017). *Practical Cardiovascular Medicine.* Wiley-Blackwell.
5. iConcept Press. (2017). *Coronary Artery Disease: Research and Practice.* iConcept Press.
6. Kaski, J.C. (2016). *Essentials in Stable Angina Pectoris.* Springer.
7. King, M.W., Bambharoliya, T., Ramakrishna, H., and Zhang, F. (2020). *Coronary Artery Disease and the Evolution of Angioplasty Devices (Briefs in Materials).* Springer.
8. Lyde, W. (2015). *Encyclopedia of Coronary Artery Disease (Physiology and Treatment): Volume III.* Hayle Medical.
9. Minatoguchi, S. (2019). *Cardioprotection against Acute Myocardial Infarction.* Springer.
10. Narila, K. (2021). *Symptoms of Coronary Artery Disease: Chest Pain, Shortness of Breath, Sweating, Palpitations, Tachycardia, Weakness, Dizziness, Nausea, Pedal Edema, Fatigue.* Narila.
11. Ostovar, L., Khadem Vatan, K., and Panahi, O. (2020). *Clinical Outcome of Thrombolytic Therapy in Patients with Acute Myocardial Infarction.* Scholars' Press.
12. Polimeni, A. (2020). *Coronary Artery Disease (Clinics Review Articles: Cardiology Clinics).* Volume 38-4. Elsevier.
13. Richardson, R.R. (2020). *Atlas of Pediatric CTA of Coronary Artery Anomalies.* Springer.
14. Shah, P.K. (2019). *Risk Factors in Coronary Artery Disease.* CRC Press.
15. Tousoulis, D. (2017). *Coronary Artery Disease: From Biology to Clinical Practice.* Academic Press.
16. Wang, M. (2020). *Coronary Artery Disease: Therapeutics and Drug Discovery (Advances in Experimental Medicine and Biology, Book 1177).* Springer.
17. Willerson, J.T., and Holmes, Jr., D.R. (2015). *Coronary Artery Disease (Cardiovascular Medicine).* Springer.

9 Myocardial Infarction

OVERVIEW

Myocardial infarction (MI), or heart attack, is caused by decreased or complete cessation of blood flow to a portion of the myocardium. MI may be "silent" and go undetected, or it could be a catastrophic event leading to hemodynamic deterioration and sudden death. Acute MI (AMI) is myocardial necrosis resulting from acute coronary artery obstruction. In severe ischemic episodes, the patient often has significant pain and feels restless and apprehensive. MI is the leading cause of death for people of most racial and ethnic groups in the United States, including African-American, American Indian, Alaska Native, Hispanic, and white men. For women from the Pacific Islands and Asian American, American Indian, Alaska Native, and Hispanic women, heart disease is second only to cancer. The prevalence of MI approaches 3 million people worldwide; every year, about 805,000 people in the United States have a heart attack. Risk factors for heart disease include hypertension, hypercholesterolemia, obesity, diabetes, smoking, unhealthy diet, physical inactivity, and excessive alcohol use. MI can lead to arrhythmia, heart failure (HF), and death.

ACUTE MYOCARDIAL INFARCTION

Myocardial ischemia develops when the ability to supply oxygen and nutrients to the myocardium is less than the oxygen and nutrient requirements of the myocardium. The heart is a primarily aerobic organ with a low threshold for a deficit in oxygen delivery. An AMI involves myocardium **necrosis** because of coronary artery obstruction (see **Figure 9.1**). It causes chest discomfort, often accompanied by dyspnea, nausea, and sweating. It is also considered to be one type of acute coronary syndrome. AMI occurs once every 40 seconds in the USA. The mortality rate of AMI remains high, and most deaths occur outside of the hospital. Prehospital care may lower the mortality rate of AMI.

EPIDEMIOLOGY

AMI is the most common form of coronary heart disease (CHD) worldwide. It causes more than 15% of all deaths annually. Prevalence is higher in men than in women. A significant proportion of the general population is affected. With metabolic syndrome or diabetes mellitus, there is an increased incidence of myocardial ischemia and MI. Incidence is lower in industrialized nations partly due to better healthcare systems, but rates are rapidly growing in Eastern Europe, Southern Asia, and Latin America. For unknown reasons, the highest prevalence of AMI in people younger than 45 is in India, Pakistan, Sri Lanka, Bangladesh, and Nepal.

In the United States, there are about 1 million MI per year, and about one American dies from MI every 40 seconds, which is approximately 518,400 annually. Of these, between 300,000 and 400,000 are fatal. However, the incidence is declining in the United States. According to the American Heart Association (AHA), the group with the highest incidence of MI is African-American men aged 75–84 (12.9 cases per 100,000 population), followed by African-American women of the same age (10.2 cases), Caucasian men (9.1 cases), and Caucasian women (7.8 cases) – see **Figure 9.2**.

ETIOLOGY AND RISK FACTORS

AMI is caused by narrowing or blockage of the coronary arteries with atherosclerotic plaque. Factors that lead to this include high low-density lipoprotein (LDL) and excessive saturated fat and trans fats in the diet. Modifiable risk factors represent over 90% of the risks for AMI. Risk

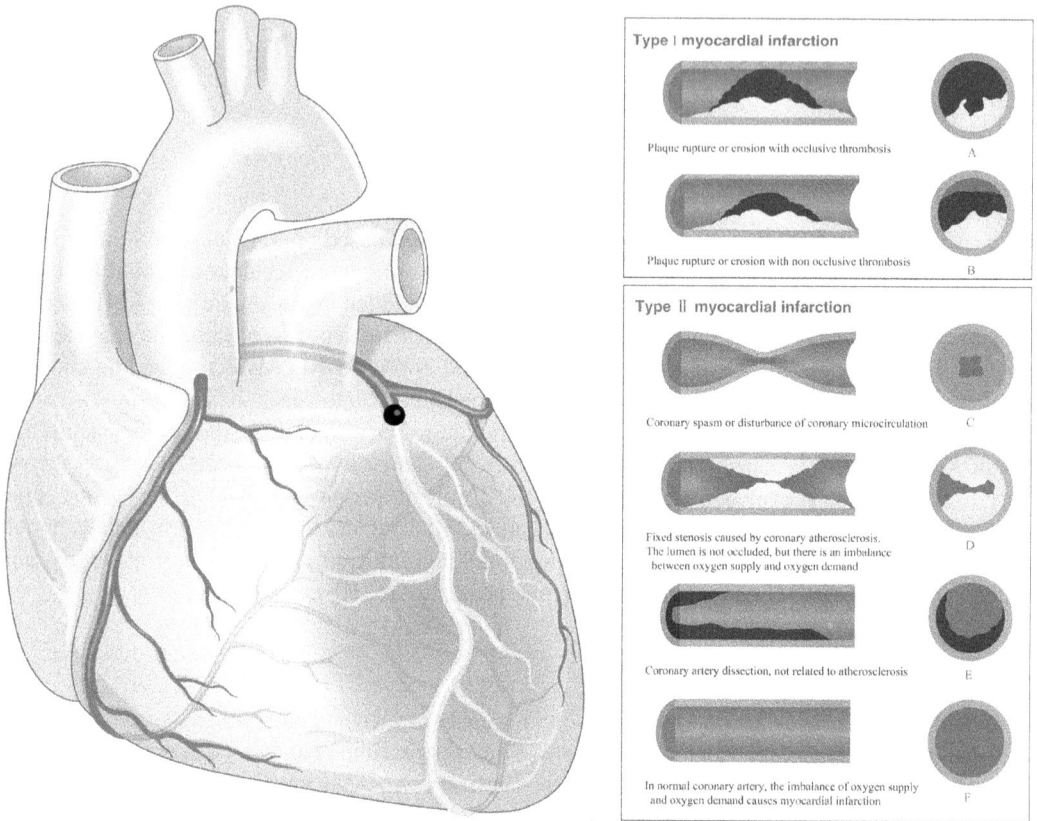

Type I myocardial infarction

Plaque rupture or erosion with occlusive thrombosis

A

Plaque rupture or erosion with non occlusive thrombosis

B

Type II myocardial infarction

Coronary spasm or disturbance of coronary microcirculation

C

Fixed stenosis caused by coronary atherosclerosis.
The lumen is not occluded, but there is an imbalance
between oxygen supply and oxygen demand

D

Coronary artery dissection, not related to atherosclerosis

E

In normal coronary artery, the imbalance of oxygen supply
and oxygen demand causes myocardial infarction

F

Pathophysiological mechanism of acute myocardial infarction
There are different mechanisms of acute myocardial infarction.

FIGURE 9.1   An AMI.

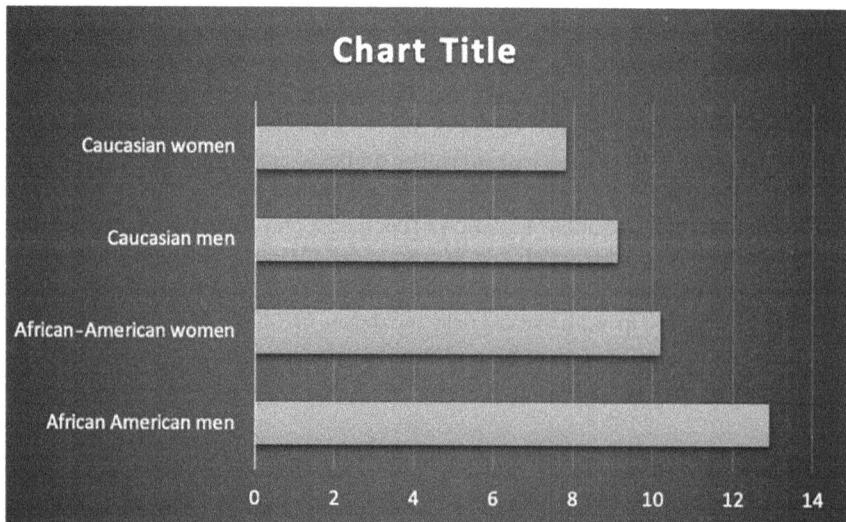

FIGURE 9.2   AMI in various individuals; cases per 100,000 population.

factors include diabetes mellitus, obesity, smoking, hypertension, high cholesterol, high triglycerides, increased age, and family history of heart disease. Additional risk factors include high-stress levels, lack of physical exercise, cigarette smoking, use of amphetamines or cocaine, and a history of **preeclampsia**.

CLINICAL MANIFESTATIONS

The majority of patients experience prodromal symptoms days to weeks before an MI. Symptoms include fatigue, dyspnea, and crescendo or unstable angina. The first MI symptom is usually deep chest pain, described as pressure or severe pain. It often radiates to the back, arms, shoulders, jaw, or all of these locations. The pain is nearly the same as that of angina pectoris but usually lasts longer and is more severe. There is often sweating, nausea, and vomiting. In some patients, the discomfort is mild. Approximately 20% of AMI cases are *silent*, with these cases more commonly seen in diabetic patients.

In silent MI, the patient may not recognize what is happening since the symptoms are vague. Some patients experience no symptoms as the MI occurs. Often, the affected person thinks they are just having indigestion, and relief of the discomfort may be incorrectly believed to be achieved by taking antacids or belching. **Syncope** is another symptom that may be seen.

Female patients often have atypical chest discomfort, and older patients may have more dyspnea than ischemic-related chest pain. The pain may be extreme if there is severe ischemia and the patient becomes apprehensive and restless. Nausea and vomiting are more familiar with *inferior MI*. Some patients' primary symptoms are dyspnea and weakness (from left ventriculi failure), pulmonary edema, significant **arrhythmia**, and shock. The patient's skin may be moist, pale, and calm, and peripheral or central cyanosis may be seen. Blood pressure can be varied, but many patients first experience early hypertension when the pain manifests. The pulse is often described as **thready**. Heart sounds are usually slightly distant, and a fourth heart sound is nearly always present.

In some cases, there is a soft systolic blowing **apical murmur**, which indicates dysfunction of the **papillary muscle** of the heart. Upon first examination, a preexisting heart condition or another type of condition may be suggested by a **friction rub** or more significant murmurs. Acute pericarditis is more likely than MI if a friction rub occurs within several hours after symptoms begin. Even so, friction rubs are usually described as transient. In about 15% of patients, the chest wall is tender when palpated. Right ventricular (RV) infarction signs include distended **jugular veins**, often with the **Kussmaul sign**, elevated RV filling pressure, clear lung fields, and hypotension.

DIAGNOSIS

The diagnosis of AMI starts with an initial and serial electrocardiogram (ECG or EKG). An EKG is crucial for diagnosis and must be done within 10 minutes of the patient's arrival. An initial EKG usually reveals an ST-segment elevation. If possible, emergency coronary angiography and percutaneous coronary intervention (PCI) are performed very soon after the onset of an AMI. Cardiac biomarker measurements help identify the present subtype of MI or distinguish between these and unstable angina. Serum levels increase within 3–12 hours from the onset of chest pain, peak at 24–48 hours, and return to baseline over 5–14 days.

Troponin levels may not be detectable for 6 hours after the onset of myocardial cell injury. The most sensitive early marker for MI is **myoglobin**. Additionally, urgent cardiac catheterization is needed for some patients. Cardiac troponin is by far the most commonly used biomarker. It has the highest known sensitivity. It enters into the bloodstream soon after a heart attack. It also stays in the bloodstream for days after all other biomarkers reach normal levels. Two forms of troponin may be measured: troponin T and troponin I. Troponin I is particular to the heart and stays higher longer than the **creatine kinase-myocardial band** (CK-MB). Current guidelines from the AHA say this is the best biomarker for finding a heart attack. The AHA says to limit the use of the other biomarkers. These include creatinine kinase, myoglobin, and CK-MB.

Creatinine kinase can also be measured several times over 24 hours. It will often at least double if a patient has had a heart attack. However, because levels of CK can go up in many conditions besides a heart attack, it is not very specific. Myoglobin is sometimes measured in addition to troponin to help diagnose a heart attack. It is also not very specific for finding a heart attack. CK-MB is more sensitive to finding heart damage from a heart attack. CK-MB rises 4–6 hours after a heart attack. But it is generally back to normal in a day or two. Because of this, it is not helpful when a healthcare provider is trying to determine whether a patient's recent chest pain was a heart attack.

TREATMENT

Emergency personnel establish a good IV route for AMI before hospitalization, give oxygen by nasal cannula, and begin continuous single-lead EKG monitoring. Medications include antiplatelet drugs, anticoagulants, and antianginal drugs. Antiplatelet drugs include aspirin, clopidogrel, prasugrel, and ticagrelor. Anticoagulants include various types of heparin and bivalirudin. Nitroglycerin is the predominant antianginal agent, and morphine is used more selectively based on the individual patient. Beta-blockers, ACE inhibitors, and statins are also given.

Fibrinolytics are most effective within a few minutes to 1 hour after the onset of AMI – the earlier, the better. Lower-risk patients usually have stress testing before discharge or soon after. Patients must be educated about closely following all medication regimens and making significant lifestyle changes. Based on any other conditions, all AMI patients remain taking antiplatelet drugs, statins, antianginals, and any other required medications. Working with physicians to manage risk factors for MI may improve their prognosis.

PREVENTION

Even if it recurs, prevention of AMI includes a heart-healthy diet with plenty of whole grains, fruits, vegetables, and lean protein. There must be significant reductions in cholesterol, saturated fat, trans fat, and sugar. This is critical for people with diabetes mellitus, high cholesterol, and hypertension. Exercising regularly and following an approved exercise plan created by a physician improves cardiovascular health. Any new exercise plan must only be started by consulting a physician. Quitting smoking significantly lowers risks for AMI and improves heart and lung health. Secondhand smoke must also be avoided.

YOU SHOULD REMEMBER

Unfortunately, about 20% of patients aged 45 and older will have another MI within 5 years of the first. MI survivors must be involved in secondary prevention measures. Five ways to lower the risks of a second MI include taking prescribed medications correctly, following up with healthcare professionals, participating in cardiac rehabilitation, managing risk factors, and getting support from family, friends, and other MI survivors.

Check Your Knowledge

1. What does an AMI involve?
2. How significant is AMI in the United States?
3. What are the prodromal symptoms before an AMI?

TYPES OF MYOCARDIAL INFARCTION

MI occurs in several different types. These include ST-segment elevation myocardial infarction (STEMI), non-ST-segment elevation myocardial infarction (NSTEMI), and **silent myocardial infarction** (SMI). STEMI occurs from the occlusion of one or more coronary arteries, usually due to plaque rupture, erosion, fissuring, or dissection. NSTEMI involves partial blockage of the coronary arteries, causing reduced flow of oxygen-rich blood to the heart muscle. SMI occurs without chest discomfort or other symptoms of angina, such as dyspnea, nausea, and sweating.

ST-Segment Elevation Myocardial Infarction

A STEMI is when **transmural myocardial ischemia** results in myocardial injury or necrosis. It is a more serious heart attack with a greater risk of severe complications and death. The clinical definition of MI requires the confirmation of the myocardial ischemic injury with abnormal cardiac biomarkers. Among heart attacks, STEMIs are typically more severe. To best understand ST elevation, it helps to know about two specific wave sections on EKG: QRS complex and ST segment. The QRS is the prominent peak that appears on a heat wave. ST segment is a short section immediately after the QRS complex (see **Figure 9.3**). Usually, there should not be any electrical activity in that segment, causing it to be flat and back to baseline.

Epidemiology

STEMI remains a significant healthcare burden in the United States, with about 750,000 cases annually. Considerable sex and gender differences exist in the presentation, pathophysiology, and outcomes of STEMI. STEMI causes 36–52 hospitalizations per 100,000 population. About 38% of

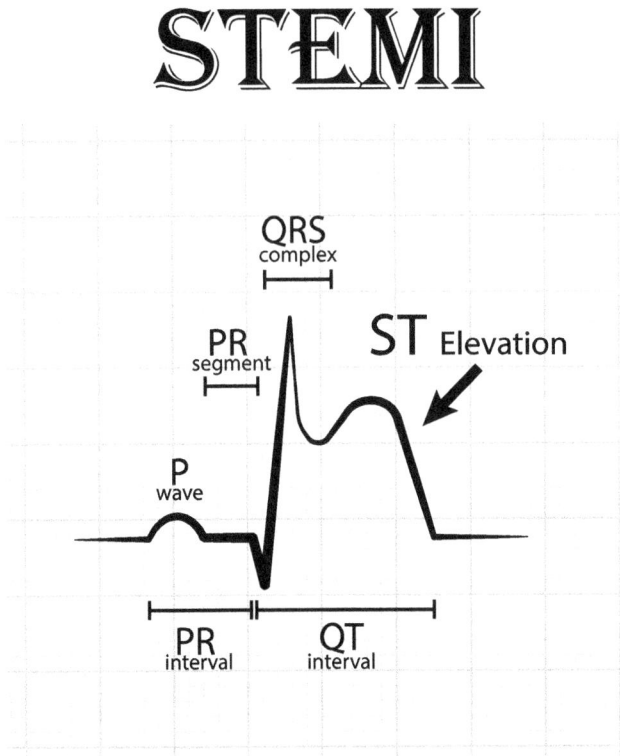

FIGURE 9.3   ST elevation on EKG.

people in the emergency room with acute coronary syndrome were diagnosed with STEMI. Males and African Americans, unmarried individuals, and veterans generally have a higher risk of MI. Mortality in STEMI ranges from 4% to 24%. It depends on the variety of patients' clinical characteristics present before and within the first hours of the onset of MI, affecting the reliability of the diagnosis.

Etiology and Risk Factors

A STEMI occurs due to the occlusion of one or more coronary arteries. It usually results from thrombosis at a ruptured or eroded plaque site. This causes transmural myocardial ischemia, resulting in myocardial injury or necrosis. Other cardiovascular pathologies that depict ST-segment elevation in an EKG include **pericarditis, myocarditis**, **right bundle branch block**, **stress cardiomyopathy**, early **repolarization**, acute vasospasm, and left ventricular hypertrophy. Major risk factors for STEMI are dyslipidemia, diabetes mellitus, hypertension, smoking, obesity, and a family history of coronary artery disease. For most patients, STEMI is a type 1 MI. Men aged 45 and older and women aged 55 and older are more likely to have a heart attack than younger men and women.

Clinical Manifestations

The main symptoms to watch for are angina or pain that radiates to the jaw, neck, back, arms, or abdomen; nausea; sweating; heart palpitations; fatigue; shortness of breath; anxiety; fainting; and dizziness.

Diagnosis

The current clinical definition of STEMI requires the confirmation of MI injury with abnormal cardiac biomarkers. Diagnosis of STEMI begins with patient and family history, physical examination, and questions about the characteristics of the pain and related symptoms, risk factors for CVD, and any recent drug use. Cocaine use can cause STEMI regardless of any other risk factors. The following diagnostic steps are EKG and assessment of troponins. EKG criteria for STEMI include the following:

- New ST-segment elevation at the **J point** in two contiguous leads, with the cutoff point as more significant than 0.1 millivolts in all leads except V2 or V3.
- In leads V2 and V3, the cutoff point is more significant than 0.2 mV in men older than 40, more meaningful than 0.25 in men younger than 40, or greater than 0.15 mV in women (see **Figure 9.4**).

Treatment

After diagnosis, STEMI is treated with IV access being obtained and cardiac monitoring started. Oxygen therapy is helpful for patients who are hypoxemic or at risk of hypoxemia. PCI should occur within 90 minutes if the facility is PCI-capable or within 120 minutes if the patient must be transferred to such a facility. If this is not possible, fibrinolytic therapy must be initiated within 30 minutes of the patient's arrival at the facility. It is essential to rule out acute aortic dissection or acute pulmonary embolism.

A beta-blocker, high-intensity statin, and aspirin are started for all patients with AMI. Nitroglycerin can reduce anginal pain but must be avoided if the patient has used a phosphodiesterase-inhibiting medication in the last 24 hours or if there is an RV infarction. Morphine can be used for pain relief, but this requires careful assessment. The choice of P2Y12-inhibiting antiplatelet medication is based on whether the patient previously had PCI or fibrinolytic therapy. Ticagrelor and prasugrel are preferred over clopidogrel for those that had PCI. Patients undergoing fibrinolytic treatment are started on clopidogrel. The relative contraindications of P2Y12 inhibitors must be considered. Prasugrel is contraindicated in patients with transient ischemic attack or stroke. Anticoagulation is

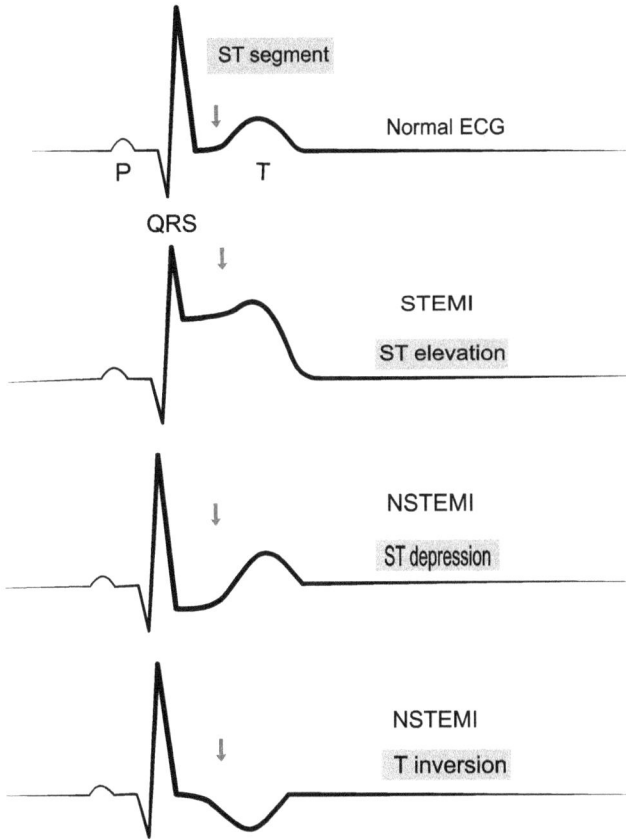

FIGURE 9.4   EKG criteria for STEMI.

started alongside unfractionated heparin, low-molecular-weight heparin (LMWH), bivalirudin, or fondaparinux.

Prevention

Though it may not be preventable, most STEMI patients require dual antiplatelet therapy for 12 months, an ACE inhibitor, a beta-blocker, and a statin. These medications have been shown to reduce the risk of MI death. Quitting or avoiding tobacco use and lowering dietary sodium, fat, and sugar are also essential.

YOU SHOULD REMEMBER

Early reports from the coronavirus disease 2019 (COVID-19) pandemic identified coronary thrombosis leading to STEMI as a complication of COVID-19 infection. However, the epidemiology of STEMI in patients with COVID-19 needs to be better characterized.

Check Your Knowledge

1. What is a STEMI?
2. What are the symptoms of STEMI?
3. What are the treatments for STEMI?

NON-ST SEGMENT ELEVATION MYOCARDIAL INFARCTION

NSTEMI, or **subendocardial MI**, is myocardial necrosis without acute ST-segment elevation. It is also evidenced by cardiac markers in the blood (with elevations of troponin I, T, and CK). On EKG, there are changes such as ST-segment depression, T-wave inversion, or both. This condition gets its name because it does not have an easily identifiable electrical pattern (ST elevation) like the other main types of heart attacks. Like different types of MI, it is a life-threatening medical emergency and needs immediate care.

Epidemiology

NSTEMI is prevalent in the United States. An estimated 780,000 cases of acute coronary syndrome are diagnosed each year. About 70%, or approximately 546,000, of those cases are NSTEMIs.

Etiology and Risk Factors

Several risk factors can increase the chances of NSTEMI. Some can be modified, while others cannot. Risk factors include diet and too much sodium, sugar, or fat. Smoking, lack of physical activity, and recreational drug use (especially stimulants like amphetamines and cocaine) are other risks. Family history, aging, and gender must also be considered.

Clinical Manifestations

The "typical" presentation of NSTEMI is pressure-like substernal pain at rest or with minimal exertion. The pain generally lasts more than 10 minutes and may radiate to either arm, neck, or jaw. It may be associated with dyspnea, chest tightness, nausea or vomiting, syncope, fatigue, or diaphoresis.

Diagnosis

NSTEMI heart attacks are diagnosed through the combination of a blood test and an EKG. Doctors use the blood test to look for indications of NSTEMI, such as higher than usual levels of CK-MB, troponin I, and troponin T.

Treatment

High-risk patients with NSTEMI should receive aggressive care, including aspirin, clopidogrel, unfractionated heparin, LMWH, IV platelet glycoprotein, calcium blockers (e.g., tirofiban, eptifibatide), and a beta-blocker. Unfractionated heparin with bolus dosing and a continuous infusion is commonly used, with most institutions having protocols available. Other strategies may include enoxaparin, bivalirudin, fondaparinux, and dual antiplatelet therapies. Fibrinolytic therapies should not be used in NSTEMI.

Prevention

A well-balanced, heart-healthy diet includes fruits, vegetables, whole grains, and healthy fats. It limits the intake of saturated and trans fats. Physical activity, at least 30 minutes five days a week, and quitting smoking are also effective.

SILENT MYOCARDIAL INFARCTION

SMI occurs in about 20% of all AMIs, with no symptoms or vague symptoms that may not be recognized as illness by the patient. They are more common in patients with diabetes mellitus. The patient often attributes the discomfort to indigestion since spontaneous relief may be incorrectly attributed to belching or consumption of antacids.

Epidemiology

The prevalence and incidence of SMI are less well-known than those of acute myocardial ischemia. Accumulating data indicate that silent ischemia is a common accompaniment of coronary artery disease. In the population at large, studies estimate that 2%–4% of middle-aged men have asymptomatic coronary artery disease and silent ischemia on treadmill testing. About 20%–30% of all MIs are quiet. In the general population, the prevalence of SMI increased markedly with age in elderly subjects. Hypertension causes only a moderate increase in prevalence, whereas underlying cardiovascular diseases and diabetes are associated with marked increases in prevalence – the incidence of silent MI changes in the same way. Studies have shown that the incidence rate of SMI is higher in men than in women. There is an increased risk of CHD deaths and all-cause mortality among both men and women with SMI. However, there is a potentially greater increased risk among women. An SMI accounts for 45% of MI and strikes men more than women.

Etiology and Risk Factors

SMIs are caused in the same ways that traditional MIs are generated. This occurs when part of the heart muscle is damaged or dies because it lacks oxygen. Risk factors for silent heart attacks include obesity, a sedentary lifestyle, smoking, diabetes, dyslipidemia, hypertension, age, gender, and a family history of heart disease.

Clinical Manifestations

A heart attack commonly does not have apparent symptoms; silent myocardial ischemia can occur in the absence of chest discomfort or other anginal equivalent symptoms, such as dyspnea, nausea, and diaphoresis, with ST-segment changes on EKG.

Diagnosis

Diagnostic tests include cardiac markers, echocardiogram, bedside ECG monitoring, ambulatory ECG (AECG) monitoring, exercise stress testing, computed tomography (CT), and radionuclide imaging techniques.

Treatment

Treatment for SMIs includes beta-blockers, monotherapy with calcium channel blockers, aspirin (antiplatelet therapy), and statin (lipid-lowering therapy).

Prevention

Preventing SMIs includes regular exercise, eating healthy foods, stopping the use of tobacco products, and staying at a healthy weight.

YOU SHOULD REMEMBER

There are three life-threatening mechanical complications of MI. These include ventricular free wall rupture, interventricular septum rupture, and acute mitral regurgitation. Ventricular free wall rupture occurs within 5 days in 50% of cases and 2 weeks in 90% of cases. It has an overall mortality rate of more than 80%.

Check Your Knowledge

1. What is a description of SMI?
2. What are the symptoms of SMI?
3. How can we diagnose the SMI?

HEART FAILURE AND MYOCARDIAL INFARCTION

Despite the remarkable advances in the treatment of coronary artery disease and AMI over the past two decades, MI remains the most common cause of HF. The factors that contribute to the **pathogenesis** of HF development at the time of the MI hospitalization include myocardial compromise due to myocardial necrosis, myocardial stunning, and mechanical complications such as papillary muscle rupture, ventricular septal defect, and ventricular free wall rupture. HF is a frequent complication of MI. Congestive HF is a long-term condition when the heart cannot pump blood well enough to give the body a regular supply. Blood and fluids collect in the lungs and legs over time. The condition may affect only the right or left side of the heart. Both sides of the heart also can be involved.

EPIDEMIOLOGY

The incidence of in-hospital HF is three times higher in patients 75–85 years old as compared with those 25–54 years of age. After hospital discharge, HF incidence is six times higher in the older age group. After MI, the incidence of HF among diabetic patients is 60%–70% higher than in patients without diabetes. Chronic kidney disease increases the risk of HF development after MI by approximately two times. COVID-19 is caused by severe acute respiratory syndrome. The coronavirus likely affects the risk of HF development after MI. However, complex clinical data are still lacking. There are several mechanisms by which the COVID-19 pandemic may influence the risk of HF development after MI. The incidence and prevalence of HF is higher among black individuals compared with other racial and ethnic groups. The majority of HF has increased among black and Hispanic individuals over time.

ETIOLOGY AND RISK FACTORS

HF is often a chronic condition, but it may come on suddenly. Many different heart problems can cause it. The most common causes of HF include CAD, AMI, arrhythmia, hypertension, myocarditis, diabetes, obesity, alcohol use, tobacco and recreational drug use, and chemotherapy. Other diseases that can cause or contribute to HF include **emphysema**, **amyloidosis**, hyperthyroidism, severe anemia, and **sarcoidosis**. The risk factors for congestive HF include having a heart attack, hypertension, CAD, family history, lack of activity, smoking, cocaine, and use of excessive alcohol.

CLINICAL MANIFESTATIONS

The clinical signs and symptoms of HF after MI include chest pain, dyspnea, persistent coughing or wheezing, edema, tiredness, fatigue, lack of appetite, nausea, nocturia, confusion, impaired thinking, tachycardia, and weight gain.

DIAGNOSIS

Tests to diagnose HF may include chest X-ray, EKG, echocardiogram, stress tests, a heart CT scan, and blood tests. The blood test is done for B-type natriuretic peptide, a protein the heart secretes to stabilize blood pressure. These levels increase with HF. Blood tests can also determine the functions of the liver and kidneys.

TREATMENT

Treatment for HF usually aims to control the symptoms for as long as possible and slow the progression of the condition. The primary medicines for HF include the following:

- *Angiotensin-converting enzyme (ACE) inhibitors* – it relax blood vessels to lower blood pressure, improve blood flow, and decrease the strain on the heart.
- *Angiotensin II receptor blockers (ARBs)* – these drugs have many of the same benefits as ACE inhibitors. They may be an option for people who cannot tolerate ACE inhibitors.
- *Angiotensin receptor plus neprilysin inhibitors (ARNIs)* – these are two blood pressure drugs used to treat HF. The combination medicine is sacubitril–valsartan.
- *Beta-blockers* – these medicines slow the heart rate, lower blood pressure, reduce HF symptoms, and help the heart work better.
- *Potassium-sparing diuretics* – also called aldosterone antagonists – help patients with severe HF with reduced ejection fraction live longer.
- *Digoxin* – it helps the heart pump blood. It also tends to slow the heartbeat. Digoxin reduces HF symptoms in patients.

PREVENTION

The best way to avoid HF is to prevent or manage the contributing conditions if they develop carefully. Stop smoking, adopt heart-healthy eating habits, exercise regularly, and lose weight.

YOU SHOULD REMEMBER

The development of HF after MI has a significant impact on outcomes, regardless of the HF type. Among patients with a history of MI, HF development increases total mortality risk threefold and cardiovascular mortality fourfold. The timing of HF development also has an impact on adverse events. HF developing more than 3 days after MI is associated with a 43% higher mortality risk as compared with patients with HF developing in the first 3 days after MI. This may be explained by different risk factors and mechanisms leading to HF at other times.

Check Your Knowledge

1. What are the causes of HF after MI?
2. What are the symptoms of HF after MI?
3. What are the treatments for HF after MI?

CLINICAL CASE STUDY 1

A 58-year-old man was brought to the local emergency department because of excessive sweating and chest pain that was centralized but radiated to his left arm. He described the pain as "crushing." It subsided after he was given oral aspirin and nitroglycerin. The patient had smoked a pack of cigarettes daily for over 20 years but had no other cardiovascular risk factors. His BP was 180/105 mmHg, heart rate was 83 bpm, and oxygen saturation was 97%. In about a half hour, the chest pain returned with greater intensity. Imaging revealed that the man's left descending coronary artery was completely occluded.

CRITICAL THINKING QUESTIONS

1. What are the three types of MI?
2. What are the etiology and risk factors for AMI?
3. How can MI be prevented?

CLINICAL CASE STUDY 2

A 66-year-old woman with a history of dyslipidemia and chronic hepatitis C virus infection was hospitalized because of extreme chest pain. She had smoked cigarettes since the age of 21. The patient was tachypneic and hypoxemic with low oxygen saturation. A nasal cannula improved this. An ECG revealed AMI and evolved anterior MI. There were extensive left ventricular wall motion abnormalities associated with severe systolic dysfunction. The patient was also positive for COVID-19 infection. The patient received empirical antibiotics but was not a candidate for surgical repair or percutaneous device closure of a post-MI septal defect (because of the presence of COVID-19). Unfortunately, she died the following day.

CRITICAL THINKING QUESTIONS

1. What is dyslipidemia a significant risk factor for?
2. How does quitting smoking relate to risks for AMI?
3. What are the effects of COVID-19 on HF after MI?

CLINICAL CASE STUDY 3

A 56-year-old man presented to an outpatient clinic for a 6-month follow-up appointment. He described shortness of breath when climbing stairs, dyspnea on exertion, and a persistent nonproductive cough. The symptoms worsened over the past 2 weeks. The patient has a history of HF with reduced ejection fraction. Physical examination reveals hypertension, pitting edema in the legs, and an increased natriuretic peptide level. Current medications include atorvastatin, carvedilol, enalapril, and furosemide.

CRITICAL THINKING QUESTIONS

1. What are the common causes of HF?
2. What are the clinical signs and symptoms of HF after MI?
3. What are the primary medicines for HF?

FURTHER READING

1. Bishop, W. (2021). *Cardiac Failure Explained: Understanding the Symptoms, Signs, Medical Tests, and Management of a Failing Heart.* Dr. Warrick Bishop.
2. Chandra, K.S. and Swamy, A.J. (2020). *Acute Coronary Syndromes.* CRC Press.
3. De Luca, G., and Lansky, A. (2010). *Mechanical Reperfusion for STEMI: From Randomized Trials to Clinical Practice.* Informa Healthcare/CRC Press.
4. Edwards, A. (2023). *Cardiomyopathy: Signs, Symptoms, Prevention, and Secrets to Maintaining a Healthy Lifestyle for Persons Living with Cardiomyopathy.* Edwards.
5. Felker, G.M., and Mann, D.L. (2019). *Heart Failure: A Companion to Braunwald's Heart Disease,* 4th Edition. Elsevier.
6. Ferrari, R., Katz, A.M., Shug, A., and Visioli, O. (2012). *Myocardial Ischemia and Lipid Metabolism.* Springer.
7. Jin, J.P. (2014). *Troponin: Informative Diagnostic Marker (Physiology: Laboratory and Clinical Research).* Nova Science Publishers, Inc.
8. Kashyap, A., and Sharma, K.N. (2023). *The Acute Myocardial Infarction Mastery Bible: Your Blueprint for Complete Acute Myocardial Infarction Management.* Virtued Press.
9. Manigault, Jr., W.M. (2021). *Pericarditis: The Unsolved Mystery.* Palmetto Publishing.
10. Morrow, D.A. (2016). *Myocardial Infarction: A Companion to Braunwald's Heart Disease.* Elsevier.
11. Niccoli, G., and Eitel, I. (2018). *Coronary Microvascular Obstruction in Acute Myocardial Infarction: From Mechanisms to Treatment.* Academic Press.
12. Steinberg, J.S. and Varma, N. (2019). *Remote Monitoring: Implantable Devices and Ambulatory ECG.* Wolters Kluwer Health.

13. Stoker, A. (2023). *Understanding Myocarditis: The Ultimate Guide to Myocarditis Diagnosis, Prevention, and Effective Treatment.* Stoker.
14. Surawicz, B., and Knilans, T. (2010). *Chou's Electrocardiography in Clinical Practice: Adult and Pediatric*, 6th Edition. Saunders/Elsevier.
15. Ungar, A., and Marchionni, N. (2017). *Cardiac Management in the Frail Elderly Patient and the Oldest Old.* Springer.
16. Walraven, G. (2016). *Basic Arrhythmias with 12-Lead EKGs*, 8th Edition. Pearson.

10 Stroke

OVERVIEW

A stroke occurs when a blood artery carrying oxygen and nutrients to the brain is blocked or ruptured. It is also called a cerebral infarction. Stroke is a leading cause of death in the United States and is a significant cause of severe disability for adults. Every 40 seconds, someone in the United States has a stroke. Individuals of Asian, African, and Latin American origin tend to have a higher frequency of primary hemorrhage than persons of European ancestry. It is also preventable and treatable. Approximately 14 million new strokes occur globally every year. Symptoms develop quickly. Most strokes are ischemic, usually caused by arterial blockage, and fewer are hemorrhagic, caused by arterial rupture. Transient ischemic attacks are like ischemic strokes, except symptoms typically resolve in less than 1 hour, and there is no permanent brain damage. Since diabetes mellitus increases risk factors for hypertension and high cholesterol, there are increased chances of having a stroke or heart attack. Adults with diabetes are about two times as likely to have a stroke or heart disease as adults without diabetes.

STRUCTURE OF THE BLOOD VESSELS IN THE HEAD AND NECK

The main blood supply to the head and neck comes from the common carotid arteries, and the main drainage is by the internal and external jugular veins. Four paired arteries supply the head and neck: the common carotid arteries and three branches from each subclavian artery (the vertebral arteries, thyrocervical trunks, and costocervical trunks) – see **Figure 10.1**. The common carotid arteries

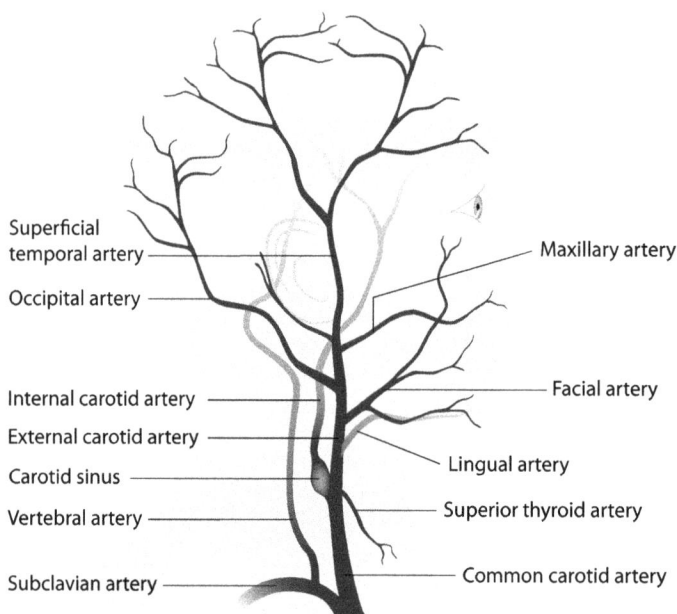

Blood Supply of the Head and Neck

FIGURE 10.1   Arteries of the head, neck, and brain.

DOI: 10.1201/9781003453376-13

have the broadest distribution. Each of the common carotid arteries is divided into two primary branches: the internal and external carotid arteries. At the point where they divide, each internal carotid artery has a slight dilation known as the **carotid sinus**. This structure contains **baroreceptors** that help in the reflex control of blood pressure. The nearby **carotid bodies** are chemoreceptors involved in controlling the respiratory rate. Suppose pressure is placed on the neck in the region of the carotid sinuses. In that case, it can result in unconsciousness since this pressure mimics hypertension and causes vasodilation that interferes with the delivery of blood to the brain. The right common carotid artery emerges from the **brachiocephalic trunk**. The left common carotid artery is the second branch of the aortic arch. Both arteries ascend through the lateral portion of the neck. At the superior border of the larynx, close to **Adam's apple**, each artery divides into its significant branches: the external and internal carotid arteries.

The external carotid arteries supply most head tissues, except the brain and eye orbits. Each external carotid artery ends after splitting into a **superficial temporal artery** that supplies the parotid salivary gland, most of the scalp, and a **maxillary artery** that supplies the jaws, chewing muscles, teeth, and nasal cavity. The *middle meningeal artery* is a branch of the maxillary artery that enters the skull via the foramen spinosum. It supplies the parietal bone's inner surface, the temporal bone's squamous area, and the dura mater below.

The ophthalmic arteries supply the eyes, orbits, forehead, and nose. Each anterior cerebral artery supplies the medial surface of the frontal and parietal lobes of the cerebral hemisphere on its side. It also anastomoses with a partner on the opposite side. The **middle cerebral arteries** continue in the **lateral sulci** of their respective cerebral hemispheres, supplying the lateral portions of the temporal, parietal, and frontal lobes.

The vertebral arteries emerge from the subclavian arteries at the root of the neck. They ascend and enter the skull via the **foramen magnum**. The right and left vertebral arteries unite in the cranium, forming the **basilary artery**. This ascends along the anterior portion of the brainstem, branching off to the cerebellum, pons, and inner ear. At the pons and midbrain border, the basilary artery divides into two posterior cerebral arteries, supplying the occipital lobes and inferior portions of the temporal lobes.

The **circle of Willis** is an anastomotic ring of arteries located at the base of the brain. This anastomotic circle connects the two major arterial systems to the brain: the internal carotid arteries and the vertebral and basilar arteries (see **Figure 10.2**). It surrounds the pituitary gland and optic chiasma while joining the brain's anterior and posterior blood supplies. The circle equalizes blood pressure (BP) in the two brain areas, providing other routes for blood to reach the brain if there is an occlusion of a carotid or vertebral artery.

The head and neck veins involve three pairs of vessels, which collect most of the blood that drains outward. These include the following:

- *The external jugular veins,* which empty into the subclavian veins
- *The internal jugular veins,* which join with the subclavian veins
- *The vertebral veins,* which drain into the brachiocephalic veins

The head and neck veins are illustrated in **Figure 10.3**.

The majority of the veins of the brain drain into the **dural venous sinuses**. These are a connected series of enlarged chambers. The superior sagittal sinuses and inferior sagittal sinuses lie within the **falx cerebri**. This continues down between the cerebral hemispheres. The inferior sagittal sinus posteriorly drains into the **straight sinus**. The superior sagittal and straight sinuses empty into the **transverse sinuses**. These continue in shallow groves on the occipital bone's internal surface. They drain into S-shaped **sigmoid sinuses**, eventually becoming the *internal jugular veins* as they exit the skill via the jugular foramen. The **cavernous sinuses** flank the sphenoid body and receive blood from the ophthalmic veins of the eye orbits and facial veins (which drain the nose and upper lip region).

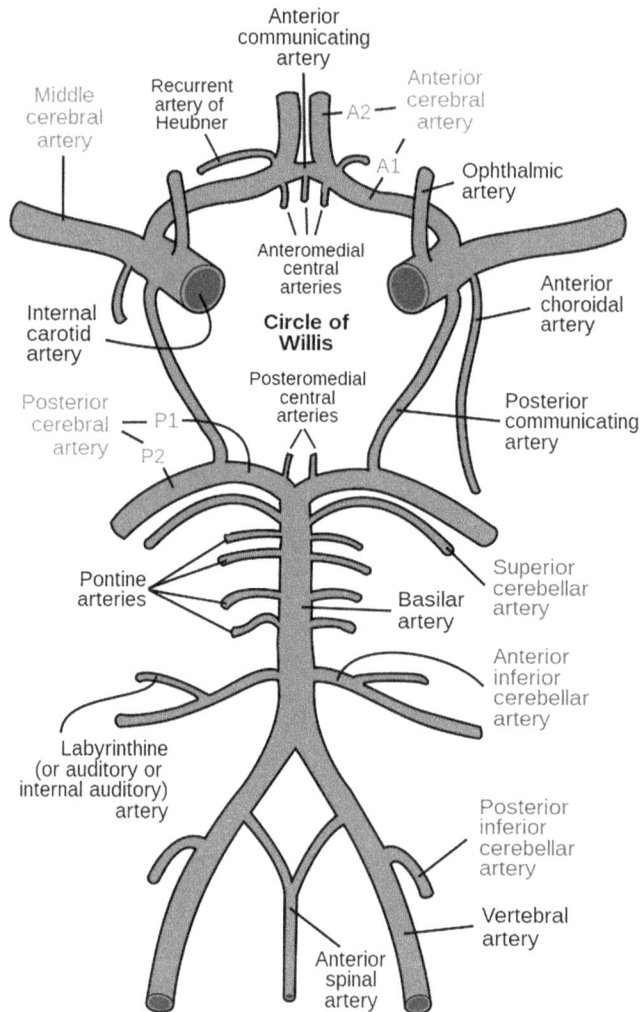

FIGURE 10.2 The circle of Willis.

The two internal jugular veins receive most of the blood from the brain. They are the most extensive paired veins that drain the head and neck. These veins arise from the dural venous sinuses and exit the skull through the *jugular foramina*. They then descend through the neck along the internal carotid arteries. At the base of the neck, the internal jugular veins join the subclavian veins on each side, forming brachiocephalic veins. The two brachiocephalic veins join to form the **superior vena cava**.

TYPES OF STROKE

A *stroke* is clinically termed a *cerebrovascular accident (CVA)*. Strokes are heterogeneous disorders signified by a focal, sudden interruption of blood flow within the cerebrum. They result in neurologic deficits. Most strokes are *ischemic*, but less often, *hemorrhagic* strokes occur. Strokes of either type constitute the 5th most common cause of death in the United States. There are approximately 14 million new strokes that occur globally every year. About one in four people over the age of 25 have some form of stroke. Nearly 60% of all strokes occur annually in people under the age of 70, with 52% occurring in men and 48% occurring in women. Strokes are also the most common cause of neurologic deficits in adults.

Head Veins

Superior Sagettal Sinus

Inferior Sagettal Sinus

Straight Sinus

Occipital

Right Transverse Sinus

Petrosal Sinus

Vertebral

Temporal

Cavernous Sinus

Maxillary

Facial

External Jugular

Internal Jugular

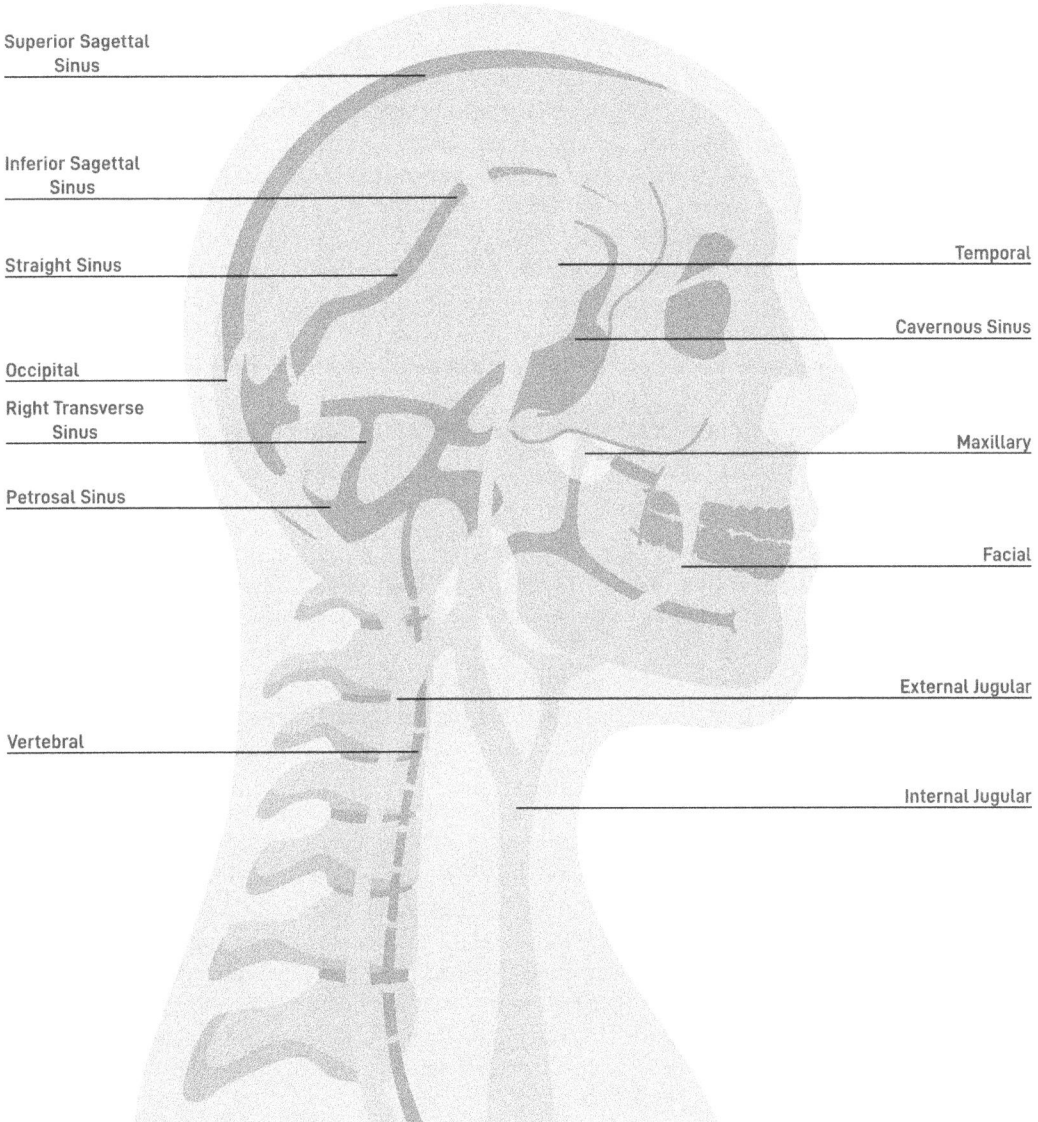

FIGURE 10.3 Veins of the head, neck, and brain.

HEMORRHAGIC STROKE

A *hemorrhagic stroke* results from cerebral vessel ruptures, such as *intracerebral* or *subarachnoid hemorrhage*. Hemorrhagic stroke makes up 20% of all cases of CVAs. Intracerebral hemorrhage is focal bleeding from a vessel within the brain's parenchyma, usually because of hypertension. This stroke usually occurs in the basal ganglia, cerebral lobes, cerebellum, or pons. However, it can occur in other areas of the brainstem or midbrain. Subarachnoid hemorrhage is sudden bleeding into the subarachnoid space, usually because of a ruptured aneurysm. Type 2 diabetes mellitus is associated with a higher incidence of hemorrhagic stroke.

Epidemiology

Hemorrhagic stroke is the second most common subtype, accounting for 10%–20% of all strokes. In contrast, it makes up 8%–15% of all strokes in the United Kingdom, the United States, and Australia. It makes up 18%–24% of all strokes in countries such as Japan and Korea. Hemorrhagic stroke is the most common type in low- and middle-income countries. It occurs mainly in older adults (over age 75), with a slight male predominance, and in people of Asian heritage. The incidence is 52 cases in every 100,000 Asians, followed by 24 per 100,000 Caucasians, 23 per 100,000 Africans, and 19.6 per 100,000 people from a Hispanic background. However, in one study in the United States, African Americans had the highest incidence, with 49 cases per 100,000.

Subarachnoid hemorrhage (SAH) caused by an aneurysm most often occurs between ages 40 and 65 but can occur at any age. Overall, it makes up about 5% of all types of stroke. Spontaneous subarachnoid bleeding occurs in about one in every 10,000 people annually, with females having 25% more cases than males. Approximately half of all patients are below 55 years of age. This is likely because most aneurysms occur relatively early, after age 40. The overall expected age range is between 40 and 65. According to the Journal of Neurology, Neurosurgery, and Psychiatry, higher rates of subarachnoid bleeding occur in the countries of Japan (23 per 100,000) and Finland (20 per 100,000), while low rates (4.2 per 100,000) in South and Central America. In the United States, SAH disproportionately affects Mexican Americans more than any other racial or ethnic group.

Etiology and Risk Factors

In most cases, hemorrhagic stroke is usually caused by a small rupture of an arteriosclerotic artery after being weakened by chronic hypertension. This type of bleeding is generally single, huge, and has severe outcomes. Less common causes include arteriovenous and other vascular malformations, congenital aneurysm, hemorrhagic brain infarction, mycotic aneurysm, excessive use of anticoagulants, primary or metastatic brain tumors, blood dyscrasia, intracranial artery dissection, bleeding of vasculitic disorder, or moyamoya disease. A lobar intracerebral hemorrhage is a **hematoma** in the cerebral lobes outside the basal ganglia. They may be caused by angiopathy from **amyloid** deposits in the cerebral arteries. This is called *cerebral amyloid angiopathy* and is most common in older adults. There can be multiple and recurring lobar hemorrhages. Modifiable risk factors related to intracerebral hemorrhage include obesity, diabetes mellitus, cigarette smoking, and a diet high in saturated and trans fats and calories. Transient severe hypertension that leads to intracerebral bleeding may sometimes be caused by cocaine or other sympathomimetic drugs.

In SAH, the bleeding is between the arachnoid and the pia mater. Head trauma is the most common cause. However, traumatic SAH is distinctly separate from non-traumatic SAH. The cause of primary subarachnoid bleeding is usually a ruptured aneurysm. In about 85% of patients, the aneurysm is a congenital intracranial saccular aneurysm. The bleeding can resolve without treatment in some patients. Less common causes include **arteriovenous malformations**, bleeding disorders, and mycotic aneurysms.

Clinical Manifestations

A hemorrhagic stroke usually starts with a sudden headache, commonly occurring during physical activity. The headache can be mild or absent in older patients. Often, the patient loses consciousness in only a few seconds or minutes. Other common symptoms include delirium, focal or generalized seizures, nausea, and vomiting. The neurologic deficits are usually sudden and very progressive. Extensive hemorrhages in the brain hemispheres cause hemiparesis. If they occur in the posterior fossa, cerebellar or brainstem deficits arise. These include conjugate eye deviation, ophthalmoplegia, pinpoint pupils, breathing that resembles snoring, and coma. In about 50% of patients, extensive hemorrhages are fatal in a few days. Those who survive experience a return to consciousness. Neurologic deficits slowly reduce as extravasated blood is resorbed. Since bleeding is not as destructive to brain tissue as an infarction, some patients have only a few neurologic deficits. If the bleeding is minor, there may be focal deficits but no impairment of consciousness. Headache or nausea may be only very slight. These hemorrhages can mimic an ischemic stroke.

With subarachnoid bleeding, the patient's headache is usually extreme and peaks within a few seconds. They may lose consciousness. This is usually immediate but can occur after several hours. Severe neurologic deficits may occur, becoming irreversible in minutes to several hours. Sensory function may be impaired. The patient may become very restless, and seizures can occur. Unless there is herniation of the cerebellar tonsils, the patient's neck is usually not stiff. Even so, aseptic meningitis causes moderate to severe meningismus within 1 day. There is generally vomiting and occasionally bilateral extensor plantar responses. There are often abnormalities in the heart or respiratory rates. During the first 5–10 days, continuing headaches, confusion, and fever are frequently seen. If there is secondary hydrocephalus, the patient may experience additional headaches, motor deficits, and obtundation over weeks. If another bleed occurs, symptoms or new ones can recur.

Diagnosis

The diagnosis of hemorrhagic stroke is based on sudden headaches, focal neurologic deficits, and, especially in high-risk patients, reduced consciousness. An intracerebral hemorrhage must be distinguished from hypoglycemia, ischemic stroke, subarachnoid hemorrhage, and seizures. Immediate blood glucose level measurement, like a quick CT or MRI, is required. Diagnosis is usually done via neuroimaging. A lumbar puncture is necessary if no bleeding is seen, but a subarachnoid hemorrhage is clinically suspected. Within hours of bleeding start, CT angiography can reveal areas where the contrast agent extravasates into the clot–a *spot sign*. This indicates continuing bleeding. The hematoma is likely to expand, worsening the outcome.

The diagnosis of subarachnoid hemorrhage is based on the symptoms. Testing must be done quickly before irreversible damage occurs. A non-contrast CT is done within 6 hours of the onset of symptoms. An MRI is just as sensitive but less likely to be available quickly. If the blood volume is small or the patient is extremely frail, with the blood being isodense with brain tissues, false-negative results can occur. When subarachnoid hemorrhage is suspected by not being seen on imaging or if neuroimaging is not available immediately, a lumbar puncture is done. This procedure is contraindicated if there is suspicion of increased intracranial pressure since a sudden decrease in cerebrospinal fluid (CSF) pressure can reduce the tamponade of a clot upon the ruptured aneurysm, resulting in additional bleeding. If subarachnoid bleeding occurs, the CSF findings include excessive RBCs, increased pressure, and **xanthochromia**.

However, RBCs in the CSF can be due to a traumatic lumbar puncture. If the RBC count is lower in CSF tubes drawn sequentially, this is suspected.

Treatment

Treating hemorrhagic stroke involves supportive measures plus control of all modifiable risk factors. Antiplatelet drugs and anticoagulants cannot be used. If the patient has taken anticoagulants previously, their effects are sometimes reversible by using fresh frozen plasma, prothrombin complex concentrate, platelet transfusions, or vitamin K. The drug called dabigatran can be 60% removed via hemodialysis. If the systolic BP is 150–220 mm Hg, it can be safely lowered to 140 mm Hg if acute antihypertensive treatment is not contraindicated for the patient. When a patient has a systolic BP higher than 220 mm Hg, a continuous intravenous (IV) infusion of an antihypertensive is aggressively administered. This requires close monitoring of systolic BP. Nicardipine is given first, increasing in dosage every 5 minutes as needed to reduce systolic BP by 10%–15%.

A midline shift or herniation can occur if a cerebellar hemisphere hematoma is more than 3 cm in diameter. Surgical evacuation often saves the patient's life. If done early for a large lobar cerebral hematoma, the outcome may be equally as successful, though rebleeding is common and may increase the neurologic deficits. Early evacuation of a deep cerebral hematoma is usually not indicated since the death rate is high during surgery, and the neurologic deficits are often severe. Antiseizure drugs are generally only used if a seizure has occurred and not as prophylactic agents.

For subarachnoid hemorrhage, comprehensive stroke centers offer the best available treatment. Hypertension is only treated if the mean arterial pressure exceeds 130 mm Hg. Intravenous nicardipine is titrated in the same way as for intracerebral hemorrhage. The patient is confined to bed rest, and there is symptomatic treatment for headaches and restlessness. Anticoagulants and antiplatelet drugs are avoided. Oral nimodipine is given every 4 hours for 21 days to prevent vasospasm. However, the BP must be kept in the desired range, usually 120–185 mm Hg systolic. Also, with an accessible aneurysm, surgery can allow it to be clipped or stented. This is especially preferred if the patient has an evacuated hematoma or acute hydrocephalus. When the patient can be aroused from unconsciousness, neurosurgeons usually operate within the first 24 hours.

Prevention

Hemorrhagic stroke is linked to chronic hypertension, so controlling BP is a critical way to reduce the risks of the condition's development. This involves managing stress, consuming a healthy diet, limiting alcohol intake, exercising regularly, avoiding smoking, and controlling diabetes mellitus. Treatment of other causative conditions can also prevent an intracerebral hemorrhage. Once intracerebral bleeding has occurred, the initial goals of treatment are to avoid the extension of the bleeding and to prevent and manage secondary brain injury as well as other complications.

YOU SHOULD REMEMBER

The recovery period of a hemorrhagic stroke is extended for many people, lasting for months or even years. However, most people with small strokes and no additional complications during the hospital stay can function well enough to live at home within weeks.

Check Your Knowledge

1. What vessels constitute the main blood supply and drainage from the head and neck?
2. What is the description of a hemorrhagic stroke?
3. How does a hemorrhagic stroke begin, and what are its other common symptoms?

ISCHEMIC STROKE

An ischemic stroke occurs when a blood clot blocks or narrows an artery leading to the brain. A blood clot often forms in arteries damaged by the buildup of plaques. It can occur in the carotid artery of the neck as well as other arteries. This is the most common type of stroke. Sudden neurologic deficits occur because of focal cerebral ischemia. This relates to permanent brain infarction, which can be positively determined via diffusion-weighted MRI.

Epidemiology

Globally, 1 in 4 adults over 25 years old will have a stroke in their lifetime. The 12.2 million people worldwide will have their first stroke this year, and 6.5 million will die. Over 110 million people in the world have experienced strokes. There were over 9.5 million new cases of ischemic stroke in 2016. However, over 67.5 million people either had a recent ischemic stroke or had one previously. Nearly 60% of these occurred among people younger than 70. Approximately 61% of people living with complications of an ischemic stroke are under 70. About 52% of cases of ischemic stroke occurred in men and 48% in women. Every 40 seconds, someone in the United States has a stroke. Every 3.5 minutes, someone dies of a stroke. More than 795,000 people in the United States have a stroke each year. About 610,000 of these are first or new strokes. The 82% and 92% of strokes in the United States are ischemic. At earlier ages, ischemic stroke causes more mortality and morbidity in men, but this reverses for women who are elderly.

Etiology and Risk Factors

The most common causes of ischemic stroke, in descending order, include *atherothrombotic occlusion of large arteries*, cerebral embolism, which is also known as an embolic infarction, non-thrombotic occlusion of small and deep cerebral arteries, which is also known as a lacunar infarction, and proximal arterial stenosis accompanied by hypotension, which decreases cerebral blood flow within arterial areas described as **watershed zones**. Diabetes is a well-known modifiable risk factor for ischemic stroke.

The other risk factors include smoking, heavy drinking, high blood pressure, and high cholesterol. The risks of having a first stroke are nearly two times higher for African Americans than for Caucasians, and African Americans also have the highest rates of death from ischemic stroke. While overall death rates have been declining over decades, Hispanic Americans have recently seen an increase in death rates.

Clinical Manifestations

The signs and symptoms of an ischemic stroke are based on the damaged area of the brain. Neurologic deficits usually indicate which artery is affected, but not precisely. The abnormalities reach their maximal levels within only several minutes. This is typical of embolic strokes. In fewer cases, deficits evolve over 24–48 hours. This is called an *evolving stroke* and is usually an atherothrombotic stroke. In most evolving strokes, unilateral neurologic dysfunction develops without fever, headache, or pain. They often begin in one arm and spread **ipsilaterally**. There is usually a step-by-step progression with periods of stability. A stroke is referred to as *submaximal* when it is over, and later, there is some residual function in the area of ischemia, indicating some tissue that is still viable but at risk of being damaged.

Embolic strokes usually occur during the day and are often preceded by a headache and neurologic deficits. Thrombi occur more at night, with the outcome of the stroke seen upon awakening. Lacunar infarcts can cause classic syndromes that involve pure motor **hemiparesis**, ataxic hemiparesis, and pure sensory hemianesthesia. Aphasia and other signs of cortical dysfunction are not present. Multiple lacunar infarcts may cause multi-infarct dementia. As a stroke begins, a seizure can occur. This is more common with embolic strokes. Seizures can also occur after months or years. Late seizures are caused by hemosiderin deposition or scarring in the area of ischemia. If the patient's condition deteriorates in 48–72 hours after clinical symptom onset–primarily progressive impairment of consciousness–this is usually due to cerebral edema and not the infarct extending in size. Function usually improves in a few days unless an infarct is extensive. Additional improvement slowly occurs for up to as long as 1 year.

Diagnosis

The diagnosis of ischemic stroke is based on sudden neurologic deficits related to a particular artery's location. Ischemic stroke is distinguished from **stroke mimics,** which cause similar deficits. A CT or MRI is done to exclude intracerebral hemorrhage, epidural or subdural hematoma, or a tumor that is quickly growing or bleeding and causing symptoms. Within a few hours, there may be only subtle CT evidence of an ischemic stroke, even when it involves the sizable anterior circulation. There may be effacement of the sulci or insular cortical ribbon. The gray-white junction between the cerebral cortex and white matter can be lost. There may also be a density in the middle cerebral artery. Once there have been 6–12 hours of ischemia, hypodensities are visible, signifying medium to large infarcts. Smaller infarcts, such as lacunar infarcts, may only be seen via MRI. Highly sensitive to early ischemia, diffusion-weighted MRI can be performed immediately after the first CT.

For all presentations of acute stroke syndrome, CT angiography immediately following non-contrast head CT is recommended. Identifying the occluded intracranial vessel and evaluating the extracranial carotid, extracranial vertebral, aortic arch, and proximal great vessels is required to manage a transient ischemic attack and significant ischemic stroke, if not immediately, over the next several days. Although MRI has greater sensitivity for the small-volume ischemia observed in a transient ischemic attack or minor stroke, it is used only when there is no time pressure to offer treatment, typically as follow-up imaging.

Blood tests can be done when an ischemic stroke causes thrombotic disorders. Routine tests usually include a complete blood count (CBC), platelet count, fasting blood glucose, lipid profile, and prothrombin /partial thromboplastin time (PT/PTT). Other tests include homocysteine measurement, antiphospholipid antibodies, antinuclear antibodies, erythrocyte sedimentation rate, rheumatoid factor, hemoglobin electrophoresis, syphilis serologic testing, and urinalysis for amphetamines or cocaine.

Treatment

Treatments for acute ischemic strokes usually require hospitalization. During the first evaluation and stabilization, various supportive measures are often needed. These include the following:

- *For decreased consciousness or bulbar dysfunction compromising the airway* – ventilatory assistance and airway support
- *If there is a need to maintain oxygen saturation above 94%* – supplemental oxygen
- *To correct hyperthermia* – an antipyretic drug is used
- *To correct hypothermia* – its cause must be ascertained as being stroke-related and then treated
- Treating hypoglycemia or hyperglycemia to normalize blood glucose levels

The perfusion of an area of the brain with ischemia may require high BP since autoregulation is lost. Therefore, the BP is not decreased except if signs of other end-organ damage or recombinant tissue plasminogen activator (tPA) with or without mechanical thrombectomy are likely needed. Signs of further end-organ damage include acute MI, aortic dissection, hypertensive encephalopathy, pulmonary edema, acute renal failure, and retinal hemorrhages. Lowering the BP by 15% within 24 hours after the onset of the stroke is done if the BP is 220/120 mm Hg or higher on two readings taken 15 minutes apart. Suppose the patient is a good candidate for acute reperfusion therapy, but the BP is higher than 185/110 mm Hg. The BP can be treated by lowering it to less than this level with labetalol, nicardipine, or clevidipine. Nicardipine is given via IV infusion, increasing doses every 5–15 minutes. Labetalol is shown in an IV bolus over 1–2 minutes and can be repeated once. Clevidipine is provided via the same method, but the dose is titrated, doubling every 2–5 minutes to reach the desired BP.

Thrombolysis-in-situ is also known as angiographically-directed intraarterial thrombolysis. It is used for thrombi and emboli and may be used for significant strokes if the symptoms started less than 6 hours previously. This is mainly for strokes caused by large occlusions of the middle cerebral artery that cannot be treated with IV recombinant tPA. Up to 12 hours after the onset of symptoms, clots in the basilar artery can be intra-arterially lysed.

Mechanical thrombectomy is also called *angiographically-directed intraarterial removal of a thrombus or embolus*, which uses a *stent retriever* device. This is done in larger stroke centers if the patient has had a recent large-vessel occlusion within the anterior circulation. It is not used in place of IV recombinant tPA within 4.5 hours of symptom onset for eligible patients with acute ischemic stroke. The newer stent retrievers can reestablish perfusion in 90%–100% of cases. Today, clinical and imaging findings suggesting many tissues are at risk for infarction can justify mechanical thrombectomy later.

For the long-term treatment of ischemic stroke, supportive care is needed. This includes controlling hyperglycemia, limiting brain damage, and improving future functionality. Before the patient eats, drinks, or attempts to swallow an oral drug, there must be screening for dysphasia. This helps identify any risks for aspiration. A speech-language pathologist or another health care practitioner trained for this must perform the screening. After an acute stroke, enteral nutrition, if required, is started within 7 days after hospitalization. Early measures are taken to prevent the development of pressure ulcers. There must be attempts to avoid any secondary strokes. There is treatment for modifiable risk factors such as diabetes mellitus, hypertension, alcoholism, smoking, dyslipidemia, and obesity. Reduction of systolic BP may be more effective if the target BP is below 120 mm Hg instead of the standard level below 140 mm Hg.

With warfarin, antiplatelet drugs have additive effects that increase bleeding risks. Aspirin is sometimes used with warfarin, but only for some high-risk patients. Clopidogrel can be used if the patient is allergic to aspirin. While taking clopidogrel, if the patient has a recurrent ischemic stroke or a coronary artery stent becomes blocked, there must be suspicion of impaired clopidogrel metabolism. During acute treatment, clopidogrel with aspirin is only given for less than 3 months. This combination is given before 30 days after stenting, usually up to a maximum of 6 months. When a patient cannot tolerate clopidogrel, ticlopidine can be used.

Prevention

The prevention of ischemic stroke includes lifestyle changes such as quitting smoking, consuming moderate amounts of alcohol, keeping weight at a healthy level, following a cardiovascular-healthy diet, regularly participating in physical exercise, attending regular medical checkups, and preventing or treating underlying risk factors such as diabetes mellitus, hypertension, and hypercholesterolemia.

Check Your Knowledge

1. How does an ischemic stroke occur?
2. What are the most common causes of ischemic stroke?
3. What does the diagnosis of an ischemic stroke require?

Transient Ischemic Attack

A **transient ischemic attack** (TIA) involves symptoms of stroke that usually last for less than 1 hour. It is defined as focal brain ischemia with sudden neurologic deficits. There is no visualization of any acute cerebral infarction when evaluation is done with diffusion-weighted MRI. The condition is similar to an ischemic stroke, except that most TIAs last less than 5 minutes. If deficits resolve in 1 hour, infarction is extremely unlikely. Deficits resolving between 1 and 24 hours usually have an infarction. At this point, they are no longer considered to be TIAs. Within the first 24 hours, TIAs significantly increase the risk of having an actual stroke. Hypertensive patients with diabetes mellitus have an increased frequency of transient ischemic attacks.

Epidemiology

Most cases of transient ischemic attacks occur in middle-aged or older adults. Global estimates are varied. For example, the estimated prevalence in the United Kingdom for a first TIA is 50 per 100,000 people. Age-adjusted incidence rates of TIA are estimated to be 72.2 per 100,000 people globally. The mean age of TIA patients is 66 years. The occurrence of TIAs is nearly even between men and women. There is no specific racial group globally with significantly higher cases of TIAs. Up to 500,000 people in the United States experience a TIA every year, and the other statistics resemble the global data–older age and no significant male/female preference. However, since African Americans have more frequent and severe hypertension, they also have the highest TIAs.

Etiology and Risk Factors

Most transient ischemic attacks are caused by emboli that usually come from the carotid or vertebral arteries. Rarely, TIAs occur from impaired perfusion caused by severe hypoxemia, a lowered oxygen-carrying capacity of the blood, or increased viscosity–especially in arteries of the brain that have become stenotic. Reduced oxygen-carrying capacity in the blood may be caused by extreme anemia or carbon monoxide poisoning. Increased viscosity may be due to severe polycythemia. Cerebral ischemia is usually not caused by systemic hypotension unless intense or preexisting arterial stenosis exists. This is because autoregulation regulates blood flow in the brain to be nearly normal over widely ranging systemic blood pressure.

Modifiable risk factors for TIAs include cigarette smoking, diabetes mellitus, insulin resistance, dyslipidemia, hypertension, abdominal obesity, excessive alcohol use, insufficient physical activity, a diet high in saturated and trans fats as well as calories, depression, and other psychosocial stress, acute myocardial infarction (MI), atrial fibrillation, infective endocarditis, hypercoagulability, and vasculitis from the use of amphetamines or cocaine. Unmodifiable risk factors for TIAs include a family history of stroke, the male gender, older age, and a previous stroke.

Clinical Manifestations

With a transient ischemic attack, the neurologic deficits resemble those of strokes. **Amaurosis fugax** is temporary blindness in one eye. This usually lasts less than 5 minutes and can occur if the TIA damages the ophthalmic artery. Symptoms of TIAs begin quickly. They commonly last between 2 and 30 minutes and then completely resolve. It is possible for an individual to have several TIAs per day or to have just 2–3 TIAs over several years.

Diagnosis

Transient ischemic attacks are diagnosed after they occur, based on the sudden neurologic deficits that indicate ischemia in an artery yet resolve within 1 hour. A TIA is not likely if the patient has isolated peripheral palsy of a facial nerve and impaired consciousness or unconsciousness. They must be distinguished from conditions that cause similar symptoms, including hypoglycemia, migraine's aura, and postictal (Todd) paralysis. Neuroimaging is needed since small hemorrhages, infarcts, and mass lesions cannot be clinically excluded. In most facilities, a CT is more immediately available. Unfortunately, CT sometimes cannot visualize an infarct for more than 24 hours. Therefore, an MRI can be used to detect evolving infarcts within hours. Though not always available, a diffusion-weighted MRI is the best method to rule out infarcts if a TIA is suspected.

The cause of a TIA is evaluated the same way as the reasons for ischemic strokes. There are tests for cardiac sources of emboli, carotid stenosis, atrial fibrillation, and hematologic abnormalities. These tests include transesophageal echocardiography, transthoracic echocardiography, cardiac CT angiography, 24-hour Holter monitoring, ultrasonography, magnetic resonance angiography, electrocardiography, event recording (also called event monitoring), implantable loop recorders, and blood tests. Stroke risk factors are screened. Evaluation continues quickly, usually with the patient being hospitalized, since the risks of an ischemic stroke are very high and often happen quickly. A patient's discharge must be carefully determined because it can be challenging to decide on the safety of doing so. Within the first 24–48 hours, the risk of a stroke, whether major or minor, is highest. If a stroke is suspected to be likely, the patient is usually admitted for evaluation and telemetry.

Treatment

The treatment of a TIA focuses on stroke prevention, using antiplatelet drugs and statins. For some patients with a high risk of stroke but no neurologic deficits, carotid endarterectomy, arterial angioplasty, and stenting can be practical. If there are cardiac sources of emboli, anticoagulation is needed. Stroke may be prevented by modifying risk factors, if this is possible.

Prevention

The best way to prevent a transient ischemic attack is to eat a healthy diet, exercise regularly, avoid smoking, and avoid excessive alcohol use. Good management of diabetes mellitus is also an essential method of preventing TIA. Anything that reduces the likelihood of developing atherosclerosis, hypertension, and high cholesterol helps prevent a TIA. If a TIA has already occurred, these changes help reduce the risk of a recurring TIA or an actual stroke.

YOU SHOULD REMEMBER

Subclavian steal syndrome involves a subclavian artery stenosed proximal to the start of the vertebral artery. The stenosed artery "steals" blood from the vertebral artery, causing blood flow to become reversed. Since the vertebral artery supplies the arms during physical exertion, there are signs of vertebrobasilar ischemia. Sometimes, a TIA can occur in a child with an extreme cardiovascular disorder, producing emboli or high hematocrit levels.

Check Your Knowledge

1. How long do most transient ischemic attacks last?
2. What are the modifiable risk factors for TIAs?
3. What does the treatment of a TIA involve?

COMPLICATIONS OF STROKE

The most common complications of the various types of stroke include encephalitis, seizures (common in larger strokes), cognitive impairment, depression, deep venous thrombosis, spasticity and hypertonicity, bedsores, hemiplegic shoulder pain, and urinary tract infections. Despite declining mortality from stroke, the annual incidence in the general population is increasing. For many stroke survivors and their families, acute stroke begins an ongoing struggle with physical impairment and subsequent disability. Over time, the immediate clinical consequences of the stroke are complicated by a variety of lesser-known medical, musculoskeletal, and psychosocial difficulties. The primary care physician is best positioned to optimize chronic disease control, reduce risk, and manage stroke complications. Early screening and appropriate management are essential. Instituting secondary prevention and attention to bowel and bladder problems can help reduce medical complications and readmissions. At the same time, adequate analgesia, positioning/splinting of limbs, and physiotherapy can lessen discomfort and prevent suffering. Primary care physicians can identify and treat post-stroke mood issues and involve psychological counseling for patients and caregivers. Adequate education and support may restore the independence of patients with strokes or minimize any resultant dependency.

Clinical Case Studies

CLINICAL CASE STUDY 1

A 52-year-old woman experienced a severe headache and collapsed at work. She was hospitalized, still unconscious. A CT scan revealed bleeding into the left parietal region. Cerebral angiography was performed to detect the cause of the sudden bleeding. There was an intracranial arteriovenous malformation that had ruptured. The bleed was likely to cause severe impairment of the patient's speech, comprehension, and right-sided body movements. Though surgery for this type of stroke can be extremely risky, the surgical team decided to evacuate the clot and excise the arteriovenous malformation. The brain was highly swollen after achieving complete microscopic excision of the arteriovenous malformation and clot evacuation. Hence, the bone flap used for access was not immediately replaced, allowing the brain to swell out to relieve pressure. The patient slowly recovered over a few weeks; fortunately, there were no neurological or movement deficits. The bone flap was replaced, and a follow-up angiography was routine.

1. Where do hemorrhagic strokes usually occur?
2. What are arteriovenous malformations?
3. What are the outcomes of extensive hemorrhages in the brain hemispheres?

CLINICAL CASE STUDY 2

A 65-year-old man presented to the emergency department with blurred vision, confusion, loss of balance, and difficulty speaking. He was transferred to the intensive care unit. Laboratory tests revealed a prolonged prothrombin time and elevated fibrinogen levels. There was central facial palsy on the left side, dysarthria, and facial drop, as well as total paralysis of the ipsilateral upper and lower limbs. A CT scan revealed lesions consistent with those of an ischemic stroke.

CRITICAL THINKING QUESTIONS

1. What causes an ischemic stroke?
2. How does a stroke occur?
3. What are the complications of strokes?

CLINICAL CASE STUDY 3

A 63-year-old woman experienced right-sided arm and leg weakness and could not explain what she was feeling to her husband. The patient was brought to the emergency department and evaluated by a neurologist, who ordered a CT scan and admitted her for observation. The imaging revealed that the patient had experienced a TIA. Soon after, the patient was discharged and given a variety of medications to prevent any possible more severe ischemic stroke. She continued to experience dysphasia and tingling in her extremities but no other symptoms.

CRITICAL THINKING QUESTIONS

1. What does a TIA involve?
2. What are most TIAs caused by?
3. How is the cause of a TIA evaluated?

FURTHER READING

1. Alexandrov, A.V., and Hacke, W. (2011). *Cerebrovascular Ultrasound in Stroke Prevention and Treatment*, 2nd Edition. Wiley-Blackwell.
2. Behrouz, R., and Birnbaum, L.A. (2019). *Complications of Acute Stroke: A Concise Guide to Prevention, Recognition, and Management*. Demos Medical.
3. Bendok, B.R., Naidech, A.M., Walker, M.T., and Batjer, H.H. (2011). *Hemorrhagic and Ischemic Stroke: Medical, Imaging, Surgical, and Interventional Approaches*. Thieme.
4. Bhalla, A., and Birns, J. (2015). *Management of Post-Stroke Complications*. Springer.
5. Boccardi, E., Cenzato, M., Curto, F., Longoni, M., Motto, C., Oppo, V., Perini, V., and Vidale, S. (2017). *Hemorrhagic Stroke: Emergency Management in Neurology*. Springer.
6. Buijck, B., and Ribbers, G. (2018). *The Challenges of Nursing Stroke Management in Rehabilitation Centres*. Springer.
7. Daniels, S.K., Huckabee, M.L., and Gozdzikowska, K. (2019). *Dysphagia Following Stroke (Clinical Dysphagia)*, 3rd Edition. Plural Publishing, Inc.
8. Ferenbach, M.J., and Herring, S.W. (2020). *Illustrated Anatomy of the Head and Neck*, 6th Edition. Elsevier/Saunders.
9. Gill, S.K., Brown, M.M., Robertson, F., and Losseff, N. (2015). *Stroke Medicine: Case Studies from Queen Square*. Springer.

10. Godefroy, O. (2013). *The Behavioral and Cognitive Neurology of Stroke*, 2nd Edition. Cambridge University Press.
11. Gupta, V.K., and Dubey, S. (2021). *Stroke: Cerebrovascular Accident (CVA)*. Lap Lambert Academic Publishing.
12. Hacein-Bey, L. (2018). *Ischemic Stroke, an Issue of Neuroimaging Clinics of North America (The Clinics: Radiology Book 28)*. Elsevier.
13. Harrigan, M.R., and Deveikis, J.P. (2018). *Handbook of Cerebrovascular Disease and Neurointerventional Technique*, 3rd Edition. Humana Press.
14. Lau, G.K.K., Pendlebury, S.T., and Rothwell, P.M. (2018). *Transient Ischemic Attack and Stroke: Diagnosis, Investigation and Treatment*, 2nd Edition. Cambridge University Press.
15. Mohr, J.P., Wolf, P.A., Grotta, J.C., Moskowitz, M.A., Mayberg, M., and von Kummer, R. (2011). *Stroke: Pathophysiology, Diagnosis, and Management*, 5th Edition. Elsevier.
16. Mokin, M., Levy, E.I., and Siddiqui, A.H. (2022). *Video Atlas of Acute Ischemic Stroke Intervention*. Thieme.
17. Norvving, B. (2014). *Oxford Textbook of Stroke and Cerebrovascular Disease (Textbooks in Clinical Neurology)*. Oxford University Press.
18. Pendlebury, S.T., Giles, M.F., and Rothwell, P.M. (2011). *Transient Ischemic Attack and Stroke: Diagnosis, Investigation and Management*. Cambridge University Press.
19. Stein, J., Harvey, R.I., Winstein, C.J., Zorowitz, R.D., and Wittenberg, G.F. (2014). *Stroke Recovery and Rehabilitation*, 2nd Edition. Demos Medical.

11 Hereditary Lipid Disorders

OVERVIEW

Hereditary lipid disorders include Niemann-Pick disease, Tay-Sachs disease, and Gaucher disease. Oils, fatty acids, waxes, and cholesterol are the various forms of lipids. A lack of specific enzymes causes hereditary lipid disorders to break down lipids, or the enzymes may not work correctly, meaning that the body cannot convert fats into energy. A harmful amount of lipids then builds up in the body. Over time, there is damage to cells and tissues, especially in the brain, peripheral nervous system, liver, spleen, and bone marrow. Many of these disorders can be very serious or even fatal. Dyslipidemias are a heterogeneous group of disorders characterized by abnormal levels of circulating lipids and lipoproteins. These abnormalities include hypercholesterolemia and hypertriglyceridemia. Their causes are complex and encompass rare monogenic disorders ranging from single-gene defects to complex polygenic basis. Monogenic hypercholesterolemias are a group of single-gene defects with Mendelian transmission. They are characterized by elevated low-density lipoprotein, cholesterol, and a high risk of premature atherosclerotic disease.

NIEMANN-PICK DISEASE

Niemann-Pick disease (NPD) is a group of autosomal recessive disorders involving splenomegaly, variable neurologic deficits, and the storage of lipids, including **sphingomyelin** and cholesterol. It is a rare, inherited disease that affects the ability to metabolize lipids within cells, causing them to malfunction and die. Affected individuals have an abnormal lipid metabolism that causes a buildup of harmful amounts of lipids in various organs. The Niemann-Pick disease primarily affects the brain, nerves, bone marrow, liver, spleen, and, in severe cases, the lungs. The disease has four types: A, B, C1, and C2. Initially, there was a type D, but research found it was a variant of type C (C1, C2).

EPIDEMIOLOGY

Niemann-Pick disease (types A and B) is estimated to affect 1 in 250,000 individuals. Niemann-Pick disease type A occurs more frequently among individuals of Ashkenazi (eastern and central European) Jewish descent than in the general population. The incidence within the Ashkenazi population is approximately 1 in 40,000 individuals. Combined, Niemann-Pick disease types C1 and C2 are estimated to affect 1 in 150,000 individuals; however, type C1 is the more common type, accounting for 95% of cases. The disease occurs more frequently in people of French-Acadian descent in Nova Scotia. In Nova Scotia, one population of affected French-Acadians was previously designated as having Niemann-Pick disease type D. However; it was later discovered that these individuals have **mutations** in the gene associated with Niemann-Pick disease type C1.

ETIOLOGY AND RISK FACTORS

Niemann-Pick disease (types A and B) is caused by gene mutations that provide instructions for producing an enzyme called *acid sphingomyelinase*. Mutations in either the NPC1 or NPC2 genes cause Niemann-Pick disease type C. The proteins produced by these genes are involved in the movement of lipids within cells. Mutations in these genes lead to a need for more functional proteins.

DOI: 10.1201/9781003453376-14

This prevents the movement of cholesterol and other lipids, leading to their accumulation in cells. Because these lipids are not correctly located in the cells, many normal cell functions that require lipids (such as cell membrane formation) are impaired. The accumulation of lipids and cellular dysfunction eventually leads to cell death, causing tissue and organ damage in Niemann-Pick disease types C1 and C2.

Risk factors include having other family members with the disease. Types A and B develop in people of Ashkenazi Jewish heritage, while type C develops in people of Nova Scotia, French-Canadian, or Spanish-American descent. Affected organs, symptoms, and treatments vary based on the type of Niemann-Pick disease. However, every class is severe and can shorten its lifespan.

CLINICAL MANIFESTATIONS

The signs and symptoms of the type A form of Niemann-Pick disease are present within the first few months of life. They include the following:

- Swelling of the abdomen (due to hepatomegaly and splenomegaly), which usually occurs around 3–6 months of age
- A cherry-red spot inside the eye
- Brain damage
- Difficulty feeding
- Hepatosplenomegaly (see **Figure 11.1**)
- Fail to gain weight and grow
- Difficulty performing basic motor skills
- Frequent respiratory infections
- Widespread lung damage (interstitial lung disease)
- Poor muscle tone
- Swollen lymph nodes

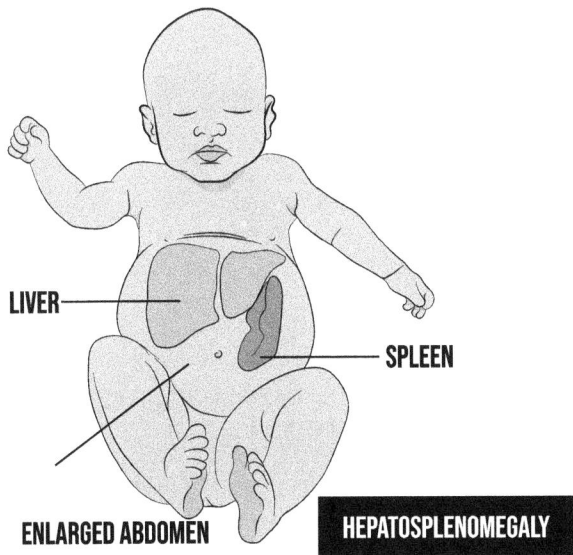

FIGURE 11.1   Hepatosplenomegaly, as part of Niemann-Pick disease.

The type B form of Niemann-Pick disease symptoms usually appear in late childhood or adolescence and typically survive into adulthood. Type B does not include the motor difficulties commonly found in type A. The signs and symptoms of type B may consist of:

- Swelling of the abdomen from enlargement of the liver and spleen, which often begins in early childhood
- Delayed growth (or failure to develop at an average rate), causing short stature as well as eye abnormalities
- High levels of blood lipids
- Low blood platelets
- Lung problems
- Mental retardation
- Dystonia
- Ataxic gait
- Vertical supranuclear gaze palsy
- Poor coordination
- Psychiatric disorders
- Respiratory infections

Symptoms of the type C form of Niemann-Pick disease usually appear around 5 years of age. However, type C can occur at any time in a person's life. The signs and symptoms of type C include:

- Difficulty moving limbs
- A decline in intellect
- A loss of muscular functioning
- A loss of vision or hearing
- An enlarged spleen or liver
- Brain damage
- Clumsiness
- Dementia
- Difficulty learning
- Difficulty moving the eyes, especially in up and down directions
- Difficulty speaking and swallowing
- Difficulty walking
- Jaundice, or yellowing of the skin after birth
- Seizures
- Tremors
- Unsteadiness

The symptoms of the type E form of Niemann-Pick disease occur in adults. This type is rare and has limited research, but the signs and symptoms include swelling of the spleen or brain and neurological problems, including swelling within the nervous system.

Diagnosis

The diagnosis of Niemann-Pick disease begins with a thorough physical exam, which can show an early warning sign such as an enlarged liver or spleen. A detailed medical history is also taken, and symptoms and family health history are discussed.

TREATMENT

Since there is currently no cure for Niemann-Pick disease, treatment is only supportive. Children usually die from an infection or progressive neurological loss. Bone marrow transplantation has been done for a few patients with type B disease, but the results were only mixed.

PREVENTION

There is no way to prevent Niemann-Pick disease because it is entirely hereditary. Even so, early diagnosis and proper treatment can improve life expectancy for some people with type B or C.

YOU SHOULD REMEMBER

The Niemann-Pick disease affects the body's ability to metabolize cholesterol and lipids in the cells. It can affect the brain, bone marrow, liver, lungs, and spleen. Type A occurs mainly in infants and usually causes death within a few years. Type B occurs later in childhood, and many people survive to adulthood. Type C is not as expected, but it eventually affects the brain.

Check Your Knowledge

1. Which organs in the body are primarily affected by Niemann-Pick disease?
2. Which is the most common type of Niemann-Pick disease?
3. What are the differences between type A and B Niemann-Pick disease?

TAY-SACHS DISEASE

Tay-Sachs disease is a rare genetic disorder passed down from parents to their children. It develops without the beta-hexosaminidase A enzyme, which is required to break down GM2 ganglioside. The enzyme helps break down **gangliosides**, which are fatty substances. When gangliosides build up to toxic levels in the CSN, the function of nerve cells is affected.

EPIDEMIOLOGY

Approximately one in every 27 Ashkenazi Jews in the United States carries the gene for Tay-Sachs disease. Non-Jewish French Canadians living near the St. Lawrence River and in the Cajun community of Louisiana also have a higher incidence. In the general population, about one in 250 people is a carrier.

ETIOLOGY AND RISK FACTORS

Tay-Sachs disease is caused by the lack of an enzyme needed to help break down **gangliosides**, which build up toxic levels in the central nervous system, affecting nerve cell function. Risk factors include having ancestors from any group with the highest disease incidence.

CLINICAL MANIFESTATIONS

In the most common and severe form, signs and symptoms start at about 3–6 months of age. With disease progression, development slows, and the muscles begin to weaken. Over time, this causes seizures, paralysis, vision and hearing loss, and other significant abnormalities. Children with this form typically live only a few years. Less often, some children have the juvenile form of the disease and may live until 10 years old. In rare cases, adults may have a late-onset form of Tay-Sachs disease, which is often less severe.

DIAGNOSIS

A thorough clinical evaluation and specialized tests confirm the diagnosis of Tay-Sachs disease. These include blood tests to measure the enzyme activity levels of hexosaminidase A. Molecular genetic testing for mutations in the HEXA gene is confirmative.

TREATMENT

Tay-Sachs disease is not curable. No treatments slow the disease's progression. Treatment goals focus on support and comfort, including medications, nutrition, respiratory care, hydration, occupational and physical therapy, and speech/language therapy. Antibiotics and anti-seizure medications may be required. Chest physiotherapy, exercise, and other techniques may help remove lung mucus. Also, drugs can be used to reduce saliva production. Positioning techniques minimize the risk of mucus accumulation, preventing aspiration pneumonia. Some patients require a nasogastric feeding tube or gastrostomy. Physical therapy helps delay joint stiffness. It reduces or delays the loss of function and pain from affected muscles. Occupational therapists often recommend activities and supportive devices. Speech and language therapists can assist with swallowing problems.

PREVENTION

There is no way to prevent Tay-Sachs disease because it is inherited. Genetic testing should be done before any pregnancies if there is a family history.

YOU SHOULD REMEMBER

Though Tay-Sachs is a fatal disease, there is some hope concerning it. Even if both parents are carriers, there is a one in four chance that a child will not be a carrier and won't have the disease.

GAUCHER DISEASE

Gaucher disease is a rare, inherited metabolic disorder in which a fat molecule called **glucocerebroside** accumulates in different organs and tissues in the body. Organs such as the spleen and liver enlarge and become dysfunctional. The fatty substances can also build up in bones, weakening them and increasing the risk of fractures. Gaucher's disease affects multiple organs and bones. More rarely, Gaucher disease affects the brain, which can cause abnormal eye movements, muscle rigidity, swallowing difficulties, and seizures. One rare subtype of Gaucher disease begins in infancy and typically results in death by 2 years of age. There are three types of Gaucher disease, as follows:

- *Type 1* is the most common type of disease reported in Western countries. It is a non-neuropathic form of the disease and is usually treatable. It affects bones and multiple organs, but the severity of the symptoms varies.

- *Type 2* is also called acute infantile neuronopathic Gaucher disease, a severe form that is usually fatal within 2 years of birth.
- *Type 3*, also called chronic neuronopathic Gaucher disease, is the most common worldwide, especially in India, the Pacific Rim, China, and the Middle East. The onset usually occurs later than in type 2 and progresses slowly into adulthood.

EPIDEMIOLOGY

The prevalence of Gaucher disease ranges from 0.70 to 1.75 per 100,000 individuals. However, the majority is higher in individuals with Ashkenazi Jewish ethnicity, with a birth incidence of approximately 1 in 850. Gaucher disease affects 1 in every 50,000–100,000 people in the general population. Type 1 is the most common disorder in Canada, Europe, Israel, and the United States.

ETIOLOGY AND RISK FACTORS

A problem with the GBA gene causes Gaucher disease, which is an autosomal recessive disorder. Each parent must pass along an abnormal GBA gene for their child to have the condition. Risk factors include being from any group with a higher disease incidence. The mutation either results in small amounts of the enzyme or its complete absence.

CLINICAL MANIFESTATIONS

Signs and symptoms include **anemia**, easy bruising, epistaxis, fatigue, and an abnormal reduction in the number of platelets. Splenomegaly and hepatomegaly develop in about 90% of Gaucher disease Type 1 patients. The fatty substances that form due to this disease can also build up in bone tissue. This occurrence weakens bones and increases the risk of fractures. It is often mild, affecting children as well as adults.

DIAGNOSIS

Gaucher disease is diagnosed with a blood test to assess enzyme levels. Carriers can be determined via a blood or saliva DNA test. The majority (68%) of patients are diagnosed between the ages of infancy and 10 years. Gaucher disease can present as **hydrops** in the perinatal period, and it must be considered a differential diagnosis of any hydrops in pregnancy.

TREATMENT

Treatments for Gaucher's disease include medications and surgery. Intravenous enzyme replacement therapy is given on an outpatient basis. Medications include eliglustat, miglustat, and osteoporosis drugs. When symptoms are severe and the patient is not a candidate for less-invasive treatments, a bone marrow transplant or splenectomy may be needed.

PREVENTION

There is no way to prevent Gaucher disease if the causative gene mutations exist. However, for at-risk individuals, genetic testing is essential since early treatment may prevent damage to bones and organs from Gaucher disease type 1. Genetic counseling concerning pregnancy is needed if a DNA test reveals a person to be a carrier.

YOU SHOULD REMEMBER

The mean life expectancy of patients with Gaucher disease type 1 is 68.2 years at birth. This is within a range of 63.9 years for splenectomized patients and 72.0 years for non-splenectomized patients.

Check Your Knowledge

1. When do clinical manifestations of Tay-Sachs disease begin?
2. What is the prevalence of Gaucher disease?
3. How is Gaucher's disease diagnosed?

GANGLIOSIDOSES

Gangliosidoses are a group of inherited metabolic diseases caused by a deficiency of different proteins required to break down lipids. Abnormal lipid buildup can permanently damage cells and tissues in the nervous system and other areas, including the liver and spleen. The disease is characterized by a generalized accumulation of GM1 ganglioside, oligosaccharides, and the mucopolysaccharide called keratan sulfate and its derivatives. It causes irreversible damage to cells in the nervous system, particularly the brain and spinal cord.

There are two distinct types of gangliosidoses, labeled GM1 and GM2, affecting males and females equally, as follows:

- *A deficiency of the enzyme beta-galactosidase causes GM1 gangliosidoses*; there are three clinical subtypes:
  - *Early infantile GM1 gangliosidosis is* the most severe form. Onset is shortly after birth. Complications include enlargement of the liver and spleen, joint stiffness, skeletal abnormalities, and a distended abdomen. Affected children may be blind and deaf by 1 year of age. They often die by age three from cardiac complications or pneumonia. Symptoms include cherry-red spots in the eyes, muscle weakness, nerve function degeneration, problems walking, and seizures.
  - *Late-infantile GM1 gangliosidosis is* – usually first seen between 1 and 3 years of age. Symptoms include an inability to coordinate movements, dementia, difficulties with speech, and seizures.
  - *Adult GM1 gangliosidosis* develops between 3 and 30 years of age. Complications include corneal cloudiness, muscle wasting, and **dystonia**. This form is usually less severe than the others and progresses more slowly.
- *GM2 gangliosidoses* – include Tay-Sachs disease and its severe form known as Sandhoff disease, both due to a deficiency of beta-hexosaminidase

EPIDEMIOLOGY

Gangliosidoses are rare disorders, and their incidence data are poorly understood. The estimated incidence is 1 of every 100,000–200,000 live births. The Tay-Sachs variant of GM2 gangliosidosis has a prevalence of 1 in 201,000 live births and an incidence of 1 in 222,000 live births. GM1 gangliosidosis occurs most commonly in the Maltese Islands (1 in 3,700), in people of Roma ancestry (1 in 10,000), and in Brazil (1 in 17,000).

ETIOLOGY AND RISK FACTORS

Gangliosidoses are caused by mutations in the GLB1 gene, resulting in a deficiency of the enzyme called *beta-galactosidase-1*, which lysosomes need to break down large sugar molecules within body cells. Risk factors include family history and being from one of the groups of people with the highest incidence and prevalence.

CLINICAL MANIFESTATIONS

Signs and symptoms of GM1 gangliosidoses include coarse facial features, hypotonia, hepatosplenomegaly, an exaggerated startle reaction, developmental regression, skeletal abnormalities, seizures, and visual impairment. Symptoms of GM2 gangliosidoses include slowed growth, a plateau of gross and fine motor development, developmental regression, hypotonia, an exaggerated **startle reaction**, seizures, visual impairment, hearing loss, and intellectual disability.

DIAGNOSIS

The diagnosis of GM1 gangliosidoses can be confirmed by measurement of acid beta-galactosidase activity in leukocytes. Patients with the infantile form have nearly no enzyme activity, while patients with the adult form may have residual activity at 5%–10% of reference values. Diagnosing GM2 gangliosidoses is aided by neuroimaging that reveals hyperdensity of the basal ganglia, which may be accompanied by other changes in the white matter and, sometimes, prominent yet non-specific cerebellar atrophy. A specific diagnosis requires the determination of HEXA and HEXB activities using artificial substrates. The diagnostic gold standard measures enzyme activity in leukocytes, **fibroblasts**, or **chorionic villi**.

TREATMENT

There are no specific treatments for gangliosidoses. Anticonvulsants can initially control seizures. Supportive therapies include hydration, proper nutrition, and keeping the airway open. Dietary restrictions do not prevent lipids from building up in the cells and tissues. For GM1, preventing irreversible neurological deficits is essential and requires an early diagnosis and management of the disease.

PREVENTION

There is currently no known way to prevent gangliosidoses.

YOU SHOULD REMEMBER

GM1 gangliosidosis is a rare condition that causes progressive degeneration of parts of the CNS. Early-onset forms are refined and usually fatal in childhood. This form is similar to Tay-Sachs disease and Sandhoff disease but is caused by different gene mutations and enzyme deficiencies. While GM1 has CNS and systemic findings, GM2 is mainly restricted to the CNS.

FARBER'S DISEASE

Farber's disease, also called *Farber's lipogranulomatosis*, is another rare, inherited lipid storage disease. Excess fat builds up in the joints, tissues, and CNS. Symptoms usually worsen over time, leading to a reduced lifespan. There are multiple subtypes, classified by severity and nervous system involvement.

EPIDEMIOLOGY

Farber's disease is sporadic, with fewer than 1,000 people in the United States having it. The overall estimated prevalence is less than 1 in 1,000,000 people. Most cases have been seen in India and the United States. Males and females are nearly equally affected.

ETIOLOGY AND RISK FACTORS

A deficiency of the enzyme ceramidase causes it. The disease is passed on to children when both parents are carriers, affecting males and females nearly equally. In its classic form, onset usually starts in infancy but can occur later in life. Risk factors are solely based on family history.

CLINICAL MANIFESTATIONS

Children with significant neurological involvement usually die early in infancy. In contrast, patients without or only mild neurological findings suffer from progressive joint deformation and contractures, subcutaneous lipogranulomas, a hoarse voice, and finally, respiratory insufficiency caused by granuloma formation in the respiratory tract and interstitial **pneumonitis,** leading to death in the third or fourth decade of life. Neurological signs and symptoms of Farber's disease include problems swallowing, increased sleepiness, lethargy, and impaired mental ability. In one of the most severe forms, hepatomegaly and splenomegaly can be diagnosed shortly after birth. Children with this form usually die within 6 months after birth.

DIAGNOSIS

The diagnosis of Farber's disease is confirmed by determining acid ceramidase activity measured in cultured skin fibroblasts, leukocytes, or amniocytes. It is done by demonstrating granulomas with macrophages that contain lipid cytoplasmic inclusions in subcutaneous nodules or by determination of ceramide accumulation. Clinical examination, assessment of symptoms, and testing of enzymes and genes are all performed.

TREATMENT

There is no specific treatment available. For pain, corticosteroids may be given. Bone marrow transplants may improve Granulomas in patients with little to no lung or nervous system complications. Older patients can have granulomas reduced or removed via surgery.

PREVENTION

Since no known prevention for Farber's disease or specific treatment exists, most children with the classic form die by age 2, usually from lung disease.

YOU SHOULD REMEMBER

Farber's disease develops when the N-acyl sphingosine *amidohydrolase 1 (ASAH1)* gene does not function normally and is inherited in an autosomal recessive pattern. As fat builds up, lipogranulomas and swollen, painful joints develop.

Check Your Knowledge

1. What are the two distinct types of gangliosidoses?
2. What are the signs and symptoms of GM1 gangliosidoses?
3. What are the neurological signs and symptoms of Farber's disease?

FABRY DISEASE

Fabry disease is an inherited neurological disorder resulting from the buildup of fat known as **globotriaosylceramide** in cells. It is also known as *alpha-galactosidase-A deficiency* and *Anderson-Fabry disease*. It increases the chances of having a heart attack, stroke, or kidney failure.

EPIDEMIOLOGY

The Fabry disease occurs in all ethnic, racial, and demographic groups. It affects approximately 1,500–4,000 males and about one in every 20,000 females. Children's mean age at the onset of this symptom is before 10 years. Data from newborn screening programs suggests that the incidence of Fabry disease is underestimated and may be higher than previously approximated.

ETIOLOGY AND RISK FACTORS

Fabry disease is a genetic condition in which affected children have a mutated gene on the X chromosome, one of two sex chromosomes in each cell. In males with a single X chromosome and a Y chromosome in each of their cells, there is a defective copy of alpha-galactosidase A (GLA), sufficient to cause Fabry disease. In females with two X chromosomes, there is a bad copy of the GLA. However, Fabry's disease will manifest only if this gene is on both of their X chromosomes. Combining a typical GLA gene on one X chromosome and a mutated GLA gene on the other X chromosome in females may result in less severe symptoms of Fabry disease. In rare cases, a female with one mutated GLA gene may have no signs or symptoms of Fabry disease. These women are called carriers, meaning their children can inherit the condition despite having no visible symptoms. Fabry disease is caused by insufficient production of normal GLA. This enzyme prevents sphingolipids from collecting in blood vessels and tissues. Risk factors for Fabry's disease are all related to family history.

CLINICAL MANIFESTATIONS

The Fabry disease starts in childhood, causing wide-ranging signs and symptoms. Characteristic features include episodes of numbness, burning or pain in the hands or feet, tingling, GI problems, heat or cold intolerance, **angiokeratomas**, a decreased ability to sweat, corneal vertillicata (opacity), tinnitus, and hearing loss. Kidney and heart disease and strokes may be observed in adults. Additional signs and symptoms include extreme pain during physical activity, dizziness, fatigue, fever, body aches, proteinuria, and edema of the legs, ankles, or feet.

DIAGNOSIS

The diagnosis of Fabry disease involves an enzyme assay, genetic testing, and newborn screenings. An enzyme assay measures the alpha-GAL enzyme in the blood, and a 1% or lower measurement indicates the disease. This test is most reliable for male patients. Since females with the condition may have normal enzyme levels, genetic testing is performed to identify the GLA gene mutation. Some states in the USA test newborns for lysosomal storage disorders such as Fabry disease, and the enzyme test is part of these routine newborn screenings.

TREATMENT

There is no cure for Fabry's disease. Treatment options include both Fabry-specific and non-Fabry-specific therapies. Treatment includes IV enzyme replacement therapy (agalsidase alfa and beta), oral chaperone therapy, and lifestyle modifications. Antihistamines are often given before these IV infusions to reduce the chance of infusion-related reactions, but they are sometimes given after the infusions. Migalastat is suitable for patients who have been tested and have gene mutations that will be responsive. At present, proteinuria and other therapies are treated to prolong kidney health.

PREVENTION

Fabry disease is inherited, so it cannot be prevented. However, an early diagnosis and multidisciplinary management can slow its progression and improve quality of life.

YOU SHOULD REMEMBER

Fabry disease is a severe genetic disorder that can lead to life-threatening heart and kidney problems. It is progressive and worsens over time. In the classic type, signs and symptoms start during childhood. In the atypical type, they begin in middle adulthood. Males usually have more severe symptoms.

KRABBE DISEASE

Krabbe disease (KD) is a rare hereditary metabolic lipid disorder that affects the brain, spinal cord, and nerves. Children with this disease are missing an important enzyme called galactocerebrosidase. This enzyme breaks down toxic chemicals in the body. Without it, toxic chemicals build up. This buildup can destroy myelin, the protective layer around the nerve cells in the body and brain. The nerves do not work correctly without this protective layer, and the brain is injured. Krabbe disease is also known as *globoid cell leukodystrophy* and usually appears during the first 6 months of life.

EPIDEMIOLOGY

In the United States, Krabbe disease affects about 1 in 100,000 individuals. A higher incidence (six cases per 1,000 people) has been reported in a few isolated communities in Israel. The mortality rate is as high as 90% in the first 2 years of life. The late-onset type has a better prognosis, and life expectancy is 5–7 years after the onset of symptoms. The average lifespan for children with infantile Krabbe disease is 13 months. Most children with late-infantile disease die within 2 years of the beginning of symptoms.

ETIOLOGY AND RISK FACTORS

Krabbe disease is another genetic disorder. It occurs when a child receives two abnormal genes from the parents, with one unnatural coming from each parent. Krabbe disease is caused by a lack of the galactosylceramidase enzyme, which helps manufacture and maintain the myelin that coats nerve cells and allows them to communicate. The disease passes from parents to children through an abnormal GALC gene; usually, the parents do not have any symptoms. Parents are considered "carriers" if they have one abnormal copy of the GALC gene and one regular document. Carriers do not have symptoms of Krabbe disease. A carrier parent has a 50% chance of passing on their abnormal copy of the GALC gene. If both parents are carriers, and both parents pass on the abnormal copy, a child will have the disease. There is a 25% chance that two carrier parents together will have a child with Krabbe disease. The only risk factors for developing Krabbe disease are parents, both carriers of the mutated gene.

CLINICAL MANIFESTATIONS

The inability to manufacture galactosylceramidase leads to a loss of myelin, followed by nerve damage. When the brain cannot send signals to the body, the symptoms of Krabbe disease manifest. The effects of this disease can be severe and lead to death. The symptoms of Krabbe disease begin in the first few months of life. They include muscle weakness, stiff limbs, loss of smiling or regular interaction, trouble walking, difficulty feeding, vision and hearing loss, muscle spasms, and seizures.

DIAGNOSIS

Many states in the U.S. include screening for Krabbe disease in a standard newborn screening protocol. The screening for Krabbe disease is a blood test. The condition is primarily diagnosed in infants less than 6 months of age. The other primary way to diagnose Krabbe disease is through imaging tests like MRIs. Children diagnosed with Krabbe disease need a hearing assessment and an eye examination to determine the degree of hearing and vision loss. This can determine what type of hearing and vision aids they need.

TREATMENT

Currently, there is no cure for Krabbe disease, which usually results in death. Hematopoietic stem cell transplants can slow the progression of Krabbe disease. This treatment helps the body replace unhealthy cells with healthy or normal cells. Hematopoietic cells are immature cells that can develop into all blood cells, including white blood cells, red blood cells, and platelets. However, treatments are available to help with a child's irritability, muscle stiffness, pain, seizures, and difficulty eating.

PREVENTION

As Krabbe disease is an inherited condition, nothing can help prevent it.

METACHROMATIC LEUKODYSTROPHY

Metachromatic leukodystrophy (MLD) is a rare hereditary lipid disorder that involves a buildup of fats called sulfatides in the cells, particularly in the brain, spinal cord, and peripheral nerves.

EPIDEMIOLOGY

The prevalence of metachromatic leukodystrophy ranges from 1 in 40,000 to 1 in 100,000 in the northern European and North American populations. The incidence is estimated to be 1 in 40,000 births in the United States of America. There is no sexual or racial predilection. The disease is categorized based on the age of onset.

ETIOLOGY AND RISK FACTORS

Metachromatic leukodystrophy is caused by a lack of the enzyme called *arylsulfatase A*, which usually breaks down sulfatides. When these fats build up in the white matter, where nerve fibers are contained, myelin is destroyed. The only risk factor for metachromatic leukodystrophy is having both parents as disease carriers.

CLINICAL MANIFESTATIONS

There are three types of MLD based on the age and symptoms that appear: late-infantile MLD, juvenile MLD, and adult MLD. All subtypes ultimately affect both intellectual and motor function. Symptoms vary by type but can include difficulty talking, seizures, difficulty walking, personality changes, and behavior and personality changes. MLD is caused by arylsulfatase-A (ARSA) or PSAP gene mutations. The symptoms include a loss of feeling in the hands and feet, seizures, trouble walking and talking, and vision or hearing loss.

DIAGNOSIS

A proper diagnosis confirms the deficiency of the missing enzyme and the resulting lowered arylsulfatase-A (ARSA) activity in the body. This diagnosis is verified and validated by several procedures, with the more common methods including blood testing, urine testing, and imaging studies.

TREATMENT

Though incurable, metachromatic leukodystrophy is treated to prevent nerve damage, slow disease progression, prevent complications, and provide supportive care. It is managed with medications (to reduce behavioral problems, seizures, sleeping difficulty, GI issues, infections, and pain), physical/occupational/speech therapy (to promote muscle and joint flexibility and maintain range of motion and functioning), nutritional assistance (to provide proper nutrition and assist with swallowing), and other treatments (wheelchairs, walkers, other assistive devices, mechanical ventilation, treatments for complications, and long-term care or hospitalization).

PREVENTION

There is no prevention or cure for metachromatic leukodystrophy, though clinical trials look promising for future treatments.

YOU SHOULD REMEMBER

Late-infantile MLD is characterized by normal development in the first 6–18 months. This is followed by a progressive regression that appears first in motor skills. The affected individual may never learn to walk or show deterioration of balance. The reversal will rapidly affect speech, overall mobility, and basic cognitive skills.

YOU SHOULD REMEMBER

Juvenile MLD is characterized by normal development with onset between ages 4 and 14 years. The beginning usually starts with either motor or cognitive symptoms, but typically not both. With motor progression, the first signs are often changes in gait (balance and walking). Mental passage usually begins with unexplainable behavioral outbursts, a lack of memory of recent events, an inability to follow simple sequences, and declining social skills. These skills continue to decline over 4–8 years, with a loss of continence control. Speech ability will also fall during this time.

YOU SHOULD REMEMBER

Adult MLD is characterized by normal development through puberty, presenting symptoms generally from the twenties through the forties. Similar to the juvenile cognitive form, the initial signs of adult-onset are often changes in mental abilities and personality. There may be poor school or work performance, anxiety, bewilderment, loss of alertness, disorganization, and poor judgment without or without declining memory. Often, this is compensated for by alcoholism or other similar behaviors. Cognition, speech, and balance/mobility skills regress along, with a loss of continence over the years.

Check Your Knowledge

1. When does Fabry's disease start to develop?
2. How much does Krabbe disease affect mortality?
3. What are the three types of metachromatic leukodystrophy?

CLINICAL CASE STUDY 1

A 38-year-old woman was diagnosed with Niemann-Pick disease type C. At the age of 8 years, she had coordination problems. By age 10, dystonia was present. By age 16, her academic performance had declined. Specialists suspected Niemann-Pick disease when the patient was 17, presenting with dystonia, ataxic gait, and vertical supranuclear gaze palsy. A brain MRI revealed atrophies of the frontal lobes, brainstem, and cerebellum—the patient presented with both hepatomegaly and splenomegaly. By age 26, a breathing tube was needed due to recurrent aspiration pneumonia, and the disease was officially diagnosed. Therapy with miglustat was undertaken, improving swallowing capacity and muscle tone.

CRITICAL THINKING QUESTIONS

1. What is Niemann-Pick disease?
2. What leads to cell death with Niemann-Pick disease?
3. What characterizes Niemann-Pick type C disease?

CLINICAL CASE STUDY 2

In 2022, the first-ever gene therapy for Tay-Sachs disease was given to two very young children. The treatment used two harmless viral vectors to bring DNA instructions to brain cells, "instructing" them to produce the missing enzyme. The DNA instruction enters the cells' nucleus and remains there, allowing for long-term hexosaminidase A (HEXA) production. The first child was 2½ years old and had late-stage disease symptoms. Within 3 months, muscle control and eye focusing had improved. By age 5, the child was stable and had no additional seizures. The second child was 7 months of age and, after 3 months of treatment, had improved brain development. By the age of 2 years, the child had no more seizures.

CRITICAL THINKING QUESTIONS

1. What does Tay-Sachs disease develop from?
2. How does Tay-Sachs disease develop in children?
3. How is the presence of Tay-Sachs disease confirmed?

CLINICAL CASE STUDY 3

A 19-year-old woman was admitted to a hospital with abdominal pain in her right upper quadrant. Physical examination detected conjunctival pallor and painful hepatomegaly below the right costal margin. An area of dullness below the left costal margin moved when the patient breathed. Ultrasound revealed hepatomegaly and splenomegaly. A bone marrow biopsy revealed hypercellularity and hyperplasia. There were abundant histiocytes with clear cytoplasm reminiscent of Gaucher cells, and the patient was subsequently diagnosed with Gaucher disease type 1.

CRITICAL THINKING QUESTIONS

1. What is the description of Gaucher disease type 1?
2. What are the three forms of Gaucher disease?
3. What clinical manifestations develop in about 90% of Gaucher disease type 1 patients?

FURTHER READING

1. Biochemical Safety Symposium. (2022). *The Control of Lipid Metabolism.* Legare Street Press.
2. Brown, R. (2022). *Lipid Metabolism and Health.* Murphy & Moore Publishing.
3. Fain, J.N. (2013). *Lipid Metabolism in Signaling Systems.* Academic Press.
4. Franz, M.J., Boucher, J.L., and Franzini Pereira, R. (2016). *Pocket Guide to Lipid Disorders, Hypertension, Diabetes, and Weight Management*, 2nd Edition. Academy of Nutrition and Dietetics.
5. Gurr, M.I., Harwood, J.L., Frayn, K.N., Murphy, D.J., and Michell, R.H. (2016). *Lipids: Biochemistry, Biotechnology, and Health*, 6th Edition. Wiley-Blackwell.
6. Jiang, X.C. (2020). *Lipid Transfer in Lipoprotein Metabolism and Cardiovascular Disease (Advances in Experimental Medicine and Biology, 1276).* Springer.
7. Li, Y. (2021). *Lipid Metabolism in Tumor Immunity (Advances in Experimental Medicine and Biology, 1316).* Springer.
8. McLean, L. (2020). *An Overview of Carbohydrate, Lipid, and Nitrogen Metabolism.* McLean.
9. Newman, C.B., and Chair, A. (2022). *Lipids: Update on Diagnosis and Management of Dyslipidemia (Endocrinology and Metabolism Clinics).* Elsevier.
10. Ntambi, J.M. (2020). *Lipid Signaling and Metabolism.* Academic Press.
11. Salway, J.G. (2017). *Metabolism at a Glance*, 4th Edition. Wiley-Blackwell.
12. Segatto, M., and Pallottini, V. (2021). *Emerging Role of Lipids in Metabolism and Disease.* International Journal of Molecular Sciences/MDPI.
13. Singh, M. (2023). *Therapeutic Platform of Bioactive Lipids: Focus on Cancer.* CRC Press.
14. Spickett, C.M., and Forman, H.J. (2015). *Lipid Oxidation in Health and Disease.* CRC Pres.
15. Thompson, D. (2015). *Handbook of Lipid Metabolism.* Callisto Reference.
16. Valenzuela Baez, R. (2013). *Lipid Metabolism.* IntechOpen.
17. Vissers, M.N., Kastelein, J.J.P., and Stroes, E.S. (2010). *Evidence-Based Management of Lipid Disorders.* TFM Publishing Ltd.
18. Yassine, H. (2015). *Lipid Management: From Basics to Clinic.* Springer.

Part IV

Disorders of Protein Metabolism

12 Protein Deficiencies

OVERVIEW

Protein deficiency due to a low protein intake in the diet is unusual in the United States. However, a lack of protein in other countries is a serious concern, especially in children. Protein deficiency can lead to malnutrition, such as kwashiorkor and marasmus, which can be life-threatening. Kwashiorkor affects millions of children worldwide. When it was first described in 1935, more than 90% of children with kwashiorkor died. Although the associated mortality is slightly lower now, most children still die after the initiation of treatment. The syndrome was named because it occurred most commonly in children who had recently been weaned from the breast, usually because another child had just been born. Children and adults with marasmus do not have enough protein in their diets or take in enough calories. Marasmus affects mainly children below the age of one in developing countries. Body weights of children with marasmus may be up to 80% less than that of an average child of the same age. Hypoalbuminemia is a common condition that various disorders may cause. Hypogammaglobulinemia may cause recurrent infections.

HYPOPROTEINEMIA

Hypoproteinemia is a condition in which a person has deficient protein levels in the blood. Protein deficiency usually occurs along with the deficiency of energy and nutrients, resulting in **protein–energy malnutrition** (PEM) or **protein-calorie malnutrition** (PCM). Many developing countries have diets low in protein and energy, so PEM is serious. It can affect people of all ages but is most severe in children. Insufficient protein and energy cause a failure of average growth, diarrhea, infections, and diseases in early life. In most cases, PEM occurs as marasmus or kwashiorkor.

EPIDEMIOLOGY

Protein malnutrition, although rare in Western societies, remains a significant cause of infant and child death in African and Asian countries. With about 156 million children malnourished throughout the world, there are 50 million that experience wasting, and 3 million that die annually. PEM is most prevalent in areas of Africa (Ethiopia, Kenya, Somalia, South Sudan, Sudan, Uganda), Southeast Asia (India, China, Bangladesh, Indonesia, Philippines, North Korea), Central America (Guatemala, Honduras, Mexico, El Salvador, Nicaragua), and South America (Peru, Bolivia, Colombia, Paraguay, Venezuela) – see **Figure 12.1**. It also occurs in specific populations within industrialized countries, including the United States. The most significant risks are among people living in poverty or isolation, substance abusers, and those with anorexia nervosa, AIDS, or cancer. In hospitals, some patients are at a higher risk of PEM because of previous unhealthy histories, low dietary intake, and more need for protein to recover from disease, trauma, or surgery. If a person is malnourished, the risks of additional complications and death are higher. Therefore, hospitals now have nutrition support teams for at-risk patients.

ETIOLOGY AND RISK FACTORS

Hypoproteinemia can be caused by malnutrition or malabsorption due to intestinal disease, excessive loss of plasma protein either into the urine (nephrotic syndrome) or into the gut lumen (protein-losing enteropathy), or hepatic failure, the liver being the site of synthesis of the plasma protein albumin.

DOI: 10.1201/9781003453376-16

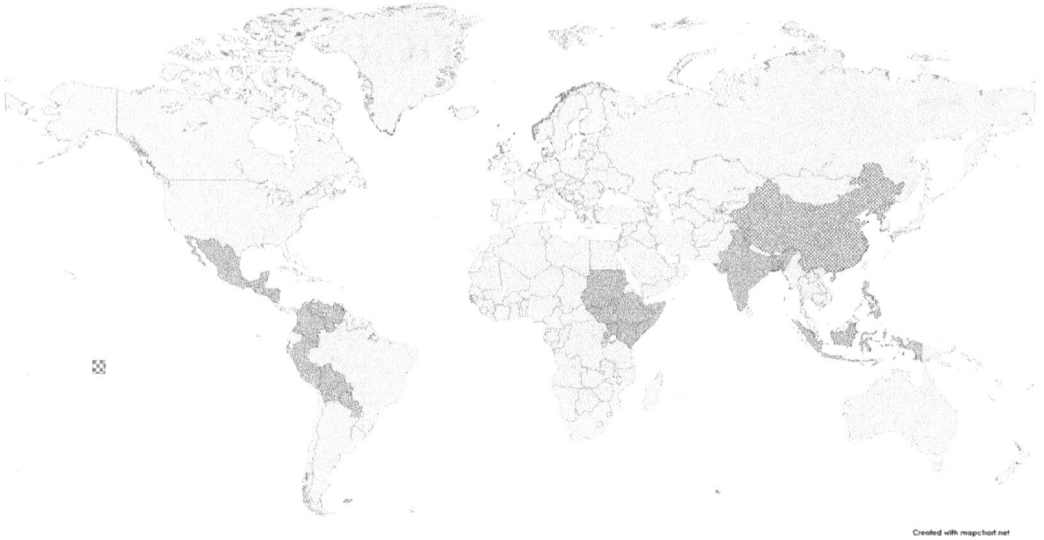

FIGURE 12.1   Countries with the highest rates of protein–energy malnutrition.

Insufficient protein may cause health problems such as kwashiorkor, marasmus, impaired mental health, edema, organ failure, wasting, muscle atrophy, and immune system weakness.

CLINICAL MANIFESTATIONS

The signs and symptoms of hypoproteinemia include edema in the face, legs, and other parts of the body, wasting muscles, growth retardation, infections, bone fractures, fatty liver, and cracking nails. Protein deficiency can also contribute to both short-term and long-term symptoms. For example, it may increase the risk of developing **cataracts**, heart problems, and muscle atrophy – these are somewhat familiar to older adults.

DIAGNOSIS

Blood tests can diagnose hypoproteinemia based on patient history and physical examination. Focusing on the cause of hypoproteinemia can also help with the diagnosis.

TREATMENT

Treatment to cure hypoproteinemia includes steroids and immune suppressors to lower intestine inflammation, antibiotics or antiparasitic drugs to counter infections, dialysis or kidney transplant for treatment of kidney disease, and treatment of liver damage with medications or surgery.

PREVENTION

Consuming enough protein can prevent hypoproteinemia. Proteins are essential for every part of the human body. Bones, muscles, skin, and nearly every vital organ or tissue contain them. The body needs protein to function and survive and must get it through food.

YOU SHOULD REMEMBER

PEM is an undesirable loss of body cell mass secondary to reduced intake or inadequate utilization of nutrients. Children (especially infants) are highly prone to developing the condition since they have fewer metabolic reserves on hand to combat illness. Calorie deprivation is often called starvation, wasting, or marasmus. PEM significantly contributes to morbidity and mortality on a global scale.

Check Your Knowledge

1. What does insufficient protein and energy cause?
2. What are the signs and symptoms of hypoproteinemia?
3. What are the treatments for hypoproteinemia?

KWASHIORKOR

Kwashiorkor is one of the two main types of severe PEM. People with kwashiorkor are significantly deficient in protein and some essential micronutrients. It is rare in developed countries and primarily found in developing countries with high rates of poverty and food scarcity. Poor sanitary conditions and a high prevalence of infectious diseases also help set the stage for malnutrition. Kwashiorkor can affect all ages, but it is most common in children, especially between the ages of 3 and 5. This is an age when many children have recently transitioned from breastfeeding to a less adequate diet – one higher in carbohydrates but lower in protein and other nutrients. The older child cannot consume enough of these foods for energy, especially protein. Kwashiorkor develops more quickly because of severe protein deficits.

EPIDEMIOLOGY

Kwashiorkor is a nutritional disease common in rural areas of developing countries. It primarily affects children in their second year of life. This typical disease of the weaning period is associated with a diet based on starchy, low-protein staple foods, such as cassava, sweet potatoes, and bananas. Kwashiorkor is more common in developing countries in Africa, Central America, and Southeast Asia. It is seen more during times of famine. Prevalent infections and parasites can elevate these needs, precipitating the development of kwashiorkor.

ETIOLOGY AND RISK FACTORS

Protein deficiency is the main feature of kwashiorkor, and many researchers believe it is the cause – but not all are convinced. Some have noted cases where dietary protein failed to prevent or improve kwashiorkor. This suggests that protein deficiency may only be part of the picture. The primary factors associated with kwashiorkor include a diet of mostly carbohydrates, inadequate food replacement during weaning, lack of essential vitamins and minerals, parasites and infectious diseases, war, and natural disasters.

CLINICAL MANIFESTATIONS

Early symptoms include fatigue, irritability, listlessness, and lethargy. As protein deprivation continues, one sees growth failure, loss of muscle mass, generalized edema, ascites, dry and brittle hair, loss of pigment in hair, and decreased immunity (see **Figure 12.2**). The hallmark sign of

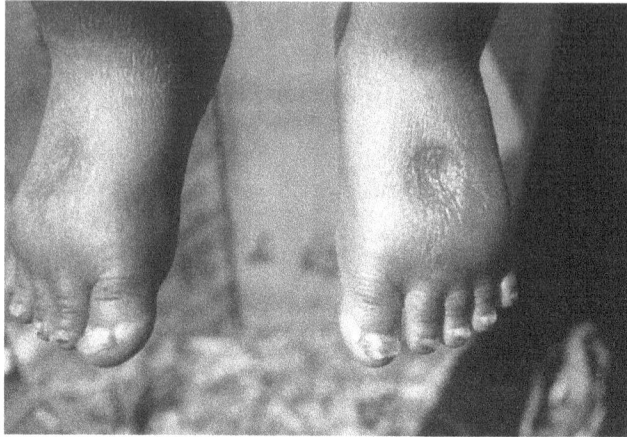

FIGURE 12.2   Edema in kwashiorkor.

kwashiorkor is edema, when there is still some remaining subcutaneous fat. Other primary symptoms include apathy, diarrhea, hepatomegaly, **fatty liver**, and infections. The symptoms complicate other concurrent diseases, such as measles, which can become severely debilitating or fatal.

Diagnosis

To diagnose kwashiorkor disease, begin with a physical examination, a history of illnesses or infections, and measuring the child's weight-to-height ratio and height-to-age score. Diagnostic tests should include a complete blood count (CBC), total protein levels, serum albumin, serum creatinine, creatinine clearance, and blood urea nitrogen (BUN). It is also required to measure serum zinc, niacin, vitamin B5 and B12, and HIV tests. Other tests are stool samples, urinalysis, and chest X-rays.

Treatment

Kwashiorkor can be corrected by eating more protein and calories, especially if treatment starts early. In cases of infection, antibiotics must be given; supplementary iron therapy is started after one week has elapsed. Vitamin A is given when severe ocular lesions are present, and whole blood transfusion may be necessary in the rare case of severe anemia.

Prevention

Kwashiorkor can be prevented by ensuring the diet has enough carbohydrates, fat (at least 10% of total calories), and protein (12% of total calories).

YOU SHOULD REMEMBER

Calories are given first in carbohydrates, simple sugars, and fats. Proteins are started after other sources of calories have already provided energy. Vitamin and mineral supplements will be given. Food must be restarted slowly since the person has been without much food for an extended period.

Check Your Knowledge:

1. Where is kwashiorkor most common?
2. What are the primary factors associated with kwashiorkor?
3. How can Kwashiorkor be corrected?

MARASMUS

Marasmus is a Greek word meaning "starvation." It is severe undernutrition – a deficiency in the body's macronutrients, including carbohydrates, protein, and fats. The affected individuals have little to no subcutaneous fat. It is most common in infants who are not breastfed or have stopped breastfeeding early in life. Weaning formulas are often not prepared correctly because of unsafe water supplies and a lack of money to buy sufficient infant formula. Parents may be forced to dilute the formula to provide more feedings, depriving the infant of nutrients, including essential calories and proteins. Large amounts of energy and protein are needed to return an infant with marasmus to average growth, development, and overall health. The child may have poor cognitive and intellectual growth when the condition affects average brain growth in the first months of life.

EPIDEMIOLOGY

Marasmus affects more than 50 million children under the age of five worldwide. It is equally distributed between genders; however, due to cultural differences in some parts of the world, women may be at an increased risk of marasmus. Marasmus is more common in developing countries, such as Asia and Africa. People in these nations are prone to having less access to food, making it difficult to get enough nutrients. A risk of certain infectious diseases can cause marasmus if left untreated. However, undernutrition in developed countries is more frequently seen in adults than children. Undernutrition is seen in 5%–10% of older adults in nursing homes and up to 50% of older adults on discharge from the hospital.

ETIOLOGY AND RISK FACTORS

The cause of marasmus is insufficient **total calorie intake**. However, it is essential to understand what precipitates a reduced calorie intake in a patient suffering from marasmus. Furthermore, the precipitating cause of a reduced calorie intake may vary between adults and children. However, the causes of marasmus can be broadly divided into social and biological causes.

The underlying social cause of marasmus in children is poverty. Poverty may occur as a result of low status and insufficient education of mothers, along with natural disasters, war, and civil instability. Poverty directly influences the ability of a household to secure a reliable food source for children, leading to an insufficient calorie supply. Unstable and unreliable childcare may occur in mothers who are unable to care for their children as a result of displacement, along with an unclean environment; this contributes to a higher frequency of infections such as diarrhea. In particular, the HIV/AIDS epidemic has been shown to create a significant burden of disease in South African households. Children who have been infected with HIV have poor nutritional outcomes compared to those who have not been infected. Breastfeeding mothers who are infected with HIV also tend to have insufficient protein and micronutrient stores compared to those who are not infected with HIV.

CLINICAL MANIFESTATIONS

Marasmus develops slowly because of severe energy, protein, and micronutrient deficiency. It leads to extreme weight loss, muscle and fat loss, and impaired growth. Marasmus in children can result in loss of fat and muscle mass. They become cachectic, with no subcutaneous fat, severe muscle atrophy, wrinkled skin, and prominence of ribs and bones. Irritability is typical, with constant weak crying. Marasmus commonly occurs due to cessation of breastfeeding before 12 months of age and replacement with diluted milk formula due to economic or sociocultural reasons. In many cultures, childhood diarrhea is treated by suppressing breastfeeding. The most common symptom of severe protein and calorie deficiency is being underweight due to malnourishment. Suppose marasmus remains untreated for a long time. In that case, the symptoms include diarrhea, dehydration, lower immunity, respiratory infection, hypotension, and bradycardia. Other symptoms include lethargy, apathy and weakness, skin atrophy, brittle hair or hair loss, and lower anterior **fontanelle** in infants.

Diagnosis

Diagnosis primarily relies on body measurements, which are then scored according to different scoring systems for children and adults. Upper arm circumference and height-to-weight ratios help healthcare providers rate the severity of undernutrition. The patient history, physical examination, and laboratory tests can confirm the diagnosis.

Treatment

The primary treatment of marasmus is to rehydrate, prevent infections, and avoid the complications of the treatment of marasmus, such as **refeeding syndrome**. The immediate treatment lasts approximately one week. Dehydration can be treated with an intravenous isotonic solution; in cases where the child is suffering from hypovolemia, plasma or blood may be used. Patients should be kept in a warm room because they may be susceptible to hypothermia. Furthermore, antibiotics can be indicated following blood cultures in the case of sepsis.

To prevent the development of refeeding syndrome, nutrition should be delivered slowly and carefully with a caloric intake between 60% and 80% of the calorie requirement for age. Vitamins such as thiamine and oral phosphate should be administered to prevent the development of hypophosphatemia associated with refeeding. Once the acute complications of marasmus have been treated and the child's appetite begins to return, there will be a gradual increase in caloric intake, vaccination, and motor activity. Children may need 120%–140% of their required caloric intake to maintain a growth rate similar to their peers. The nutritional rehabilitation phase may last from 2 to 6 weeks.

Prevention

Prevention and safety measures for marasmus include drinking boiled water and staying hydrated. Maintain good sanitation and hygiene, and have a healthy and well-balanced diet.

YOU SHOULD REMEMBER

Infections and diseases caused by viruses, bacteria, parasites, and other pathogens can cause loss of appetite. This can lead to a low intake of essential nutrients in infected children and adults. Diseases such as HIV/AIDS and malaria in rural areas can cause marasmus. It can also be caused by poor absorption of nutrients due to celiac disease and pancreatic problems.

YOU SHOULD REMEMBER

Marasmus and Kwashiorkor are two different variations of severe PEM. Marasmus is a deficiency of all macronutrients, while kwashiorkor is predominantly a protein deficiency. Kwashiorkor occurs in people who may have access to carbohydrates – bread, grains, or starches – but lack protein. Marasmus has a wasted and faded appearance, while kwashiorkor is known for causing edema – swelling with fluid, especially in the belly and the face.

Check Your Knowledge

1. How common is marasmus?
2. How does Marasmus develop?
3. What is the primary treatment for marasmus?

PLASMA PROTEINS

Plasma carries nutrients, hormones, and proteins to different body parts. It also removes waste products of cell metabolism from various tissues to the organs responsible for detoxifying and excreting them. In addition, plasma is the vehicle for transporting the blood cells through the blood vessels. Plasma contains about 90% water, with 10% comprising ions, proteins, dissolved gases, nutrient molecules, and wastes. The proteins in plasma include the antibody proteins, coagulation factors, and the proteins albumin and fibrinogen, which maintain serum **osmotic pressure**. Each can be separated using different techniques to form various blood products to treat other conditions. For instance, clotting factors treat coagulation disorders like **hemophilia** or **disseminated intravascular coagulation**.

Plasma proteins are the most abundant substances in the plasma and are present in three major types: albumin, globulins, and fibrinogen. They play specialized roles as follows:

Albumin helps maintain the **colloid osmotic pressure** of the blood. It is the smallest in size among the plasma proteins but makes up the most significant percentage. The colloid osmotic pressure of the blood is essential in maintaining a balance between the water inside the blood and that in the tissue fluid around the cells. When the plasma proteins are deficient, the water in the plasma leaks out into the space around the blood vessels. It may result in **interstitial edema**, a feature of liver disorders, kidney disease, and malnutrition. Albumin also helps transport many substances, such as drugs, hormones, and fatty acids.

Globulins are of three types, alpha, beta, and gamma, from smallest to largest. Gamma globulins are called **antibodies**. The alpha globulins include the High-density lipoprotein (HDL) essential in carrying fats to the cells for building various substances and energy metabolism. HDL is best known for preventing plaque formation by transporting cholesterol within the blood. Low-density lipoproteins (LDL) are beta globulins that transport fat to the cells for steroid and cell membrane synthesis. It also promotes cholesterol plaque formation, an arterial and heart disease risk factor.

Antibodies (gamma globulins) are also called **immunoglobulins**. The B lymphocytes, a subset of the immune cells, produce them. Antibodies are responsible for the body's humoral immune function, recognizing and neutralizing **pathogens** via specific receptors.

Fibrinogen is a necessary soluble plasma clotting factor precursor converted to a threadlike protein called **fibrin** on contact with a sticky surface. The fibrin threads formed in this way trap platelets to form the primary platelet clot on which a stable blood clot is formed by coagulation. The clotting factors in plasma cause a blood clot to start at the site of any break in the smooth endothelial lining of the blood vessels. This not only prevents blood loss but protects the body against invading microbes.

HYPOALBUMINEMIA

Albumin has several physiological roles. One of the most important is maintaining the osmotic pressure within the vascular compartments, preventing fluids from leaking into the extravascular spaces. It accounts for around 80% of the colloid osmotic pressure. Additionally, albumin functions as a low-affinity, high-capacity carrier of several different endogenous and exogenous compounds, acting as a depot and a carrier for these compounds. Binding compounds to albumin may reduce their toxicity, such as in the case of unconjugated bilirubin and drugs in the neonate. Also, albumin binds at least 40% of the circulating calcium and is a transporter of hormones such as thyroxine, cortisol, and testosterone. Albumin also is the primary carrier of fatty acids and has significant anti-oxidant properties. Albumin also maintains an acid-base balance as it acts as a **plasma buffer**. Albumin markers nutritional status and disease severity, particularly in chronic and critically ill patients. Renal and Gastrointestinal (GI) tract loss of albumin may account for around 6% and 10% of albumin loss in healthy individuals, respectively – a decrease in serum albumin levels below the reference interval is termed **hypoalbuminemia**.

Epidemiology

Hypoalbuminemia is a common problem among persons with acute and chronic medical conditions. At the time of hospital admission, 20% of patients have hypoalbuminemia.

The prevalence of hypoalbuminemia is higher among hospitalized, critically ill, and older patients. The prevalence of hypoalbuminemia is 19% on admission and 35.7% during hospitalization. Hypoalbuminemia dose-dependently increases the risk of severity, mortality, local complications, and organ failure and is associated with more extended hospital stays.

Etiology and Risk Factors

Hypoalbuminemia may result from decreased albumin production, increased loss of albumin via the kidneys, GI tract, skin, or extravascular space, or increased albumin catabolism or a combination of two or more mechanisms. Hypoalbuminemia is a feature of chronic and advanced hepatic cirrhosis. The risk factors include nephrotic syndrome, chronic kidney disease, kwashiorkor, diabetes mellitus, essential hypertension, cardiac failure, protein-losing enteropathy, sepsis, and patients with burn wounds.

Clinical Manifestations

Hypoalbuminemia's symptoms are typically related to conditions affecting the liver, kidneys, and heart, as well as nutritional deficiencies. Patients with hypoalbuminemia present with peripheral and central edema and **anasarca**. They may also complain of fatigue, excessive weakness, jaundice, loss of appetite, polyuria, dyspnea, and other related nutritional deficiencies, such as iron deficiency anemia in celiac disease.

Diagnosis

Hypoalbuminemia is often a finding in routine laboratory testing following the presentation of patients for other primary medical conditions or diseases. The principal value of **protein electrophoresis** in a patient with low serum albumin is with the differential diagnosis of hypoalbuminemia. Hypoalbuminemia will be present in acute inflammation with an increase in alpha-1 and alpha-2 globulins and normal gamma globulins. The protein electrophoresis pattern in chronic inflammation will show hypoalbuminemia with a polyclonal increase in gamma globulins. In the presence of nephrotic syndrome, hypoalbuminemia with an increase in alpha-2 globulins due to increased macroglobulin and low gamma globulins are the typical patterns in serum protein electrophoresis. With chronic liver disease, hypoalbuminemia with increased gamma globulins and beta–gamma bridging is standard.

Specific tests include alpha-1-antitrypsin clearance to determine protein loss via gut distal to the pylorus. This involves a timed collection of stool together with a serum sample. Alpha-1-antitrypsin is resistant to degradation by digestive enzymes. It is used as an endogenous marker for the presence of blood proteins in the intestinal tract. Elevated **alpha-1-antitrypsin** clearance suggests excessive GI protein loss.

Treatment

Treatment is directed at the cause of hypoalbuminemia since it is a consequence of some diseases. In the critically ill, in particular, burn patients, albumin infusions may be given. It is controversial whether albumin infusions are of clinical benefit to other groups of critically ill patients. It also has some value in patients with cirrhosis with certain complications.

Prevention

Prevention of hypoalbuminemia includes eating a balanced diet full of dairy, protein, and whole-grain carbohydrates or taking supplements to increase the amount of protein and calories in the diet, removing foods high in sodium (salt) from the diet, and using medicine to manage underlying health conditions.

Check Your Knowledge

1. What are examples of plasma proteins?
2. In which individuals is hypoalbuminemia a common problem?
3. How is hypoalbuminemia prevented?

HYPOGAMMAGLOBULINEMIA

Hypogammaglobulinemia is a disorder caused by low serum immunoglobulin (Ig) or antibody levels. Igs are the main components of the humoral immune response and can recognize antigens to trigger a biological response and eradicate the infectious source. There are two main types of hypogammaglobulinemia: primary and secondary. Various Igs exist (IgA, IgM, IgG, and IgE). Primary hypogammaglobulinemia may have a delay of several years between clinical presentation and diagnosis. The most common cause is common variable immunodeficiency.

Epidemiology

The most common Ig deficiency is IgA, with an incidence of approximately 1 in 700 Caucasian individuals. Primary immunodeficiencies are the most prevalent after IgA deficiency (1:1,000 individuals). A prevalence rate of 1:66,000–75,000 in Brazil has been estimated. These data exhibit significant variability in several countries, likely due to healthcare accessibility, time to diagnosis, or even lack of patient identification.

Etiology and Risk Factors

Hypogammaglobulinemia occurs with either inadequate production or excess loss of antibodies. The causes are typically either primary or secondary. Primary causes are genetic conditions that affect the production of antibodies. In contrast, secondary causes are external factors that affect the levels of antibodies. B lymphocytes are special immune cells responsible for producing antibodies. Chromosomal and genetic mutations that affect B lymphocytes may affect the production of antibodies. Transient hypogammaglobulinemia of infancy is a primary hypogammaglobulinemia. It occurs at birth and during the first few months of life. However, the antibody levels tend to return to normal when the infant gradually produces antibodies. This typically occurs during the first or second year of life.

Reduced Ig levels characterize secondary hypogammaglobulinemia due to a medication or a disease process, leading to decreased antibody production or increased antibody loss. People with medical conditions such as nephrotic syndrome, hematologic malignancy, or gastrointestinal diseases that lead to protein loss or use drugs such as immunosuppressants (corticosteroids or chemotherapy) and some anti-seizures may develop this condition. Patients can be predisposed to recurrent upper and lower respiratory tract infections.

Clinical Manifestations

Patients with mild hypogammaglobulinemia may be asymptomatic, but those with more severe hypogammaglobulinemia usually present with a history of recurrent infections. A detailed clinical history should emphasize family history, age of onset, recurrent infections, type of microorganisms, and site of infections. Common illnesses associated with hypogammaglobulinemia include ear infections, sinusitis, bronchitis, pneumonia, meningitis, and skin infections. When IgG levels are below the normal range, it can also cause recurrent infections, allergies, asthma, and a weakened immune system. The most commonly recognized clinical feature is recurrent infection. IgA deficiency is a separate diagnosis, but it can eventually lead to a loss of IgG or may occur concurrently.

Diagnosis

Laboratory studies may be helpful, including CBC, serum Ig levels (IgA, IgG, and IgM), and antibody response for recall antigens. Chest radiography and high-resolution computed tomography (HRCT) are used to evaluate for **bronchiectasis** and lymph node biopsy is used to rule out infection or malignancy.

Treatment

Watchful waiting is encouraged in slightly low IgG cases with intact antibody production. Infants with transient hypogammaglobulinemia often have a resolution of this finding without intervention. Some patients will have low Ig without disrupting the ability to produce antibodies and require no intervention. Replacement therapy with IgG administered intravenously (IVIG) or subcutaneously (SCIG) is the treatment of choice for most primary immunodeficiency syndromes.

If poor T-cell function is also a part of the immune deficiency (severe or combined immune deficiency), a stem cell transplant or bone marrow transplant may be the definitive treatment. It may replace B-cell function, so IgG replacement is no longer necessary. Treatment of secondary hypogammaglobulinemia is directed at the underlying cause.

Prevention

Though there is no prevention against hypogammaglobulinemia, proper hand hygiene, sanitation, early detection of infections, and compliance with treatments can improve symptoms and long-term outcomes. Any medications or underlying diseases influencing the condition should be discussed.

Check Your Knowledge

1. What is the most common Ig deficiency?
2. What are the primary and secondary causes of hypogammaglobulinemia?
3. What common illnesses are associated with hypogammaglobulinemia?

PROTEIN ALLERGIES

Dietary protein intolerance is a clinical syndrome resulting from an individual's sensitization to one or more proteins that have been absorbed via a permeable mucosa in the small intestine. Intolerance to various food proteins, mainly to cows' milk, has been recognized in children for many years. It develops through immunological, non-immunological, metabolic, genetic, and pharmacological mechanisms. It is often associated with gastrointestinal symptoms. With early identification of the condition and intervention, the disorder is manageable and has a favorable prognosis.

EPIDEMIOLOGY

In the United States, it is estimated that 3.5%–4% of the general population exhibits IgE-mediated food allergy or sensitivity. A large study of almost 40,000 children found that 8% have an allergy to a food, and 30% have multiple food allergies. Furthermore, more than a third of children with a food allergy have a history of severe allergic reactions. Peanuts are the most prevalent food allergen, followed by milk and shellfish. The severity of these allergies can vary significantly, and some individuals may not experience significant effects with dietary intake, although a sensitive response is observed in an experimental testing environment.

Non-Hispanic White individuals across all ages had the lowest rate of self-reported or parent-reported food allergies (9.5%) compared with Asian (10.5%), Hispanic (10.6%), and non-Hispanic Black (10.6%) individuals.

ETIOLOGY AND RISK FACTORS

Protein intolerance is caused by the inability to digest or effectively break down amino acids. When food proteins are not digested well, they can act as antigens, resulting in food protein allergies. Most frequently, cow's milk proteins cause food intolerance during infancy. Food protein-induced enterocolitis syndrome (FPIES) is also commonly attributed to intolerance to cow's milk proteins. The affected individuals present with diarrhea, edema, and hypoalbuminemia. With an increase in age and the introduction of different foods, egg protein intolerance and soy and peanut allergies have become more prevalent.

CLINICAL MANIFESTATIONS

Clinical features of food protein allergies involve various organ systems and vary among different disorders. However, patients primarily present with gastrointestinal manifestations. In non-immunological food protein allergies, the amount of food ingested tends to be more directly related to the severity of symptoms. Excessive intestinal gas, bloating, abdominal pain, and diarrhea are common presenting symptoms. In immunological food protein allergies, trace amounts of the sensitized food protein can trigger an explosive reaction and may involve the blood vessels and skin. The IgE-mediated reactions occur within minutes to an hour of food protein ingestion, and symptoms range from skin rashes, urticaria, angioedema, and wheezing to anaphylaxis (see **Figure 12.3**). In contrast, non-IgE-mediated reactions may occur in hours to days.

DIAGNOSIS

No perfect test is used to confirm or rule out a food allergy. A family history of allergies and a careful exam can often identify or exclude other medical problems. However, a blood test can measure the immune system's response to particular foods by measuring the allergy-related antibody known as IgE. A skin prick test also can determine the reaction to a specific food.

TREATMENT

Mothers should avoid cow's milk and dairy products in breastfed infants. Extensively hydrolyzed formula with documented hypoallergenicity must be recommended for treating cow's milk allergy, especially in non-breastfed infants and young children. Amino acid formulas can also be recommended for patients with more severe symptoms. Steroids are the mainstay treatment in

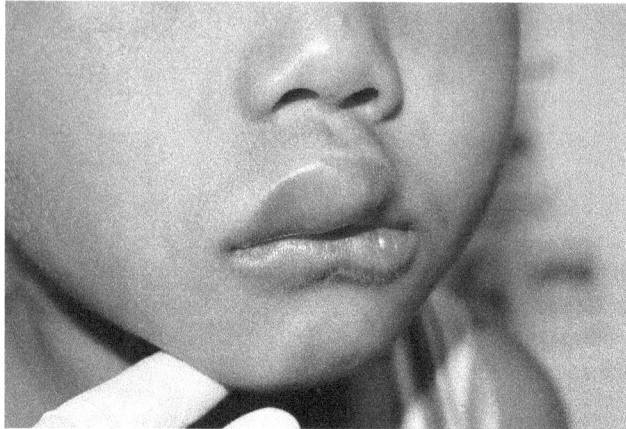

FIGURE 12.3   Angioedema.

IgE-mediated immunological food protein allergies, including eosinophilic gastrointestinal disorders. If acute allergic reactions or anaphylaxis is suspected, the probable offending food must be immediately avoided, and emergency medical care should be provided. They may be given a prescription for an auto-injectable epinephrine device and instructed to use it properly.

PREVENTION

The only definitive prevention of food protein intolerance is the strict elimination of the offending food protein in the diet. Patients should be counseled on monitoring manufactured food ingredients and compliance with the elimination diet. Patients on long-term elimination diets should also have access to appropriate diet counseling, ideally by a nutritionist or dietitian, and regular growth monitoring, especially in children.

YOU SHOULD REMEMBER

FPIES is a type of non-IgE-mediated food allergy that can present with severe vomiting, diarrhea, and dehydration. Like other food allergies, FPIES reactions are triggered by eating a particular food. The most common triggers include cow milk, soy, and grains (rice, barley, oats). The most severe forms of FPIES can lead to a drop in energy, a change in body temperature, and low blood pressure, leading to hospitalization.

Check Your Knowledge

1. What is protein intolerance caused by?
2. What are the clinical features of food protein allergies?
3. How can a protein allergy be prevented?

Clinical Case Studies

CLINICAL CASE STUDY 1

A 6-year-old boy was brought to the local hospital with excessive skin lesions and loss of appetite that had persisted for months. The child's condition was recognized as PEM, and he was treated with increased nutritive intake, micronutrients, and trace elements. The child responded well and soon showed signs of recovery. The parents were counseled about their financial needs and instructed on improving the child's protein and calorie intake for the future.

CRITICAL THINKING QUESTIONS

1. Where in the world is PEM most prevalent?
2. What are the causes of hypoproteinemia?
3. What treatments are available for hypoproteinemia?

CLINICAL CASE STUDY 2

A 2-year-old girl was diagnosed as having marasmus complicated by tuberculosis. The family was impoverished; the only regular dietary components included cassava, corn, peppers, and tomatoes. The child had severe anemia as well as mild diarrhea and vomiting. She had been exclusively breastfed for her first year, having no appetite for any other food sources. She then began eating cereal-based products, mashed yams, and small fish. Treatment for the marasmus began with regular food supplements, which increased the child's caloric intake. Soon, her diarrhea and vomiting subsided, and she began to have an excellent appetite. Treatment was then started for anemia and tuberculosis.

CRITICAL THINKING QUESTIONS

1. What is the definition of "marasmus"?
2. What is the underlying social cause of marasmus?
3. What is the primary treatment of marasmus?

CLINICAL CASE STUDY 3

A 56-year-old man with a history of hypertension, fibromyalgia, and colonic polyps presented with extensive warts on his hands and feet, which caused pain when they came into contact with objects. Laboratory testing revealed the presence of hypogammaglobulinemia as well as hypoalbuminemia and lymphopenia. The patient started treatment for his multiple conditions.

CRITICAL THINKING QUESTIONS

1. In which groups is hypoalbuminemia most common?
2. What is hypogammaglobulinemia caused by?
3. What are the primary and secondary causes of hypogammaglobulinemia?

FURTHER READING

1. Arpilor, L. (2023). *Protein Deficiency Symptoms: Understand the Body's Signals when Lacking Adequate Protein Intake and How It Can Impact Overall Health*. Arpilor.
2. Ayre, J. (2017). *Practical Observations on the Nature and Treatment of Marasmus, and of Those Disorders Allied To It: Which May Be Strictly Denominated Bilious*. Forgotten Books.
3. Ben Rabeh, R. (2023). *Cow's Milk Protein Allergy: Diagnostic Approach and Management Strategy*. Our Knowledge Publishing.
4. Bouchetara, A. (2021). *Cow's Milk Protein Allergy in Children*. Our Knowledge Publishing.
5. Doley, J., and Marian, M.J. (2022). *Adult Malnutrition: Diagnosis and Treatment*. CRC Press.
6. Ekanem, E., and James, M. (2022). *Kwashiorkor is Back!* Ekanem.
7. Franco-Paredes, C. (2016). *Core Concepts in Clinical Infectious Diseases (CCCID)*. Academic Press.
8. Goswami Vachani, J. (2023). *Failure to Thrive and Malnutrition: A Practical, Evidence-Based Clinical Guide*. Springer.

9. Icon Group International. (2010). *Hypoproteinemia: Webster's Timeline History (1943–2007).* Icon Group International, Inc.

10. Icon Group International (2007). *Hypoalbuminemia: Webster's Timeline History (1953–2007).* Icon Group International, Inc.

11. Lonsdale, D., and Marrs, C. (2017). *Thiamine Deficiency Disease, Dysautonomia, and High Calorie Malnutrition.* Academic Press.

12. Lundblad, R.L. (2012). *Biotechnology of Plasma Proteins (Protein Science Series).* CRC Press.

13. Sivaramanan, S. (2016). *Poverty, Disease, Disability and Malnutrition: Complete Environmental Review and Essay.* Sivaramanan.

14. Taha, H., and Habeeb, S. (2014). *Main Electrolytes Derangement in Re-feeding Syndrome.* Lap Lambert Academic Publishing.

15. Tappan, J. (2017). *The Riddle of Malnutrition: The Long Arc of Biomedical and Public Health Interventions in Uganda (Perspectives on Global Health).* Ohio University Press.

13 Protein Misfolding Diseases

OVERVIEW

Protein misfolding is believed to be the primary cause of Alzheimer's disease, Parkinson's disease, Huntington's disease, Creutzfeldt–Jakob disease, and many other degenerative and neurodegenerative disorders. The accumulation of misfolded and aggregated proteins in the brain is a hallmark shared by several neurodegenerative disorders. Most protein molecules must fold into defined three-dimensional structures to acquire functional activity. However, protein chains can adopt many conformational states, and their biologically active conformation is often only marginally stable. Metastable proteins tend to populate misfolded species prone to forming toxic aggregates, including soluble oligomers and fibrillar amyloid deposits, linked with neurodegeneration in Alzheimer's and Parkinson's disease and many other pathologies. All cells contain an extensive protein homeostasis network comprising molecular chaperones and other factors to prevent or regulate protein aggregation. These defense systems tend to decline during aging, facilitating the manifestation of aggregate deposition diseases. Protein misfolding diseases are rare worldwide. Chaperones have been suggested as potential therapeutic molecules for target-based treatment among therapeutic approaches to treating various protein-misfolding diseases.

ALZHEIMER'S DISEASE

Alzheimer's disease (AD) is the most common cause of dementia and is a neurocognitive disorder. Between 60% and 80% of dementia in older adults involve AD. This disease causes progressive atrophy and the death of brain cells, resulting in a continuous decline in cognition and behavioral and social skills. The affected individual becomes unable to function independently. There is altered processing of the amyloid precursor protein, resulting in deposition and fibrillar aggregation of **beta-amyloid**, the primary component of **senile plaques**. These plaques contain degenerated axonal or dendritic processes, astrocytes, and glial cells surrounding an amyloid core. Beta-amyloid may change kinase and phosphatase activities, leading to tau hyperphosphorylation, the protein stabilizing microtubules. Soon, neurofibrillary tangles form. Other determinants of AD include the **apolipoprotein epsilon** (apo E) alleles. These proteins influence beta-amyloid deposits, the integrity of the cytoskeleton, and just how well neuronal repair can occur.

EPIDEMIOLOGY

AD is more common in women than men, partially because women live longer. Prevalence in industrialized countries will likely increase as the population ages. There is a rapid increase globally in people living with AD. About 44 million people are now estimated to live with AD or a related form of dementia globally. *Vascular dementia* is more common when there are vascular risk factors such as diabetes mellitus, hypertension, hyperlipidemia, and smoking, as well as after multiple strokes.

AD accounts for 60%–80% of dementia in older adults. In the United States, about 10% of people aged 65 or older have AD. The percentage of adults with AD increases with age – 65–74 years (3%), 75–84 years (17%), and age 85 or older (32%). *Vascular dementia* usually begins after age 70 and is more common in men. AD is responsible for approximately 122,000 deaths annually in the United States. There are about 1.62 million deaths related to dementia per year globally, and 60%–80% of these are associated with AD.

DOI: 10.1201/9781003453376-17

Etiology and Risk Factors

Most AD cases are sporadic, with onset after age 65 or older and an unclear cause. Even so, 5%–15% of patients are familial and have an early start, before age 65 – usually related to gene mutations. There are five or more distinct genetic loci on chromosomes 1, 12, 14, 19, and 21. Autosomal dominant forms of AD, usually with early onset, are caused by gene mutations of the amyloid precursor protein, presenilin I, and presenilin II. There is altered processing of the amyloid precursor protein, resulting in deposition and fibrillar aggregation of beta-amyloid, the primary component of senile plaques. These plaques contain degenerated axonal or dendritic processes, astrocytes, and glial cells surrounding an amyloid core. Beta-amyloid may change kinase and phosphatase activities, leading to tau hyperphosphorylation, the protein stabilizing microtubules. Soon, neurofibrillary tangles form.

Other determinants of AD include the apolipoprotein epsilon (apo E) alleles. These proteins influence beta-amyloid deposits, the integrity of the cytoskeleton, and just how well neuronal repair can occur. The risk of AD is much higher when there are two epsilon-4 alleles but decreases if the epsilon-2 allele is present. If an individual has two epsilon-4 alleles, AD risks by age 75 are 10–30 times higher. Chances can be increased by diabetes mellitus, hypertension, dyslipidemia, and smoking. Aggressive treatment of these factors before middle age can reduce risks for cognitive impairment later on.

Clinical Manifestations

The first sign of AD is the loss of short-term memory. The affected individual asks questions repeatedly, often misplaces items, and needs to remember meetings or appointments. Additional problems with cognition may involve difficulty with complicated tasks, impaired reasoning, poor judgment, language dysfunction, and an inability to recognize faces or everyday objects. The disease progresses slowly and can plateau occasionally. Common behavioral disorders include agitation, feelings of persecution, wandering, and yelling.

Diagnosis

The diagnosis of AD is similar to how other dementias are diagnosed. Even though imaging studies are helpful, a definitive diagnosis of AD is only confirmed by evaluating brain tissue after death. A thorough history is taken, and a standard neurological examination is performed. The clinical criteria are 85% accurate for diagnosing and differentiating AD from other dementias. The traditional diagnostic criteria include all of the following factors:

- There are deficits in two or more areas of cognition.
- Dementia is clinically established and documented via a formal mental status examination.
- Onset occurs over months to years, with progressive memory decline and other cognitive functions.
- There is no disturbance of consciousness.
- There are no brain or systemic disorders such as stroke or tumors.
- Onset is after age 40, but usually after age 65.

Deviations do not exclude an AD diagnosis because *mixed dementia* may be present. Biomarkers include low levels of beta-amyloid in the cerebrospinal fluid (CSF) and beta-amyloid deposits in the brain visible via positron emission tomography (PET) imaging. Downstream neuronal degeneration or injury is signified by increased levels of tau protein in the CSF, tau deposits in the brain seen in PET imaging with a specific radioactive tracer, reduced cerebral metabolism in the temporoparietal cortex (measured with PET using fluorodeoxyglucose), and local atrophy of the medial,

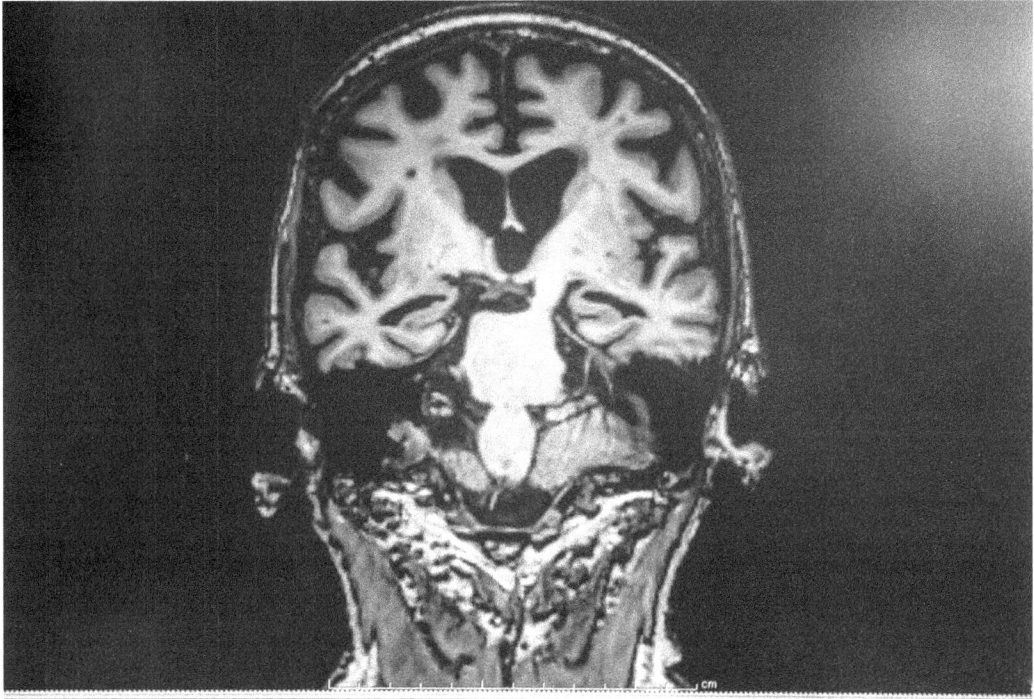

FIGURE 13.1   MRI imaging showing changes in tau deposits in the brain of an Alzheimer's disease patient.

basal, and lateral temporal lobes plus the medial parietal cortex. A critical factor in these imaging studies is the assessment of Pittsburgh compound B (PiB). These results increase the likelihood of AD, but the biomarkers are not standardized or highly available. Routine testing for the apo epsilon-4 allele is not recommended. Laboratory tests and neuroimaging are performed to assess other treatable causes of dementia and disorders that may worsen the symptoms. Tests for diseases such as HIV or syphilis are sometimes indicated. An MRI of the brain of a patient with AD is shown in **Figure 13.1**.

TREATMENT

AD requires the same safe and supportive treatments as other dementias. Environments should be well-lit, colorful, and familiar to help with orientation. Large clocks and calendars are recommended. Signal monitoring systems should be implemented for patients who wander. Caregivers may need much help and must be educated about the disease and how to care for the patient. Healthcare providers must monitor caregiver stress and burnout, and support measures must be suggested. Drugs used for AD include cholinesterase inhibitors such as donepezil, galantamine, and rivastigmine. Donepezil is taken once daily and is generally well tolerated, but it has side effects such as diarrhea, nausea, dizziness, and cardiac arrhythmias. Memantine is an N-methyl-D-aspartate (NMDA) receptor antagonist that improves cognition and can be used with one of the cholinesterase inhibitors. *Aducanumab* is a human IgG1 anti-amyloid monoclonal antibody now available as a monthly infusion for AD. It has reduced brain beta-amyloid plaques in clinical trials. Adverse effects include MRI-visualized signal changes of cerebral edema, microhemorrhage, and hemosiderosis. A few clinical test patients had severe adverse effects, including confusion, disorientation, ataxia, gait disturbance, headache, visual disturbances, nausea, and falling.

PREVENTION

AD risks may be decreased by a diet rich in omega-3 fatty acids and low in saturated fats, challenging mental activities such as puzzles and learning new skills, controlling hypertension, drinking alcohol only in modest amounts, exercising, and lowering cholesterol levels. Once dementia has developed, drinking alcohol can worsen the symptoms.

YOU SHOULD REMEMBER

AD risks may be decreased by a diet rich in omega-3 fatty acids and low in saturated fats, challenging mental activities such as puzzles and learning new skills, controlling hypertension, drinking alcohol only in modest amounts, exercising, and lowering cholesterol levels. Once dementia has developed, drinking alcohol can worsen the symptoms.

Check Your Knowledge

1. What are examples of neurodegenerative disorders?
2. Are most cases of AD sporadic or familial?
3. What is the first sign of AD?

PARKINSON'S DISEASE

Parkinson's disease (PD) is a degenerative disorder that progresses slowly. Cognitive deterioration is characterized by Lewy bodies in the substantia nigra, developing late during PD. The condition is chronic, global, and usually irreversible. PD is caused by the destruction of the nerve cells that make dopamine. Therefore, the risk factors include longstanding nerve cell destruction, increased age, male gender, presence of visual hallucinations, family history of dementia, and severe motor symptoms.

EPIDEMIOLOGY

PD dementia develops in about 40% of patients with PD about 10–15 years after it is diagnosed. Lewy body dementia is estimated to have an incidence of 0.1% annually in the global population but makes up about 3.2% of all new dementia cases. It affects slightly more men than women. There are about 1 million cases of Lewy body dementia in the United States. **Frontotemporal dementia** makes up as much as 10% of all dementia. It affects men and women nearly equally. Incidence is 2.7–4.1 out of every 100,000 people. The prevalence of *HIV-associated dementia* in the later disease stages ranges between 7% and 27%, though 30%–40% of patients may have less severe forms. The incidence is inversely proportional to the patient's CD4 count. Before developing better medications for HIV/AIDS, 21%–25% of patients develop dementia. Regardless of severity, about 3% of athletes with multiple concussions develop *chronic traumatic encephalopathy.*

PD dementia usually develops after age 70. Lewy body dementia often starts to manifest after age 50–60. Frontotemporal dementia usually begins early, between ages 40 and 65, but can occur later in life. Since HIV diagnoses are highest in people aged between 25 and 29, *HIV-associated dementia* takes months to years to develop. This means it is seen in younger patients than other dementias, but after symptoms of HIV infection develop. This is the variable point of development since signs of the disease can start within 1–4 weeks but then become dormant for 10 years or more. *Chronic traumatic encephalopathy* can develop at any time during life but is often seen in younger adults. However, it can also develop in older adults – the patient's age is directly linked to the amount of causative trauma and when it occurs.

ETIOLOGY AND RISK FACTORS

The actual cause of PD is largely unknown. *PD dementia* is caused by the destruction of the nerve cells that make dopamine. Therefore, the risk factors include longstanding PD, increased age, male gender, whether visual hallucinations are present, older age of onset of PD, family history of dementia, and severe motor symptoms. Lewy's body dementia is caused by the buildup of Lewy's body in the areas of the brain that control memory, thinking, and movement. Risk factors include age, sex, heredity, and exposure to toxins such as insecticides, rotenone, organochlorines, and beta-hexachlorocyclohexane.

CLINICAL MANIFESTATIONS

PD has various manifestations based on the age of onset. The juvenile and early-onset forms progress more slowly than later-onset PD. A resting tremor of one hand is often the initial symptom. It is slow, coarse, and most evident while resting, yet absent during sleep. The amplitude is increased by fatigue or emotional tension. The wrist and fingers are often affected, and sometimes, the thumb moves against the index finger in a **pill-rolling movement**. The hands or feet are affected first. The jaw and tongue may be affected, but the voice is not, though it may become **hypophonic**. There is a characteristic of **monotonous** and sometimes **stuttering dysarthria**. As rigidity progresses, the tremor may become less noticeable. Resting tremors are slight or absent in the rigid-akinetic forms of PD. In many patients, rigidity develops independently of the quake. If a rigid joint is moved, semi-rhythmic jerks occur because the intensity of the rigidity is varied. This causes a ratchet-like effect known as **cogwheel rigidity**.

It results in resting tremors, rigidity, **bradykinesia**, and, over time, gait instability, postural instability, or both. The initial tremor of one hand may be barely noticeable. In the early stages of PD, the patient's face often has little expression. Though incurable, medications have evolved well and can significantly improve symptoms.

PD begins with cognitive impairment, with actual dementia beginning 10–15 years after motor symptoms appear. Executive dysfunction usually occurs earlier. A motor decline occurs quicker, and falls are more frequent than in PD when the patient does not have dementia.

Bradykinesia is constant, and repeated motor activities cause a progressive or sustained decrease in movement amplitude, known as **hypokinesia**. Actions become hard to initiate, known as **akinesia**. Muscle aches and fatigue may result from rigidity and hypokinesia. The face develops a mask-like appearance called **hypomimic**, with the mouth open and blinking reduced. Excessive drooling may occur. Hypokinesia and impaired control of the distal muscles results in writing in tiny letters, known as micrographia, compromising activities of daily living.

Later in the disease course, postural instability may develop in a **stooped position**, with the patient having problems initiating walking, turning, and stopping (see **Figure 13.2**). Short steps are taken, and the walk is described as *shuffling*. The arms are flexed to the waist and swing very little or not at all with each step. Some patients experience an accidental quickening of steps, with progressive shortening of the stride length. This is **festination**, which often precedes freezing of the gait. With no warning, voluntary movements such as walking may suddenly stop. When the center of gravity is displaced, the patient tends to fall forward or backward. Dementia develops in about 33% of patients, usually late in the disease course.

DIAGNOSIS

Making an accurate diagnosis of PD can be complicated. To conclude, the clinician must carefully weigh symptoms, family history, and other factors. The standard diagnosis of PD is clinical. No lab or imaging test is recommended or definitive for PD. However 2011, the U.S. Food and Drug Administration approved an imaging scan called the DaTscan. This technique lets clinicians see detailed pictures of the brain's dopamine system.

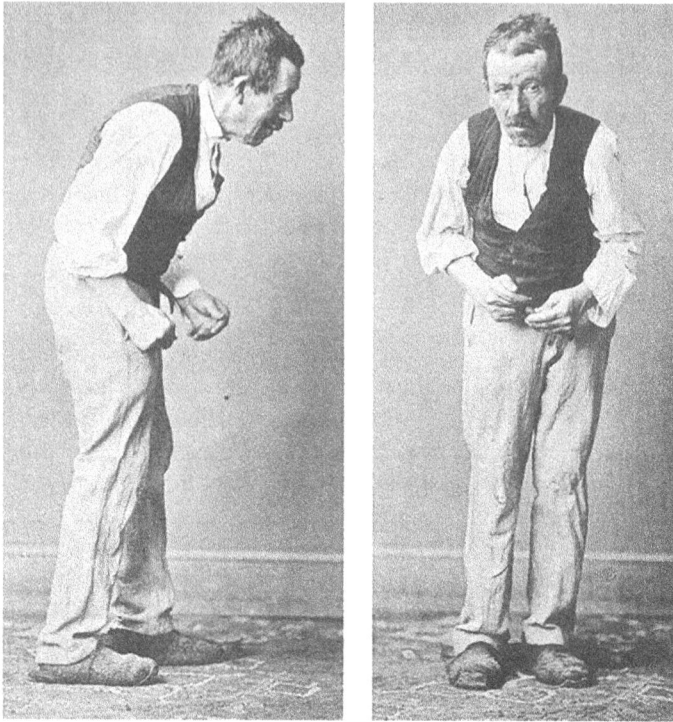

FIGURE 13.2   A patient with Parkinson's disease.

TREATMENT

PD is best treated with carbidopa/levodopa. Levodopa is the metabolic precursor of dopamine. Coadministration with carbidopa prevents levodopa from being decarboxylated into dopamine outside the brain. Levodopa is highly effective at relieving bradykinesia and rigidity while significantly reducing tremors. Cholinesterase inhibitors may improve cognitive function. Pimavanserin is a nondopaminergic selective inverse agonist of the serotonin 5-HT-2A receptor. It is used to treat delusions and hallucinations.

PREVENTION

So far, only two theories have shown to be helpful: exercise and diet. According to studies, physical activity is an excellent way to treat patients with PD and appears to help prevent or delay the onset. Getting the body moving helps build strength, balance, endurance, and coordination. Aim for a balanced diet of whole foods, like vegetables and fruits, lean protein, beans and legumes, whole grains, and the right balance between omega-3 and omega-6 fatty acids. It is also essential to stay hydrated.

YOU SHOULD REMEMBER

PD is a brain condition that causes problems with movements, mental health, sleep, pain, and other health issues. The condition worsens over time, and there is no cure. However, therapies can reduce symptoms such as painful muscle contractions and difficulty speaking. Many people with PD also develop dementia, and men are affected more than women.

Check Your Knowledge

1. How does cognitive deterioration with PD come about?
2. Which gait changes are expected with PD?
3. What are the best treatments for PD?

HUNTINGTON'S DISEASE

Huntington's disease is an autosomal dominant disorder with features of **chorea**, neuropsychiatric symptoms, and cognitive deterioration that usually begins in middle age and progressively worsens. Because of a gene mutation, neurons in the brain degenerate gradually. Due to the severity of the phenotype, Huntington's disease starts insidiously and lasts forever.

EPIDEMIOLOGY

Huntington's disease affects men and women equally. Globally, about one in every 10,000 people has the disease. In the United States, about 30,000 people are affected every year. The condition is not prevalent within any particular population.

ETIOLOGY AND RISK FACTORS

A faulty gene causes Huntington's disease. Cells in parts of the brain are susceptible to the effects of the defective gene. This makes them function poorly and eventually die. A parent with the Huntington's disease gene has one good copy of the gene and one bad copy. Some populations have a slightly higher incidence of Huntington's disease, but no lifestyle factors or habits have been shown to either cause the condition or help prevent it.

CLINICAL MANIFESTATIONS

Before or along with the movement abnormalities, dementia or psychiatric disturbances develop. These may include **apathy**, depression, **anhedonia**, irritability, antisocial behaviors, and fully developed bipolar or schizophreniform disorder. The patient will likely have suicidal thoughts and attempts more often than the general public. Abnormal movements include athetosis, chorea, myoclonic jerks, and pseudo-tics, which manifest **tourettism**. Affected people may walk strangely, resembling the walk of a marionette puppet. There is facial grimacing, an inability to move the eyes quickly without blinking or thrusting the head (known as *oculomotor apraxia*), and an inability to stick the tongue out or grasp objects intentionally. Over time, Huntington's disease makes walking impossible. Swallowing becomes difficult. The dementia that develops becomes severe, and most patients must be institutionalized. There is often depression, anxiety, and **obsessive-compulsive disorder**. Some patients with a history of long periods of anxiety with obsessional preoccupations develop psychosis with clinical **lycanthropy**, in which they have a prominent delusional idea of being "a werewolf."

DIAGNOSIS

Huntington's disease is diagnosed based on its well-understood symptoms and a positive family history, which is confirmed by genetic testing. Neuroimaging identifies caudate atrophy and, in many patients, some of the frontal-predominant cortical atrophy.

TREATMENT

There is no cure for *Huntington's disease*. It is treated supportively to help manage some symptoms. Antipsychotic medications may partially suppress the chorea and agitation. Doses of antipsychotics are increased until symptoms are controlled or unwanted adverse effects such as lethargy or parkinsonism develop. Alternative medications include vesicular monoamine transporter type 2 inhibitors, such as tetrabenazine or deutetrabenazine. They deplete dopamine and help reduce chorea and dyskinesias.

PREVENTION

Because Huntington's disease is genetic, there is no prevention. If you have a history of Huntington's disease in your family, you may wish to have genetic counseling before having children.

Check Your Knowledge

1. What is the description of Huntington's disease?
2. What are the psychiatric disturbances of Huntington's disease?
3. How is Huntington's disease diagnosed?

CREUTZFELDT–JAKOB DISEASE

Creutzfeldt–Jakob disease (CJD) is a rare brain disorder leading to dementia. It belongs to a group of human and animal diseases known as **prion disorders**. Symptoms of CJD can be similar to those of AD. But CJD usually gets worse much faster and leads to death. CJD received public attention in the 1990s when some people in the United Kingdom became sick with a form of the disease. They developed variant CJD (vCJD) after eating meat from diseased cattle. However, most cases of CJD haven't been linked to eating beef.

EPIDEMIOLOGY

All types of CJD are serious but are very rare. About one to two cases of CJD are diagnosed per million people worldwide each year. The disease most often affects older adults. Most cases of CJD (about 85%) are believed to occur sporadically, caused by the spontaneous transformation of normal prion proteins into abnormal prions. This sporadic disease occurs worldwide, including in the United States, at a rate of roughly one to two cases per 1 million population per year.

ETIOLOGY AND RISK FACTORS

CJD and related conditions appear to be caused by changes to a prion protein (see **Figure 13.3**). These proteins are typically produced in the body. But when they encounter infectious prions, they fold and shape differently. They can spread and affect processes in the body.

  Prions are proteins that occur naturally in the brains of animals and people. Usually, the proteins are harmless, but when they are misshapen, they can cause devastating illnesses such as cow disease and CJD in humans. The risk of getting CJD is low. The disease can't be spread through coughing, sneezing, touching, or sexual contact.

CLINICAL MANIFESTATIONS

Changes in mental abilities mark CJD. Symptoms get worse quickly, usually within several weeks to a few months. Early symptoms include:

PrP^C
is a normal protein

PrP^Sc
the disease-causing form of the
prion protein

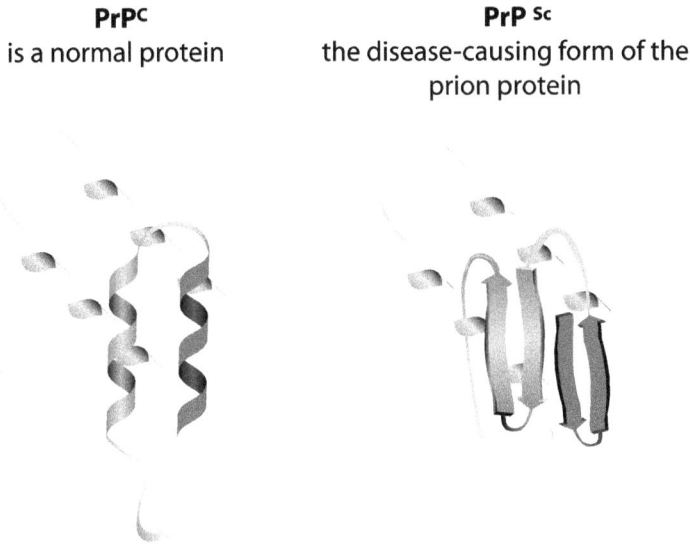

FIGURE 13.3   Creutzfeldt–Jakob disease and changes to a prion protein.

- Personality changes
- Depression, mood swings, and anxiety
- Memory loss
- Impaired thinking
- Blurry vision or blindness
- Problems with coordination
- Trouble speaking
- Difficulties with walking and balance
- Insomnia
- Confusion
- Trouble swallowing
- Sudden, jerky movements
- Coma

Death usually occurs within a year. People with CJD typically die of medical issues associated with the disease. They might include having trouble swallowing, falls, heart issues, lung failure, pneumonia, or other infections. In people with vCJD, changes in mental abilities may be more apparent at the beginning of the disease. In many cases, dementia develops later in the illness. Symptoms of dementia include losing the ability to think, reason, and remember.

Another rare form of prion disease is variably **protease-sensitive prionopathy**. It can mimic other forms of dementia. It causes changes in mental abilities and problems with speech and thinking. The course of the disease is longer than that of other prion diseases – about 24 months.

DIAGNOSIS

A few tests can help diagnose CJD, including electroencephalography, MRI, and cerebrospinal fluid tests. However, the only way to confirm a diagnosis of CJD is by brain biopsy or an autopsy. In a brain biopsy, a neurosurgeon removes a small piece of tissue from a living person's brain so a neuropathologist can examine it. This procedure may be dangerous for the individual and is generally discouraged unless it is needed to rule out a treatable disorder. In an autopsy, the whole brain is examined after death.

TREATMENT

CJD has no cure, although some drugs are being tested to control it. Today's treatments aim to make the person comfortable and ease symptoms. Medications may help relieve pain and muscle jerks. During later stages of the disease, intravenous fluids and machine feeding may also be used.

PREVENTION

There is no known way to prevent sporadic CJD. If you have a family history of neurological disease, you may benefit from talking with a genetics counselor. A counselor can help you sort through your risks.

YOU SHOULD REMEMBER

CJD has severe effects on the brain and body. The condition usually progresses quickly. Over time, people with CJD withdraw from friends and family. They also lose the ability to care for themselves. Many slip into a coma. The disease is always fatal.

Check Your Knowledge

1. What type of disorder is CJD classified as?
2. How quickly does CJD cause death?
3. How can CJD be confirmed?

Clinical Case Studies

CLINICAL CASE STUDY 1

A 69-year-old man was assessed because his wife noticed worsening difficulties with verbal communication. He also had begun asking his wife for instructions on how to do specific household tasks that he previously knew how to do. The patient also had short-term memory loss and was unable to remember conversations that had happened just a few days before. He also became irritable quite quickly, unlike how he had been throughout his life. The patient's wife explained that her husband's mother had dementia up until she died at age 78 in a nursing home. An electroencephalogram of the patient's brain activity revealed slowed functionality, consistent with diffuse mild brain dysfunction. A diagnosis of AD was made based on his severe memory impairment and prominent language problems.

CRITICAL THINKING QUESTIONS

1. What is the description of the beta-amyloid plaques that accumulate in AD?
2. How common is AD?
3. What are the clinical manifestations of AD?

CLINICAL CASE STUDY 2

A 69-year-old woman was diagnosed with PD. She lived independently with support from a home healthcare organization, receiving assistance with meal preparation and household chores. Occupational therapy was also provided to help the patient reduce her fall risk and maintain her muscle strength and coordination. Over time, the patient was convinced to allow a caregiver to live in her home so that she would have assistance 24/7. As her condition worsened, this became extremely important and helpful, and the patient greatly benefited from the care she received.

CRITICAL THINKING QUESTIONS

1. What are the causes and risk factors of PD?
2. What is the best treatment for PD?
3. What may happen late in the disease course of PD?

CLINICAL CASE STUDY 3

A 64-year-old man had been diagnosed with Huntington's disease and admitted to an inpatient mental health unit. After this, he was transferred to a specialist inpatient neuropsychiatry unit. He had a history of anxiety, obsessional preoccupations, and, eventually, psychosis. He was almost always mentally and physically agitated, with severe choreiform movements that affected his upper body. He also repeatedly stated that he was "turning into a werewolf." The patient also described wanting to strangle his wife and cannibalize her, as well as to burn down churches. Before his institutionalization, the patient had not improved even though various antidepressants and antipsychotics were tried.

CRITICAL THINKING QUESTIONS

1. Who does Huntington's disease affect?
2. What are the psychiatric disturbances of Huntington's disease?
3. How is Huntington's disease treated?

FURTHER READING

1. Beller, J. (2020). *Creutzfeldt-Jakob Disease: The Best Science in Everyday Language! (Dementia Types, Symptoms, Stages, and Risk Factors).* Jerry Beller Health Research Institute.
2. Bird, T.D. (2019). *Can You Help Me? Inside the Turbulent World of Huntington Disease.* Oxford University Press.
3. Graff-Radford, J., and Lunde, A.M. (2020). *Mayo Clinic on Alzheimer's Disease and Other Dementias (A Guide for People with Dementia and Those Who Care For Them),* 2nd Edition. Mayo Clinic Press.
4. Hetz, C. (2018). *Protein Misfolding Disorders: A Trip into the ER.* Bentham Books.
5. Hewitt, J., and Gabata, M. (2011). *Huntington's Disease: Causes, Tests, and Treatments.* CreateSpace Independent Publishing Platform.
6. Lewis, P.A., and Spillane, J.E. (2018). *The Molecular and Clinical Pathology of Neurodegenerative Disease.* Academic Press.
7. Pocchiari, M., and Manson, J. (2018). *Handbook of Clinical Neurology, 153: Human Prion Diseases.* Elsevier.
8. Prusiner, S.B. (2017). *Prion Diseases (Perspectives in Medicine).* Cold Spring Harbor Laboratory Press.
9. Sabat, S.R. (2018). *Alzheimer's Disease and Dementia: What Everyone Needs to Know.* Oxford University Press.
10. Vine, J.M. (2017). *A Parkinson's Primer: An Indispensable Guide to Parkinson's Disease for Patients and Their Families.* Paul Dry Books.
11. Weiner, W.J., Shulman, L.M., and Lang, A.E. (2013). *Parkinson's Disease: A Complete Guide for Patients and Families,* 3rd Edition. Johns Hopkins University Press.

12. Wu, K.C. (2023). *Biological Impermanence: Protein Misfolding: In Situ Electromagnetic Origin of Diseases.* BookBaby.
13. Agronin, M.E. (2014). *Alzheimer's Disease and Other Dementias: A Practical Guide*, 3rd Edition. Routledge.
14. Ahlskog, J.E. (2013). *Dementia with Lewy Bodies and Parkinson's Disease Dementia: Patient, Family, and Clinician Working Together for Better Outcomes.* Oxford University Press.
15. Ali, I. (2009). *HIV Associated Dementia: Dopaminergic Neuronal Apoptosis and Future Implications for Clinical Intervention.* Null.
16. Beller, J. (2020). *Dementia with Lewy Bodies: Guide for Doctors, Nurses, Patients, Families, & Caregivers.* Jerry Beller Health Research Institute.
17. Libon, D.J., Lamar, M., Swenson, R.A., and Heilman, K.M. (2020). *Vascular Disease, Alzheimer's Disease, and Mild Cognitive Impairment: Advancing an Integrated Approach.* Oxford University Press.
18. Miller, B.L. (2013). *Frontotemporal Dementia (Contemporary Neurology Series, 85).* Oxford University Press.
19. Rahman, S. (2020). *Essentials of Delirium: Everything You Need to Know for Working in Delirium Care.* Jessica Kingsley Publishers.
20. Turan Isik, A., and Grossberg, G.T. (2018). *Delirium in Elderly Patients.* Springer.
21. Walter, L.C., and Chang, A. (2020). *Current Diagnosis and Treatment: Geriatrics*, 3rd Edition. McGraw-Hill/Lange.

14 Hereditary Protein Disorders

OVERVIEW

Hereditary protein disorders occur when parents pass the defective genes that cause these disorders on to their children. In most hereditary metabolic diseases, both parents of the affected child carry a copy of the abnormal gene. Because two copies of the abnormal gene are usually necessary for the confusion, neither parent has the condition. Some hereditary metabolic disorders are X-linked, which means only one copy of the abnormal gene can cause the disease in boys. Because these disorders cause symptoms early in life, newborns have several common amino acid disorders. In the United States, newborns are commonly screened for phenylketonuria, maple syrup urine disease, tyrosinemia, and homocystinuria.

Phenylketonuria is a rare inherited disorder that causes phenylalanine to build up in the body. Maple syrup urine disease is a severe but rare inherited condition. Tyrosine is an amino acid that is found in most proteins. When people with tyrosinemia break down protein, abnormal toxic breakdown products of tyrosine build up in their bodies. This causes progressive damage to the liver and kidneys.

PHENYLKETONURIA

Phenylketonuria (PKU) is a disorder involving an inborn error of amino acid metabolism. It causes a clinical syndrome that leads to intellectual defects and behavioral and cognitive abnormalities caused by elevated serum phenylalanine. It is usually due to deficient phenylalanine hydroxylase (PAH) activity. Inheritance is autosomal recessive.

EPIDEMIOLOGY

PKU occurs in all ethnic groups but is less common in Ashkenazi Jews and people of African descent. Incidence is approximately 1 in every 10,000–15,000 newborns. Most cases of PKU are detected shortly after birth by newborn screening, and treatment is started promptly. The prevalence in the general US population is approximately four cases per 100,000 individuals, and the incidence is 350 cases per million live births. About 0.04%–1% of the residents in intellectual disability clinics are affected by PKU. Globally, 450,000 individuals have PKU, with a global prevalence of 1 of every 23,930 live births (within a range of 1 in 4,500 [Italy] to 1 in 125,000 [Japan]).

ETIOLOGY AND RISK FACTORS

PKU is caused by an inherited change in the PAH gene, which helps create the enzyme required to break down phenylalanine. PKU is passed down in a recessive pattern, meaning that for a child to develop PKU, both parents must contribute a mutated version of the PAH gene. If both parents have PKU, their child will have it as well. Sometimes, a parent does not have PKU but is a carrier, which means the parent carries a mutated PAH gene. If only one parent carries the mutated gene, the child will not develop PKU. Even if both parents carry the mutated PAH gene, their child may not develop PKU. A child's parents each have two versions of the PAH gene, only one of which they will pass on during conception. If both of a child's parents are carriers, there is a 25% chance that each parent will pass on the normal PAH gene. In this case, the child will not have the disorder.

DOI: 10.1201/9781003453376-18

Conversely, there is also a 25% chance that the carrier parents will pass along the mutated gene, causing the child to have PKU. However, there is a 50% chance that a child will inherit one normal gene from one parent and one abnormal one from the other, making the child a carrier. Risk factors for inheriting PKU include having both parents with the gene mutation and being of a particular racial or ethnic descent.

CLINICAL MANIFESTATIONS

Newborns with PKU seem normal during the first days of life. However, without treatment, nervous system damage progresses gradually and becomes apparent over several months. The primary sign of untreated PKU is severe intellectual disability. There is also significant hyperactivity, gait disturbances, **microcephaly**, seizures, and psychoses. Often, there is a musty odor in the breath, skin, or urine because of too much phenylalanine in the body. This is due to the breakdown product of phenylalanine, known as phenylacetic acid, in the sweat and urine. Affected children usually have lighter eyes, hair, and skin color than their family members who do not have the disease (see **Figure 14.1**). Some individuals develop a rash that mimics infantile eczema.

DIAGNOSIS

The early diagnosis of PKU before the end of the first month of life is critical to controlling hyperphenylalaninemia. In many developed countries (including the United States), neonates are routinely screened for PKU 24–48 hours after birth via blood tests. Abnormal results are confirmed

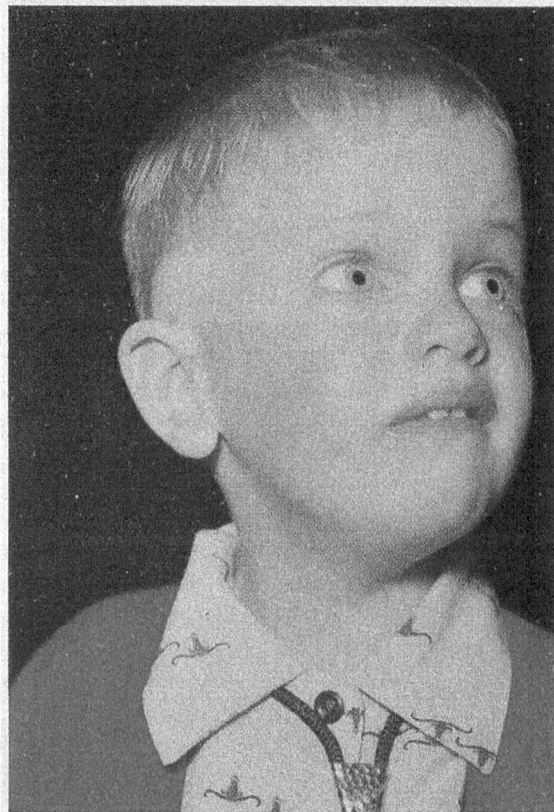

FIGURE 14.1   A child with phenylketonuria.

by direct measurement of phenylalanine levels. In the classic form of PKU, neonates usually have phenylalanine levels higher than 20 mg/dL (1.2 mM/L). If the deficiency is partial, these levels are below 8–10 mg/dL if the diet is regular. However, levels higher than 6 mg/dL require treatment. The distinction from classic PKU is made via a mutation analysis that identifies mild gene mutations, or less commonly; liver PAH activity assays that reveal activity between 5% and 15% of normal.

A Tetrahydrobiopterin (BH4) deficiency is distinguished from other types of PKU by elevated concentrations of biopterin or neopterin in the blood, cerebrospinal fluid, or urine (or all three of these). Genetic testing is also valuable. It is essential to recognize the deficiency. The urine biopterin profile must be determined at the initial diagnosis since standard PKU treatment will not prevent neurological damage. If the child is part of a family with a positive PKU history, diagnosis can be made prenatally via direct mutation studies after amniocentesis or chorionic villus sampling.

TREATMENT

The treatment of PKU is a lifelong restriction of dietary phenylalanine. All-natural protein contains approximately 4% phenylalanine. This means that the diet requires low-protein natural foods such as certain cereals, plus fruits and vegetables, phenylalanine-free elemental amino acid mixtures, and protein hydrolysates that are treated to remove phenylalanine. There are a variety of commercially available phenylalanine-free products for infants and children. Some amount of phenylalanine is needed for growth and metabolism. The requirement is met by measuring natural protein levels from low-protein or milk foods.

Plasma phenylalanine levels must be frequently monitored. Target levels for all children are between 2 and 6 mg/dL. Dietary planning and management must be started before pregnancy for women of childbearing age. Tyrosine supplements are used more today because this is an essential amino acid in patients with PKU. Also, all patients with PAH deficiency must be given a trial of sapropterin to determine if this will be beneficial. For BH4 deficiency, treatment additionally includes tetrahydrobiopterin, 1–5 mg/kg orally, three times per day, plus levodopa, carbidopa, 5-OH tryptophan, and folinic acid 10–20 mg once per day (if there is a dihydropyridine reductase deficiency). Treatment goals and approaches are the same as those used for PKU.

PREVENTION

There is no way to prevent or avoid PKU since it is a genetic condition. Genetic testing is the only way to determine if the defective gene exists. Some people carry the gene but do not have the disease.

YOU SHOULD REMEMBER

PKU is an inborn error of metabolism that can be diagnosed during the first days of life with routine newborn screening. It is characterized by the absence or deficiency of an enzyme called PAH, which is responsible for processing the amino acid phenylalanine.

Check Your Knowledge

1. When are most cases of PKU usually diagnosed?
2. What happens if a newborn with PKU is not treated?
3. What is the treatment for PKU?

MAPLE SYRUP URINE DISEASE

Maple syrup urine disease (MSUD) is a rare but severe and life-threatening inherited condition. It means the body cannot process certain amino acids, causing a harmful build-up of substances in the blood and urine. The disease is due to an inborn error of branched-chain amino acid metabolism. It impairs the metabolism of amino acids such as isoleucine, leucine, and valine. The classical clinical variant of the order develops in the neonatal period. It can lead to severe complications if not recognized and treated within the first week of life.

EPIDEMIOLOGY

MSUD occurs in about 1 of every 86,800–185,000 live births worldwide. About 2,000 people in the United States live with MSUD. It affects males and females equally. Incidence is 1 in 200 live births in specific **Mennonite populations** in Pennsylvania and other locations due to a founder variant in the branched-chain ketoacid dehydrogenase complex gene.

ETIOLOGY AND RISK FACTORS

A branched-chain alpha-ketoacid dehydrogenase deficiency causes MSUD. If both parents are carriers, the offspring has a 25% chance of receiving the two mutated genes and, therefore, having the disease. There is a 50% chance of receiving only one defective gene and being a carrier. There is also a 25% chance of receiving one normal gene from each parent.

CLINICAL MANIFESTATIONS

Patients with severe neonatal MSUD are usually typical for the first 2 or 3 days of life. They then develop lethargy, hypertonia with authoritarian **opisthotonic posturing**, loss of appetite, poor feeding, vomiting, seizures, respiratory failure, and coma that can lead to death. Usually, the disease does not produce lactic acidemia, metabolic acidosis, hyperammonemia, hypoglycemia, abnormal **acylcarnitines**, or ketosis. Without treatment, however, it can lead to hypoglycemia and ketoacidosis. Patients that recover from an initial episode can experience growth failure, mental retardation, and recurring metabolic decompensation. The four main types of MSUD are:

- *Classic* – Classic MSUD is the most severe type of MSUD. It is also the most common. Symptoms usually develop within the first 3 days of birth.
- *Intermediate* – This type of MSUD is less severe than classic MSUD. Symptoms typically appear in children between 5 months and 7 years old.
- *Intermittent* – Children with intermittent MSUD develop as expected until an infection or period of stress causes symptoms to appear. People with intermittent MSUD usually tolerate higher levels of the three amino acids than those with classic MSUD.
- *Thiamine-responsive* – This type of MSUD responds to treatment using high doses of vitamin B1 (thiamine) and a restricted diet. People with thiamine-responsive MSUD have a higher tolerance for the three amino acids with treatment.

DIAGNOSIS

Newborn screening programs for MSUD are based on detecting **hyperleucinemia**. For healthy full-term infants, false-positive results are rare. Mass spectrometry technology has reduced the rate of false-positive and false-negative results, which concurrently measures concentrations of isoleucine, leucine, and valine. This allows the use of amino acid ratios to identify better newborns that are at risk. However, a positive newborn screening result is sometimes not received until after the patient is ill and within the neonatal intensive care unit. Regardless, a response to a positive screening result must occur quickly.

Bedside detection of a characteristic maple syrup odor may be the first clue aiding diagnosis. If suspected, the diagnosis can be partially confirmed by a rapid screening test called the dinitrophenylhydrazine (DNPH) test. This detects the alpha-ketoacids formed from isoleucine, leucine, and valine. Diagnosis is then established via plasma amino acid analysis and urine organic acid analysis. Characteristic findings are increased leucine, isoleucine, valine, and alloisoleucine (its presence is pathognomonic for the disease), plus the distinct urinary organic acid pattern. MSUD is not related to abnormal carnitine metabolism. Definitized enzyme analysis may be performed with leukocytes or cultures of skin fibroblasts. However, treatment must not be delayed while awaiting a definitive diagnosis.

TREATMENT

Treatment of an acutely ill newborn with MSUD includes hypercaloric nutritional support (high glucose concentrations, an insulin infusion to avoid hyperglycemia, and a source of leucine, isoleucine, and valine-free protein). Protein catabolism must be suppressed, and an anabolic state must be induced. Via this regimen, concentrations of isoleucine, valine, or both may become too low, limiting the rate of new protein synthesis. Treatment progress must be monitored frequently to determine when the branched-chain amino acids must be added to the diet. They must be carefully reintroduced (orally or parenterally). For extreme cases, the approach may not reduce the leucine concentration or correct the other metabolic abnormalities quickly enough. This means that hemodialysis is required.

PREVENTION

There is no method of preventing MSUD because it is inherited. A genetic counselor can help determine the risks of having an infant with the disease. It also informs parents if either or both are carriers of the disease.

YOU SHOULD REMEMBER

MSUD is a rare inherited disorder caused by the body's inability to properly process amino acids, leading to a characteristic odor of maple syrup in the urine. If not diagnosed and treated soon after birth, it can be life-threatening – as early as the first 2 weeks of life.

Check Your Knowledge

1. What are the four central MSUD types?
2. What are newborn screening programs for MSUD based on?
3. What are the treatments for MSUD?

TYROSINEMIA

Tyrosinemia is a genetic disorder characterized by multistep disruptions that break down the amino acid tyrosine. If untreated, tyrosine and its byproducts build up in tissues and organs. Tyrosine is also a precursor of neurotransmitters, hormones, and melanin. The neurotransmitters involved include dopamine, epinephrine, and norepinephrine, while the hormone is thyroxine. Deficiency of enzymes involved in the metabolism of tyrosine results in various syndromes. The multiple forms of tyrosinemia include the following:

- *Transient tyrosinemia of the newborn*
- *Tyrosinemia type I*
- *Tyrosinemia type 2*
- *Tyrosinemia type 3*

EPIDEMIOLOGY

Up to 10% of newborns have transient tyrosinemia, which is benign and resolves without sequelae. Tyrosinemia type 1 affects males and females equally. Prevalence is estimated to be 1 of every 100,000–120,000 births worldwide. For unknown reasons, it is much more common in Quebec, Canada, with a birth prevalence of 1 in 16,000. The Saguenay–Lac-Saint-Jean region of Quebec has the highest prevalence, affecting 1 of every 1,850 births. Tyrosinemia type 2 is much rarer, with an estimated prevalence of less than 1 in every 1,000,000 births. Less than 150 cases have been reported, though it occurs most often in Arab and Mediterranean populations. Alkaptonuria is a rare disease but occurs everywhere worldwide, affecting 1 in every 100,000–250,000 births. In the United States, prevalence is 1 case per 1,000,000 people. While classic albinism affects about 18,000 people in the United States, oculocutaneous albinism (type 1) affects about 1 out of every 40,000 individuals in most populations. The type 2 form of oculocutaneous albinism is widespread among African Americans and Africans.

ETIOLOGY AND RISK FACTORS

Tyrosinemia is caused by mutations in the fumarylacetoacetate hydrolase (FAH) gene responsible for producing the FAH enzyme. Deficiency of FAH leads to elevation of plasma tyrosine levels, usually in premature infants and especially in those receiving high-protein diets. Tyrosinemia type 1 is an autosomal recessive condition caused by FAH deficiency, an important enzyme needed for tyrosine metabolism. Tyrosinemia type 2 is rarer and caused by tyrosine transaminase deficiency. Alkaptonuria is another rare autosomal recessive condition caused by homogentisic acid oxidase deficiency. The only risk factor for various forms of tyrosinemia is receiving a gene mutation from each parent.

CLINICAL MANIFESTATIONS

With transient tyrosinemia of the newborn, most infants are asymptomatic. However, some develop lethargy, poor feeding, failure to gain weight and grow at the expected rate, fever, diarrhea, vomiting, hepatomegaly, and jaundice. Tyrosinemia type 1 may manifest as fulminant liver failure in the neonatal period or as indolent subclinical hepatitis, painful peripheral neuropathy, or in older infants and children, as renal tubular disorders (hypophosphatemia, metabolic acidosis, or rickets). Children who do not die of related liver failure during infancy have a much higher risk of developing liver cancer – accumulation of tyrosine results in cutaneous and oral ulcers. Secondary elevation of phenylalanine (though mild) can cause neuropsychiatric abnormalities without treatment. With alkaptonuria, homogentisic acid oxidation products accumulate in the skin, darkening it. Also, crystals collect in the joints. Signs and symptoms of tyrosinemia type 2 often begin in early childhood, including excessive tearing, nystagmus, **photophobia**, eye pain and redness, and **palmoplantar hyperkeratosis**. Tyrosinemia type 3 is the rarest of the three types. The characteristic features of this type include intellectual disability, seizures, and periodic loss of balance and coordination.

DIAGNOSIS

With transient tyrosinemia of the newborn, metabolites may appear on routine neonatal screening for PKU. Tyrosinemia is distinguished from PKU by elevated plasma levels of tyrosine. Diagnosis of tyrosinemia type 1 is suggested by elevated tyrosine in the plasma and confirmed by genetic testing or a high level of succinylacetone in the plasma or urine. It may also be diagnosed by low fumarylacetoacetate hydroxylase activity in blood cells or specimens taken as part of a liver biopsy. Diagnosis of tyrosinemia type 2 is via elevated plasma tyrosine, lack of succinylacetone in the plasma or urine, and genetic testing. There is usually no need to measure decreased enzyme activity as part of a liver biopsy. Alkaptonuria is generally diagnosed in adults from the presence of **ochronosis** and arthritis. The urine turns dark when exposed to air due to oxidation products of homogentisic acid. Diagnosis involves finding elevated urinary levels of homogentisic acid higher than 4–8 g over 24 hours.

TREATMENT

Most cases of transient tyrosinemia of the newborn resolve spontaneously. Symptomatic patients should have dietary tyrosine restriction to 2 g/kg/day and receive 200–400 mg of oral vitamin C once daily. For tyrosinemia type 1, treatment with nitisinone is effective for acute episodes and slows disease progression. A diet low in phenylalanine and tyrosine is recommended, and liver transplantation is also effective. Tyrosinemia type 2 is easily treated with restriction (mild to moderate) of dietary tyrosine and phenylalanine. There is no effective treatment for alkaptonuria, though ascorbic acid (1 g orally once per day) may reduce pigment deposition by increasing the renal excretion of homogentisic acid.

PREVENTION

Since it is inherited, tyrosinemia cannot be prevented. However, a special low-protein diet and certain medications can adequately help to manage the condition in its various manifestations.

YOU SHOULD REMEMBER

Liver transplantation is still the only way to correct tyrosine metabolism, but this is rarely necessary nowadays. More than 90% of children respond very well to Nitisinone and diet. At present, liver transplantation is only needed where children with the acute form do not react to nitisinone rapidly or where liver cancer is suspected. After receiving a transplant, children can eat a regular diet and lead healthy, active lives.

Check Your Knowledge

1. What are the causes and risk factors for tyrosinemia?
2. What are the clinical manifestations of tyrosinemia?
3. What is the diagnosis of tyrosinemia?

HOMOCYSTINURIA

Homocystinuria is a rare but potentially severe inherited condition. This means that the body cannot process the amino acid methionine. This causes a harmful build-up of substances in the blood and urine. Various defects in methionine metabolism result in the accumulation of *homocysteine* and its dimer. There are various methionine and sulfur metabolism disorders, plus many other amino acid and organic acid metabolism disorders. Homocysteine is an intermediate in the metabolism of methionine. It is remethylated to regenerate methionine or combined with serine in various transsulfuration reactions, forming cystathionine, followed by cysteine. Eventually, cysteine is metabolized to glutathione, sulfite, and taurine. Defects in remethylation or transsulfuration may cause homocysteine to collect, causing the disease. The initial step in methionine metabolism is conversion to adenosylmethionine. This requires the enzyme called methionine adenosyltransferase. When this enzyme is deficient, methionine becomes elevated in the blood, which can sometimes cause false-positive neonatal screening results for homocystinuria. There are the following classifications of homocystinuria:

- *Classic homocystinuria*
- *Other forms of homocystinuria*
- *Cystathioninuria*
- *Sulfite oxidase deficiency*

EPIDEMIOLOGY

The most common form of homocystinuria affects at least 1 in 200,000–335,000 people worldwide. The disorder appears to be more common in some countries, such as Ireland (1 in 65,000), Germany (1 in 17,800), Norway (1 in 6,400), and Qatar (1 in 1,800). Classic homocystinuria is estimated to affect 1 in every 100,000–200,000 individuals in the United States. Worldwide prevalence is estimated to be 0.82 of every 100,000 (via clinical records) and 1.09 of every 100,000 (via neonatal screening). The epidemiology of the other forms of homocystinuria needs to be better documented, with no accurate figures available. Cystathioninuria has a prevalence of 1–9 in every 100,000 people. Most sulfite oxidase deficiency is unknown, with only 50 documented cases.

ETIOLOGY AND RISK FACTORS

Classic homocystinuria is caused by an autosomal recessive deficiency of cystathionine beta-synthase (which catalyzes the formation of **cystathionine** from homocysteine and serine). Various defects in remethylation can cause homocystinuria. Defects include the following:

- *Deficiencies of methionine synthase and MS reductase (MSR)*
- *Delivery of methylcobalamin and adenosylcobalamin*
- *Deficiency of methylenetetrahydrofolate reductase* (which is needed to generate the 5-methyltetrahydrofolate required for the methionine synthase reaction)

These forms of homocystinuria have no methionine elevation, so they cannot be detected by neonatal screening. The disorder known as *cystathioninuria* is caused by a deficiency of cystathionase, which converts cystathionine to cysteine. Accumulation of cystathionine causes increased urinary excretion without any clinical symptoms. *Sulfite oxidase* converts sulfite to sulfate in the last step of cystine and methionine degradation, requiring a molybdenum factor. A deficiency of the enzyme or the cofactor causes a similar disease. The disorder is autosomal recessive in inheritance. The only risk factors for all forms of homocystinuria involve having gene defects that both parents pass on to their children.

CLINICAL MANIFESTATIONS

In classic homocystinuria, excess homocysteine adversely affects connective tissue, which may involve **fibrillin**, especially in the eyes and skeleton. Neurological abnormalities may be caused

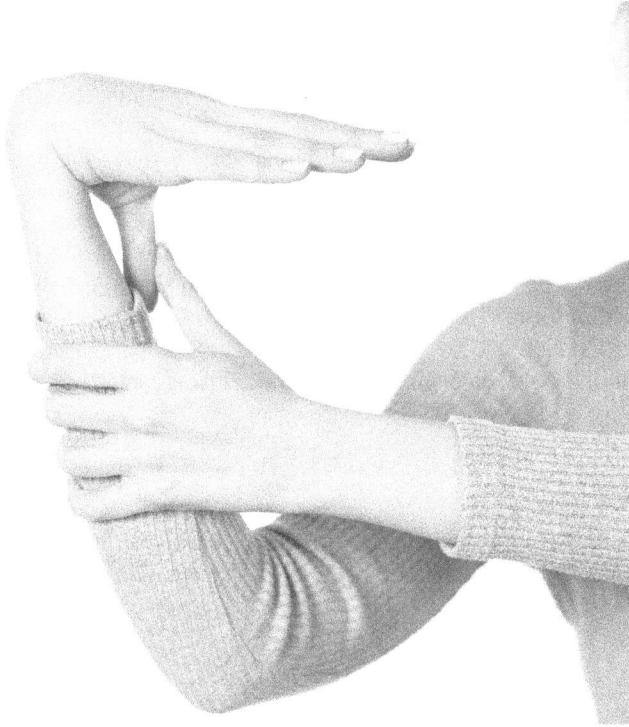

FIGURE 14.2   Hyperlaxity, as part of homocystinuria.

by thrombosis or a direct effect. Arterial and venous thromboembolic signs can occur at any age. Often, **ectopia lentis** develops, as well as intellectual disability and osteoporosis. Though affected individuals are not usually tall, they can have a **marfanoid habitus**. This describes symptoms resembling *Marfan syndrome*, including a long arm span, crowded oral maxilla, sometimes a high palate arch, **arachnodactyly**, and **hyperlaxity** (see **Figure 14.2**).

The signs and symptoms of the "other" forms of homocystinuria resemble those of classic homocystinuria. Also, methionine synthase and MSR deficiencies involve neurological deficits and **megaloblastic anemia**. Clinical manifestations of methylenetetrahydrofolate reductase deficiency are varied but include ataxia, intellectual disability, psychosis, spasticity, and weakness. The most severe form of *sulfite oxidase deficiency* appears in neonates, causing hypotonia, myoclonus, and seizures that progress to early death. If the state of the disease is less severe, signs are similar to those of cerebral palsy, or there may be **choreiform movements**.

DIAGNOSIS

Diagnosis of classic homocystinuria is via neonatal screening for elevated serum methionine. Raised total plasma homocysteine levels, DNA testing, or both will confirm the disease. An enzymatic assay in skin fibroblasts is also available. Diagnosis of MS and MSR deficiencies is suggested by homocystinuria and **megaloblastic anemia**. It is confirmed by DNA testing. Patients with cobalamin defects have megaloblastic anemia plus methylmalonic acidemia. Methylenetetrahydrofolate reductase deficiency is diagnosed by DNA testing. Diagnosis of sulfite oxidase deficiency is suggested by elevated urinary sulfite. It is confirmed by measurement of enzyme levels in fibroblasts and cofactor levels in liver biopsy specimens, genetic testing, or both.

TREATMENT

There is no cure for homocystinuria. However, classic homocystinuria can be treated with a low-methionine diet with L-cysteine supplementation. This is combined with high doses of pyridoxine (100–500 mg orally, once per day). Since about 50% of patients respond to high-dose pyridoxine (vitamin B6) independently, methionine intake may not need to be restricted. Trimethylglycine enhances remethylation and can help lower homocysteine. The dosage usually begins at 100–125 mg/kg orally, twice daily, and then titrated as needed. Some patients require 9 g per day or more. Also, folate (1–5 mg orally, once per day) is given. The intellectual outcome is normal or nearly normal when treatment is started early. Oral vitamin C (100 mg, once daily) can help prevent thromboembolism. Treatment of the other forms of homocystinuria involves replacing hydroxocobalamin (vitamin B12) intramuscularly daily for patients with **multiple sclerosis** (MS) and cobalamin defects. Folate supplementation is also given. Treatment of sulfite oxidase deficiency is supportive.

PREVENTION

While homocystinuria is not preventable, it is possible to control homocysteine levels in some infants with pyridoxine. If this is successful, the child will need vitamin B6 supplements throughout life.

YOU SHOULD REMEMBER

In classic homocystinuria, homocysteine accumulates and dimerizes, forming disulfide homocysteine excreted in the urine. Since remethylation is intact, some additional homocysteine is converted to methionine and accumulates in the blood. Excessive homocysteine predisposes to thrombosis.

Check Your Knowledge

1. What is the characteristic of homocystinuria?
2. What is the cause of classic homocystinuria?
3. What is the marfanoid habitus?

LESCH–NYHAN SYNDROME

Lesch–Nyhan syndrome (LNS) is a sporadic inborn error of purine metabolism and an X-linked recessive disorder. Females carry it, pass it on to male children, and present at birth – average life expectancy, with treatment, is into the early- to mid-20s. There can be an increased risk of sudden death because of respiratory problems, though many patients live longer with good medical and psychological care.

EPIDEMIOLOGY

LNS usually first affects babies between 3 and 12 months of age. The estimated prevalence is 1 in every 235,000–380,000 births. It occurs relatively equally in all populations. Although it is an X-linked disorder manifesting primarily in males, a few females with LNS have been reported.

Etiology and Risk Factors

LNS is caused by a deficiency of hypoxanthine-guanine phosphoribosyl transferase (HPRT). The degree of the deficiency and its resulting manifestations vary between the specific gene mutations that are present. The HPRT deficiency causes a failure of the salvage pathway for guanine and hypoxanthine, which are instead degraded to uric acid. A decrease in guanosyl monophosphate and inositol monophosphate causes an increase in the conversion of 5-phosphoribosyl-1-pyrophosphate (PRPP) to 5-phosphoribosylamine. This results in uric acid overproduction. Risk factors include the male gender and having male family members on the mother's side with the syndrome.

Clinical Manifestations

LNS causes brain and behavior problems, including severe arthritis, poor muscle control, and mental disability. A key symptom is uncontrollable self-injury. Hyperuricemia predisposes patients to gout and its complications. An orange, sandy precipitate known as xanthine appears in infants' urine. This progresses to central nervous system (CNS) involvement, with intellectual disability, involuntary movements, spastic cerebral palsy, and self-mutilating behaviors such as biting. Later in the disease course, chronic hyperuricemia causes gouty arthritis, nephropathy, tophi, and urolithiasis.

Diagnosis

A thorough clinical evaluation, including a detailed patient history and specialized blood tests, may confirm the diagnosis of LNS. It is based on dystonia, intellectual disability, and self-mutilation. There are usually elevated serum uric acid levels. Diagnostic confirmation is via DNA analysis.

Treatment

Treatment for LNS is symptomatic. Gout can be treated with allopurinol to control excessive amounts of uric acid. Kidney stones may be treated with **lithotripsy** or laser beams. There is no standard treatment for the neurological symptoms of LNS, so management of the disease is supportive. Physical restraints, dental extractions, and drug therapy may be needed for self-mutilation. Hyperuricemia is treated with a low-purine diet, which avoids beans, organ meats, and sardines. The xanthine oxidase inhibitor called allopurinol prevents the conversion of collected hypoxanthine to uric acid. Since hypoxanthine is highly soluble, it is excreted.

Prevention

There is no way to prevent LNS due to gene mutations during gestation, but prenatal testing to detect the gene mutations may be possible in some cases.

YOU SHOULD REMEMBER

LNS is characterized by the overproduction of uric acid, leading to gouty arthritis and **nephrolithiasis**. As the body collects too much uric acid, it clumps together, forming tiny stones or crystals (urate) in the skin, hands, and feet. The crystals may irritate the joints and cause gout.

Check Your Knowledge

1. What are the signs and symptoms of LNS?
2. How can it be diagnosed with LNS?
3. What is the prevention of LNS?

FRIEDREICH ATAXIA

Friedreich ataxia is an autosomal recessive disease in terms of its inheritance. It causes progressive damage to the nervous system, resulting in movement problems. Nerve fibers in the spinal cord and peripheral nerves degenerate and become thinner.

EPIDEMIOLOGY

Friedreich ataxia is the most common inherited ataxia, affecting 1in 50,000 people in the United States. Rates are highest in people of Western European descent, the Middle East, South Asia, and North Africa. The disease has not been seen in Southeast Asians, sub-Saharan Africans, or Native Americans. Global prevalence is 2–4 per 100,000 people, though the carrier frequency is 1 every 60–100.

ETIOLOGY AND RISK FACTORS

Friedreich ataxia is caused by a gene mutation that results in abnormal repetition of the DNA sequence "GAA" (alpha-glucosidase) in the FXN gene on the long arm of chromosome 9. The FXN gene codes for the mitochondrial protein called **frataxin**. Risk factors for Friedreich ataxia involve parents carrying the disease's defective gene.

CLINICAL MANIFESTATIONS

In Friedreich ataxia, gait unsteadiness starts between the ages of 5 and 15. This is followed by arm ataxia, **dysarthria**, and **paresis**, though paresis alone is more common in the legs. Mental function usually declines. If tremors are present, they are only minimal. Reflexes and the senses of position and vibration are lost. Common signs and symptoms include progressive cardiomyopathy, scoliosis, and **talipes equinovarus** (see **Figure 14.3**). Initial symptoms include unsteady posture, frequent falling, and progressive difficulty in walking due to impaired ability to coordinate voluntary movements. Patients often use a wheelchair by their late 20s. Death is usually caused by arrhythmia or heart failure and most often occurs in middle age.

DIAGNOSIS

Diagnosis of Friedreich ataxia requires a careful medical examination, medical history, assessment of balance difficulty, loss of joint sensation, absence of reflexes, and signs of neurological problems. Diagnostic tests are made to confirm a physical examination such as electromyogram, nerve conduction studies, electrocardiogram, echocardiogram, blood tests for elevated glucose levels and vitamin E levels, a genetic test, and scans such as MRI and CT scans of brain and spinal cord are done to rule out other neurological conditions.

TREATMENT

There is no effective treatment for Friedreich ataxia. Therapy's main goal is to treat the symptoms and complications to maintain optimal function for as long as possible. Treatment options include

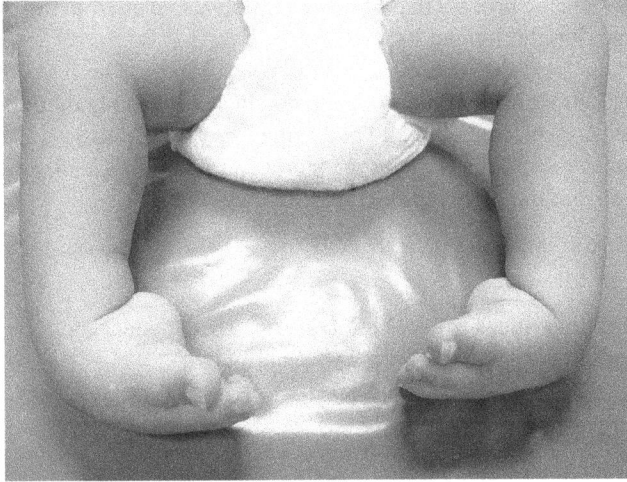

FIGURE 14.3   Talipes equinovarus.

physical therapy, speech therapy, corrective braces or surgery, medications for present heart conditions, medications for present diabetes, pain medications, antibiotics, mobility support devices, and heart transplantation if the disease coexists with significant cardiomyopathy.

PREVENTION

There is no way to prevent Friedrich ataxia. Genetic counseling and screening are recommended if the disease is present and an individual plans to have children.

YOU SHOULD REMEMBER

The exact role of frataxin remains unclear. Frataxin assists iron-sulfur protein synthesis in the electron transport chain to generate adenosine triphosphate, the energy molecule necessary to perform cell metabolic functions. It also regulates iron transfer in the mitochondria by providing a proper amount of reactive oxygen species to maintain normal processes. One result of frataxin deficiency is mitochondrial iron overload, which damages many proteins due to its effects on cellular metabolism.

Check Your Knowledge

1. What is the characteristic of Friedreich ataxia?
2. What are the clinical manifestations of Friedreich ataxia?
3. What are the treatments for Friedreich ataxia?

UREA CYCLE DISORDERS

Urea cycle disorders (UCD) are a group of genetic conditions that affect the function of proteins and enzymes that move ammonia out of the blood. **Ammonia** is toxic and can cause life-threatening side effects if the body cannot get rid of it. Limiting the amount of protein we eat and taking medicine or supplements can help treat this condition. UCD involves hyperammonemia that develops under catabolic or protein-loading conditions.

The urea cycle is a filtering process that removes toxic substances from the body and keeps other suitable substances moving throughout it.

The liver makes urea, and the urea cycle begins when we eat. The body breaks down protein from food in the diet and turns it into amino acids, which help the body build muscle, transport nutrients, and keep the organs functioning. Digestion of proteins leads to waste products that turn into ammonia. Enzymes move urea through the blood and kidneys. The final step of the urea process is to excrete urea from the body in the urine.

EPIDEMIOLOGY

The incidence in the United States is predicted to be one UCD patient for every 35,000 births, presenting about 113 new patients per year across all age groups.

ETIOLOGY AND RISK FACTORS

UCDs are caused by a genetic mutation. These genes produce proteins and enzymes that move urea through the body. A genetic mutation causes the body to lack the proteins or enzymes needed to function. The risk factors include when a person inherits a changed gene from both parents.

CLINICAL MANIFESTATIONS

Signs and symptoms of UCDs range from mild to severe. They are usually present soon after birth but could happen at any age. Mild manifestations include failure to thrive, episodic hyperammonemia, nausea, vomiting, tachypnea, confusion, and intellectual disability. Severe manifestations include altered mental status, spasticity, seizures, coma, and death.

DIAGNOSIS

A physical exam, complete medical history, and blood and urine tests must be performed. An amino acid profile, liver biopsy, and genetic test can confirm the diagnosis of UCD.

TREATMENT

Treatment for UCD focuses on lowering the amount of ammonia in the blood, including eating a diet low in protein, hemodialysis, taking amino acid supplements, and medications such as sodium phenylacetate and sodium benzoate to remove ammonia from the blood. In severe cases of hyperammonemia, a liver transplant must be done.

PREVENTION

Dietary restrictions can help prevent or control UCD symptoms. Protein intake is closely monitored, and protein restriction is advised while balancing protein, fats, and carbohydrates to ensure essential amino acids are adequately ingested, and calorie intake matches the body's energy requirements. Children are treated with a low-protein and high-calorie diet that includes a lot of vegetables, fruits, and other starchy foods that are high in calories but low in protein.

Clinical Case Studies

CLINICAL CASE STUDY 1

A 24-year-old pregnant woman and her husband were evaluated for PKU. Both were diagnosed to carry a mutated PAH gene. Upon deciding to have the child, they were given gestation planning that aimed at reducing phenylalanine levels into a manageable range. The couple's baby was delivered at week 34 of gestation via cesarean section, and the newborn had PKU.

CRITICAL THINKING QUESTIONS

1. What does PKU cause?
2. What are the signs of PKU?
3. What is the treatment for PKU?

CLINICAL CASE STUDY 2

An 11-day-old baby girl was assessed in a hospital because of lethargy and refusing to nurse. Her elder brother had died in the neonatal period, and another brother had developmental delays with seizures. The baby has one healthy brother. The baby was found to be breathing very shallowly, showing signs of intermittent dystonic posturing, and had a "fruity" body odor. Respiratory support and a large glucose infusion were given. Blood tests suggested MSUD. The baby improved with a special diet plus mega doses of thiamine.

CRITICAL THINKING QUESTIONS

1. How does MSUD develop?
2. What is the most severe form of MSUD?
3. What does MSUD treatment in an acutely ill infant require?

CLINICAL CASE STUDY 3

A 2-month-old male infant was hospitalized because of feeding difficulties, vomiting, and excessive crying. Masses were palpable on his feet and hands, and the infant cried when they were touched. Tests revealed elevated uric acid and creatinine concentrations. The infant had metabolic acidosis plus respiratory alkalosis. Urinalysis revealed that glucose, lactic acid, and ketones were positive. Tubulopathy was considered, and renal failure was impending. Ultrasound revealed enlargement of both kidneys. Brain MRI showed increased white matter water content. The infant was given oral sodium bicarbonate and allopurinol, which normalized blood levels. The official diagnosis was LNS.

CRITICAL THINKING QUESTIONS

1. What is the cause of LNS?
2. What are the clinical manifestations of LNS?
3. What are the treatments for LNS syndrome?

FURTHER READING

1. Al Mosawi, A. (2018). *Lesch Nyhan Syndrome.* Lap Lambert Academic Publishing.
2. Ananda, A.N., and Green, M. (2011). *Maple Syrup Urine Disease.* CreateSpace Independent Publishing Platform.
3. Andrews, G. (2024). *Rare Genetic Disorders: A Practical Guide to Progeria and Lesch-Nyhan Syndrome.* Andrews.
4. Blau, N., Burlina, A.B., Burton, B.K., and Cannet, C. (2021). *Phenylketonuria and BH4 Deficiencies,* 4th Edition. UNI-MED Verlag AG.
5. Burlina, A.P. (2018). *Neurometabolic Hereditary Diseases of Adults.* Springer.
6. Donev, R. (2022). *Advances in Protein Chemistry and Structural Biology: Disorders of Protein Synthesis,* Volume 132. Academic Press.
7. Jones, P., Patel, K., and Rakheja, D. (2020). *A Quick Guide to Metabolic Disease Testing Interpretation: Testing for Inborn Errors of Metabolism,* 2nd Edition. Academic Press.
8. Kelly, E.B. (2013). *Encyclopedia of Human Genetics and Disease,* 2 Volumes. Greenwood.
9. Khan, I.A., and Nadeem, A. (2023). *Friedreich's Ataxia and Disability.* Khan.
10. Lopez, J. (2023). *Ataxia: Diagnosis and Treatment.* American Medical Publishers.
11. Monch, E. (2014). *Deficiencies of the Urea Cycle: Clinical Significance and Therapy.* Uni-Med Verlag AG.
12. Nyhan, W.L., Hoffmann, G.F., Al Aqueel, A., and Barshop, B.A. (2020). *Atlas of Inherited Metabolic Diseases,* 4th Edition. CRC Press.
13. Qoronfleh, M.W., Essa, M.M., and Babu, C.S. (2022). *Proteins Associated with Neurodevelopmental Disorders (Nutritional Neurosciences).* Springer.
14. Rubinstein, J., Rakic, P., Chen, B., and Kwan, K.Y. (2020). *Neurodevelopmental Disorders: Comprehensive Developmental Neuroscience.* Academic Press.
15. Sadick, T.L. (2019). *Genetic Diseases and Development Disabilities: Aspects of Detection and Prevention.* Routledge.
16. Tabbouche, O. (2018). *Identification of Three Novel Mutations: By Studying the Molecular Genetics of Maples Syrup Urine Disease (MSUD).* Scholars' Press.
17. Tanguay, R.M. (2017). *Hereditary Tyrosinemia: Pathogenesis, Screening, and Management (Advances in Experimental Medicine and Biology 959).* Springer.
18. Trang, T., Nguyen, T.H., Vu, C.D., Nguyen, N.K., Huong, M., Che, K., Nguyen, D., Chi, Q., and Huong, N. (2023). *Hear Our Stories: Rare Diseases, Amino Acid Metabolism Disorders, Urea Cycle Disorders, Prader-Willi, Osteogenesis Imperfecta.* Trang.
19. U.S. Department of Health and Human Services and Agency for Healthcare Research and Quality. (2013). *Adjuvant Treatment for Phenylketonuria: Future Research Needs: Number 21.* CreateSpace Independent Publishing Platform.
20. Vance, D.J. (2013). *Treatment of Homocystinuria due to Cystathionine Beta Synthase Deficiency: Including Use of Low-Methionine Natural-Food Diet with Supplementary Cysteine.* Multifactor Health and Education Initiative.
21. Verbeek, M.M., de Waal, R.M., and Vinters, H.V. (2013). *Cerebral Amyloid Angiopathy in Alzheimer's Disease and Related Disorders.* Springer.
22. Wu, G. (2021). *Amino Acids: Biochemistry and Nutrition,* 2nd Edition. CRC Press.

Part V

Vitamin Deficiency and Toxicity

15 Fat-Soluble Vitamins

OVERVIEW

Vitamins A, D, E, and K are called fat-soluble vitamins because they are soluble in organic solvents and absorbed and transported like fats. Fat-soluble vitamins are integral to many physiological processes, such as vision, bone health, immune function, and coagulation. Sometimes, these vitamins may result in keratomalacia syndromes or potential toxicities. The body stores fat-soluble vitamins. Night blindness and keratomalacia can result in vitamin A deficiency. Vitamin D is found primarily in two forms: vitamin D2 (ergocalciferol) and vitamin D3 (cholecalciferol), which are synthesized in the skin after exposure to sunlight. Rickets, osteomalacia, and osteoporosis are caused by vitamin deficiency. The predominant form of vitamin E is a-tocopherol. However, other tocopherols and tocotrienols are also in circulation, such as the alpha, gamma, beta, and delta forms. Vitamin K has two primary forms: vitamin K1 and vitamin K2. The large intestine microflora synthesizes vitamin K2. Despite structural differences between fat-soluble vitamins, they are absorbed and transported similarly due to their low solubility in hydrophilic media.

VITAMIN A DEFICIENCY

Vitamin A is a fat-soluble vitamin that is naturally present in many foods. Vitamin A is essential for normal vision, the immune system, reproduction, and growth and development. Vitamin A also helps the heart, lungs, and other organs work properly. More than 90% of vitamin A is stored in the liver. Smaller amounts are in the adipose tissue, eyes, bone marrow, kidneys, and testicles. Most vitamin A is excreted in the urine, while carotenoids are excreted in the bile and eliminated with the feces. Diets rich in carotenoids may decrease risks for eye diseases, cancers, and cardiovascular disease. Beta-carotene has the most vitamin A activity and may act as an antioxidant in tissues, protecting them from damage from **free radicals**. People with high blood levels of antioxidant nutrients have a decreased risk of **cataracts**. The carotenoids called lutein and zeaxanthin may protect against age-related **macular degeneration** of the eyes in certain people, but more studies are continuing (see **Figure 15.1**). Night blindness, keratomalacia, and hyperkeratosis commonly develop in vitamin A deficiency.

NIGHT BLINDNESS

Night blindness may develop because of the effects of vitamin A deficiency on the retina. It is one of the first signs of vitamin A deficiency. In its more severe forms, vitamin A deficiency contributes to blindness by making the cornea very dry, characterized by marks called **Bitot's spots**, thus damaging the retina and cornea with poor vision in the dark (see **Figure 15.2**).

Epidemiology

Vitamin A deficiency is rare in the United States, but it can affect people who do not get enough vitamin A in their diets. It also affects people with certain liver disorders and conditions affecting their bodies' absorption of vitamins. In developing countries around the world, many people do not get enough vitamin A. Infants, children, and people who are pregnant or breastfeeding are the most at risk. Vitamin A deficiency is the leading cause of blindness in children worldwide. Every year, between 250,000 children and 500,000 children worldwide become blind because of vitamin A deficiency. Vitamin A deficiency occurs in Asia, Africa, and South America, where foods

DOI: 10.1201/9781003453376-20

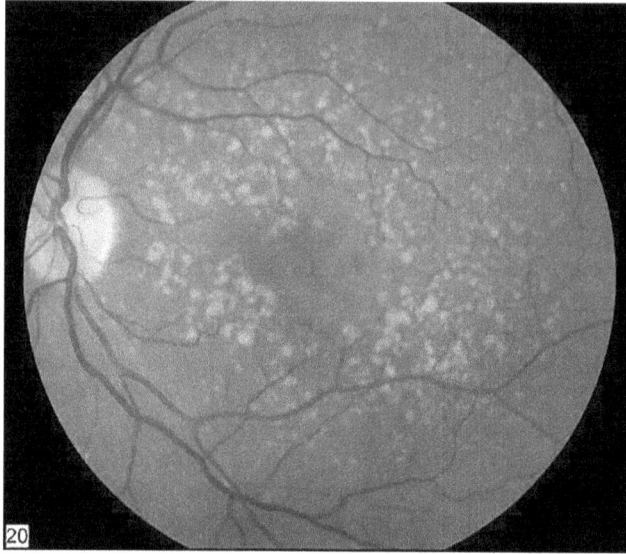

FIGURE 15.1   Macular degeneration of the eyes in vitamin A deficiency.

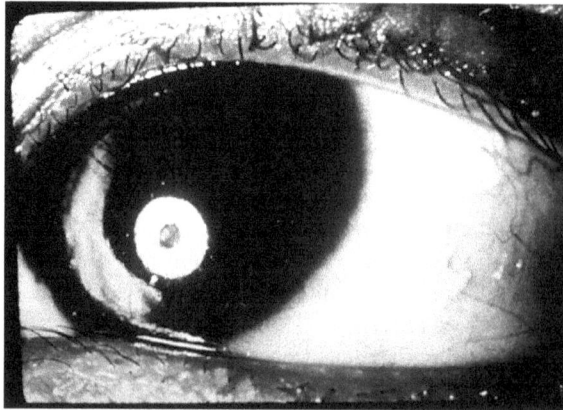

FIGURE 15.2   Bitot's spots due to vitamin A deficiency in the eyes.

containing no vitamin A are found. The countries with the highest rates of vitamin A deficiency include India, Pakistan, Bangladesh, Afghanistan, Sri Lanka, Zambia, Bhutan, Nepal, Mexico, Haiti, Peru, Honduras, Argentina, Ecuador, and Brazil (see **Figure 15.3**).

Etiology and Risk Factors

Vitamin A deficiency happens when a diet lacks vitamin A for a long time. Risk factors include celiac disease, cystic fibrosis, chronic diarrhea, bile duct blockage, zinc or iron deficiency, and alcohol use disorder.

Clinical Manifestations

Vitamin A deficiency can result in eye changes, and night blindness is an early symptom. The corneas become dry and damaged, and infections develop more often. As a result, **conjunctival xerosis** may develop. Skin irritation and **follicular hyperkeratosis frequently** occur. Hair follicles become blocked with keratin, and the skin's surface condition becomes dry and rough, with a sandy feel. In infants and young children, vitamin A deficiency can impair growth.

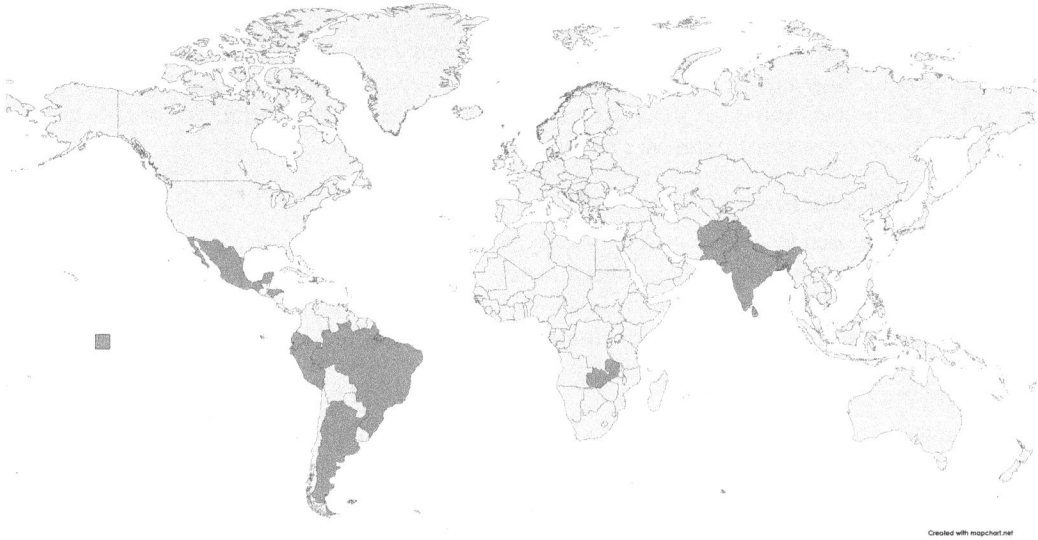

FIGURE 15.3 Countries with the highest rates of vitamin A deficiency.

Diagnosis

Blood plasma concentrations of retinol are used to assess subclinical vitamin A deficiency. In children and adults, a plasma retinol concentration of less than 0.70 µmol/L indicates subclinical vitamin A deficiency and a concentration of less than 0.35 µmol/L indicates severe vitamin A deficiency.

Treatment

Vitamin A deficiency is traditionally treated with vitamin A palmitate in oil 60,000 mcg (200,000 IU), which has been shown to reduce child mortality rates by 35%–70%—orally once a day for 2 days, followed by 4,500 units once a day.

Prevention

To prevent vitamin A deficiency, people should eat dark green leafy vegetables, yellow and orange fruits (such as papayas and oranges), carrots, and yellow vegetables (such as squash and pumpkin). Other food sources include milk and cereals fortified with vitamin A, liver, egg yolks, and fish liver oils.

Check Your Knowledge

1. What are the risk factors for vitamin A deficiency?
2. What are the early symptoms of vitamin A deficiency?
3. What are the treatments for vitamin A deficiency?

KERATOMALACIA

Keratomalacia is an ocular condition usually affecting bilaterally and resulting from a severe vitamin A deficiency. It may dry and cloud the cornea due to vitamin A deficiency, sometimes leading to corneal ulcers and bacterial infections. The tear glands are also affected, resulting in an inadequate tear film and dry eyes. People with extreme eye dryness can develop foamy spots on the conjunctiva.

Epidemiology

Vitamin A deficiency diseases are uncommon in developed countries because of the abundance of the vitamin in the food supply. However, this is different in underdeveloped or developing countries. The effect of chronic vitamin A deficiency is increased severity and mortality risk of infections (particularly measles and infection-associated diarrhea).

Etiology and Risk Factors

Keratomalacia, caused by a vitamin A deficiency, is characterized by diffuse, excessive keratinization of all mucous membrane epithelia, including the cornea and conjunctiva (xerophthalmia). Risk factors include a family history, vigorous rubbing of the eyes, and having certain conditions, such as **retinitis pigmentosa**, Down syndrome, **Marfan syndrome**, hay fever, and asthma.

Clinical Manifestations

Early symptoms may include poor vision at night or in dim light (night blindness) and xerophthalmia, followed by wrinkling, progressive cloudiness, and increasing corneal softening. With advancing vitamin A deficiency, dry, "foamy," silver-gray deposits may appear on the delicate membranes covering the whites of the eyes. Without adequate treatment, increasing corneal softening may lead to corneal infection, perforation, and degenerative tissue changes, resulting in blindness. In addition, vitamin A deficiency may have additional effects in some cases, particularly during infancy and childhood.

Diagnosis

The diagnosis of keratomalacia is based on the presence of a dry or ulcerated cornea in an underweight person. Eye examination, **electroretinography**, and blood tests are also helpful.

Treatment

Along with increasing vitamin A consumption, people who suffer from keratomalacia are typically prescribed lubricating and antibiotic eye drops or ointments. In cases where the cornea has been sufficiently damaged, **keratoplasty** is recommended.

Prevention

An adequate and varied diet of good sources of vitamin A includes liver, beef, chicken, eggs, fruit, and vegetables (especially orange and green vegetables).

YOU SHOULD REMEMBER

In North America, vitamin A deficiency is more commonly seen in poor people, older adults, alcoholics, and people with cystic fibrosis, celiac disease, chronic diarrhea, Crohn's disease, pancreatic insufficiency, and acquired immunodeficiency syndrome (AIDS).

YOU SHOULD REMEMBER

Keratomalacia is a progressive disease that starts as xerophthalmia. Caused by a vitamin A deficiency, xerophthalmia is an eye disease that, if left untreated, can progress to keratomalacia. It is characterized by abnormal dryness of the eyes. The condition starts with dryness of the conjunctiva, also known as conjunctival xerosis. It then progresses to dryness of the cornea or corneal xerosis. In its late stages, xerophthalmia develops into keratomalacia.

Check Your Knowledge

1. What are the characteristics of keratomalacia?
2. What countries have the highest rates of vitamin A deficiency?
3. What are the early symptoms of keratomalacia?

VITAMIN A TOXICITY

Vitamin A toxicity can be caused by ingesting high doses of vitamin A – usually accidentally by children or chronically, such as through megavitamin therapy or treatment for skin disorders. There are three types of vitamin A toxicity as follows:

- *Acute* – it is caused by ingestion of a single massive dose of vitamin A or several large doses over a few days, which is about 100 times the recommended dietary allowance (RDA); effects include GI tract upset, blurred vision, headache, and poor muscle coordination; these disappear once dosing stops; and substantial doses (10 g in adults and 500 mg in children) can be fatal.
- *Chronic* – it is caused by repeated ingestion of at least ten times the RDA; effects include joint pain, loss of appetite, headache, skin disorders, liver damage, reduced bone minerals, double vision, hemorrhage, and coma; the supplement must be discontinued; symptoms will decrease over a few weeks; and chronic ingestion of high amounts can cause permanent liver, bone, and eye damage.

EPIDEMIOLOGY

Infants and children are at a higher risk of toxicity due to their smaller body size and reduced tolerance for high doses. Accidental ingestion of vitamin A supplements by children is a common cause of acute toxicity. There is no substantial difference in the occurrence of vitamin A toxicity between men and women. However, pregnant women are at risk if they take high doses of vitamin supplements. However, the prevalence of vitamin A toxicity is unknown. Excessive supplement intake typically occurs in developed countries when individuals exceed the RDA. Supplementation programs have been implemented in regions where vitamin deficiency is a significant public health concern. Moreover, toxicity can arise if dosing guidelines are not carefully followed.

ETIOLOGY AND RISK FACTORS

The toxicity of vitamin A is relatively uncommon and usually arises from excessive supplementation or medication usage. The primary cause of toxicity is the consumption of substantial quantities of vitamin A through dietary supplements and foods. This usually occurs when individuals consume high doses of vitamin A without proper medical supervision. Most diets contain a combination of preformed vitamin A and provitamin A carotenoids. Preformed vitamin A is derived from animal sources and is found in egg yolks, butter, chicken, beef, organ meats, fish, fish oils, and fortified foods. Preformed vitamin A is readily absorbed in the small intestine and stored in the liver. Therefore, excessive dietary preformed vitamin A from animal-based sources and supplements can contribute to the risk of toxicity.

CLINICAL MANIFESTATIONS

Common signs and symptoms of accidentally ingesting a megadose of vitamin A include headaches, rashes, drowsiness, irritability, nausea, vomiting, and stomach pain. In acute vitamin A toxicity, symptoms can be resolved over time. In chronic vitamin A toxicity, symptoms include severe headaches, intracranial hypertension, **alopecia** of eyebrows, pruritus, bone fractures, **arthralgia**, splenomegaly, hepatomegaly, and **anorexia**.

DIAGNOSIS

A patient's history and physical examination findings guide the selection of diagnostic studies. Patients with persistent headaches while taking vitamin A medications should be evaluated for increased intracranial pressure and **pseudotumor cerebri syndrome**. Laboratory findings include serum vitamin A levels, hematological abnormalities (leukocytosis, thrombocytopenia, and anemia), liver function tests, serum lipids, and renal function.

TREATMENT

Vitamin A toxicity is treated by stopping the use of vitamin A supplements. Generally, signs and symptoms will resolve independently within 1–4 weeks, depending on their severity. Congenital disabilities caused by vitamin A toxicity during pregnancy are irreversible. Patients with dry or peeling skin should use moisturizers or emollients to alleviate discomfort and facilitate skin healing. For patients experiencing dry eyes, artificial tears and lubricating eye drops, including those containing methylcellulose, can be beneficial.

PREVENTION

Hypervitaminosis A can be prevented by not ingesting more than the recommended amount. This level is for synthetic and natural vitamin A.

YOU SHOULD REMEMBER

Pregnant women should avoid using oral retinoid medications and excessive vitamin A supplements to reduce the risk of vitamin A-related malformations. Prescribers should only recommend oral retinoids to women of childbearing age who are not pregnant and use reliable birth control methods to prevent the potential risk of vitamin A-related teratogenic effects.

Check Your Knowledge

1. What are the common signs and symptoms of vitamin A toxicity?
2. How could you diagnose vitamin A toxicity?
3. What are the treatments for vitamin A toxicity?

VITAMIN D DEFICIENCY

Vitamin D deficiency may cause health problems like brittle bones and muscle weakness. The two primary forms of vitamin D are D2 and D3. **Ergocalciferol** (vitamin D2) is mostly human-made and added to foods. In contrast, cholecalciferol (vitamin D3) is synthesized in the skin of humans from 7-dehydrocholesterol and is also consumed in the diet via animal-based foods. Therefore, vitamin D is better classified as a hormone or **prohormone**. Without enough UV-light exposure, adequate dietary intake of vitamin D is required. Most fortified foods and supplements that contain vitamin D have it in the form of ergocalciferol. This is also the form found naturally in food sources.

Sun exposure generally provides 80% of the vitamin D3 needed by the body. The sun exposure required is based on time of day, geographic location, seasons, individual age, skin color, and use of sunscreen. People in more northern areas generally do not produce enough vitamin D3 during winter. For people of any size, the production of vitamin D3 in the skin decreases by approximately 70% by age 70. Therefore, older people should get small amounts of sun exposure in the early morning and late afternoon, minimizing skin cancer risks or taking vitamin D supplements to avoid deficiency.

RICKETS

Rickets is a metabolic disease of childhood, characterized by softening of the bones as a result of inadequate intake of vitamin D and insufficient exposure to sunlight, also associated with impaired calcium and phosphorus metabolism. It was a common metabolic disease of bone a century ago in North America, Europe, and East Asia (mainly due to vitamin D deficiency). Vitamin D deficiency remains the most common form of metabolic bone disease, entirely preventable and treatable. It is a childhood disease characterized by imperfect calcification, softening, and distortion of bone bending and breaking more easily (see **Figure 15.4**).

Epidemiology

Rickets is a sporadic epidemic, and despite the introduction of numerous preventive strategies, vitamin D deficiency has remained a global health problem among children. Moreover, developed countries such as the United States, Canada, the United Kingdom, and Australia have not been exempt from this. Rickets affects an estimated one in 200,000 children. The condition is most often caused by a lack of vitamin D in the diet or insufficient sun exposure rather than genetic mutations.

Etiology and Risk Factors

Nutrition problems or genetics usually cause rickets – insufficient exposure to sunlight and lack of vitamin D in children's diet. Genetic diseases interfere with the body's absorption of vitamin D. The risk factors are age (newborns and infants), children who do not get enough sunlight outdoors, and darker-skinned children who take longer to absorb vitamin D.

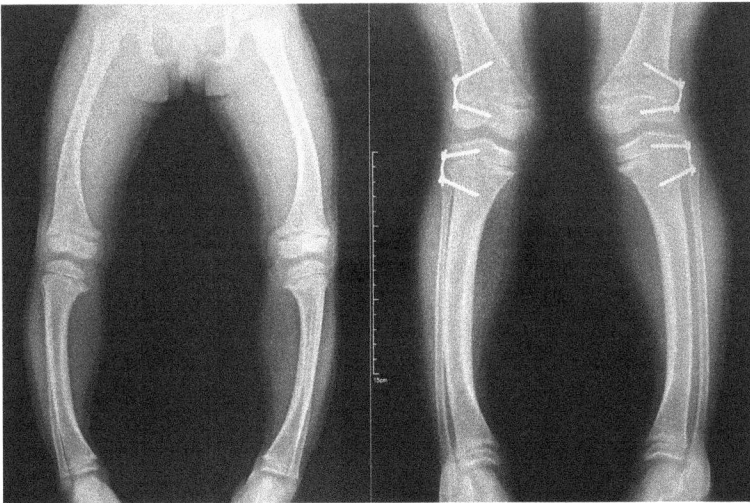

FIGURE 15.4 X-ray of a child showing rickets.

Clinical Manifestations

Signs and symptoms of rickets include bone pain, bowing of keg bones, swelling of the ends of ribs (**rachitic rosary**), and **pigeon chest**. Growth delays, cavities in teeth, and seizures may also be seen. Rickets in developed countries are usually due to fat malabsorption, such as cystic fibrosis.

Diagnosis

A diagnosis of rickets is based on a physical examination or symptoms; X-rays of the affected bones can reveal bone deformities. Blood and urine tests can confirm a diagnosis of rickets and monitor treatment progress. Genetic testing (for inherited rickets) may also be needed.

Treatment

For most children, rickets can be successfully treated by ensuring they eat foods containing calcium and vitamin D or taking vitamin supplements. A combination of phosphate supplements and a particular form of vitamin D is required to treat **hypophosphatemic rickets**, where a genetic defect causes abnormalities in how the kidneys and bones deal with phosphate.

Prevention

Rickets can be prevented and treated by having safe daily sun exposure and eating foods containing vitamin D and calcium.

YOU SHOULD REMEMBER

Intrauterine fractures due to congenital rickets may occur. The last trimester bears the burden of fetal skeletal mineralization as approximately 80% is deposited then. A fetus that has vitamin D deficiency during pregnancy will likely be taken with a near-normal serum calcium concentration and normal skeletal morphology but risks developing rickets within the first weeks and months of life, especially if exclusively breastfed. The skull is the best location to seek radiographic evidence of congenital and nutritional rickets in infants under 3 months of age, as the skull is the most affected bone at this age, reflective of rapid brain growth.

Check Your Knowledge

1. What are the causes and risk factors of rickets?
2. What are the clinical manifestations of rickets?
3. What are the treatments for rickets?

OSTEOMALACIA

Osteomalacia occurs in adults because of insufficient calcium and phosphorus, making the bones soft and deformed. The diet usually causes low levels of vitamin D, inadequate sunlight, or a problem with how the body uses vitamin D. There is poor calcification of newly synthesized bone. Hence, fractures of the hips or spine are common. Osteomalacia is most common with kidney or liver disease, which impairs calcitriol synthesis or intestinal infections. Osteomalacia will be discussed in **Chapter 18** in detail.

OSTEOPOROSIS

Osteoporosis is a medical condition in which the bones become brittle and fragile from tissue loss, typically due to hormonal changes or deficiency of calcium or vitamin D. Around the world, one in three women and one in five men over the age of 50 will suffer a broken bone due to osteoporosis. Throughout life, bone is constantly being renewed, with new bone replacing old bone, which helps keep the skeleton strong. But for people with osteoporosis, more and more bone is lost and not replaced. Osteoporosis will be discussed in **Chapter 18** in detail.

YOU SHOULD REMEMBER

There is controversy about whether vitamin D may protect against infections such as COVID-19. Some experts believe that the vitamin can protect against the disease or decrease the severity of the illness, but studies are ongoing. So far, results have shown just a slightly better set of outcomes in patients with moderate to severe COVID-19 when vitamin D, specifically D3, was administered.

VITAMIN D TOXICITY

The main consequence of vitamin D toxicity is hypercalcemia, which can cause nausea and vomiting, weakness, and frequent urination. Vitamin D toxicity might progress to bone pain and kidney stones. Hypervitaminosis D is rare and usually caused by excessive doses of vitamin D due to misuse of over-the-counter supplements or erroneous prescriptions. Less commonly, poisoning from exposure to rodenticides containing cholecalciferol can also lead to vitamin D toxicity.

EPIDEMIOLOGY

Vitamin D toxicity is rare, but it may happen at high doses. There are around 4,500 cases per year in the United States. Vitamin D toxicity remains an ongoing issue, and its incidence is likely to continue increasing, owing to the widespread availability of over-the-counter preparations and public interest. Long-term high-dose D supplement intake may result in adverse health effects, increase in mortality, greater risk of pancreatic cancer, cardiovascular events, and increased falls and fractures in older adults. Hypervitaminosis D has been associated with dental enamel hypoplasia and focal pulp calcification in children.

ETIOLOGY AND RISK FACTORS

Vitamin D toxicity can result from excessive vitamin D supplementation, knowingly or accidentally. Prescription errors without frequent monitoring of vitamin D levels can also result in toxicity. Toxicity resulting from lack of monitoring is frequently seen in patients requiring high doses to treat ailments like osteoporosis, renal osteodystrophy, psoriasis, gastric bypass surgery, celiac disease, or inflammatory bowel disease. People who take prescription-strength vitamin D are at risk of vitamin D toxicity due to the high dose of the medication unless they check their levels periodically.

CLINICAL MANIFESTATIONS

The clinical signs and symptoms of vitamin D toxicity manifest from hypercalcemia's effects. Often, symptoms can be nonspecific and subtle, such as weakness, fatigue, anorexia, and bone pains. More severe symptoms include neurological symptoms like confusion, apathy, agitation, irritability, and, sometimes, ataxia, stupor, and coma. Gastrointestinal symptoms include abdominal pain, nausea, vomiting, constipation, peptic ulcers, and pancreatitis. Renal symptoms manifest as polyuria, polydipsia, and nephrolithiasis. Severe hypercalcemia can also lead to cardiac arrhythmias.

DIAGNOSIS

A detailed history is essential in making a diagnosis of vitamin D toxicity. A thorough review of the medication list, including the use of over-the-counter supplements, is pertinent. History should also focus on acquiring details of chronic medical ailments that require high doses of vitamin D supplementation, such as osteoporosis, renal osteodystrophy, psoriasis, gastric bypass surgery, and celiac or inflammatory bowel disease. A dietary history is essential, especially the excessive use of vitamin D-fortified milk and supplementary vitamin D. Laboratory evaluation includes measuring serum calcium, ionized calcium, phosphate levels, calcium in the urine, and parathyroid hormone.

Imaging studies are usually not required to diagnose vitamin D toxicity but can reveal incidental findings of chronic toxicity due to pathologic calcifications. Skeletal radiographs typically show periosteal calcifications. Abdomen and pelvic CT scans can reveal nephrolithiasis. In addition, other pathologic calcifications may be observed in the blood vessels, myocardium, lung, and skin. When a patient presents with significant alteration in mental status upon admission, it is advisable to perform a baseline brain CT scan to assess for possible intracranial pathologies or alternative causes.

TREATMENT

Treatment of vitamin D toxicity is mainly supportive and focuses on lowering calcium levels. In severe cases, calcitonin and bisphosphonates can be used. Patients may need hemodialysis due to renal failure or correct refractory hypercalcemia.

PREVENTION

Individuals should not take more vitamin D supplements than recommended to avoid toxicity. Many combination vitamin supplements contain vitamin D, so check the labels of all the supplements you are taking for vitamin D content.

Check Your Knowledge

1. What are the signs and symptoms of vitamin D toxicity?
2. How can we approach the assessment of vitamin D toxicity?
3. How can we prevent vitamin D toxicity?

VITAMIN E DEFICIENCY AND TOXICITY

Vitamin E is essential to vision, reproduction, blood, brain, and skin. It also has antioxidant properties. Antioxidants might protect the cells against the effects of free radicals. Vitamin E deficiency is extremely rare in humans as it is unlikely to be caused by a diet of low vitamin E. Rather, it tends to be caused by irregular dietary fat absorption or metabolism. It is a lipid-soluble nutrient. Vitamin E may have a role in reducing atherosclerosis and lowering rates of ischemic heart disease. Premature infants have low vitamin E reserves due to vitamin E only being able to cross the placenta in small amounts. The two types of vitamin E include **tocopherols** and **tocotrienols**. The most active form is *alpha-tocopherol*. It is found in foods and vitamin supplements. *Gamma-tocopherol* does not have as much physical activity but is a potentially beneficial form of vitamin E in many vegetable oils. Good sources of vitamin E include canola, cottonseed, safflower, sunflower oils, avocado, wheat germ, almonds, peanuts, and sunflower seeds. Products from plant oils, including margarine, salad dressings, and shortenings, are also good sources.

The early breakdown of red blood cells and hemolytic anemia signifies vitamin E deficiency. This is very serious in preterm infants, so they are given supplemental vitamin E and specialized infant formula containing it. Vitamin E deficiency can reduce immune function and cause neurological changes in the spinal cord and peripheral nervous system. These have occurred when the deficiency resulted from a genetic abnormality of lipoprotein synthesis that decreases vitamin E transport and distribution.

EPIDEMIOLOGY

Serum alpha-tocopherol levels in 0.1% of United States adults over 20 are deficient. The prevalence of vitamin E deficiency includes 89.8% of men and 96.3% of women 19 or older having insufficient alpha-tocopherol intake. The deficiency prevalence reached 67% and 80% in infants and children.

ETIOLOGY AND RISK FACTORS

Vitamin E deficiency is extremely rare in humans as it is unlikely to be caused by a diet of low vitamin E. Rather, it tends to be caused by irregular dietary fat absorption or metabolism. It is a lipid-soluble nutrient. The highest risk is for people who have cystic fibrosis or Crohn's disease. Preterm infants are highly susceptible to vitamin E deficiency. Because they are born with only limited amounts of stored vitamin E and often have poor intestinal absorption of the vitamin. Short bowel syndrome patients may take years to develop symptoms. Surgical resection, mesenteric vascular thrombosis, and pseudo-obstruction are also causative. Smokers are also at risk since oxidative stress and lipid peroxidation from cigarette smoke make their bodies require more vitamin E. In developing countries, the most common cause is inadequate vitamin E intake.

CLINICAL MANIFESTATIONS

Vitamin E deficiency may be associated with several neurologic manifestations. Clinical features may only appear many years after the onset of deficiency. The onset of symptoms tends to be gradual, and progression is slow. The main clinical features are **spinocerebellar ataxia** and polyneuropathy. Patients presenting early may show **hyporeflexia**, difficulty walking, weak muscles, decreased night vision, and loss of vibratory sense; however, they have normal cognition. A more moderate stage of this deficiency may show limb and **truncal ataxia**, profuse muscle weakness, and limited upward gaze. Late presentations may show cardiac arrhythmias with reduced cognition. Ataxia is the most common examination finding. Premature infants with the deficiency may develop a severe form of anemia.

DIAGNOSIS

The diagnosis is based on symptoms and results of a physical examination with laboratory assistance. A low alpha-tocopherol level or low serum alpha-tocopherol to serum lipid measurement ratio is the mainstay of diagnosis. In addition, we can observe increased stool fat and decreased serum carotene levels as additional markers of intestinal malabsorption in patients with vitamin E deficiency. Spine MRIs in patients with myeloneuropathy may reveal increased signal in the dorsal cervical spine region. In adults, alpha-tocopherol levels should be less than 5 mcg/mL. In an adult with hyperlipidemia, the abnormal lipids may affect the vitamin E levels and a serum alpha-tocopherol to serum lipid level, needing to be less than 0.8 mg/g, which is more accurate.

TREATMENT

Treatment is based on the underlying cause of the deficiency, such as fat malabsorption and fat metabolism disorders. Also, a diet modification can assist in supplementation; increasing intake of leafy vegetables, whole grains, nuts, seeds, vegetable oils, and fortified cereals is highly recommended.

Though generally presented in our diets, adults need 15 mg of vitamin E daily. A supplement of 15–25 mg/kg once per day or mixed tocopherols 200 IU can both be used.

PREVENTION

To prevent vitamin E deficiency, individuals must consume large amounts of potatoes, bread, and meat. To increase vitamin E levels, replace some of the saturated fats in the diet with polyunsaturated fats from vegetable oils, nuts, and seeds.

YOU SHOULD REMEMBER

Vitamin E is a popular supplement, along with other antioxidants, to help prevent cancer, cardiovascular disease, and other chronic diseases linked to free radical damage. However, studies have reported that vitamin E, selenium, or both do not decrease the risk of various cancers, though the effects of vitamin E may vary based on the stage of prostate cancer and blood levels of the form of vitamin E known as alpha-tocopherol. Similar outcomes have been reported with vitamin E to decrease risks for *atherosclerosis*.

YOU SHOULD REMEMBER

Antioxidants protect other compounds by becoming oxidized. Therefore, a better name for them is *redox agents* since they can undergo oxidation, the loss of an electron, and then reduction and regaining the electron. *However, antioxidant* is still the more common term.

YOU SHOULD REMEMBER

Vitamin E toxicity is rare, but occasionally, high doses can cause bleeding, muscle weakness, fatigue, nausea, and diarrhea. The most significant risk of vitamin E toxicity is bleeding. Diagnosis is based on a person's symptoms.

Check Your Knowledge

1. Why is vitamin E essential for the human body?
2. What are the neurologic manifestations of vitamin E deficiency?
3. What are the treatments for vitamin E deficiency?

VITAMIN K DEFICIENCY AND TOXICITY

Vitamin K is needed for blood clotting and the building of bones. **Prothrombin** is a vitamin-dependent protein involved with blood clotting. Osteocalcin is another protein that requires vitamin K to produce healthy bone tissue. There are two primary forms of vitamin K, also known as *quinones*. They include vitamin K1 (phylloquinone) in plant foods like leafy greens and vitamin K2 (menaquinone) in animal and fermented foods. The most biologically active form is phylloquinone, the primary dietary form.

Vitamin K is required for blood clotting factors to be synthesized by the liver and for pre-pro-thrombin to be converted into prothrombin, an active blood clotting factor. Vitamin K is converted to an inactive form after activating clotting factors. Warfarin and similar drugs significantly inhibit this reactivation process, acting as potent anticoagulants. People who take warfarin to reduce blood clotting must maintain a regular dietary intake of vitamin K but avoid supplements with vitamin K. Bone metabolism is also affected by vitamin K.

EPIDEMIOLOGY

Early and classical vitamin K deficiency affects an estimated 1 in 60 to 1 in 250 newborns in the United States. Late vitamin K deficiency is less common and affects an estimated 1 in 14,000 to 1 in 25,000 infants in the United States. Although vitamin K deficiency may be commonly observed in 8%–31% of typically healthy adults, it rarely causes clinically significant bleeding. Bleeding naturally occurs in individuals with malabsorption syndromes and liver disease or those receiving medications that interfere with vitamin K metabolism. The incidence of early vitamin K deficiency without prophylactic neonatal vitamin K is as high as 12%. Without vitamin K supplementation, the current incidence of classic deficiency is estimated to be 0.25%–1.7%.

ETIOLOGY AND RISK FACTORS

Vitamin K deficiency may be caused by insufficient consumption of vitamin K-rich foods, includ-ing leafy greens and fermented products. Certain medical conditions that affect fat absorption, such as celiac disease or inflammatory bowel diseases, can also delay or prevent vitamin K absorption. Furthermore, prolonged use of antibiotics can disrupt the GI bacteria responsible for synthesizing vitamin K. Medications that interfere with vitamin K metabolism, such as blood thinners, can also contribute to deficiency. The risk factors include if the newborns did not receive the vitamin K shot at birth. Infants are 80 times more likely to develop late vitamin K deficiency than infants who do receive a vitamin K shot at birth. People are taking certain medications that can cause vitamin K deficiency as a side effect.

CLINICAL MANIFESTATIONS

The typical presentation in the newborn includes bleeding, which can be spontaneous or associ-ated with surgery. There is often a history of easy bruising, mucosal bleeding, and developmental and skeletal anomalies. In adults, vitamin K deficiency may manifest as bleeding at venipuncture sites or after minor trauma. Patients may also administer antibiotics, anticonvulsants, warfarin, or other prescription medications interfering with vitamin K metabolism. Physical examination often reveals the presence of **ecchymoses** or **petechiae** (see **Figure 15.5**).

DIAGNOSIS

Laboratory tests can diagnose vitamin K deficiency, including the prothrombin time test, which helps identify the time the plasma takes in the blood to clot. Prothrombin is a component that is involved in the process of blood clotting. The average time taken by the blood plasma to solidify is around 11–13 seconds. Any delay in these levels might be noted as vitamin K deficiency. The coagulation test helps identify the clotting ability of the blood. This helps in assessing the risk of many severe health conditions.

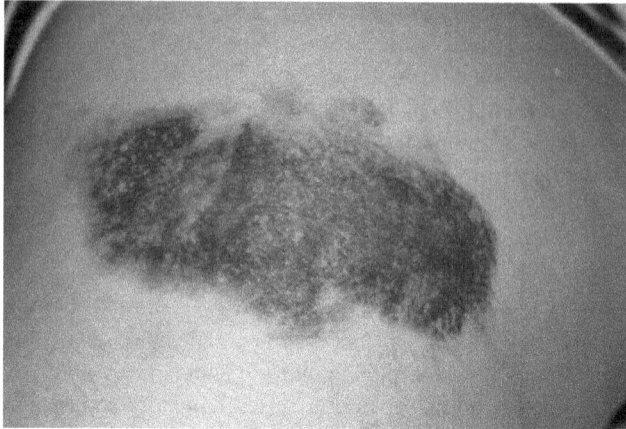

FIGURE 15.5   Ecchymoses.

TREATMENT

Intramuscular vitamin K injection is the recommended prophylactic method for all newborns and infants due to its increased efficacy compared to oral administration. If a newborn vomits or regurgitates an oral dose of vitamin K within 1 hour, it is recommended to give them another dose. Oral vitamin K should be avoided in preterm infants and neonates with cholestasis or intestinal conditions that may interfere with absorption. For adults, oral vitamin K supplementation or occasional subcutaneous injection is the preferred method of maintaining adequate vitamin K levels and treating minor bleeding. IV administration is typically reserved for cases of severe bleeding.

PREVENTION

Green beans, avocados, kiwifruit, vegetable oils (especially soybean and canola oils), yogurt, fermented food and drinks, and some cheeses are good sources of vitamin K. Eating these foods can help prevent vitamin K deficiency.

YOU SHOULD REMEMBER

Vitamin K stores are low at birth because the newborn intestinal tract does not have the bacteria needed to synthesize the vitamin. Because defective blood clotting can cause bleeding, newborns in North America are given vitamin K injections within 6 hours after birth.

YOU SHOULD REMEMBER

Vitamin K toxicity is extremely rare. No known adverse effects are associated with excessive dietary intake of vitamin K. The only reported toxicity comes from menadione, which has no use in humans. Its toxicity is thought to be associated with its water-soluble properties. When toxicity does occur, it manifests with signs of jaundice, hyperbilirubinemia, hemolytic anemia, and kernicterus in infants.

Check Your Knowledge

1. What are the causes of vitamin K deficiency?
2. What are the signs and symptoms of vitamin K deficiency?
3. Why is intramuscular vitamin K injection recommended for all newborns?

Clinical Case Studies

CLINICAL CASE STUDY 1

A 5-year-old girl who lived in Central Africa was brought to a pediatrician because of chronic diarrhea and recurring infections. The child also had vision problems. A blood test revealed that her serum retinol was low, and she was diagnosed with vitamin A deficiency. A thorough diet review was conducted, and the child was started on oral vitamin A supplementation.

CRITICAL THINKING QUESTIONS

1. What is vitamin A essential for?
2. What are the risk factors for vitamin A deficiency?
3. What does the prevention of vitamin A deficiency involve?

CLINICAL CASE STUDY 2

A 22-year-old man with diabetes mellitus went to see his physician because of severe fatigue, bone pain, and muscle cramps. The patient had suffered from these symptoms for a few months and admitted to feeling somewhat depressed about his health situation. The physician discussed the patient's diet, and the patient stated that he never ate fish because he could not tolerate the taste. He was also allergic to cow's milk. Blood tests revealed his vitamin D levels were much lower than usual. The patient was given oral ergocalciferol supplements for 8 weeks. His blood levels normalized, and he was then started on maintenance doses of vitamin D3 (cholecalciferol).

CRITICAL THINKING QUESTIONS

1. What is the definition of the vitamin D-related disease known as rickets?
2. In which individuals do osteomalacia occur?
3. What is the description of osteoporosis?

CLINICAL CASE STUDY 3

An infant, 6 weeks old, was brought to the emergency department for ecchymosis of his bilateral testis. He was born at home by a midwife. His mother noted that 2 days before admission, the discoloration of his left testicle expanded to the right testicle. Pregnancy was uncomplicated. The infant did not receive vitamin K prophylaxis at birth, though his mother was taking oral vitamin K; the physical examination of the infant revealed pale, weak, and jaundiced. Based on the severely abnormal coagulation studies, the infant was treated acutely for suspected vitamin K-deficiency-related bleeding. The patient received three IV doses of vitamin K.

CRITICAL THINKING QUESTIONS

1. What are the clinical manifestations of vitamin K deficiency?
2. How can we diagnose vitamin K deficiency?
3. What is the prophylactic method of vitamin K deficiency in newborns?

FURTHER READING

1. Abd Muid, S., Froemmino, G.R.A., Ali, A.M., and Nawawi, H.M. (2018). *Pure Tocotrienols and Tocotrienol-Tocopherol Mixed Fraction as Anti-Atherosclerotic Agents.* Abd Muid.
2. Alex, B. (2023). *The Vitamin D Essence: How to Identify Vitamin D Deficiencies and Easily Resolve Them.* Alex.
3. Anderson, D.C. and Grimes, D.S. (2020). *Vitamin D Deficiency and COVID-19: Its Central Role in a World Pandemic.* Tennison Publishing.
4. Combs, Jr., G.F., and McClung, J.P. (2023). *The Vitamins: Fundamental Aspects in Nutrition and Health*, 5th Edition. Academic Press.
5. Eugenia, S. (2023). *Vitamin A Deficiency: Insights, Interventions, and Innovations (Medical Care and Health).* Eugenia.
6. Grayson, T. (2021). *Overcoming Osteomalacia: A Unique Guide to Understanding, Symptoms, Diagnosis, Treatment of Osteomalacia with Medical and Alternative Forms of Treatment.* Grayson.
7. Halliwell, B., and Gutteridge, J.M.C. (2017). *Free Radicals in Biology and Medicine*, 5th Edition. Oxford University Press.
8. Hoshino, A., and Lindberg, I. (2012). *Peptide Biosynthesis: Prohormone Convertases 1/3 and 2 (Colloquium Series on Neuropeptides).* Morgan & Claypool Life Sciences.
9. Purser, D. and Larkin, J. (2019). *Vitamin Deficiency Symptoms and Cures: Modern Deficiency Illness: Using Intracellular Micronutrient Results.* Purser and Larkin.
10. Rheaume-Bleue, K. (2013). *Vitamin K2 and the Calcium Paradox: How a Little-Known Vitamin Could Save Your Life.* Harper.
11. Rydon, R. (2016). *Profiles of the Nutrients: Book 3. Water-Soluble and Fat-Soluble Vitamins.* Lulu.com.
12. Singh, P. (2023). *Osteoporosis, Osteoarthritis, and Rheumatoid Arthritis: An Agonizing Skeletal Triad.* Bentham Books.
13. Slovik, D.M., and Underwood, A. (2019). *Osteoporosis: A Guide to Prevention and Treatment (Special Health Report).* Harvard Medical School.
14. Taylor, L. (2023). *Fat-Soluble Vitamins: Biochemistry and Clinical Applications.* American Medical Publishers.

16 Water-Soluble Vitamins

OVERVIEW

Water-soluble vitamins, like fat-soluble vitamins, are essential organic substances that are also needed in small amounts. They include thiamin, riboflavin, niacin, pantothenic acid, pyridoxine, folacin, vitamin B12, biotin, and ascorbic acid. All water-soluble vitamins play a different role in energy metabolism; they are required as functional parts of enzymes involved in energy release and storage. They are referred to as coenzymes and cofactors, respectively. They assist in converting a substrate to an end product. Coenzymes and cofactors are essential in catabolic pathways and also play a role in many anabolic pathways. At insufficient levels in the diet, these vitamins may impair the typical blood and, consequently, the delivery of nutrients and wastes. Vitamin C deficiency causes scurvy and, if advanced, psychological problems. Water-soluble vitamins, except B12, can be supplied by plants in the diet. These vitamins are stored in the body for a short time. Therefore, it needs to be consumed regularly.

VITAMIN B1 DEFICIENCY

Vitamin B1 (thiamine) acts as a coenzyme for transketolase reactions in the form of thiamine pyrophosphate. Thiamine also plays an unidentified role in propagating nerve impulses and taking part in **myelin sheath** maintenance. Vitamin B1 deficiency can affect the cardiovascular, nervous, and immune systems, as commonly seen in wet or dry Beriberi and Wernicke–Korsakoff syndrome (cerebral Beriberi). Worldwide, it is most widely reported in populations where polished rice and milled cereals are the primary food source and in patients with chronic alcohol use disorder.

EPIDEMIOLOGY

The prevalence is highest in cultures that depend on a high proportion of their calories from foods with poor thiamine content, such as milled rice. Beriberi can affect both genders, although alcoholism is more prevalent in males. However, beriberi is much less common today but persists in some Asian countries, mainly among refugees and poorer people of all ages.

ETIOLOGY AND RISK FACTORS

The causes of thiamine deficiency include individuals whose diets are primarily high in polished rice or processed grains, chronic alcoholism, gastric bypass surgery, and parenteral nutrition without adequate thiamine supplementation. It might also be caused by malnutrition, malabsorption syndrome, diarrhea, diuretic use, pregnancy, and lactation. Risk factors include alcohol dependence, malabsorption, and a diet low in thiamine.

CLINICAL MANIFESTATIONS

Initial symptoms of thiamine deficiency include anorexia, irritability, and difficulties with short-term memory. With prolonged thiamine deficiency, patients may endorse loss of sensation in the extremities. Dry beriberi presents as symmetrical peripheral neuropathy, while wet beriberi presents with heart failure. Wernicke–Korsakoff syndrome can manifest with central nervous system (CNS) symptoms such as gait changes, double vision, crossing of the eyes, rapid eye movements, apathy, **ataxia**, confusion, hallucinations, and **confabulation**. Overall, beriberi is signified

DOI: 10.1201/9781003453376-21

by **peripheral neuropathy**, muscle wasting, pain, tenderness, cardiomegaly, dyspnea, anorexia, edema, poor memory and confusion, weight loss, and convulsions.

Infantile beriberi in children younger than 4 months of age typically presents first with nonspecific signs and symptoms, including irritability, refusal to breastfeed, tachycardia and tachypnea, vomiting, and constant crying or aphonia. As the disease progresses, signs and symptoms of congestive heart failure begin to appear, such as tachypnea, tachycardia, pulmonary edema, hepatomegaly, and, sometimes, **cyanosis**.

Diagnosis

Diagnosing thiamine deficiency relies on patient history, physical examination findings, and follow-up with laboratory testing for confirmation—measurement of thiamine in the blood, urinalysis, and functional enzymatic assay of transketolase activity.

Treatment

Treatment for thiamine deficiency includes administration of parenteral thiamine. The recommended dose is 50 mg, given intravenously or intramuscularly for several days. The duration of therapy depends on the symptoms, and treatment is indicated until all symptoms have disappeared. Maintenance is recommended orally at 2.5–5 mg daily unless malabsorption syndrome is suspected. Thiamine, even at high doses, is not toxic in a person with normal renal function. No cases of thiamine toxicity have been reported from the use of thiamine at the dosages indicated, even in patients in critical condition.

Prevention

To prevent beriberi, eat a nutrient-dense, balanced diet with thiamine-rich foods, such as groundnuts, soybeans, beans, and legumes.

YOU SHOULD REMEMBER

Vitamin B1 is an essential micronutrient; deficiency can result in distinct clinical presentations. Acute deficiency can present as Wernicke encephalopathy, with ocular abnormalities, mental state changes, and ataxia. Acute or chronic deficiency can also lead to wet beriberi (which shows as high-output cardiac failure with edema and orthopnea) or low-output cardiac failure with lactic acidosis and peripheral cyanosis. Dry beriberi occurs with chronic deficiency and is characterized by distal peripheral polyneuropathy.

YOU SHOULD REMEMBER

Wernicke's encephalopathy is most common in alcoholics, as chronic alcoholism impairs both intestinal thiamine absorption and increases thiamine requirements for metabolism. Wernicke's encephalopathy can also occur in HIV-infected patients, pregnant women suffering from hyperemesis gravidarum, and postoperative bariatric patients.

Check Your Knowledge

1. What are the functions of thiamine in the body?
2. What are the causes of thiamine deficiency?
3. What are the initial symptoms of thiamine deficiency?

VITAMIN B2 DEFICIENCY

Vitamin B2 (riboflavin) is essential for energy production, red blood cell generation, enzyme function, and ordinary fatty acid and amino acid synthesis. In addition to producing energy for the body, riboflavin is an antioxidant and necessary for producing glutathione, a free radical scavenger. Additionally, it is essential for normal development, growth, reproduction, lactation, physical performance, and well-being. A small amount is stored in the liver, kidneys, and heart. Excessive amounts are excreted in the urine. If excessive riboflavin supplements are taken, the urine becomes yellow and glows under a black light. Riboflavin is a component of the coenzymes needed for energy metabolism.

EPIDEMIOLOGY

Vitamin B2 is relatively uncommon in the developed world, but mild deficiency can affect up to 50% of the population in developing countries.

ETIOLOGY AND RISK FACTORS

Riboflavin deficiency can be associated with inadequate dietary intake and malabsorption. Pregnant and breastfeeding women may require higher riboflavin intake, and deficiency can occur if dietary intake is insufficient. Chronic alcohol consumption can interfere with the absorption and utilization of vitamin B2. Some medications, particularly those used to treat migraines, may interfere with the absorption or utilization of riboflavin. The risk of riboflavin deficiency also includes alcoholics and people with very poor diets. Certain GI disorders, such as Crohn's disease, celiac disease, and irritable bowel syndrome, can impair the body's ability to absorb nutrients from this vitamin. Long-term use of phenobarbital also affects riboflavin levels since the drug increases its breakdown, along with other nutrients in the liver.

CLINICAL MANIFESTATIONS

The signs and symptoms of riboflavin deficiency (**ariboflavinosis**) include fatigue, sore throat, **angular stomatitis**, **cheilosis**, anemia, disorders, blurred vision, hair loss, and reproductive problems. Skin cracking around the corners of the mouth and seborrheic dermatitis (see **Figure 16.1**) are also symptoms. Some people also experience confusion, sensitivity to light, headaches, and poor growth.

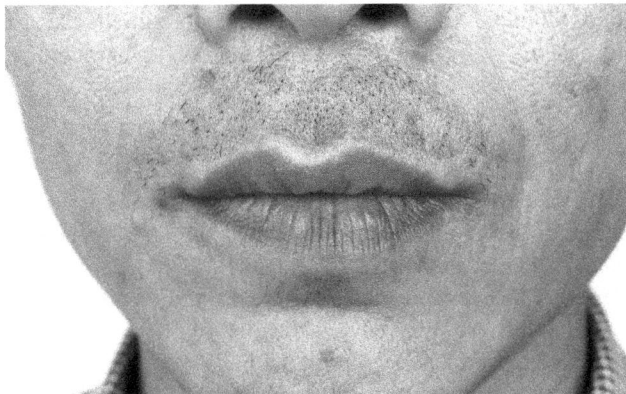

FIGURE 16.1   Angular stomatitis.

DIAGNOSIS

The diagnosis is based on symptoms, urine tests, and response to riboflavin supplements. Patients have painful cracks in the corners of the mouth and lips, scaly patches on the head, and a magenta mouth and tongue.

TREATMENT

Treatment of riboflavin deficiency includes riboflavin 5–30 mg orally once a day in divided doses given until recovery. Sometimes, riboflavin is given parenterally as one vitamin in a multivitamin preparation.

PREVENTION

As a preventive measure, people undergoing hemodialysis or peritoneal dialysis or who have a malabsorption disorder should take riboflavin supplements or a daily multivitamin. Patients with riboflavin deficiency are given high doses of riboflavin, taken by mouth until symptoms resolve.

YOU SHOULD REMEMBER

Exposure to ultraviolet radiation in daylight causes riboflavin to break down quickly. Therefore, paper and plastic containers should be used for milk, milk products, and cereals, and glass containers should be avoided.

Check Your Knowledge

1. What are the functions of riboflavin in the body?
2. What are the risk factors for riboflavin deficiency?
3. What are the signs and symptoms of riboflavin deficiency?

VITAMIN B3 DEFICIENCY

Vitamin B3 (niacin) deficiency is a condition known as **pellagra**. A niacin deficiency is rare because it is found in many foods, both from animals and plants. Niacin is available as a supplement in nicotinic acid or nicotinamide. Sometimes, the amounts in supplements are far beyond the recommended daily allowance (RDA), causing unpleasant flushing side effects. Niacin supplements are also available as a prescription medicine used to treat high cholesterol; this typically comes in an extended-release form of nicotinic acid that allows slower, more gradual absorption so that it does not cause flushing. Because of the very high doses of nicotinic acid needed, up to 2,000 mg daily, this supplement should only be used when monitored by a physician.

EPIDEMIOLOGY

Historically, pellagra has occurred in poor populations throughout the world, including Europe, Africa, Asia, and the Southern United States. It usually occurs in populations with minimal diet, especially where protein is scarce, and corn is the staple food. Today, pellagra in the United States is rare, occurring in less than 1%, and is usually due to secondary causes, such as alcohol use. The same is true in other industrialized Western nations, many of which have adopted the practice of fortifying bread and cereal products. However, primary pellagra still exists in less developed regions, especially tribal populations where corn remains the staple. Today, it is most commonly found in India, China, and sub-Saharan Africa.

ETIOLOGY AND RISK FACTORS

The primary cause of pellagra is an inadequate diet. Drugs, alcoholism, GI tract diseases, and malignancies are the common causes of secondary pellagra. Excessive and chronic alcohol intake can induce pellagra due to reducing the absorption of niacin. Niacin is primarily absorbed in the small intestine; therefore, malabsorptive disorders such as chronic diarrhea, inflammatory bowel disease, and malignancy can impair niacin absorption. Also, a drug used for tuberculosis, such as isoniazid, may cause an increase in the risk of niacin deficiency.

CLINICAL MANIFESTATIONS

The signs and symptoms of severe niacin deficiency lead to pellagra, a condition that causes chronic diarrhea, sometimes bloody, nausea, vomiting, and loss of appetite. Dermatology symptoms include a thick, scaly, pigmented rash on skin areas exposed to sunlight (see **Figure 16.2**). Neurological symptoms of severe niacin deficiency include fatigue, headache, apathy, depression, memory loss, and hallucinations.

DIAGNOSIS

Medical history and diet are essential to diagnose pellagra. Clinical symptoms may be straight-forward when skin and mouth lesions, diarrhea, delirium, and dementia co-occur. However, the presentation could be more specific more often. Laboratory testing should be completed to confirm the results, and it should include testing for tryptophan, NAD, NADP, and niacin levels. Urinary excretion of N1-methyl nicotinamide (NMN) of less than 5.8 μmol (0.8 mg/day) may suggest niacin deficiency.

TREATMENT

The RDA for niacin is 16 mg daily for men and 14 mg for women. Good sources of niacin include red meat, fish, poultry, fortified bread and cereals, and enriched pasta and peanuts. Food items should be consumed in their fresh form rather than in processed form, such as canning, milling, and freezing. Boiling food should be avoided as vitamin B5 is water-soluble, and its content is lost in cooked food. Vitamin B5 can be taken as a supplement with other B-complex vitamin formulations.

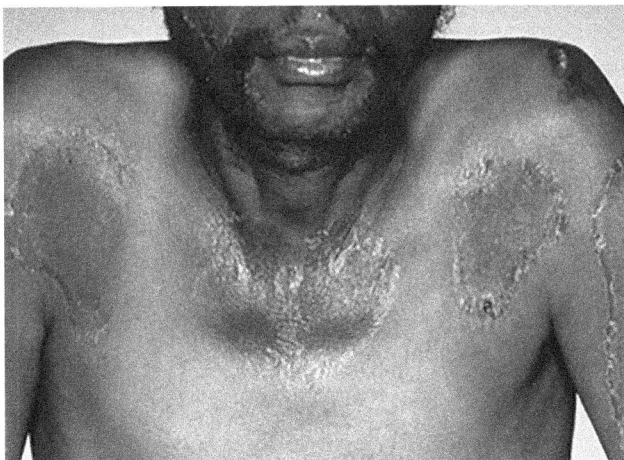

FIGURE 16.2 Skin rash of pellagra.

PREVENTION

A well-balanced diet is the simplest way to ensure adequate nutrition. When food choices are limited, enriched foods and dietary supplements can help. Vitamin B-complex supplement provides enough niacin for most healthy adults. The recommended daily dose of niacin is about 15 mg.

YOU SHOULD REMEMBER

Although there is no evidence of toxic levels for consuming niacin through foods, niacin consumption in heavily fortified foods, pharmacological or supplemental levels can result in adverse events. High levels of niacin (3,000 mg/day) may cause flushing, jaundice, impaired vision, and abdominal discomfort, and a sustained high level can cause hepatotoxicity. The tolerable upper intake level of 35 mg/day of niacin in adults 19 or older may cause adverse effects.

Check Your Knowledge

1. Which countries are most commonly found in pellagra today?
2. What are the neurological symptoms of severe niacin deficiency?
3. What is the recommended daily allowance for vitamin B3?

VITAMIN B5 DEFICIENCY

Vitamin B5 (pantothenic acid) is naturally present, added to foods, and available as a supplement. It makes coenzyme A (CoA), a chemical compound that helps enzymes build and break down fatty acids. Pantothenic acid is used for energy metabolism. Because pantothenic acid is found in a wide variety of foods, a deficiency is rare except in people with other nutrient deficiencies, as seen with severe malnutrition.

ETIOLOGY AND RISK FACTORS

Usually, vitamin B5 deficiency is caused by a genetic mutation where pantothenic acid cannot be metabolized. The disorder is known as pantothenate kinase-associated neurodegeneration. Malnourishment also results in vitamin B5 deficiency. Risk factors for pantothenate deficiency include acetylcholine deficiency, myelin loss, and age-related dementias like Huntington's disease. The risk factors include women on oral contraceptives, alcoholics, people with impaired absorption, and patients with insufficient food intake (elderly and postoperative).

CLINICAL MANIFESTATIONS

Symptoms of pantothenic acid deficiency include headache, restlessness, fatigue, insomnia, depression, irritability, nausea or vomiting, stomach pains, muscle cramps, burning feet, and upper respiratory infections. These symptoms of vitamin B5 deficiency in adults are also the same in children. A toxic level of pantothenic acid has not been observed from food sources. With substantial daily doses of 10 g/day, stomach upset, or mild diarrhea has been reported.

TREATMENT

To treat pantothenic acid deficiency in the body, a diet rich in meat, vegetables, eggs, milk, cereal grains, and legumes should be consumed. All these food items are rich sources of vitamin B5.

PREVENTION

If pantothenic acid is deficient, a diet rich in meat, vegetables, eggs, milk, cereal grains, and legumes should be consumed. All these food items are rich sources of vitamin B5.

VITAMIN B6 DEFICIENCY

Vitamin B6 (pyridoxine) is present in many foods, including meat, fish, beans, grains, fruits, vegetables, and nuts. As a coenzyme, vitamin B6 is a cofactor in over 100 enzymatic reactions. It contributes to neurotransmitter synthesis, interleukin-2 production, and hemoglobin formation. Pyridoxine supports normal immune function and gene expression regulation. Low levels of pyridoxine have been seen in cardiovascular disease, diabetes mellitus, inflammatory bowel disease, and rheumatoid arthritis. Excess vitamin B6 is mainly excreted in the urine. Seizures, mental status changes, anemia, rashes, and glossitis may cause vitamin B6 deficiency.

EPIDEMIOLOGY

Vitamin B6 deficiency is rare in most countries. The CDC has estimated that 10% of the United States population has low concentrations. It is most prominent in women, older adults, African Americans, smokers, women taking oral contraceptives, alcoholics, underweight people, or those consuming a poor diet.

ETIOLOGY AND RISK FACTORS

The causes of vitamin B6 deficiency include chronic alcohol dependence, obesity, protein-energy malnutrition, pregnancy, preeclampsia and eclampsia, malabsorptive states, and **bariatric surgery** predispose to vitamin B12 deficiency. Certain conditions can increase the risk of developing a deficiency by interfering with the absorption of vitamin B6. These conditions include kidney disease, celiac disease, ulcerative colitis, Crohn's disease, and rheumatoid arthritis. Some anticonvulsants, including valproic acid, carbamazepine, and phenytoin, can increase the catabolism of vitamin B6 and lead to a deficiency. In patients with tuberculosis, isoniazid competitively inhibits the action of pyridoxine, and routine supplementation is recommended.

CLINICAL MANIFESTATIONS

Typical signs and symptoms of moderate deficiency, such as glossitis, stomatitis, cheilosis, mental status changes, and peripheral neuropathy, may occur in other medical conditions and are not unique to vitamin B6 deficiency. Severe deficiency can result in **microcytic hypochromic anemia**, seizures, **seborrheic dermatitis**, depression, and confusion (see **Figure 16.3**).

DIAGNOSIS

Early vitamin B6 deficiency may have minimal or vague symptoms or none at all. The beginning of new symptoms such as anemia, sensory neuropathy, altered mental status, dermatitis in adults, or seizures in infancy should raise suspicion of deficiency. Direct biomarkers measure B6 vitamers in blood and urine must be done. However, the assay is only sometimes widely available, and results may be delayed. Erythrocyte transaminase activity is a functional test of pyridoxine status and can be more accurate for vitamin B6 deficiency.

TREATMENT

Vitamin B6 supplements have long been used to treat carpal tunnel syndrome, premenstrual syndrome, and pregnancy-related nausea. Though evidence for its effectiveness is unproven, the Food

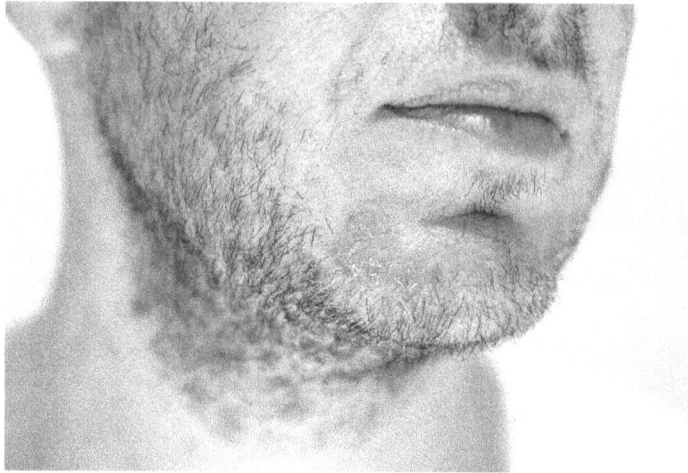

FIGURE 16.3   Seborrheic dermatitis.

and Drug Administration has approved a medication that contains vitamin B6 to treat mild to moderate pregnancy-related nausea. Another consideration is the ingestion of megadoses of this vitamin, which can lead to peripheral neuropathy. Infants diagnosed with pyridoxine-dependent seizures require lifelong treatment. A wide range of dosing has been recommended, from 5–20 mg/kg/day to 500 mg/day.

Prevention

A varied and adequate diet can prevent vitamin B6 deficiency. Fish, poultry, organ meats, fortified cereals, grains, potatoes, soy products, and legumes are all excellent sources of vitamin B6.

YOU SHOULD REMEMBER

Marginal biotin deficiency is common in pregnancy and could be attributable to an increased demand for biotin. Likewise, lactation can lead to an increased demand for biotin. Clinical data show that patients with MS, when treated with daily biotin doses of up to 300 mg, respond positively, with a reversal in disease progression and a reduction in chronic disability.

Check Your Knowledge

1. What are the functions of pyridoxine in the body?
2. What are the causes of vitamin B6 deficiency?
3. What are the signs and symptoms of severe vitamin B6 deficiency?

VITAMIN B7 DEFICIENCY

Vitamin B7 (biotin) is a coenzyme that participates in carboxylation reactions to add carbon dioxide to compounds. Nutrient databases concerning biotin still need to be completed, and its content is only known for a few foods. Since humans excrete more biotin than is consumed, large intestine bacteria are believed to synthesize this vitamin. Biotin is absorbed most efficiently from the small intestine. Biotin acts as a coenzyme for carboxylase enzymes, adding carbon dioxide to various compounds. The enzymes are needed to metabolize carbohydrates, fats, and proteins. Biotin deficiencies are rare.

EPIDEMIOLOGY

A biotin deficiency in the United States is rare, as most people eat enough biotin in a varied diet. A suboptimal biotin level is standard in pregnancy. Despite an average dietary biotin intake, about 50% of US pregnant women are marginally deficient. About 1 of every 60,000 infants has a genetic defect, resulting in a low amount of biotinidase, meaning they cannot break down biocytin in foods for absorption. According to the worldwide neonatal screening survey, profound biotin deficiency is about 1 in 112,000, and partial deficiency is 1 in 129,282. The combined incidence of profound and partial deficiency is 1 in 60,089 live births. Biotinidase deficiency has been diagnosed more commonly in children of the White race. Research has observed a higher incidence of biotin deficiency in Brazil, Turkey, and Saudi Arabia. People who excessively consume alcohol have a relatively higher incidence of low biotin levels compared to the general population. The prevalence is higher in countries with higher rates of biotin deficiency, such as Saudi Arabia and Turkey.

ETIOLOGY AND RISK FACTORS

There are many causes of biotin deficiency. It can occur in rare inborn errors of metabolism, namely holocarboxylase synthetase deficiency or biotinidase deficiency. Biotinidase deficiency is an autosomal recessive disorder. It can present as severe biotin deficiency with both neurological and dermatological features. It affects endogenous recycling and failure in releasing biotin from dietary protein. Gastrointestinal tract bacterial imbalances resulting from broad-spectrum antibiotics or inflammatory bowel disease can affect biotin synthesis in the intestine and thus lead to biotin deficiency. Alcoholism can increase the risk of biotin deficiency and many other nutrients as alcohol can block their absorption, and also because alcohol abuse is generally associated with poor dietary intake. About a third of pregnant women show a mild biotin deficiency despite eating adequate intakes, though the exact reason is not apparent. Anticonvulsants have caused biotin deficiency because of malabsorption from severe intestinal diseases.

CLINICAL MANIFESTATIONS

Biotin deficiency leads to variable clinical presentations, mainly neurological and dermal abnormalities. The dermal symptoms include hair loss, dry skin, and skin rash. Neurological symptoms include hypotonia, seizures, ataxia, numbness, and tingling of the extremities, mental retardation, and developmental delay in children. No evidence in humans has shown biotin toxicity, even with high intakes. Because it is water-soluble, any excess amount will leave through the urine. There is no established upper limit or toxic level for biotin. Children with hereditary disorders of biotin deficiency, such as biotinidase deficiency, may also show impaired immune system function, leading to increased susceptibility to infections.

DIAGNOSIS

The diagnostic tests for biotin deficiency are urinary 3-hydroxyisovaleric acid and biotin and the status of propionyl-CoA carboxylase in lymphocytes. The most reliable marker of biotin deficiency is the increased excretion of 3-hydroxyisovaleric acid in the urine. Evidence shows that serum biotin concentration does not decrease in biotin deficiency patients receiving biotin-free total parenteral nutrition. Therefore, serum biotin levels are not reliable indicators of marginal biotin deficiency.

TREATMENT

The most important aspects of medical care in patients with biotin deficiency include early diagnosis and prompt institution of therapy with 5–10 mg daily of oral biotin. Some experts suggest increasing the dose to 15–20 mg daily at the onset of puberty. The infant is usually treated with regular biotin supplements, which have to continue throughout life in most cases.

PREVENTION

To prevent biotin deficiency, individuals must eat various whole foods, quit smoking, limit alcohol consumption, treat inflammatory bowel disease to improve absorption, and be aware of medication use or supplements that may interact with biotin.

YOU SHOULD REMEMBER

Biochemical abnormalities are seen with folic acid deficiency. However, a lack of folate can lead to macrocytic anemia. In addition, lack of folate raises the levels of homocysteine, which is associated with atherosclerotic disease. Lack of folate causes several pregnancy-related complications, including placenta abruption, spontaneous abortion, neural tube defects, and severe language deficits in the offspring.

Check Your Knowledge

1. What are the neurological symptoms of biotin deficiency?
2. What are the dermal symptoms of biotin deficiency?
3. What are the diagnostic tests for biotin deficiency?

VITAMIN B9 DEFICIENCY

Vitamin B9, also known as folic acid or *folate*, was named because it is present in large amounts in leafy green vegetables, and *folium* is the Latin word meaning "leaf." Folate coenzymes are essential for the synthesis and maintenance of new cells. Normal cell division requires folate, which functions very similar to vitamin B12. Folate is necessary for pregnant people. Folate deficiency initially affects cells that actively synthesize DNA since they have a short lifespan and rapid turnover of erythrocytes. When a pregnant woman is deficient in folate, **neural tube defects** in the fetus are much more likely. The most common defects are **spina bifida** and **anencephaly** (see **Figure 16.4**

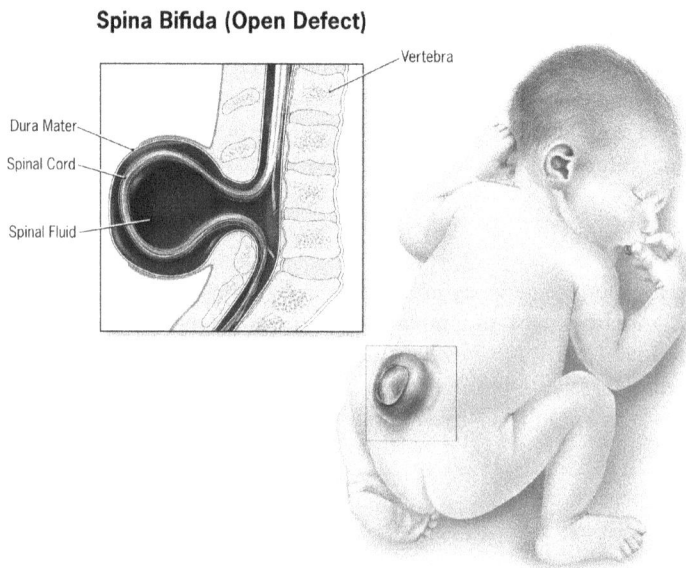

FIGURE 16.4   Spina bifida.

and **Figure 16.5**). Folate deficiency can also increase the chances of **placental abruption**. In addition, the newborn baby may be premature. Studies have also shown that low folate during pregnancy could lead to the development of **autism** in children.

EPIDEMIOLOGY

Vitamin B9 deficiency used to be expected in the United States, but fortification of the food supply has dramatically decreased its prevalence. Women of childbearing age and non-black Hispanic women were at high risk of folic acid deficiency due to inadequate folic acid intake. Today, less than 1% have folate deficiency. However, this condition can occur from low intake, malabsorption, and increased requirements for the vitamin. Folate deficiency is much more common in countries that do not have mandatory folic acid fortification measures in place, such as China, the Netherlands, Australia, New Zealand, Norway, Italy, Germany, the United Kingdom, France, Austria, Brazil, Algeria, Belgium, India, Moldova, Malaysia, Pakistan, the Philippines, Portugal, Georgia, Singapore, Sri Lanka, and Slovakia.

ETIOLOGY AND RISK FACTORS

One of the most common causes of folate deficiency is not eating a balanced diet. A healthy diet includes foods that naturally contain folate or are enriched with folic acid. Other causes of folate deficiency can include Crohn's disease, celiac disease, excessive alcohol use, hemolytic anemia, kidney dialysis, and overcooking fruits or vegetables. Pregnancy or lactation is also at risk for folic acid deficiency. Some anti-seizure drugs interfere with the proper absorption of folate.

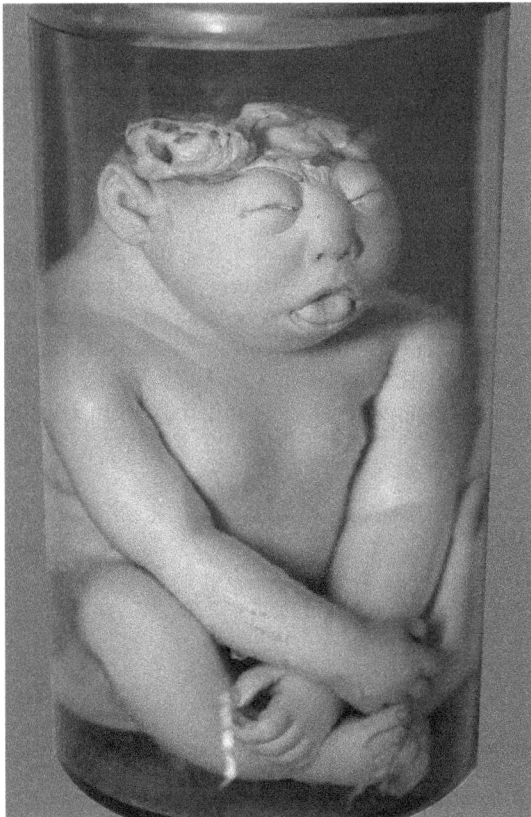

FIGURE 16.5   Anencephaly.

CLINICAL MANIFESTATIONS

At an early stage, a person may not have apparent symptoms of folate deficiency anemia. Still, as it becomes more severe, patients may complain of fatigue, dyspnea, paleness, headache, dizziness, irritability, trouble concentrating, reduced sense of taste, and sores in the mouth or tongue. **Megaloblastic anemia** diarrhea becomes persistent, causes abnormal liver function, and reduces immune function. A deficiency of folate can lead to cognitive dysfunction and encephalopathy.

DIAGNOSIS

Patients with a folic acid deficiency should also be evaluated for vitamin B12 deficiency, as both cause macrocytic anemia. Initial laboratory tests should include a complete blood count (CBC) and a peripheral smear. Laboratory tests for folic acid deficiency would reveal anemia, manifesting as a decrease in hemoglobin and hematocrit levels. The mean corpuscular volume (MCV) would be increased to a level greater than 100, consistent with a diagnosis of macrocytic anemia.

TREATMENT

All patients with folate deficiency should receive supplemental folic acid to correct the deficiency. Oral folic acid (1–5 mg daily) treats folate deficiency. Parenteral administration of folic acid can be used for patients unable to tolerate oral medications. Patients with malabsorption or short gut syndromes may typically require long-term treatment.

PREVENTION

The best way to prevent folate deficiency is to eat a healthy diet with folate or folic acid. Folate can be found naturally in liver, seafood, eggs, dairy products, meat, citrus fruits, dark green leafy vegetables, and beans.

YOU SHOULD REMEMBER

Pernicious anemia, one of the causes of vitamin B12 deficiency, is an autoimmune condition that prevents the body from absorbing vitamin B12. Left untreated, pernicious anemia can cause serious medical issues, including irreversible damage to the nervous system. Most patients begin feeling better shortly after starting treatment. Pernicious anemia cannot be cured, but increasing vitamin B12 intake may eliminate most symptoms. The neurologic complications of pernicious anemia, however, can persist even after B12 stores are entirely replaced.

Check Your Knowledge

1. Why is folic acid necessary for pregnant people?
2. What are the risk factors for folate deficiency?
3. What are the clinical manifestations of folic acid?

VITAMIN B12 DEFICIENCY

Vitamin B12 (**cobalamin**) is the only vitamin that incorporates the mineral called *cobalt* into its molecule. It plays an essential role in RBC formation, cell metabolism, nerve function, and the production of DNA, the molecules inside cells that carry genetic information. Vitamin B12 deficiency is uncommon in the United States. However, people who follow a vegetarian or vegan diet might be prone to deficiency because plant foods do not contain vitamin B12. Older adults and people with digestive tract conditions that affect nutrient absorption are also susceptible to vitamin B12 deficiency. Selective vitamin B12 absorption is a multistep process that involves the stomach, pancreas, and small intestine. Absorption of vitamin 12 requires an **intrinsic factor,** which is a protein made in the stomach, and hydrochloric acid in the gastric juice. Free B12 combines with an intrinsic factor, enhancing the absorption of the vitamin in the ileum. Some people with Crohn's disease may surgically remove part or all of the ileum, which can also lead to difficulty absorbing vitamin B12. The deficiency of intrinsic factors and vitamin B12 can result in **pernicious anemia.**

EPIDEMIOLOGY

The epidemiology of vitamin B12 deficiency varies based on the etiology. Vitamin B12 deficiency is prevalent primarily in older adults, children, and women of reproductive age, with prevalence ranging from 10% to 40%. In general, no relationship between vitamin B12 status and geographic distribution of the population can be claimed. The condition has the potential to be a worldwide public health problem. Any person can develop vitamin B12 deficiency at any age. People 60 years or older are more likely to have vitamin B12 deficiency than other age groups. In the United States and the United Kingdom, approximately 6% of adults younger than 60 have vitamin B12 deficiency, but the rate is closer to 20% in those older than 60.

ETIOLOGY AND RISK FACTORS

Vitamin B12 deficiency has three primary causes: autoimmune (pernicious anemia), malabsorption, and dietary insufficiency. It also occurs because of Chron's disease or certain medications. Deficient intake of animal food products also causes B12 deficiency. Severe deficiency causes megaloblastic anemia. The effects of low levels of B12, folate, and even B6 can cause high blood levels of **homocysteine**, which increases the risks of heart attack and stroke. Homocysteine can damage the endothelial cells of the arterial linings.

CLINICAL MANIFESTATIONS

A vitamin B12 deficiency can lead to anemia, fatigue, muscle weakness, intestinal problems, nerve damage, and mood disturbances. There are sensory disturbances in the legs, including burning, prickling, tingling, and numbness of fingertips. Walking and balance become affected. Mental problems include loss of concentration and memory, disorientation, and dementia. Bowel and bladder control is eventually lost, and visual disturbances are common. Gastrointestinal problems include tongue soreness and constipation.

DIAGNOSIS

The tests used to diagnose vitamin B12 deficiency are a CBC and a vitamin B12 blood test level. A person is diagnosed with vitamin B12 deficiency if the amount of vitamin B12 in their blood is less than 150 per mL. In patients deficient in vitamin B12, the CBC would show anemia, which manifests as a decrease in hemoglobin and hematocrit. In addition, the MCV, which measures the size of red blood cells, would be increased to a level greater than 100. This is consistent with a diagnosis of **macrocytic anemia**. A peripheral blood smear would show hypersegmented neutrophils, with a portion having greater than or equal to five lobes.

TREATMENT

The treatment of vitamin B12 deficiency involves replacement with vitamin B12. However, depending on the etiology of the deficiency, the duration and route of treatment vary. In patients who are deficient due to a strict vegan diet, an oral supplement of vitamin B12 is adequate for repletion. In patients with a deficiency in intrinsic factors, either due to pernicious anemia or gastric bypass surgery, a parenteral dose of vitamin B12 is required, as oral vitamin B12 will not be fully absorbed due to the lack of intrinsic factors. A dose of 1,000 mcg of vitamin B12 via the intramuscular route is recommended monthly. In newly diagnosed patients, 1,000 mcg of vitamin B12 is given intramuscularly weekly for 4 weeks to replenish stores before switching to once-monthly dosing.

Routine monitoring of vitamin B12 should be performed in patients at risk of developing a vitamin B12 deficiency, such as Crohn's or celiac disease. If the severity of the illness worsens and vitamin B12 levels begin to decline, treatment is then started. However, prophylactic treatment before vitamin B12 levels fall is not indicated.

PREVENTION

Most people can prevent vitamin B12 deficiency by consuming foods and drinks that contain it. Options for consuming vitamin B12 include red meat, fish, poultry, eggs, milk, and other dairy products.

YOU SHOULD REMEMBER

Smokers need more vitamin C because smoking creates oxidative stress, increasing the turnover of the vitamin. Women taking oral contraceptives may also need more vitamin C. Obese people often have low serum vitamin C, in part due to a poor diet and the body's faster use of the vitamin to try to reduce inflammation. Burn and trauma patients also need more vitamin C because it is linked to **collagen** synthesis, which significantly increases as tissues are rebuilt.

Check Your Knowledge

1. What are the causes of pernicious anemia?
2. What are the clinical manifestations of vitamin B12 deficiency?
3. How can be diagnosed vitamin B12 deficiency?

VITAMIN C DEFICIENCY

Vitamin C (ascorbic acid) is involved in multiple body functions, mainly as a donor of electrons. It is the least stable of all vitamins and is lost during storage, processing, and cooking. Higher doses of vitamins may cause bloating, gastritis, diarrhea, kidney stones, and excessive iron absorption. High doses also give false medical test results for blood in the stool. Vitamin C is also believed to have additional roles in immune function. The vitamin C deficiency disease is known as **scurvy**.

EPIDEMIOLOGY

Scurvy (severe vitamin C deficiency) is rare as most people get enough vitamin C in their diet. In the United States, scurvy most commonly affects babies, children, and older adults who do not get enough vitamin C in their diet. Globally, scurvy is linked to poverty. The rates of vitamin C deficiency around the world vary. In the United States, 7.1% of people may develop a deficiency. In north India, the rate is 73.9%.

ETIOLOGY AND RISK FACTORS

The most likely people include those with an overall poor diet, those with kidney disease who get dialysis, heavy drinkers, and smokers. People at most significant risk are poor people with low incomes, alcoholics, smokers, and anyone with a poor diet.

CLINICAL MANIFESTATIONS

Acute vitamin C deficiency leads to scurvy. The timeline for the development of scurvy varies, depending on vitamin C body stores, but signs can appear within 1 month of little or no vitamin C intake. Initial symptoms can include fatigue, malaise, and inflammation of the gums. As vitamin C deficiency progresses, collagen synthesis becomes impaired, and connective tissues weaken, causing petechiae, ecchymoses, purpura, joint pain, poor wound healing, hyperkeratosis, and corkscrew hairs. Additional signs of scurvy include depression, **gingivitis**, bleeding gums, and loosening of teeth due to tissue and capillary fragility (see **Figure 16.6**). Iron deficiency anemia can also occur due to increased bleeding and decreased nonheme iron absorption secondary to low vitamin C intake. Taking too much vitamin C can cause nausea, vomiting, heartburn, diarrhea, headache, insomnia, and skin flushing.

DIAGNOSIS

The diagnosis of scurvy is usually made clinically in a patient with skin or gingival signs and is at risk of vitamin C deficiency. Laboratory confirmation may be available. A complete blood count is done, often detecting anemia. Bleeding, coagulation, and **prothrombin times** are standard.

TREATMENT

With immediate treatment, the symptoms of scurvy should start to pass within 24–48 hours. Some symptoms may take longer to go away. Dental and gum issues and corkscrew hairs may take weeks to months to disappear. Severe gum disease may cause permanent damage. The treatment is essential to avoid further complications. The condition is easily treatable by consuming more vitamin C. The patients should maintain a nutritious diet that includes one to two times their recommended amount of vitamin C. They can do so by adding fresh fruits and vegetables to every meal. Children with scurvy can take a supplement of up to 300 mg daily. Adults must take between 500 and 1,000 mg. Untreated, scurvy is eventually fatal.

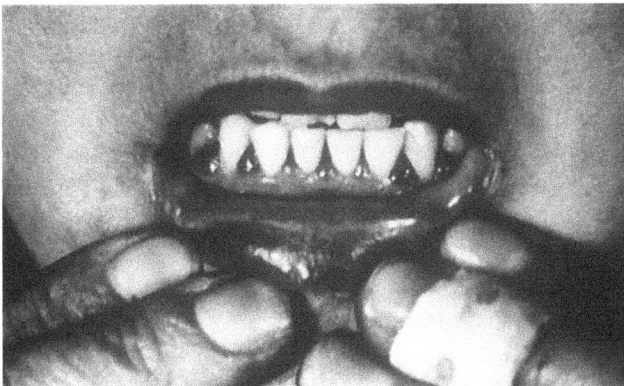

FIGURE 16.6 The gingivitis of scurvy.

PREVENTION

Individuals can prevent scurvy by getting the recommended daily allowance of vitamin C in their diet. The best sources of the nutrient are fresh fruits and vegetables.

YOU SHOULD REMEMBER

Vitamin C is under continued study concerning its possible preventive effects against cancer of the mouth, esophagus, stomach, and lungs. Some studies also suggest that good vitamin C status offers some protection against heart disease and stroke. Some evidence exists that high vitamin C intake may sometimes prevent or treat the common cold.

Check Your Knowledge

1. What are the causes of scurvy?
2. What are the clinical manifestations of vitamin C deficiency?
3. How can vitamin C be diagnosed?

Clinical Case Studies

CLINICAL CASE STUDY 1

A 53-year-old male with a history of heavy alcohol consumption for 15 years went to his family physician. He stated that his eyes were burning and his tongue was sore. The patient was added to mild abdominal pain with no appetite. The physical examination revealed cracks on the lips and the corners of the mouth. The skin was oily, the hair lacked moisture and natural shine, and the finger-nails were split—the physician diagnosed vitamin B2 deficiency.

CRITICAL THINKING QUESTIONS

1. What are the functions of vitamin B2 in the body?
2. What are the causes of vitamin B2 deficiency?
3. What are the clinical manifestations of vitamin B2 deficiency?

CLINICAL CASE STUDY 2

A 27-year-old female farmer presented to the federal medical clinic with a 10-week history of dark-ening and thickening of the neck, hands, feet, and upper trunk region, including the upper chest. The affected skin area was exacerbated after exposure to sunlight. The lesions were accompanied by itching and burning sensations following exposure to the sun. She also complained of diarrhea. Cognitive abilities did not reveal remarkable disorientation. She had no history of severe anger, rage, delusions, or seizures. There was no history of tuberculosis treatment. Her dietary history revealed a persistent intake of corn, the household's essential meal. The patient was worried and less active as the disease condition worsened. After laboratory tests, she was diagnosed with pellagra.

CRITICAL THINKING QUESTIONS

1. What are the causes of pellagra?
2. What are the clinical manifestations of pellagra?
3. How can we diagnose pellagra?

CLINICAL CASE STUDY 3

A 78-year-old white man comes to a neurologist with progressive neuropathy and declining mental status over several months. The patient initially developed numbness in his fingertips, the toes, and the arch of his feet. He began to lose motor control of his hands, which manifested as dropping objects. As signs and symptoms progressed, he had visual tracking problems that were severe enough to interfere with driving a car, and he developed short-term memory loss and slowing of cognitive function.

CRITICAL THINKING QUESTIONS

1. What are the functions of vitamin B12 in the body?
2. What are the causes of vitamin B12 deficiency?
3. What are the clinical manifestations of vitamin B12 deficiency?

FURTHER READING

1. Allison-Francis, E. (2011). *Correcting the Vitamin D Deficiency Epidemic: Strategies to Fight Diseases and Prolong Life.* Dare Books.
2. Arpilor, L. (2023). *Pellagra Symptoms, Causes, and More.* Arpilor.
3. Donofrio, P.D. (2012). *Textbook of Peripheral Neuropathy.* Demos Medical.
4. Dutta, P. (2023). *Vitamin B2: The Power of Riboflavin and Its Impact on Health.* Apricot Publications.
5. Eskin, M.N.A. (2018). *Advances in Food and Nutrition Research: New Research and Developments of Water-Soluble Vitamins,* Volume 83. Academic Press.
6. Florkin, M., and Stotz, E.H. (2014). *Comprehensive Biochemistry,* Volume 11: Water-Soluble Vitamins, Hormones, Antibiotics. Elsevier.
7. Ghazanfar, A., and Elya, R. (2014). *The B12 Deficiency Survival Handbook: Fix Your Vitamin B12 Deficiency before any Permanent Nerve and Brain Damage.* CreateSpace Independent Publishing Platform.
8. Hoffbrand, V. (2023). *The Folate Story: A Vitamin under the Microscope.* Matador.
9. Icon Group International. (2010). *Seborrheic Dermatitis: A Medical Dictionary, Bibliography, and Annotated Research Guide to Internet References,* 2nd Edition. Icon Group International, Inc.
10. Persky, W. (2014). *Vitamin D and Autoimmune Disease: How Vitamin D Prevents Autoimmune Disease.* Persky Farms.
11. Purser, D., and Larkin, J. (2019). *Vitamin Deficiency Symptoms and Cures: Modern Deficiency Illness: Using Intracellular Micronutrient Results: Vitamin Deficiencies Can Cause Diabetes, Infertility, Anxiety, Fatigue, Depression.* Purser.
12. Rapha Publishing and McFarlane, S. (2023). *Vitamin C Deficiency Symptoms and Treatment (Supplements).* Rapha Publishing.
13. Rydon, R. (2016). *Profiles of the Nutrients: 3. Water-Soluble and Fat-Soluble Vitamins.* Lulu.com.
14. Stanger, O. (2012). *Water Soluble Vitamins: Clinical Research and Future Application (Subcellular Biochemistry, 56).* Springer

Part VI

---

*Mineral Deficiency and
Toxicity Disorders*

17 Natremia, Chloremia, and Kalemia

OVERVIEW

Sodium and potassium levels in the blood are essential. The correct ratio of these elements to the body's total water must stay balanced to ensure each person remains healthy. Hyponatremia is an excess of water with sodium. It can be induced by marked polydipsia and impaired water excretion due to kidney failure or persistent release of antidiuretic hormone. Hypernatremia refers to levels of sodium in the blood being too high. It typically occurs when a person has a reduced fluid intake or excessive fluid loss. Acute hypernatremia is associated with a rapid decrease in intracellular water content and brain volume caused by an osmotic shift of free water out of the cells. Within 24 hours, electrolyte uptake into the intracellular compartment results in partial restoration of brain volume. Hypochloremia results from excessive gastric secretions or urine loss, resulting in hypochloremic alkalosis. Hyperchloremia usually occurs due to dehydration or excess administration of sodium or other chlorides. Hypokalemia refers to a lower-than-normal potassium level in the blood. Potassium helps carry electrical signals to cells in the body. It is critical to the functioning of nerve and muscle cells, particularly heart muscle cells. Hyperkalemia is a potentially life-threatening metabolic problem caused by the inability of the kidneys to excrete potassium, impairment of the mechanisms that move potassium from circulation into the cells, or a combination of these factors.

HYPONATREMIA

Hyponatremia represents a relative excess of water to sodium. It can be induced by a marked increase in water intake and impaired water excretion due to kidney failure or persistent release of **antidiuretic hormone**. It occurs when the concentration of sodium in the blood is abnormally low. Sodium is an electrolyte that helps regulate the amount of water in the interstitial tissues.

EPIDEMIOLOGY

Hyponatremia is the most common electrolyte condition in clinical practice, occurring in 15%–30% of hospitalized patients. Post-operative hyponatremia develops in 4.4% of patients within the first week of surgery. Globally, the prevalence of hyponatremia among patients aged 18 years old and above varies depending on the studied population. It is estimated to range from 1.72% to 17.5% in the United States and 32.5% in hospitalized patients in China and Switzerland, respectively. The association between hyponatremia and patient characteristics such as age and gender has been investigated thoroughly. The results have shown that the prevalence of hyponatremia increases with age. However, there are conflicting results regarding the association between gender and the prevalence of hyponatremia.

ETIOLOGY AND RISK FACTORS

Hyponatremia can be caused by excessive fluid loss due to sweating or burns, severe vomiting, diarrhea, poor nutrition, alcohol use disorder, overhydration, chronic hypothyroidism, **diabetes insipidus**, adrenocortical deficiency, use of certain diuretics or seizure medications, antidepressants and pain medication, and liver, congestive heart failure, or kidney failure.

DOI: 10.1201/9781003453376-23

CLINICAL MANIFESTATIONS

Signs and symptoms may include nausea and vomiting, headache, fatigue, hypotension, irritability, lethargy, muscle weakness or muscle cramps, seizures, confusion, and coma.

Hyponatremia is very dangerous for many organs, especially for the brain.

DIAGNOSIS

The diagnosis of hyponatremia includes a medical history and a physical exam—blood tests that indirectly show total body water, sodium levels, and, in some cases, hormones that regulate water uptake by the kidneys.

TREATMENT

Hyponatremia is a common water balance disorder that often leads to a diagnostic or therapeutic challenge. Treatment is based on the cause and the seriousness of hyponatremia. The mainstay of management is rehydration with sodium chloride (0.9% solution) and discontinuation of diuretic therapy where appropriate. Correction or maintenance of other serum electrolytes is vital. Correction of hypokalemia is significant because low potassium can impair correction of hyponatremia.

PREVENTION

To prevent hyponatremia, people should not drink too much beer and other forms of alcohol. Drink enough water, but only a little water. Healthcare providers must manage the underlying condition and maintain a balanced diet.

YOU SHOULD REMEMBER

Hyponatremia often occurs in patients with intracranial hemorrhage, encephalitis, meningitis, concussion, and brain tumors. Cerebral salt wasting is due to decreased sympathetic nervous system function or secretion of a circulating factor that decreases renal sodium reabsorption.

Check Your Knowledge

1. What are the causes of hyponatremia?
2. What are the clinical symptoms of hyponatremia?
3. What is the treatment of hyponatremia?

HYPERNATREMIA

Hypernatremia refers to a high concentration of sodium in the blood. Sodium is essential for many bodily functions. However, when it is too much, it can result in an imbalance in the body's electrolytes and serious problems. Sodium helps regulate the blood volume, blood pressure, body pH, and cells' electrical conductivity. This means that sodium helps balance the amount of water on the inside or outside of the cells, and it is also critical for how muscles and nerves work. The kidneys help regulate how much sodium is in the body – most of it is removed through urine, and a small amount comes out in sweat.

Hypernatremia due to dehydration is a common health condition that can affect anyone regardless of age, sex, race, or ethnicity. Severe hypernatremia mainly affects infants, older adults, and debilitated and hospitalized patients.

EPIDEMIOLOGY

Hypernatremia is primarily seen in infants and the elderly population. Infants receiving inadequate water replacement in the setting of gastroenteritis or ineffective breastfeeding is a common scenario. Premature infants are at higher risk due to their relatively small mass to surface area and their dependency on the caretaker to administer fluids. Patients with neurologic impairment are also at risk due to impaired thirst mechanisms and lack of water availability. Hypernatremia can occur in the hospital setting due to hypertonic fluid infusions, especially when combined with the patient's inability to have adequate water intake. Hypernatremia occurs in approximately 1% of hospitalized patients. The condition usually develops after hospital admission. An incidence closer to 2% has been reported in debilitated elderly persons and breastfed infants.

ETIOLOGY AND RISK FACTORS

Hypernatremia may be caused by insufficient water consumption, severe dehydration, excessive loss of body fluids, and use of corticosteroids. **Conn's disease** may also cause it. Hypernatremia represents a relative free water deficit, possibly from renal water loss, diuretics, vomiting, diarrhea, and surgical drains. Hypernatremia can be very serious, especially in small children. It can be caused by dehydration due to diarrhea, vomiting, excessive sweating, significant burns, or other systemic problems. It can also cause severe problems in older people. Sometimes, as the brain ages, it does not quickly pick up on electrolyte imbalances, leading to hypernatremia. Older people can also have kidney impairments that can contribute to this condition.

CLINICAL MANIFESTATIONS

Primary symptoms of hypernatremia are extreme thirst, dry skin, dry mouth, **oliguria**, and dark urine. Other clinical manifestations are headache, fainting, tachycardia, confusion, lethargy, irritability, seizures, and coma.

DIAGNOSIS

Hypernatremia is diagnosed by findings from the history, physical examination, laboratory studies, and evaluation of blood volume status. Measuring serum and urine electrolytes, determining osmolality, and evaluating renal, adrenal, thyroid, hepatic, and cardiac function are valuable approaches.

TREATMENT

Treatment of hypernatremia may include replacing the water deficit over 48 hours, daily maintenance with IV sodium chloride 0.9% and glucose 5%, and treating the underlying cause. It is important to remember that rapid correction of hypernatremia can lead to cerebral edema because water moves from the serum into the brain cells. Untreated hypernatremia could result in complications like brain hemorrhage, permanent brain damage, and death.

PREVENTION

To prevent hypernatremia, a person must drink plenty of water to stay hydrated. They should also increase their fluid intake in hot climates or during physical activity and have a healthy diet. A low-sodium diet will reduce oral solute intake and decrease renal water loss.

YOU SHOULD REMEMBER

One of the most severe complications of hypernatremia is a subarachnoid or subdural hemorrhage, which can cause permanent brain damage or death.

YOU SHOULD REMEMBER

About 80% of the sodium in U.S. diets comes not from the salt shaker but from packaged processed restaurant and store-bought foods. Only about 5% comes from salt added during cooking; approximately 6% comes from salt added at the table. Using a high amount of sodium causes hypertension.

HYPOCHLOREMIA

Hypochloremia is an electrolyte imbalance that occurs when the blood's chloride level is low. Chloride is the major anion associated with sodium in the extracellular fluid compartment (ECF). It is an essential electrolyte that helps muscles and nerves function. It also keeps the blood's pH regular and maintains fluid balance.

EPIDEMIOLOGY

Little is known about the clinical effects of chloride on critically ill patients. However, studies have reported incidence rates of hypochloremia in the general intensive care unit (ICU) from 6.7% to 35.1%. Among patients with heart failure, the reported incidence rate of hypochloremia ranges from 7.4% to 23%.

ETIOLOGY AND RISK FACTORS

Hypochloremia is caused by excessive use of **loop diuretics**, nasogastric suction, or vomiting. **Metabolic alkalosis** is typically present with hypochloremia. Vomiting causes a loss of hydrochloric acid and certain drugs, such as antacids.

CLINICAL MANIFESTATIONS

There usually are not any symptoms or signs of hypochloremia. However, there may be associated symptoms from underlying causes of hypochloremia. The signs and symptoms of hypochloremia include diarrhea or vomiting, dehydration, fluid loss, fatigue, and dyspnea.

DIAGNOSIS

The diagnosis of hypochloremia is based on the patient's history or medication causing the imbalance, along with the laboratory assessment of chloride values. A chloride blood test can detect abnormal concentrations of chloride. As hypochloremia co-exists with other electrolyte imbalances, such as hyponatremia and hypokalemia, blood tests for other electrolytes are also performed to screen for various conditions.

TREATMENT

Several chloride-containing solutions can be used to correct total body chloride depletion, including isotonic sodium chloride (normal saline, physiologic saline) for replacement of just sodium and chloride; potassium chloride for replacement of potassium and chloride; and lysine monochloride, arginine monochloride, ammonium chloride, or HCl when acid replacement is necessary for conditions associated with chloride depletion and severe metabolic alkalosis.

PREVENTION

Preventing hypochloremia depends on the etiology, such as kidney disease, heart disease, liver disease, or diabetes. These conditions must be treated promptly. Drinking enough fluid and avoiding excessive salt consumption can also prevent this electrolyte imbalance.

Check Your Knowledge

1. What are the causes of hypochloremia?
2. What is the diagnosis of hypochloremia?
3. What is the treatment of hypochloremia?

HYPERCHLOREMIA

Hyperchloremia is an electrolyte imbalance that occurs when there's too much chloride in the blood. Chloride is an essential electrolyte that maintains the body's acid-base (pH) balance, regulates fluids, and transmits nerve impulses.

EPIDEMIOLOGY

The prevalence of hyperchloremia is unknown. The disease's exact frequency and distribution depend on its etiology, morbidity, and mortality rates.

ETIOLOGY AND RISK FACTORS

Hyperchloremia may be caused by severe dehydration, frequent vomiting, diarrhea, excessive salt, respiratory alkalosis, renal acidosis, renal failure, or dialysis. It may also be caused by administering medications or fluids with a lower sodium-to-chloride ratio than average. The standard sodium-to-chloride ratio is approximately 3:2.

CLINICAL MANIFESTATIONS

The signs and symptoms of hyperchloremia are fatigue, muscle weakness, fatigue, dry mouth, polydipsia, edema, arrhythmia, hypertension, and confusion; the symptoms of hyperchloremia and electrolyte imbalances are so general that it is impossible to diagnose this syndrome based on symptoms alone.

DIAGNOSIS

Hyperchloremia is typically diagnosed by a chloride blood test, usually part of a more extensive metabolic panel. A metabolic panel measures the levels of several electrolytes in the blood, including carbon dioxide or bicarbonate.

TREATMENT

The exact treatment for hyperchloremia depends on its cause. Treatment for dehydration will include hydration. If the patient receives too much saline, the supply of saline will be stopped until the patient recovers. If medications are causing the issue, stop the medication.

PREVENTION

Preventing hyperchloremia is simply drinking enough fluid and avoiding excessive salt consumption, which can prevent this electrolyte imbalance.

HYPOKALEMIA

Hypokalemia is an electrolyte with low serum potassium concentrations. Severe and life-threatening hypokalemia is defined when potassium levels are less than 2.5 mEq/L. In general, hypokalemia is associated with the diagnoses of cardiac disease, renal failure, malnutrition, and shock.

EPIDEMIOLOGY

One of the most common electrolyte disturbances seen in clinical practice is hypokalemia. It is more prevalent than hyperkalemia, and most cases are mild. Hypokalemia prevalence in the United States rose from 3.78% to 11.06%. This is higher in non-Hispanic blacks than in non-Hispanic white persons. Hypokalemia is also prevalent in hospitalized patients, in particular, pediatric patients, those who have a fever, and those who are critically ill. The prevalence of hypokalemia in hospitalized patients is between 6.7% and 21%. Additionally, in developing countries, an increased risk of mortality is observed in children when severe hypokalemia is associated with diarrhea and severe malnutrition.

ETIOLOGY AND RISK FACTORS

In general, hypokalemia is associated with diagnoses of cardiac disease, renal failure, malnutrition, and shock. Hypokalemia may be caused by excessive sweating, severe vomiting or diarrhea, dehydration, consuming excessive alcohol, excessive laxatives, diabetic ketoacidosis, chronic kidney disease, **Cushing's syndrome**, hyperaldosteronism, hypomagnesemia, specific diuretics, and corticosteroids. Hypomagnesemia often occurs with and may worsen hypokalemia, especially in the presence of chronic diarrhea, alcoholism, genetic disorders, diuretic use, and chemotherapy. Both promote the development of cardiac arrhythmias.

CLINICAL MANIFESTATIONS

Clinical symptoms of hypokalemia become evident once the serum potassium level is less than 3 mEq/L unless there is a sudden severe fall or the patient has a process that is potentiated by hypokalemia. The severity of symptoms also tends to be proportional to the degree and duration of hypokalemia. Clinical manifestations include muscle cramps, severe muscle weakness (leading to paralysis of gastrointestinal (GI)muscles), hypotension, faintness, polyuria, and polydipsia. Severe hypokalemia can also lead to muscle cramps, **rhabdomyolysis**, and resultant **myoglobinuria**. Hypokalemia can result in a variety of cardiac dysrhythmias. Although dysrhythmias are more likely to be associated with moderate to severe hypokalemia, there is a high degree of individual variability, and it can occur with even mild decreases in serum levels. Affected muscles can include the muscles of respiration, which can lead to respiratory failure and death.

DIAGNOSIS

Diagnostic evaluation of hypokalemia involves measuring urinary potassium excretion and assessing acid-base status. Measuring urinary potassium excretion can help distinguish renal losses from other causes of hypokalemia. Ideally, potassium excretion is measured via a 24-hour urine collection. After determining the presence or lack of renal potassium wasting, acid–bas status should be assessed.

TREATMENT

The goals of therapy for hypokalemia are to prevent or treat life-threatening complications, replace the potassium deficit, and diagnose and correct the underlying cause. Therapeutic urgency depends on the severity of hypokalemia, the existence of comorbid conditions, and the rate of decline of serum potassium levels. Potassium replacement is indicated in most cases of hypokalemia, especially in renal or GI loss cases. The presence of concomitant hypomagnesemia should also be investigated and corrected if present. Hypokalemia can be refractory to potassium replacement alone in the presence of hypomagnesemia. Hypokalemia is treated with oral or intravenous potassium.

PREVENTION

To prevent dEll of potassium. Foods that prevent hypokalemia contain potassium, including many fruits and vegetables, lean meat and fish, dairy, and legumes.

YOU SHOULD REMEMBER

In the context of renal or GI losses, potassium replacement aims to immediately raise serum potassium concentration to a safe level and then replace the remaining deficit over days to weeks. A potassium-sparing diuretic should also be considered when the etiology of hypokalemia involves renal potassium wasting, as potassium replacement therapy alone may not suffice.

Check Your Knowledge

1. What are the causes of hypokalemia?
2. What are the clinical manifestations of hypokalemia?
3. What is the diagnostic evaluation of hypokalemia?

HYPERKALEMIA

Hyperkalemia is a common and potentially life-threatening disorder occurring in hospitalized patients. Potassium is a chemical critical to the function of nerve and muscle cells, including the myocardium. The blood potassium level is typically 3.6–5.2 mEq/L.

A potassium level above 5.2–5.5 mEq/L is considered hyperkalemia.

EPIDEMIOLOGY

In the general U.S. population, hyperkalemia is rare. It is estimated that 2%–3% of people have high potassium levels in the blood. However, they are up to three times more likely to have hyperkalemia if they have chronic kidney disease. Hyperkalemia is unusual in the general population, reported in less than 5% worldwide, but may affect up to 10% of all hospitalized patients. Most cases in hospitalized patients are due to medications and renal insufficiency. Diabetes, malignancy, extremes of age, and acidosis are other essential causes in inpatients. Hyperkalemia is rare in children but may occur in up to 50% of premature infants. It is more commonly reported in men than women, perhaps due to increased muscle mass rates of rhabdomyolysis and increased prevalence of the neuromuscular disease. Other factors include non-Black patients and older age.

ETIOLOGY AND RISK FACTORS

The most common cause of hyperkalemia is kidney disease – a high-potassium diet, including potassium supplements. Hyperkalemia may also occur more in patients with diabetes mellitus and heart failure due to renal impairment. It may also be caused by severe dehydration, severe acidosis, certain blood pressure medications or diuretics, and adrenal insufficiency (Addison's disease). Today, there is a risk that the use of Angiotensin-converting enzyme (ACE) inhibitors may cause hyperkalemia, which can be of concern in high-risk populations like people with diabetes, heart failure, and peripheral vascular disease.

CLINICAL MANIFESTATIONS

Patients with chronic hyperkalemia may be asymptomatic at increased levels, while patients with acute hyperkalemia may develop severe symptoms. Infants have higher baseline levels than children and adults. Signs and symptoms of hyperkalemia include fatigue, lethargy, muscle weakness, loss of appetite, nausea and vomiting, increased thirst, craving for salty foods, depression, irritability, polyuria, and poor concentration. Dangerously high potassium levels affect the heart and cause sudden chest pain, palpitations, dyspnea, **paresthesias**, and arrhythmia, which are life-threatening problems. People with Addison's disease may also have a darkening of their skin. This darkening is most visible on scars, skin folds, and pressure points such as the elbows, knees, knuckles, toes; the lips; and mucous membranes such as those lining the cheeks (see **Figure 17.1**).

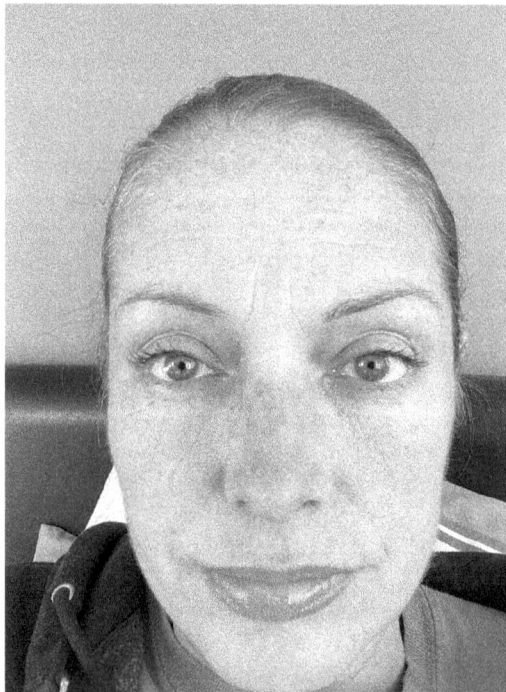

FIGURE 17.1   Addison's disease.

DIAGNOSIS

The first test that must be done in a patient with suspected hyperkalemia is an ECG since the most lethal complication of hyperkalemia is cardiac condition abnormalities, which can lead to dysrhythmias and death. An ECG shows changes in the heart rhythm. T wave elevation is the earliest sign of hyperkalemia in an ECG. Laboratory testing includes serum blood urea nitrogen and creatinine to assess renal function and urinalysis to screen for renal disease. Urine potassium, sodium, and osmolality may also help evaluate the cause. Early ECG hyperkalemia changes are typically seen as tall, peaked T waves with a narrow base, best seen in precordial leads, shortened QT interval, and ST-segment depression (see **Figure 17.2**).

In patients with renal disease, the serum calcium level should also be checked because hypocalcemia may exacerbate the cardiac effects of hyperkalemia. A complete blood count to screen for leukocytosis or thrombocytosis may also be helpful. Serum glucose and blood gas analysis should be ordered in diabetics and patients with suspected acidosis. Lactate dehydrogenase should be ordered in patients with suspected **hemolysis**. **Creatinine phosphokinases** and urine myoglobin should be ordered in patients with suspected rhabdomyolysis. Uric acid and phosphorus should be

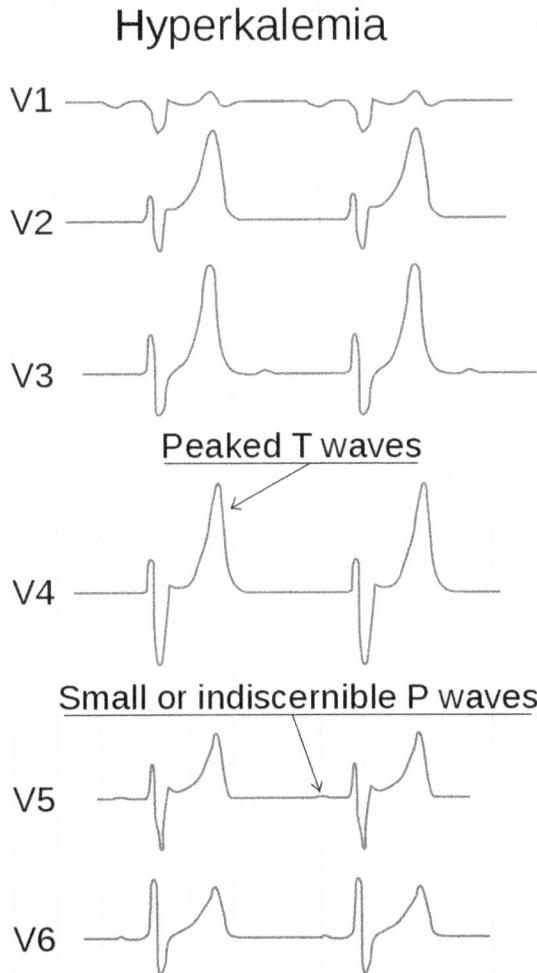

FIGURE 17.2   ECG changes because of hyperkalemia.

ordered in patients with suspected **tumor lysis syndrome**. Digoxin toxicity may cause hyperkalemia, so serum levels should be checked in patients on digoxin. If no other cause is found, consider cortisol and aldosterone levels to assess for mineralocorticoid deficiency.

TREATMENT

Treatment of hyperkalemia includes discontinuing sources of potassium intake. Calcium therapy will stabilize the cardiac response to hyperkalemia and should be initiated first in the setting of cardiac toxicity. Calcium does not alter the serum concentration of potassium but is a first-line therapy in hyperkalemia-related arrhythmias and ECG changes. Calcium chloride contains three times more elemental calcium than calcium gluconate. Still, it is more irritating to peripheral vessels and more likely to cause tissue necrosis with extravasation, so it is usually only given through central venous lines or peripherally in cardiac arrest. Thus, calcium gluconate is the usual initial drug of choice in patients with evidence of cardiac toxicity. Beta-2 adrenergic drugs such as albuterol will also shift potassium intracellularly. Loop or thiazide diuretics may help enhance potassium excretion, and hemodialysis should be performed in patients with end-stage renal disease or severe renal impairment.

PREVENTION

The best way to prevent hyperkalemia is to be aware of kidney health, reduce dietary potassium, carefully dose hyperkalemia-inducing medications, and use diuretics that promote renal extraction of hyperkalemia. Foods that should be avoided include winter squash, asparagus, avocados, potatoes, tomatoes, pumpkin, and spinach. People with hyperkalemia must avoid oranges, nectarines, kiwifruit, bananas, cantaloupe, honeydew, prunes, and raisins.

YOU SHOULD REMEMBER

The early-onset hyperkalemia may have been caused by the accumulation of potassium ions transported through the placenta, the shift of potassium ions from the intracellular to the extracellular space in the infant due to the malfunctioning of the Na^+/K^+ pump, and the inhibition of renal distal tube potassium ion secretion; there is a possibility that these mechanisms are induced by maternal and fetal hypermagnesemia after maternal magnesium sulfate administration.

YOU SHOULD REMEMBER

Pseudohyperkalemia is common and represents a false elevation in measured potassium due to specimen collection, handling, or other causes. Hyperkalemia should always be confirmed before aggressive treatment in cases where the serum potassium is elevated without explanation. True hyperkalemia may be caused by increased potassium intake, transcellular movement of intracellular potassium into the extracellular space, and decreased renal excretion. The urgency of therapy depends on symptoms, serum levels, and causes of hyperkalemia.

Check Your Knowledge

1. What are the most common causes of hyperkalemia?
2. What are the clinical manifestations of hyperkalemia in the heart?
3. What is the first test to be done to evaluate hyperkalemia?

Clinical Case Studies

CLINICAL CASE STUDY 1

An 8-month-old infant was brought to the emergency department with high fever, diarrhea, and vomiting. The infant had tachycardia, tachypnea, and lethargy. Initial serum sodium was 197 mmol/L. Ultimately, the infant was diagnosed with diabetes insipidus complicated by severe dehydration secondary to a viral infection.

CRITICAL THINKING QUESTIONS

1. What are the causes of hyponatremia?
2. What are the clinical manifestations of hyponatremia?
3. What are the treatments for hyponatremia?

CLINICAL CASE STUDY 2

A 28-year-old patient was admitted to the hospital with generalized weakness and myalgias. Three weeks before, she had abdominal pain, loss of appetite, nausea, and vomiting. Five days before admission, she developed muscle weakness that worsened until she was unable to get out of bed without assistance. Her medical history was unremarkable. She denied illegal drug abuse and alcohol. Initial laboratory tests showed average blood cell counts, severe hypokalemia (potassium, 1.6 mEq/L), and metabolic acidosis. The ECG showed flattened T waves in lateral leads. She was given 120 mEq of potassium overnight, and the day after admission, her blood potassium level increased to 2.2 mEq/L.

CRITICAL THINKING QUESTIONS

1. What are the causes of hypokalemia?
2. What are the signs and symptoms of hypokalemia?
3. What is the diagnosis of hyponatremia?

CLINICAL CASE STUDY 3

A neonate born at 30 weeks of gestation developed hyperkalemia (K^+ 6.4 mmol/L) immediately 2 hours after birth. Despite sound urine output, the neonate's blood potassium concentration reached 7.0 mmol/L 4 hours after birth. The neonate and his mother had severe hypermagnesemia caused by an intravenous infusion of magnesium sulfate given for prolonged gestation due to pre-term labor.

CRITICAL THINKING QUESTIONS

1. What are the signs and symptoms of hyperkalemia?
2. What is the diagnosis of hypernatremia?
3. What are the treatments for hypernatremia?

FURTHER READING

1. Arpilor, L. (2023). *Symptoms of Too Much Potassium: Recognize the Symptoms of Hyperkalemia and Its Potential Impact on Heart and Muscle Function.* Arpilor.
2. Blevins, L.S. (2012). *Cushing's Syndrome,* 2nd Edition. Springer Science-Business Media, LLC.
3. Healy, Z. (2021). *Critical Concept Mastery Series: Acid-Base Disturbance Cases.* McGraw-Hill/Medical.

4. Icon Group International. (2011). *Hypernatremia: Webster's Timeline History, 1952–2007.* Icon Group International, Inc.
5. Kamoi, K. (2011). *Diabetes Insipidus.* IntechOpen.
6. Kellerman, R.D., and Rakel, D.P. (2023). *Conn's Current Therapy.* Elsevier.
7. Leigh, R.M. (2022). *Hyperchloremia: TSYK (Questions and Answers).* Leigh.
8. Leigh, R.M. (2022). *Hypochloremia: TSYK (Questions and Answers).* Leigh.
9. Lippi, G., Cervellin, G., Favaloro, E.J., and Plebani, M. (2012). *In Vitro and In Vivo Hemolysis: An Unresolved Dispute in Laboratory Medicine (Patient Safety Book 4).* De Gruyter.
10. Luyase, N. (2021). *Causes of Paresthesia: Frostbite, Hypothyroidism, Multiple Sclerosis, Hyperventilation Syndrome, Pressure-induced Paresthesia, Reactive Hyperemia, Malnutrition, Rheumatoid Arthritis.* Luyase.
11. McAninch, J.W., and Lue, T.F. (2012). *Smith and Tanagho's General Urology,* 18th Edition. McGraw-Hill/Lange.
12. Ramos, M. (2019). *Hypokalemia for Everyone (Medicine for Everyone, Book 2).* Second Medical Opinions PLC.
13. Simon, E.E. (2014). *Hyponatremia: Evaluation and Treatment.* Springer.

18 Calcemia and Phosphatemia

OVERVIEW

Calcium and phosphate are oppositely related within the body; as blood calcium levels rise, phosphate levels fall. This is because phosphate binds to calcium, reducing the available free calcium within the bloodstream. By precipitating calcium, decreasing vitamin D production, and interfering with PTH-mediated bone resorption, hyperphosphatemia can cause hypocalcemia, which can be life-threatening in severe cases. Having too much phosphorus in the body is more common and problematic than having too little. Too much phosphorus is generally caused by kidney disease, excessive dietary phosphorus, and insufficient calcium. A higher phosphorus intake is associated with an increased risk of cardiovascular disease. As the amount of phosphorus people eat rises, so does the need for calcium. The delicate balance between calcium and phosphorus is necessary for proper bone density and the prevention of osteoporosis. The kidneys, bones, and intestines tightly regulate calcium and phosphorus levels in the body. Conditions related to calcium and phosphate levels include hypocalcemia, hypercalcemia, hypophosphatemia, and hyperphosphatemia.

HYPOCALCEMIA

Calcium has a vital role in skeletal mineralization. More than 99% of the calcium in the body is stored in bone as hydroxyapatite. In this form, calcium provides skeletal strength and a reservoir to release calcium into the blood circulation. Calcium homeostasis is maintained by hormones regulating calcium transport in the small intestine, kidneys, and bone. The primary hormones are parathyroid hormone, **calcitonin**, and vitamin D-3. The calcium in the blood helps the nerves' actions, supports the muscles' movement, helps the blood clot to prevent bleeding, and helps the heart work properly. Hypocalcemia can hinder the body's ability to perform these crucial functions.

Hypocalcemia may be caused by kidney failure, hypoparathyroidism, vitamin D deficiency, pancreatitis, prostate cancer, malabsorption, and the use of heparin or antiepileptic drugs. Signs and symptoms of hypocalcemia most commonly include paresthesias, muscle spasms, cramps, tetany, circumoral numbness, and seizures. Oral calcium supplements are the most common treatment for hypocalcemia. Treating the cause is just as important as treating the hypocalcemia itself. Synthetic forms of parathyroid hormone, vitamin D supplements, and IV calcium gluconate are used.

Hypocalcemia is a treatable condition that happens when the calcium levels in the blood are too low. Many health conditions can cause hypocalcemia, often caused by hypoparathyroidism, vitamin D, pancreatitis, prostate cancer, malabsorption, and the use of heparin or antiepileptic drugs. A chronic calcium deficiency can lead to dental changes, cataracts, alterations in the brain, osteoporosis, and bone fractures. A calcium deficiency may cause no early symptoms. It is usually mild, but without treatment, it can become life-threatening. A discussion of osteoporosis, osteomalacia, and bone fracture is as follows.

OSTEOPOROSIS

Osteoporosis is a bone disease that develops when bone mineral density and mass decrease or when the structure and strength of bones change. Decreased bone strength can increase the risk of fractures.

DOI: 10.1201/9781003453376-24

Epidemiology

Osteoporosis is a primary non-communicable disease and the most common bone disease, affecting one in three women and one in five men over the age of 50 worldwide. In 2018, osteoporosis prevalence was higher among women than men. The **age-adjusted prevalence** of osteoporosis at either the femur neck, lumbar spine, or both was 12.6% among adults aged 50 and over and higher among adults aged 65 and over (17.7%). Osteoporosis affects women and men of all races and ethnic groups. For many women, the disease begins to develop a year or two before menopause. It is the most common among non-Hispanic white and Asian women. African American and Hispanic women have a lower risk of developing osteoporosis, but they are still at significant risk. Among men, osteoporosis is more common in non-Hispanic whites. The cost associated with osteoporosis carries a substantial burden in our society.

Etiology and Risk Factors

Osteoporosis occurs when too much bone mass is lost, and changes occur in the structure of bone tissue. Many people with osteoporosis have several risk factors, but others who develop osteoporosis may not have any specific risk factors. There are some risk factors that we cannot change and others that we may be able to change. However, understanding these factors may prevent the disease and fractures. The risk factors include age, sex, race, family history, body size, and hormone changes. Examples of modifications to hormones include low estrogen levels in women after menopause, low levels of estrogen from the abnormal absence of menstrual periods in premenopausal women due to hormone disorders, extreme levels of physical activity, and low levels of testosterone in men.

The risk of osteoporosis is higher in people who have some medical issues, including celiac disease, inflammatory bowel disease, **rheumatoid arthritis**, kidney or liver disease, and **multiple myeloma**.

Clinical Manifestations

Osteoporosis is called a "silent" disease because there are typically no symptoms until a bone is broken. Symptoms of a spine fracture include severe back pain, loss of height, or spine malformations such as **kyphosis** (see **Figure 18.1**). Bones affected by osteoporosis may become so fragile that fractures occur spontaneously or result from minor falls, such as a fall from a standing height that would not usually cause a break in a healthy bone. Fractures may occur from everyday stresses such as bending, lifting, or coughing. Osteoporosis-related breaks most commonly occur in the hip, wrist, or spine.

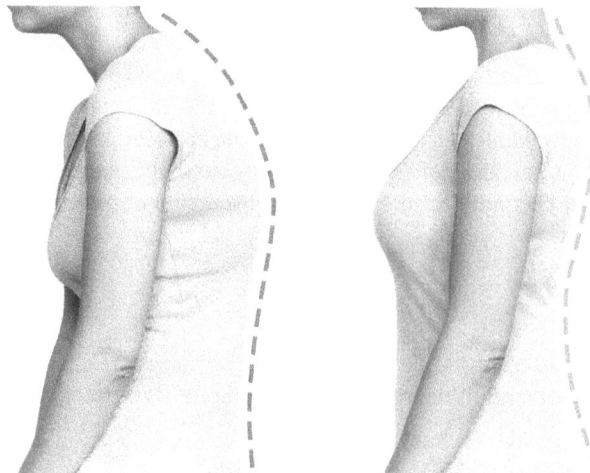

FIGURE 18.1   Kyphosis in comparison to normal spinal curvature.

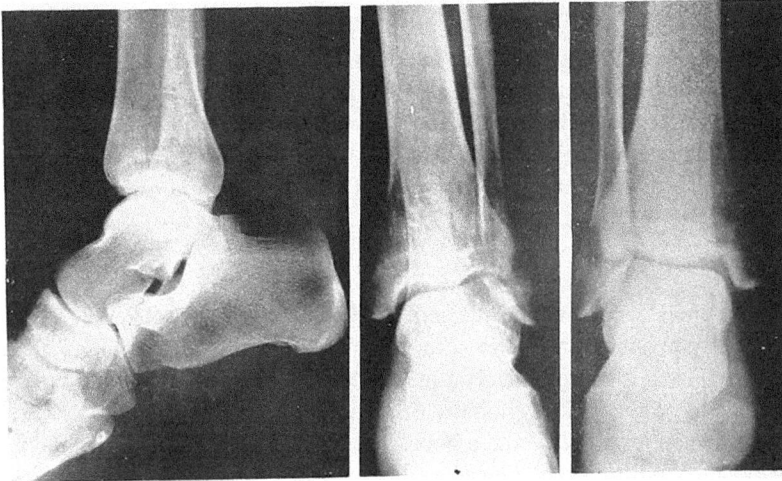

FIGURE 18.2 Decreased bone density in osteoporosis (seen in X-ray).

Diagnosis

Osteoporosis is a common disease that affects the older population. It usually goes undiagnosed for an extended period. Bone density is measured by dual-energy X-ray absorptiometry (DXA) at the hip and spine (see **Figure 18.2**). It is generally considered the most reliable way to diagnose osteoporosis and predict fracture risk. Some people have a peripheral DXA, which measures bone density in the wrist and heel. This type of DXA is portable and may make screening more accessible.

Treatment

The goals for treating osteoporosis are to slow or stop bone loss and prevent fractures.

Proper nutrition, lifestyle changes, exercise, and medications. The U.S. Food and Drug Administration (FDA) has approved bisphosphonates, calcitonin, combined estrogen, progestin therapy, human parathyroid hormone, and calcium with vitamin D.

Prevention

A healthy lifestyle can be essential for keeping bones strong. Factors contributing to bone loss include low levels of physical activity and prolonged periods of inactivity, which can contribute to an increased rate of bone loss. Chronic heavy drinking of alcohol is a significant risk factor for osteoporosis. Medicines, a healthy diet, and weight-bearing exercise can help prevent bone loss or strengthen weak bones. Men and women between the ages of 18 and 50 need 1,000 mg of calcium a day. This daily amount increases to 1,200 mg when women turn 50, and men turn 70.

YOU SHOULD REMEMBER

Long-term use of oral or injected corticosteroid medicines, such as prednisone and cortisone, interferes with the bone-rebuilding process. Osteoporosis has also been associated with medications used to combat or prevent cancer, seizures, gastric reflux, and transplant rejection.

Check Your Knowledge

1. What are the etiology and risk factors of osteoporosis?
2. What are the clinical symptoms of osteoporosis?
3. What is the treatment for osteoporosis?

Osteomalacia

Osteomalacia is a "bone softening" disorder in adults, usually caused by prolonged vitamin D deficiency. This results in abnormal osteoid mineralization. Osteomalacia most often occurs because of a problem with vitamin D, which helps the body absorb calcium. Populations at risk include homebound older adults with little sun exposure and insufficient dietary calcium and vitamin D. Osteomalacia can also result from hypocalcemia, hypophosphatemia, or direct inhibition of the mineralization process.

Epidemiology

There is a growing prevalence of vitamin D deficiency in many countries. People who live in cooler climates, particularly people with darker skin, are more at risk of developing osteomalacia. The incidence of osteomalacia is approximately 1 in 1,000 people. However, the true incidence of osteomalacia still needs to be recognized globally. It is more common in individuals with limited sun exposure, low socioeconomic status, and a poor diet. The risks vary worldwide and are contingent on geographic location, cultural preferences, and ethnicity.

Etiology and Risk Factors

A lack of the proper amount of calcium in the blood can lead to weak and soft bones. Severe and prolonged vitamin D deficiency can result in osteomalacia. Populations at risk include homebound older adults with little sun exposure and insufficient dietary calcium and vitamin D, patients with malabsorption, and those with limited sun exposure due to clothing covering most of the body or restrictions related to skin conditions. In older adults, vitamin D production decreases, and in general, the storage of vitamin D declines. Other causes of osteomalacia include **nephrotic syndrome**, which leads to the pathologic excretion of vitamin D binding protein, which binds to serum **calcidiol**. Liver disease (cirrhosis, non-alcoholic fatty liver disease, non-alcoholic **steatohepatitis**) leads to deficient production of calcidiol. Some medications, such as antiepileptic drugs (phenobarbital, phenytoin, and carbamazepine), long-term steroid use, and antifungal agents (ketoconazole), have implications in vitamin D deficiency,

Clinical Manifestations

The most common symptoms of osteomalacia are pain in the bones and hips, bone fractures, and muscle weakness. Patients can also have difficulty walking. People with this condition may easily have broken bones, tiredness, stiffness, and trouble getting up.

Diagnosis

No single laboratory finding is specific to osteomalacia. However, patients with osteomalacia will usually have hypophosphatemia or hypocalcemia. Additionally, increased alkaline phosphatase activity is typically characteristic of diseases with impaired osteoid mineralization. Some sources believe that hypophosphatemia, hypocalcemia, and increased bone alkaline phosphatase levels are necessary even to suspect osteomalacia. Measuring the level of vitamin D, X-rays, bone mineral density scans, and bone biopsy are helpful to diagnose osteomalacia.

Treatment

Treatment should focus on reversing the underlying disorder and correcting vitamin D and other electrolyte deficiencies. Treatment may involve oral vitamin D, calcium, and phosphorus supplements. People who cannot absorb nutrients well through the intestines may need more vitamin D and calcium doses. Other treatments to relieve or correct osteomalacia symptoms may include wearing braces to reduce or prevent bone irregularities, surgery to correct bone deformities (in severe cases), and adequate exposure to sunlight. The healing of osteomalacia is achieved when there are increases in urine calcium excretion and bone mineral density. Serum calcium and phosphate may normalize after a few weeks of treatment, but normalization of bone alkaline phosphatase lags, which may stay elevated for months.

Prevention

Osteomalacia is a preventable metabolic bone disorder. Most cases are related to vitamin D deficiency, so it can usually be treated appropriately and cured. If other clinical factors have contributed to the development of osteomalacia, then treatment will need to be tailored and adjusted as necessary. Eating a diet rich in vitamin D and calcium, along with sufficient exposure to sunlight, can help prevent osteomalacia due to vitamin D deficiency.

YOU SHOULD REMEMBER

Osteoclasts, bone-resorbing cells, break down bone by secreting collagenase. Osteoblasts deposit the osteoid matrix, a collagen scaffold in which inorganic salts are deposited to form mineralized bone. This intricate process is directly and indirectly influenced by hormonal signals, namely parathyroid hormone and calcitonin, which act in response to serum calcium levels.

Check Your Knowledge

1. What are the etiology and risk factors of osteomalacia?
2. What are the clinical symptoms of osteomalacia?
3. What is the treatment for osteomalacia?

BONE FRACTURES

Fractures occur in individuals of all ages. However, the type and body location vary widely depending on different factors, mainly related to individual bone quality and the nature of the trauma. Bone fractures are a common injury that can affect anyone at any age. A bone density screening is required for older adults over 50 or those with a family history of osteoporosis. There are many different types of fractures. They include greenstick, open (compound), oblique, transverse, spiral, comminuted, compression, stress, and segmental fractures (see **Figure 18.3**).

Epidemiology

The overall incidence was 1,229 fractures per 100,000 individuals per year. Fractures occur at an annual rate of 2.4 per 100 people. Men are more likely to experience fractures (2.8 per 100

TYPES OF BONE FRACTURES

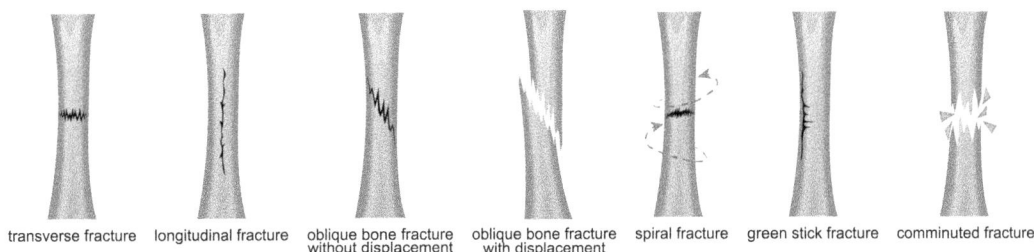

transverse fracture   longitudinal fracture   oblique bone fracture without displacement   oblique bone fracture with displacement   spiral fracture   green stick fracture   comminuted fracture

FIGURE 18.3   Types of fractures.

population) than women (2.0 per 100). Approximately 6.3 million fractures occur each year in the United States. Fractures account for 16% of all musculoskeletal injuries in the U.S. annually. More than 40% of fractures occur at home (22.5% inside and 19.1% outside). However, after age 45, fracture rates become higher among women. Among persons 65 and over, fracture rates are three times higher among women than men. Approximately 3.5 million visits are made to emergency departments for fractures each year.

The most common fracture before age 75 is a wrist fracture. In those over 75, hip fractures become the most common broken bone. Fractures are a common and significant injury in childhood, but information about the pattern of fractures among children is scarce. The incidence of fractures in many locations has been reported to increase, which could mainly be attributed to an increase in the number of fragility fractures in a growing older adult population. It is estimated that worldwide, one in three women and one in five men over the age of 50 will experience osteoporosis fractures in their remaining lifetimes.

Etiology and Risk Factors

Bone fractures can be caused by falls, sports injuries, and car accidents; overuse or repetitive motions can tire muscles and put more pressure on the bone. Risk factors include advanced age, gender, low body weight, cigarette smoking, excessive alcohol consumption, and glucocorticoid therapy.

Clinical Manifestations

Bone fractures are a common injury that can affect anyone at any age. The most common bone fracture symptoms include intense pain, bruising, edema and tenderness around the injury, and deformity.

Diagnosis

Along with a complete medical history and physical exam, other tests to diagnose bone disorders include laboratory tests on blood, urine, and other body fluids. Imaging, such as an X-ray, CT scans, an MRI, a radionuclide bone scan, and a biopsy are used.

Treatment

Depending on where the fracture is and how severe, treatment may include:

- *Splints are* to stop the movement of the broken limb.
- *Braces are* to support the bone.
- *Plaster cast is used* to provide support and immobilize the bone.
- *Traction is* a less common option.
- *They surgically inserted metal rods or plates*–to hold the bone pieces together.

Surgical treatment for fractures aims to reposition the broken pieces of bone to their normal alignment and stabilize them so they heal in the appropriate position. Various specialized implants, typically made of stainless steel or titanium, can be used for the internal fixation of such fractures.

Prevention

Getting enough calcium and vitamin D can help keep your bones strong. So can staying active. Try to get at least 150 minutes/week of physical activity. Other ways to maintain bone health include quitting smoking and avoiding or limiting alcohol use.

YOU SHOULD REMEMBER

The severity of a fracture generally depends on the force that caused the break. If the bone's breaking point has been exceeded only slightly, the bone may crack rather than breakthrough. If the force is extreme, such as that caused by an automobile crash or gunshot, the bone may shatter.

Check Your Knowledge

1. How common are bone fractures in the United States?
2. How can we diagnose bone fractures?
3. What is the treatment for bone fractures?

HYPERCALCEMIA

Hypercalcemia occurs when the calcium level in the blood is above average. Too much calcium in the blood can weaken bones, create kidney stones, and interfere with the heart and brain's functioning.

EPIDEMIOLOGY

Hypercalcemia affects approximately 1% of the general population and about 2% of patients with cancer. The annual incidence of hypercalcemia is 0.09%–0.6%, varying by population screened. Approximately 90% of people with hypercalcemia have primary hyperparathyroidism or cancer. The incidence of hyperparathyroidism alone is about one to two cases per 1,000 adults. Mild cases are often not diagnosed. Hypercalcemia can affect anyone at any age, but it's most common in people assigned female at birth over age 50 (after menopause).

ETIOLOGY AND RISK FACTORS

Hypercalcemia may be caused by primary hyperparathyroidism and lung and breast cancers. Kidney stones, hyperthyroidism, excessive use of antacids, excessive use of calcium or vitamin D supplements, and use of lithium, theophylline, or certain diuretics. Calcium is one of the most critical and common minerals in the body. Most of the body's calcium is stored in the bones. It is needed for blood coagulation—parathyroid hormone and calcitonin control calcium levels in the blood and bones. Vitamin D also plays an essential role in maintaining calcium levels because the body needs it to absorb calcium from foods. Treatment of hypercalcemia depends on the cause and severity of the condition. In mild cases of hypercalcemia, more water must be consumed, and any calcium-rich antacid tablets or supplements must be stopped. If the hypercalcemia is due to an overactive parathyroid gland, surgery is done.

CLINICAL MANIFESTATIONS

Most cases of hypercalcemia are not life-threatening, and many people do not have any symptoms. The symptoms of hypercalcemia range from mild to severe. They may include increased thirst and urination, headaches, abdominal pain, nausea, vomiting, constipation, loss of appetite, bone pain, muscle pain, irritability, confusion, and fatigue. However, severe hypercalcemia can reveal more serious signs and symptoms, including arrhythmia, kidney failure, depression, forgetfulness, and coma.

Diagnosis

Hypercalcemia is a fairly common finding on routine blood tests. Blood calcium levels indicate different levels of diagnosis and severity of hypercalcemia – a hypercalcemic crisis is a medical emergency of 14.0–16.0 mg/dL. The following tests help diagnose hypercalcemia and its cause: calcium blood tests, vitamin D blood tests, parathyroid hormone blood tests, and calcium urine tests. If primary hyperparathyroidism is causing hypercalcemia, ultrasound, CT scans, and nuclear medicine imaging are helpful.

Treatment

Initial therapy for severe hypercalcemia includes the simultaneous administration of intravenous isotonic saline, subcutaneous calcitonin, and bisphosphonate. If high levels of vitamin D cause hypercalcemia, short-term use of steroids such as prednisone is usually helpful. Problems associated with overactive parathyroid glands can often be cured by surgery to remove the tissue causing the pain.

Prevention

Not all cases of hypercalcemia can be prevented, but avoiding excess intake of calcium pills and calcium-based antacid tablets can help.

Check Your Knowledge

1. What are the etiologies and risk factors for hypercalcemia?
2. What are the signs and symptoms of hypercalcemia?
3. How can we diagnose hypercalcemia?

Nephrolithiasis

Nephrolithiasis is the term employed for kidney stones, also known as renal calculi, and they are crystal concretions formed typically in the kidney. Calculi usually start in the kidneys and ideally leave the body via the urethra without pain. Larger stones are painful and may need surgical intervention. There are different types of kidney stones. The cause of the problem depends on the type of stone. Stones can form when urine contains too much of certain substances that form crystals. These crystals can develop into stones over weeks or months. The common types include calcium, oxalate, and uric acid (see **Figure 18.4**).

Epidemiology

The prevalence of nephrolithiasis is approximately 3% in the general population, and the estimated lifetime risk of developing a kidney stone is about 12% for white males. Although nephrolithiasis may occur at any age, its onset is more common in young and middle-aged adults. Lifetime prevalence is estimated at 13% for men and 7% for women. The spontaneous 5-year recurrence rate is 35%–50% following an initial stone event. Roughly 50% of patients with previous urinary calculi have a recurrence within 10 years. Kidney stones are two to three times more common in males than females. It occurs more often in adults than in elderly persons, and more often in elderly persons than in children. Whites are affected more often than people of Asian ethnicity, who are affected more often than blacks. In addition, nephrolithiasis occurs more frequently in hot, arid areas than temperate regions.

Uric acid nephrolithiasis accounts for 8%–10% and is increasing globally. It mainly presents in obese cases or individuals with metabolic syndrome, and its growing incidence corresponds to the increasing prevalence of metabolic syndrome, obesity, and diabetes worldwide.

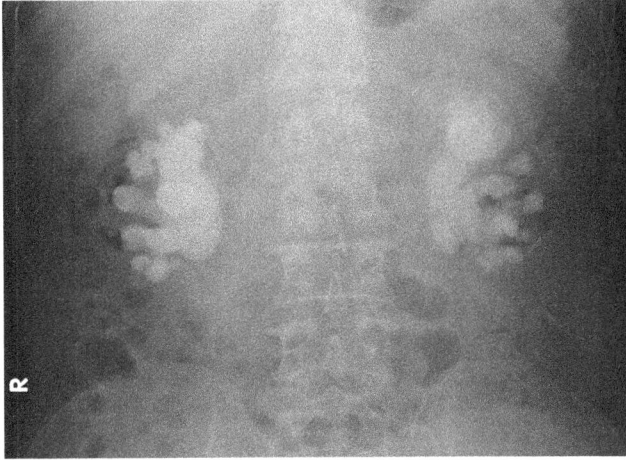

FIGURE 18.4   Bilateral kidney stones, with the letter "R," signifying the right side.

Etiology and Risk Factors

Most kidney stones are calcium stones, usually in calcium oxalate. Oxalate is a substance made daily by your liver or absorbed from your diet. Certain fruits, vegetables, nuts, and chocolate have a high oxalate content. Dietary factors, high doses of vitamin D, intestinal bypass surgery, and several metabolic disorders can increase the concentration of calcium or oxalate in urine. Calcium stones may also occur in the form of calcium phosphate. This type of stone is more common in metabolic conditions, such as **renal tubular acidosis**. It may also be associated with certain medications used to treat **migraines** or seizures.

Uric acid stones can form in people who lose too much fluid because of chronic diarrhea or malabsorption, those who eat a high-protein diet, and those with diabetes or metabolic syndrome. Certain genetic factors may also increase your risk of uric acid stones. **Cystine stones** form in people with a hereditary disorder called cystinuria, which causes the kidneys to excrete too much of a specific amino acid. The risk factors include family or personal history, dehydration, obesity, and certain supplements and medications, such as vitamin C, dietary supplements, laxatives (when used excessively), and calcium-based antacids, which can increase the risk of kidney stones.

Clinical Manifestations

A kidney stone usually will not cause symptoms until it moves around within the kidney or passes into one of the ureters. The ureters are the tubes that connect the kidneys and bladder. If a kidney stone becomes lodged in the ureters, it may block the flow of urine and cause the kidney to swell and the ureter to spasm, which can be very painful. At that point, the patient may experience sharp pain in the side and back below the ribs. Pain that radiates to the lower abdomen and groin comes in waves and fluctuates in intensity. Other signs and symptoms may include cloudy or foul-smelling urine, hematuria, nausea, vomiting, fever, and chills.

Diagnosis

Clinical guidelines recommend laboratory evaluation of patients who experience kidney stones. Testing may include an analysis of stone composition and biochemical blood evaluations for calcium, albumin, creatinine, uric acid, potassium, and bicarbonate. Urinalysis can assess pH, volume, calcium, creatinine, uric acid, oxalate, citrate, and sodium. An abdominal X-ray, CT scan, or ultrasound will complete the diagnosis.

Treatment

If you can pass a kidney stone, it may pass through the urinary tract without treatment. Larger kidney stones or kidney stones that block the urinary tract or cause great pain may need urgent treatment. Therefore, a kidney stone may be treated with **shockwave lithotripsy**, ureteroscopy, percutaneous nephrolithotomy, or **nephrolithotripsy**. The procedure involves surgically removing a kidney stone using small telescopes and instruments inserted through a small incision in the back.

Prevention

In most cases, drinking enough liquids daily is the best way to help prevent most kidney stones. Drinking enough fluids dilutes the urine and helps flush away minerals that might form stones. Although water is best, other beverages like citrus may help prevent kidney stones. Some studies show that citrus drinks, such as lemonade and orange juice, protect against kidney stones because they contain citrate, which stops crystals from turning into stones.

YOU SHOULD REMEMBER

The classic characteristic of the pain with nephrolithiasis is severe ureteral colic. It is often of sudden onset and intensifies over time into an intense, severe flank pain that may resolve with stone passage or removal. The pain may migrate anteriorly along the abdomen and inferiorly to the groin as the stone moves toward the ureterovesical junction. Gross hematuria, frequency, urinary urgency, nausea, and vomiting may also be present.

Check Your Knowledge

1. What are the common types of nephrolithiasis?
2. What are the causes of nephrolithiasis?
3. What are the signs and symptoms of nephrolithiasis?

HYPOPHOSPHATEMIA

Hypophosphatemia refers to abnormally low levels of phosphate in the blood. Often, a person is unaware of this condition and may not present with symptoms. Phosphate plays a role in nearly every cellular function. Variations in phosphate levels can affect many parts of a person's body.

EPIDEMIOLOGY

Hypophosphatemia is typically asymptomatic and is present in up to 5% of patients. It is much more prevalent in alcoholism, diabetic ketoacidosis, or sepsis, with a frequency of up to 80%. The morbidity of hypophosphatemia is highly dependent on its etiology and severity.

ETIOLOGY AND RISK FACTORS

Acute alcohol abuse, vitamin D deficiency, severe burns, hyperparathyroidism, starvation, intravenous iron administration, or certain antacids usually cause hypophosphatemia. Besides the causes mentioned, risk factors include chronic vomiting or diarrhea, long-term use of diuretics, and Cushing's syndrome.

CLINICAL MANIFESTATIONS

The signs and symptoms of hypophosphatemia include muscle weakness, softening of bones, bone pain and fractures, appetite loss, myalgia, tiredness, numbness, seizures, confusion, tooth decay or late baby teeth eruptions, and heart failure. Hypophosphatemia affects the entire body, even on an intracellular level. The complications of hypophosphatemia include rhabdomyolysis, hemolytic anemia, arrhythmias, and respiratory failure.

DIAGNOSIS

Hypophosphatemia can be diagnosed with a simple blood test that measures phosphate levels. It can be confirmed if the blood phosphate concentration is less than 2.5 mg/dL.

TREATMENT

Oral phosphate replacement medications are usually used to treat mild to moderate hypophosphatemia. If hypophosphatemia is severe, phosphate replacement through an IV is prescribed. A diet high in phosphorus to correct phosphate levels is recommended.

PREVENTION

Add more phosphate to the diet to correct mild symptoms and prevent low phosphate in the future. Milk and other dairy foods are good sources of phosphate. Taking a phosphate supplement is also helpful. If vitamin D levels are low, the patient needs to increase this vitamin's intake.

Check Your Knowledge

1. What are the causes of hypophosphatemia?
2. What are the signs and symptoms of hypophosphatemia?
3. How can hypophosphatemia be prevented?

HYPERPHOSPHATEMIA

Phosphate is an abundant mineral found in the body. The body stores about 85% of the total body phosphate in hydroxyapatite crystals in the bone—nearly 10% is found in muscles. The rest is in various compounds in the extracellular and intracellular fluids. Phosphate is predominantly an intracellular **anion**. It is essential in many biological functions, such as adenosine triphosphate (ATP) formation and protein phosphorylation. It is also in nucleic acids and is an important intracellular buffer.

EPIDEMIOLOGY

Hyperphosphatemia is rare in the general population, but in patients with advanced chronic kidney disease, the rate of hyperphosphatemia can be 70%. However, it is a significant complication for patients with peritoneal dialysis, leading to increased morbidity and mortality.

ETIOLOGY AND RISK FACTORS

Hyperphosphatemia is usually caused by low calcium levels, metabolic or respiratory acidosis, chronic kidney disease, hypoparathyroidism, severe muscle injury, and excessive use of laxatives that contain phosphate. Renal failure is the most common cause of hyperphosphatemia. Other less common causes include a high intake of phosphorus or increased renal reabsorption. High phosphate can result from excessive use of phosphate-containing laxatives or enemas. Hypoparathyroidism, acromegaly, and thyrotoxicosis enhance renal phosphate reabsorption, resulting in hyperphosphatemia. Diabetic ketoacidosis, septicemia, crush injuries, and **tumor lysis syndrome** are also caused by hyperphosphatemia. The risk factors for hyperphosphatemia include obesity, renal stones, hypercholesterolemia, hypocalcemia, diabetes, and autoimmune disease.

CLINICAL MANIFESTATIONS

Most patients with hyperphosphatemia are asymptomatic. However, it may cause tetany, muscle cramps, and perioral numbness or tingling. Other symptoms include bone and joint pain, pruritus, and a rash. Soft-tissue calcifications are common among patients with chronic kidney disease; they manifest as quickly palpable, hard, subcutaneous nodules, often with overlying scratches.

DIAGNOSIS

To diagnose hyperphosphatemia, a physical exam, urinalysis, blood test, and X-ray are used. An X-ray is essential if the patient shows signs of mineral and bone disorders. The X-ray helps reveal calcium deposits in organs or veins and any changes in the structure of a person's bones.

TREATMENT

Treatment includes eliminating phosphate intake and administering phosphate-binding antacids like calcium carbonate. The mainstay of therapy in patients with advanced chronic kidney disease is the reduction of phosphate intake, usually accomplished by avoiding foods containing high amounts of phosphate and using phosphate-binding medications taken with meals. Although quite effective, aluminum-containing antacids should not be used as phosphate-binding agents in patients with end-stage renal disease because of the possibility of aluminum-related dementia and osteomalacia. Saline diuresis can enhance phosphate elimination in cases of acute hyperphosphatemia in patients with intact kidney function. Hemodialysis can lower phosphate levels in cases of severe acute hyperphosphatemia.

PREVENTION

The best way to prevent hyperphosphatemia is to be aware of kidney health and to limit the amounts of phosphate and calcium input in the body.

Clinical Case Studies

CLINICAL CASE STUDY 18.1

A 73-year-old female was brought to the emergency department after falling from the stairs at home. She had severe pain and could not move her right leg. Her past medical history revealed hypertension and chronic heart failure. The patient is married with five children. She smokes one pack of cigarettes every day and occasionally drinks alcohol. She does not exercise and is fully mobile with no disabilities. The patient does not report symptoms of orthopnea, weakness, chest pain, palpitation, paroxysmal nocturnal dyspnea, or excessive bleeding. After the blood test and MRI, she was diagnosed with a right femur fracture due to osteoporosis.

1. What are the causes of osteoporosis?
2. What are the clinical manifestations of osteoporosis?
3. What are the treatments for osteoporosis?

CLINICAL CASE STUDY 18.2

A 64-year-old male with acute left-side pain presented to the emergency department. A ureteric calculus with associated hydronephrosis was identified, and he was prescribed pain medications and discharged to pass the stone naturally. Three days later, he returned to the emergency department with severe pain, hematuria, and a fever. A urologist was treated with a temporary ureteric stent and antibiotics.

CRITICAL THINKING QUESTIONS

1. What are the risk factors for kidney stones?
2. What are the clinical manifestations of nephrolithiasis?
3. What are the treatments for nephrolithiasis?

CLINICAL CASE STUDY 18.3

A 62-year-old female with underlying type 2 diabetes mellitus, hypertension, and chronic kidney disease presented emergently with general weakness and altered mental status. The creatinine level was 14 mg/dL (high) 2 months before consultation, and he was advised of the initiation of hemodialysis, which she refused. After that, the patient stopped taking all prescribed medications and self-medicated with honey and persimmon vinegar, in the false belief that it was detoxifying. At the time of admission, she was delirious. Her laboratory results showed a blood urea nitrogen level of 183.4 mg/dL (very high), a serum creatinine level of 26.61 mg/dL (0.5–1.3 mg/dL), a serum phosphate level of 19.3 mg/dL (2.5–5.5 mg/dL), a total calcium level of 4.3 mg/dL (8.4–10.2 mg/dL), a vitamin D level of 5.71 ng/mL (30–100 ng/mL), and a parathyroid hormone level of 401 pg/ml (9–55 pg/mL). Brain computed tomography revealed a non-traumatic spontaneous subdural hemorrhage, presumably due to uremic bleeding. Physical exams, urinalysis, blood tests, and X-rays were used to diagnose hyperphosphatemia.

CRITICAL THINKING QUESTIONS

1. What are the causes of hyperphosphatemia?
2. What are the clinical manifestations of hyperphosphatemia?
3. What are the treatments for hyperphosphatemia?

FURTHER READING

1. Belinaye, H. (2022). *Compendium of Lithotripsy.* Legare Street Press.
2. Bilezikian, J.P. (2018). *Primer on the Metabolic Bone Diseases and Disorders of Mineral Metabolism,* 9th Edition. Wiley-Blackwell.
3. Chew, F.S., Maldijian, C., and Mulcahy, H. (2016). *Broken Bones: The Radiologic Atlas of Fractures and Dislocations,* 2nd Edition. Cambridge University Press.
4. Coe, F.L., Worcester, E.M., Evan, A.P., and Lingeman, J.E. (2019). *Kidney Stones: Medical and Surgical Management,* 2nd Edition. Jaypee Brothers Medical Publishers Ltd.
5. Donovan Walker, M. (2022). *Hypercalcemia: Clinical Diagnosis and Management (Contemporary Endocrinology).* Humana Press/Springer.
6. Grayson, T. (2021). *Overcoming Osteomalacia: A Unique Guide to Understanding, Symptoms, Diagnosis, Treatment of Osteomalacia with Medical and Alternative Forms of Treatment.* Grayson.

7. Hewitt, J., and Gabata, M. (2011). *Nephrotic Syndrome.* CreateSpace Independent Publishing Platform.

8. Jackson, H. (2022). *What Is Hypocalcemia?* Jackson.

9. Kaneko, K. (2016). *Molecular Mechanisms in the Pathogenesis of Idiopathic Nephrotic Syndrome.* Springer.

10. Kearns, A.E. (2021). *Mayo Clinic on Osteoporosis: Keep Your Bones Strong and Reduce Your Risk of Fractures.* Mayo Clinic Press.

11. Long, L. (2017). *Updates and Advances in Nephrolithiasis: Pathophysiology, Genetics, and Treatment Modalities.* IntechOpen.

12. Munoz, R. (2022). *Renal Tubular Acidosis in Children: New Insights in Diagnosis and Treatment.* Springer.

13. Paloian, N.J., and Penniston, K.L. (2022). *Diagnosis and Management of Pediatric Nephrolithiasis.* Springer.

14. Roussouly, P., Pinheiro-Franco, J.L., Labelle, H., and Gehirchen, M. (2019). *Sagittal Balance of the Spine: From Normal to Pathology: A Key for Treatment Strategy.* Thieme.

15. Sayre, L.A. (2018). *Spinal Disease and Spinal Curvature: Their Treatment by Suspension and the Use of the Plaster of Paris Bandage.* Forgotten Books.

16. Schmutz, R., Birkhauser, F., and Zehnder, P. (2019). *Extracorporeal Shock Wave Lithotripsy in Clinical Practice.* Springer.

17. Slovik, D.M., and Underwood, A. (2019). *Osteoporosis: A Guide to Prevention and Treatment.* Harvard Health Publishing.

19 Iron Deficiency and Toxicity

OVERVIEW

Iron is essential for several metabolic pathways and delivers oxygen to organs and tissues. A deficiency can result in a wide range of nonspecific symptoms that may not be initially recognized due to iron deficiency. Iron deficiency is the most common cause of anemia worldwide, affecting approximately 20% of the world's population. Iron deficiency anemia produces microcytic and hypochromic red cells on the peripheral smear. It is usually due to blood loss, but malabsorption, such as celiac disease, is a much less common cause. The symptoms of iron deficiency are generally nonspecific. Iron deficiency, without anemia, is even more common. Patients may present with unexplained, nonspecific symptoms. Anemia is highly prevalent in indigenous communities. The goal of treatment is to replenish iron stores and improve symptoms. Management should initially involve dietary counseling and oral supplements. The management of iron deficiency requires identification and investigation. Oral iron is readily available, effective, safe, convenient, and cost-effective for uncomplicated iron deficiency. For those patients intolerant of oral iron or with conditions where oral iron is likely ineffective or harmful, the intravenous route is preferred. Iron poisoning is most common in children and is usually accidental and particularly dangerous. Iron tablets may adhere to the stomach and duodenum, causing irritation, hemorrhagic necrosis, and perforation in severe cases.

IRON-DEFICIENCY ANEMIA

Iron deficiency anemia develops when the body's iron stores drop too low to support average RBC production. Inadequate dietary iron, impaired iron absorption, bleeding, or loss of body iron in the stool may be the cause. Iron equilibrium in the body is usually regulated carefully to ensure that sufficient iron is absorbed to compensate for body losses of iron. Iron deficiency occurs in stages, which include the following:

- *Iron requirement exceeds intake*–this causes progressive depletion of bone marrow iron stores.
- *As stores decrease,* the absorption of dietary iron increases to compensate.
- *Later stages,* deficiency impairs red blood cell synthesis, and anemia results.

EPIDEMIOLOGY

Iron deficiency anemia is the most common nutritional deficiency globally. About 30% of the population is affected. The condition is more common in infants, children, and women. However, adult men are also susceptible based on their health conditions and socioeconomic status. In neonates, breastfeeding is protective against iron deficiency due to the higher bioavailability of iron in breast milk compared to cow's milk; iron-deficiency anemia is the most common form of anemia in young children on cow's milk. In developing countries, the iron-deficiency rate is higher than in the United States, where the prevalence of iron-deficiency anemia in men under 50 is 1%. For women of child-bearing age, the rate is 10%.

In comparison, 9% of children ages 12–36 months are iron-deficient, and one-third develop anemia. While the rate of iron-deficiency anemia is low in the United States, low-income families are particularly at risk. Iron deficiency anemia also has a high prevalence in hospitalized patients.

DOI: 10.1201/9781003453376-25

ETIOLOGY AND RISK FACTORS

Several causes of iron deficiency vary based on age, gender, and socioeconomic status. The primary cause of iron deficiency is blood loss (especially in older patients), insufficient iron intake, or decreased absorption. In males and postmenopausal women, the most common cause is chronic occult bleeding that is usually from the GI tract, such as due to malignancies, peptic ulcers, hemorrhoids, or **vascular ectasias**. In poorer countries, intestinal bleeding caused by **hookworm** infection is a common cause of iron-deficiency anemia. In premenopausal women, cumulative menstrual blood loss is a common cause, with a mean amount of 0.5 mg of iron lost daily. Less common causes include recurrent **hemoptysis** and **hematuria**.

Iron deficiency also occurs because of increased iron requirements. Dietary intake of iron is often insufficient from birth to 2 years of age and during adolescence. In pregnancy, the fetal iron requirement increases the iron requirements of the mother, even though menses are not occurring. Lactation increases the iron requirement even more. Causes of decreased iron absorption include **gastrectomy**, **atrophic gastritis**, **achlorhydria**, and short-bowel syndrome. Risk factors for iron deficiency anemia include women, infants, children, vegetarians, frequent blood donors, poor diet, celiac disease, Crohn's disease, cancer, kidney failure, certain medications, and older adults.

CLINICAL MANIFESTATIONS

Initially, iron deficiency anemia can be so mild that it goes unnoticed. However, the signs and symptoms can intensify as the body becomes more deficient in iron and anemia worsens. Most iron deficiency symptoms are related to anemia. They include extreme fatigue, loss of stamina, dyspnea, chest pain, tachycardia, headache, dizziness, pale skin, **brittle nails**, and weakness (see **Figure 19.1**). Restless legs syndrome is another common symptom, an urge to move the legs while remaining inactive.

DIAGNOSIS

Iron deficiency anemia is suspected if there is chronic blood loss. The red blood cells are typically **microcytic** and **hypochromic** (see **Figure 19.2**). A complete blood count, serum iron and iron-binding capacity, serum ferritin, transferrin saturation, and reticulocyte count must be obtained. Serum iron level and hemoglobin (Hb) are low for iron deficiency. The iron-binding capacity increases in iron deficiency, but the transferrin saturation decreases.

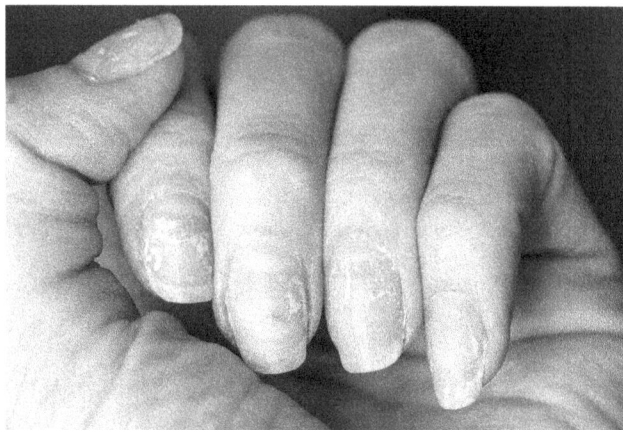

FIGURE 19.1   Brittle nails caused by iron deficiency anemia.

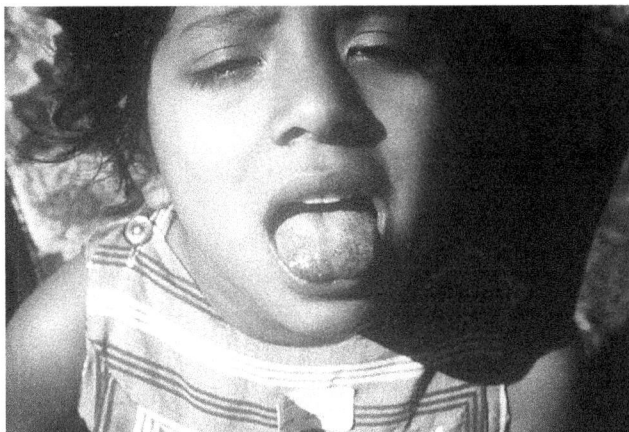

FIGURE 19.2   Microcytic and hypochromic red blood cells.

TABLE 19.1
Diagnostic Stages of Iron Deficiency Anemia

Stage	Description
1	Decreased bone marrow iron stores. Serum iron and Hb are normal, but serum ferritin levels fall to less than 30 ng/mL. A compensatory increase in iron absorption causes an increase in iron-binding capacity (the transferrin level).
2	Erythropoiesis is impaired (when serum iron falls to less than 50 mcg/dL) and transferrin saturation is less than 16%. Though the transferrin level is increased, the serum iron level decreases, as does transferrin saturation. The serum transferrin receptor level increases to more than 8.5 mg/L.
3	Anemia with normal red blood cells (RBCs) and indices develops.
4	Microcytosis develops, followed by hypochromia.
5	Iron deficiency begins to affect the tissues, becoming symptomatic.

Low serum ferritin levels are specific to iron deficiency. The reticulocyte count is low in iron deficiency, and a peripheral smear usually shows hypochromic red cells with significant **anisopoikilocytosis**. **Table 19.1** summarizes the diagnostic stages of iron-deficiency anemia.

The diagnosis of iron-deficiency anemia is based on its cause, and many patients require no further testing once this is determined. Men and postmenopausal women with no apparent blood loss should have their GI tract evaluated since anemia can be the only indication of an occult GI cancer. In rare cases, the patient underestimates any chronic epistaxis or genitourinary bleeding. If so, this requires evaluation even if the GI study results are expected.

TREATMENT

Oral iron can be provided via iron salts or saccharated iron 30 minutes before meals. Iron salts include ferrous sulfate, ferrous gluconate, and ferrous fumarate. The dosing schedule is because food or antacids can reduce iron absorption. A typical initial dose is 65 mg of elemental iron, such as 325 mg of ferrous sulfate, once per day or every other day. Larger doses are mostly unabsorbed because of increased hepcidin production. However, they have adverse effects such as constipation and other GI upsets. Ascorbic acid in pill form (500 mg) or orange juice enhances iron absorption without increasing gastric distress.

Parenteral iron provides a faster therapeutic response but can cause adverse effects. These are usually allergic reactions or infusion-related fevers, arthralgias, and myalgias. Parenteral iron is reserved for those who cannot tolerate oral iron, those for whom oral iron is ineffective, patients losing significant amounts of blood due to capillary or vascular disorders, and those with a need for fast iron repletion because of severe anemia, elective surgery, or pregnant women during the third trimester. Though the dose of parenteral iron is based on weight and current Hb levels, the initial amount of 1,000 mg is usually sufficient.

Oral iron therapy usually lasts six or more months after Hb levels have been corrected and tissue stores have been replenished. Iron studies are rechecked at least 4 weeks after treatment to ensure sufficient repletion. Serial Hb measurements assess responses until average RBC values are present. Anemia should be corrected within 2 months. If there is a subnormal response, this suggests ongoing hemorrhage, underlying infection, cancer, insufficient iron intake, or malabsorption of oral iron. If fatigue, weakness, and shortness of breath do not subside after the anemia is resolved, a different cause should be evaluated.

PREVENTION

The prevention of iron-deficiency anemia requires eating iron-rich foods. These include red meat, pork, poultry, beans, seafood, dark green leafy vegetables, dried fruit, iron-fortified breads, cereals, pastas, and peas. Meat is the best source of absorbable iron. Those who do not eat meat must increase their intake of iron-rich plant-based foods. Iron absorption is enhanced by consuming foods rich in vitamin C simultaneously. These include citrus juices, broccoli, grapefruit, kiwi, leafy greens, melons, oranges, peppers, strawberries, tangerines, and tomatoes. In infants, iron deficiency is prevented by the use of human breast milk or iron-fortified formula for the first year. Cow's milk is not a good source of iron. After 6 months, infants can start eating iron-fortified cereals or pureed meats at least twice daily. After 1 year, children should not drink more than 20 ounces of milk daily because it often replaces other foods richer in iron.

YOU SHOULD REMEMBER

To prevent iron deficiency anemia in infants, feed the baby breast milk or iron-fortified formula for the first year. Cow's milk is not a good source of iron for babies and is not recommended for infants under 1 year. After the age of 6 months, start feeding the baby iron-fortified cereals or pureed meats at least twice daily to boost iron intake. After 1 year, be sure children drink at most 20 ounces (about 600 mL) of milk daily. Too much milk often replaces other foods, including those rich in iron.

Check Your Knowledge

1. What are the causes of iron deficiency?
2. What are the clinical manifestations of iron deficiency?
3. What is the best way to prevent iron deficiency in young children?

PEDIATRIC IRON POISONING

Iron poisoning is one of the most common toxic ingestion and one of the deadliest among children. Failure to diagnose and treat iron poisoning can have severe consequences, including multi-organ loss and death. It is signified by acute gastroenteritis, then a quiet, nearly asymptomatic period, and finally shock and liver failure. Iron tablets may look like candy to children, and prenatal multivitamins are the source of iron in most fatal childhood iron ingestions.

Iron is toxic to the GI, the heart, the lungs, and the brain. Excess-free iron is a mitochondrial toxin that leads to derangements in energy metabolism. It interferes with oxidative phosphorylation, which causes metabolic acidosis. Additionally, iron catalyzes the formation of free radicals and acts as an oxidizer. If plasma protein binding is saturated, it combines with water, forming iron hydroxide and free hydrogen ions and worsening metabolic acidosis.

EPIDEMIOLOGY

In 2018, the American Association of Poison Control Centers reported 4,459 single exposures to iron and iron salts: 2,173 were in children aged five and younger, 156 were in patients aged 6–12, and 540 were in patients aged 13–19. If no symptoms develop within the first 6 hours after ingestion, the risk of severe toxicity is minimal. If shock and coma develop within the first 6 hours, the mortality rate is about 10%.

ETIOLOGY AND RISK FACTORS

The cause and risk factors for pediatric iron poisoning are based on the amount of elemental iron consumed. Ingestion of less than 20 mg/kg of iron is non-toxic. Ingestion of 20–60 mg/kg results in moderate symptoms. Ingestion of more than 60 mg/kg can result in severe toxicity and lead to severe morbidity and mortality. The amount of elemental iron ingested differs depending on the formulation of iron salts. The most common iron formulations are 325 mg ferrous sulfate tablets, which contain 65 mg of essential iron per tablet; 300 mg ferrous gluconate tablets, which include 36 mg of elemental iron per tablet; and 100 mg ferrous fumarate tablets, which contain 33 mg of essential iron per tablet. Prenatal vitamins may have 60–90 mg of elemental iron per tablet. Children's vitamins vary from 5 to 19 mg of elemental iron per tablet.

CLINICAL MANIFESTATIONS

Children may show signs of toxicity with ingestions of 10–20 mg/kg of elemental iron. Severe toxicity is likely with ingestions of more than 50 mg/kg. Symptoms of iron poisoning occur in five stages with various symptoms and progression, as follows:

- *Stage 1 (within 6 hours)*–vomiting, hematemesis, irritability, explosive diarrhea, abdominal pain, lethargy (if toxicity is severe), tachycardia, tachypnea, hypotension, metabolic acidosis, coma (NOTE: the severity of symptoms is usually based on the overall severity of the poisoning, with late-stage symptoms only developing if the symptoms of this stage are moderate or severe; if no symptoms develop within 6 hours, the risk of severe toxicity is slight, but if shock and coma develop within 6 hours, the mortality rate is approximately 10%)
- *Stage 2 (within 6–48 hours)*–up to 24 hours of apparent improvement, known as the latent period
- *Stage 3 (within 12–48 hours)*–shock, seizures, fever, coagulopathy, metabolic acidosis
- *Stage 4 (2–5 days)*–jaundice, coagulopathy, hypoglycemia, liver failure
- *Stage 5 (2–5 weeks)*–gastric outlet or duodenal obstruction that is secondary to scarring

DIAGNOSIS

The diagnosis of iron toxicity is based on the history and clinical presentation. Serum iron levels are used to determine a patient's potential for toxicity. A serum iron level measured at its peak, 4–6 hours after ingestion, is the most helpful laboratory test. Sustained-release or enteric-coated preparations may have erratic absorption, and therefore, a second level of 6–8 hours post-ingestion should be checked.

Peak serum iron levels below 350 mcg/dL are associated with minimal toxicity. Levels between 350 and 500 mcg/dL are associated with moderate toxicity. Levels above 500 mcg/dL are associated with severe systemic toxicity. Iron is rapidly cleared from the serum and deposited in the liver. Therefore, the iron level drawn after ingestion may be deceptively low if measured after its peak.

Other laboratory tests include electrolytes, kidney function, serum glucose, coagulation studies, a complete blood count, and liver function. Plain radiographs may reveal iron in the GI tract, but many iron preparations are not radiopaque. Normal radiographs do not exclude iron ingestion. X-rays may show the radiopaque iron tablets for 2–6 hours post-ingestion. One may see the iron tablets on the kidney, ureter, and bladder (KUB) film.

TREATMENT

Patients who remain asymptomatic 4–6 hours after ingestion or those who have not ingested a potentially toxic amount do not require any treatment for iron toxicity. Patients with GI symptoms that resolve quickly and have typical vital signs require supportive care and an observation period, as it may represent the second stage of iron toxicity. Patients who are symptomatic or demonstrate indications of hemodynamic instability require aggressive management and admission to an intensive care unit. The following is used for the treatment of iron toxicity:

1. Deferoxamine is a chelating agent that can remove iron from tissues and free iron from plasma.
2. An Intravenous crystalloid infusion is administered to correct hypovolemia and **hypoperfusion.**
3. Whole-bowel irrigation with a polyethylene glycol solution may clear the GI tract of iron pills before absorption.

Patients with iron bezoars may require surgery. In severe cases, hemodialysis can also be effective.

PREVENTION

The prevention of iron poisoning includes sufficient storage, containers, consultations with health professionals, and careful use of iron-containing supplements. Store all iron-containing supplements and multivitamins out of reach and sight of children. Replace child-resistance closures tightly after every use – they help slow children down should they try to open the containers. Consult health professionals before taking any iron-containing multivitamins or supplements. Never take more than one iron supplement before consulting with a physician.

YOU SHOULD REMEMBER

Approximately 10% of ingested iron is absorbed from the intestine and subsequently bound to transferrin. Normal serum iron levels range from 50 to 150 mcg/dL, and total iron-binding capacity (TIBC) ranges from 300 to 400 mcg/dL. When iron levels rise after significant ingestion, transferrin becomes saturated. Excess iron circulates in the blood as free iron, which is directly toxic to target organs.

Check Your Knowledge

1. Which organs of the body are more damaged by iron poisoning?
2. What are the clinical manifestations of iron poisoning?
3. What is the treatment for iron poisoning?

PLUMMER-VINSON SYNDROME

Plummer-Vinson syndrome (PVS) is defined by the classic triad of dysphagia, iron-deficiency anemia, and **esophageal webs**. Even though the syndrome is rare nowadays, its recognition is essential because it identifies a group of patients at increased risk of squamous cell carcinoma of the pharynx and the esophagus.

EPIDEMIOLOGY

Exact data about the incidence and prevalence of the syndrome are not available. PVS is common among Caucasians in Northern countries, particularly in middle-aged women. The syndrome has also been described in children and adolescents. The rapid fall in the prevalence of the syndrome correlates with the improvement of nutritional status and the disappearance of widespread iron deficiency in countries where the syndrome had been previously described, particularly in Africa, where both iron deficiency and malnutrition are common.

ETIOLOGY AND RISK FACTORS

The pathogenesis is unknown. The PVS's most important possible etiological factor is iron deficiency. This theory is primarily based on the finding that iron deficiency is a part of the classic triad of PVS, together with dysphagia and esophageal webs. Dysphagia can be improved by iron supplementation. Indeed, impaired esophageal motility has been described in PVS, which was corrected by iron treatment. It has been shown that iron deficiency can precede dysphagia. Other risk factors include malnutrition, genetic predisposition, or even autoimmune processes. The latter is based on the association between PVS and certain autoimmune disorders, such as celiac disease, thyroid disease, and rheumatoid arthritis. The other risk factors include severe menorrhagia, hematuria, hematomas, and GI bleeding.

CLINICAL MANIFESTATIONS

The main clinical features of PVS are dysphagia, upper esophageal webs, and iron-deficiency anemia. The dysphagia is usually painless and intermittent or progressive over years, limited to solids, and sometimes associated with weight loss. Symptoms resulting from anemia, such as weakness, pallor, fatigue, and tachycardia, may dominate the clinical picture. Furthermore, it is characterized by **glossitis**, **angular cheilitis**, and **koilonychia**. Spleen and thyroid enlargement may also be observed (see **Figures 19.3 and 19.4**).

PVS has been identified as a risk factor for developing squamous cell carcinoma of the upper gastrointestinal tract. The 3%–15% of the patients with PVS, primarily women between 15 and 50 years of age, have been reported to develop esophageal or pharyngeal cancer. A decreasing trend in the overall incidence of hypopharyngeal cancer in women was demonstrated, probably due to the diminished prevalence of PVS.

DIAGNOSIS

The diagnosis is based on the evidence of iron-deficiency anemia and one or more esophageal webs in a patient with postcricoid dysphagia. Barium swallow X-rays can detect esophageal webs, but videofluoroscopy is the best way to demonstrate this. Esophageal strictures are also detectable by upper GI endoscopy. They appear smooth, thin, and gray, with a central lumen. Esophageal webs typically occur in the proximal part of the esophagus and may be missed and accidentally ruptured unless the endoscope is introduced under direct visualization.

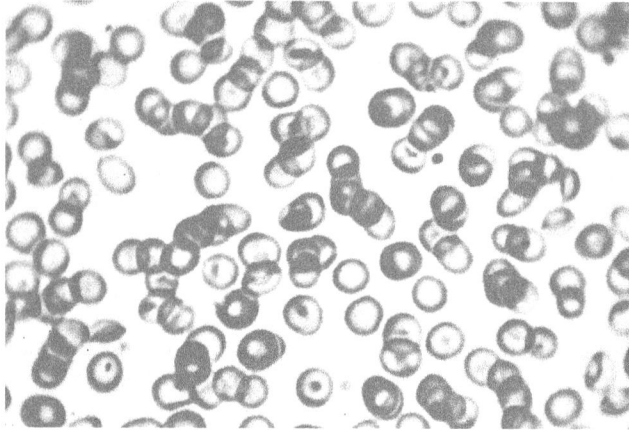

FIGURE 19.3   A patient with glossitis.

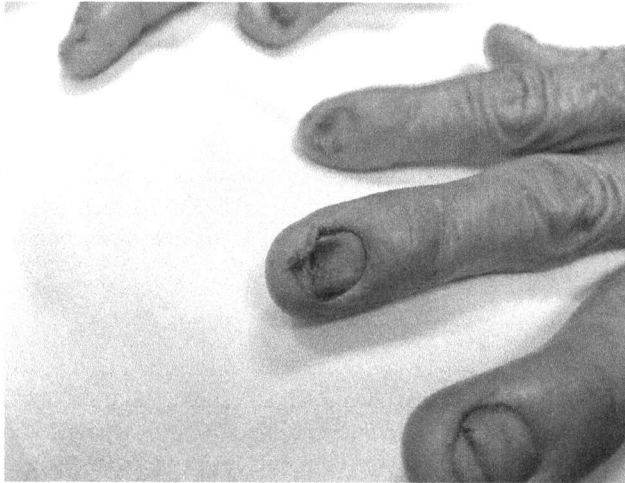

FIGURE 19.4   A patient with koilonychia.

The esophageal webs, which can also occur without anemia and PVS, are characterized by one or more thin membranes of squamous epithelium and submucosa. They usually protrude from the anterior wall, extending laterally but not to the posterior wall, meaning they rarely encircle the lumen. Laboratory examinations typically reveal iron-deficiency anemia with decreased Hb, hematocrit, mean **corpuscular** volume, serum iron and ferritin, and increased total **iron-binding capacity**.

TREATMENT

PVS can be treated effectively with iron supplementation and mechanical dilation. Iron supplementation alone can resolve dysphagia in many patients. However, rupture and dilation of the web should be performed in cases of significant obstruction of the esophageal lumen by the esophageal web and persistent dysphagia despite iron supplementation. Usually, only one dilation is enough to relieve dysphagia, but occasionally, multiple sessions are required. Also, successful balloon dilation has been described. Since PVS is associated with an increased risk of **squamous cell carcinoma** of the pharynx and the esophagus, patients should be followed closely. A surveillance upper GI endoscopy is recommended every year, even though the effectiveness of this recommendation has yet to be definitively confirmed.

PREVENTION

The best way to prevent PVS is to get enough iron in the diet and supplements. Evaluation for a source of blood loss or not absorbing it from their diet. This may include an upper endoscopy or a colonoscopy.

Check Your Knowledge

1. What is the classic triad of PVS?
2. What are the risk factors for PVS?
3. What are the main clinical features of PVS?

HEREDITARY HEMOCHROMATOSIS

Hemochromatosis is a metabolic disorder in which the organs accumulate excess iron, leading to organ damage (see **Figure 19.5**). It causes the body to absorb too much iron from food. Excess iron is stored in various organs, especially the liver, heart, pancreas, joints, and pituitary gland. There are a few types of hemochromatosis, but a gene change causes the most common type, which is passed down through families. Types 1, 2, and 3 hemochromatosis are inherited.

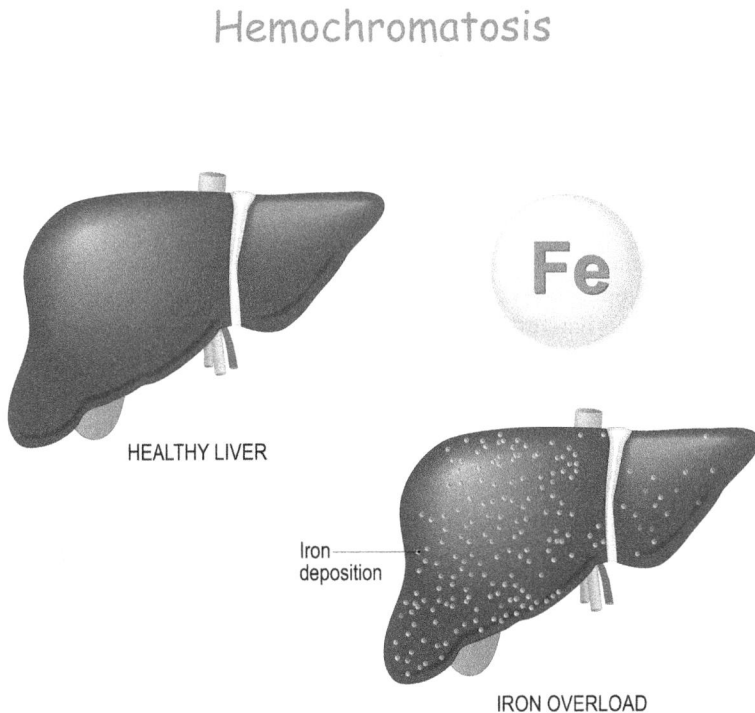

FIGURE 19.5 Hemochromatosis of the liver.

EPIDEMIOLOGY

Hereditary hemochromatosis is the most common autosomal recessive disorder in whites, with a prevalence of 1 in 300–500 children. In the United States, about 1 in 300 non-Hispanic white people has hereditary hemochromatosis, with lower rates among people of other races and ethnicities. Type 1 (classic form) of hemochromatosis is most common in Caucasians of Northern European descent. Most patients with hemochromatosis have an average life expectancy. Survival may be shortened for people who are not treated and develop cirrhosis or diabetes mellitus.

ETIOLOGY AND RISK FACTORS

Hemochromatosis can cause severe damage to the body, including the heart, liver, and pancreas. Juvenile hemochromatosis is a genetic condition inherited in an autosomal recessive manner. The risk factors are family history and genetic disorders. In secondary hemochromatosis, medical treatments or other medical conditions cause iron overload. Examples include blood transfusions, taking executive iron supplements, kidney dialysis, hepatitis C infection, or fatty liver disease. Other factors that increase the chances of developing hemochromatosis include alcohol abuse and a family history of arthritis, diabetes, erectile dysfunction, or heart attack.

CLINICAL MANIFESTATIONS

Some patients with hemochromatosis never have symptoms. Early symptoms often overlap with those of other common conditions. The signs and symptoms include fatigue, weakness, arthralgia, abdominal pain, diabetes, **impotence**, loss of sex drive, liver failure, bronze skin color, heart failure, and memory fog.

DIAGNOSIS

Many patients with hemochromatosis do not exhibit any symptoms. The disease is usually diagnosed due to family screening (genetic testing) or after a blood test indicates a high iron level or abnormal liver enzymes. Blood tests, including ferritin transferrin saturation, are the most critical initial tests. If there is concern for organ injury, an MRI and liver biopsy can also be performed.

TREATMENT

Early diagnosis and treatment of the disorder are important. Treatment may help prevent, delay, or sometimes reverse the complications of the disease. It may also lead to higher energy levels and a better quality of life. Patients have different responses to treatment. Some people who have frequent therapeutic **phlebotomy** may feel exhausted. People with advanced diseases or getting intense treatment that weakens them may need help with daily tasks and activities. At first, the patients may need to have therapeutic phlebotomy often. After the initial treatment period, they may require ongoing treatment two to six times a year. This will help prevent the iron from building up again. Iron chelation therapy removes extra iron from the body. The medication is taken by mouth at home or injected into the blood by a healthcare provider.

PREVENTION

To help maintain normal iron levels, the patients must avoid iron supplements and raw shellfish and restrict vitamin C, red meat, and alcohol intake. They must also screen the liver for possible hepatocellular carcinoma. If hemochromatosis has caused advanced cirrhosis, then an evaluation for liver transplantation may be necessary. A liver transplant cures hemochromatosis, and patient outcomes are excellent.

YOU SHOULD REMEMBER

A child who inherits two copies of a mutated gene (one from each parent) is highly likely to develop the disease. However, not all people with two mutated copies establish signs and symptoms of hemochromatosis. People who inherit only one copy of the mutated gene are carriers but usually have no or mild symptoms since one correct copy appears to regulate iron absorption adequately. "Silent" carriers, without signs of the disease, can still pass on the defect to their children.

Check Your Knowledge

1. What are the causes of hemochromatosis?
2. What are the symptoms of hemochromatosis?
3. What are the treatments for hemochromatosis?

Clinical Case Studies

CLINICAL CASE STUDY 1

A 17-year-old girl was evaluated because of persistent anemia, which caused her to be tired and weak. Her Hb, mean corpuscular volume and ferritin levels were below average. She reported having regular menstrual periods. The patient received a blood transfusion and was given iron supplements, which increased her Hb level to normal. She remained on iron supplementation for 1 year. After it was stopped, her Hb again dropped to lower than average. An endoscopy revealed the cause of her condition, which was a hemangioma in the small intestine. It was resected, and the patient's condition normalized permanently.

CRITICAL THINKING QUESTIONS

1. How does iron-deficiency anemia develop?
2. What are the three stages of iron-deficiency anemia?
3. What are the most common symptoms of iron deficiency?

CLINICAL CASE STUDY 2

A 15-month-old baby boy was brought to the emergency department after he had ingested a significant amount of elemental iron contained in his mother's iron supplements. He showed signs of hypotension, recurrent vomiting, metabolic acidosis, and excessive irritability. His serum iron levels were very high but insufficient for an exchange transfusion. The baby was given oxygen, fluid therapy, IV antiemetics, and antacids. He was then transferred to the pediatric ICU, where a whole bowel irrigation was performed. The baby started passing clear stools within 3 hours. He was then given IV deferoxamine and began to return to normal.

1. What causes pediatric iron poisoning?
2. How is pediatric iron poisoning diagnosed?
3. What are the steps required for the treatment of pediatric iron poisoning?

CLINICAL CASE STUDY 3

A 78-year-old woman was hospitalized because of dysphagia, vomiting, shortness of breath, and chronic weight loss. The patient also had conjunctival pallor, koilonychia, angular cheilitis, and signs of microcytic hypochromic anemia with iron deficiency. Via endoscopy and esophagography, a web was detected that prevented the passage of the endoscope into the upper esophagus. Oral iron therapy was given daily for 2 weeks, and the patient's symptoms improved.

CRITICAL THINKING QUESTIONS

1. What signs and symptoms define Plummer-Vinson syndrome?
2. What may the anemia of Plummer-Vinson syndrome cause?
3. Which type of cancer is related to Plummer-Vinson syndrome?

FURTHER READING

1. Agarwal, N., Gupta, M., and Agarwal, A. (2021). *Iron Deficiency Anemia in Pregnancy.* Lap Lambert Academic Publishing.
2. Bouhdjila, A. (2023). *Iron Deficiency in Children Under Five Years Old: Prevalence, Risk Factors and Prevention Methods.* Our Knowledge Publishing.
3. Dincer, Y. (2013). *Iron Deficiency and Its Complications (Nutrition and Diet Research Progress).* Nova Science Publishers, Inc.
4. Elliott, P. (2023). *The Complete Heavy Metal Healthy Detox Guide: Detoxify, Removing Poisoning Chemicals and Toxins to Improve and Promote Our Wellness.* Elliott.
5. Food and Nutrition Board. (2023). *Iron Deficiency Anemia.* Legard Street Press.
6. Garrison, C. (2011). *The Iron Disorders Institute Guide to Hemochromatosis: Symptoms, Relief, and Support for Sufferers,* 2nd Edition. Cumberland House.
7. Gunther, K. (2023). *Diet for Iron Deficiency.* Springer.
8. Ishmael, D. (2022). *Countering Hemochromatosis: Ultimate Guide: Step-by-Step Guide on Healing Strategies, Remedies, Natural Remedies, Treatments & More.* Ishmael.
9. Lazarus, H.M., and Schmaier, A.H. (2019). *Concise Guide to Hematology.* Springer.
10. McCalvert, J. (2022). *Hemochromatosis: A Comprehensive Strategy for the Management of Hemochromatosis.* McCalvert.
11. Meselson, A. (2013). *The Complete Guide on Anemia: Learn Symptoms, Causes, and Treatments.* Meselson.
12. Miller, E.M. (2023). *Thicker Than Water: A Social and Evolutionary Study of Iron Deficiency in Women.* Oxford University Press.
13. Nabil-Savari, M., and Jabali, A. (2023). *Theranostic Iron-Oxide Based Nanoplatforms in Oncology: Synthesis, Metabolism, and Toxicity for Simultaneous Imaging and Therapy (Nanomedicine and Nanotoxicology).* Springer.
14. Sharp, M. (2022). *Iron Deficiency Anemia.* American Medical Publishers.
15. Shatzel, J. (2021). *Iron Deficiency: A Patient's Guide to the Most Common Nutrient Deficiency in the World.* Shatzel.
16. Silva, R. (2012). *Quick & Easy Diet Cures 4 Iron Deficiency Anemia.* CreateSpace Independent Publishing Platform.
17. Yehuda, S., and Mostofsky, D.I. (2011). *Iron Deficiency and Overload: From Basic Biology to Clinical Medicine (Nutrition and Health).* Humana Press.

20 Iodine Deficiency

OVERVIEW

Iodine is an essential trace element in the thyroid hormones thyroxine and triiodothyronine. Its deficiency occurs most frequently in areas with little iodine in the diet – typically, these are remote inland areas where no marine foods are eaten.

The thyroid hormone is vital for the growth of bones and nerves and for knowing how proteins, fats, and carbohydrates are used in the body. Iodine is critical before birth and in babies and young children. It is crucial during pregnancy and can help prevent certain health conditions later in life. The thyroid takes up iodine in small amounts to make thyroid hormones. Without iodine, thyroid hormone production can decrease. A low thyroid hormone can lead to hypothyroidism. Iodine-deficiency (ID) disorders describe the conditions known as endemic goiter. They occur from insufficient iodine in the diet. Simple, nontoxic goiter is a noncancerous thyroid gland enlargement that does not involve over- or underproduction of thyroid hormones. Noncancerous thyroid enlargement can occur because of a lack of iodine in the diet or ingesting certain substances or medications. Patients often have no symptoms.

IODINE DEFICIENCY AND GOITER

ID is considered a significant public health problem worldwide, affecting all groups of people. Children and lactating women are the most vulnerable categories. At a global scale, approximately 2 billion people are suffering from ID, and about 50 million present with clinical manifestations. Iodine is primarily involved in synthesizing the thyroid hormones T4 and T3 – approximately 80% of iodide is absorbed by the thyroid gland in an adult. Pregnant and lactating women need more iodine. ID is uncommon in areas where iodized salt is used, yet it is relatively common worldwide.

With mild to moderate ID, the thyroid gland is influenced by **thyroid-stimulating hormone** (TSH). The gland hypertrophies to concentrate iodide inside of itself, causing a colloid goiter. While most patients remain **euthyroid**, a severe ID in an adult can cause **hypothyroidism**. This condition can decrease fertility or increase risks for stillbirth, spontaneous abortion, and prenatal and infant mortality. Severe maternal ID can harm the fetus, causing congenital **cretinism**, low birth weight, impaired mental function, neurological disorders, poor physical development, problems walking, a short stature, and death (see **Figure 20.1**). Cretinism is a restriction of brain development and growth, characterized by severe intellectual disability, hearing problems, loss of speech abilities, muscle spasticity, and short stature.

ID disorders can start before birth, jeopardizing children's mental health and often their very survival. During the neonatal period, childhood, and adolescence, ID diseases can lead to hypothyroidism. Severe ID during pregnancy can result in **stillbirth**, spontaneous abortion, and congenital abnormalities such as cretinism – a grave disease, an irreversible form of intellectual disability that affects people living in ID areas of Africa and Asia. The less visible yet pervasive cognitive impairment that reduces intellectual capacity at home, school, and work is of even greater significance.

SIMPLE NONTOXIC GOITER

A goiter may be an overall enlargement of the thyroid or result from irregular cell growth that forms one or more nodules in the thyroid. A goiter may be associated with no change in thyroid function or an increase or decrease in thyroid hormones. **Simple, nontoxic goiter** is benign thyroid hypertrophy

DOI: 10.1201/9781003453376-26

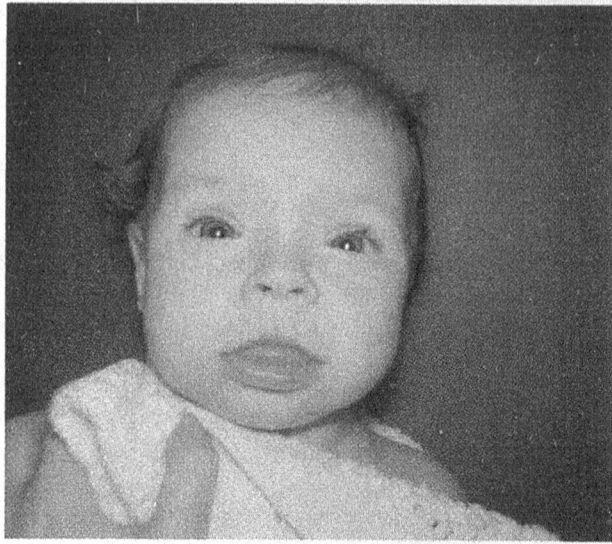

FIGURE 20.1 Cretinism.

that may be diffuse or nodular thyroid hypertrophy. There is no **hyperthyroidism**, hypothyroidism, or inflammation. Except in cases of severe ID, thyroid function is normal. The patient is asymptomatic, except for an apparent nontender enlargement of the thyroid. Simple, nontoxic goiter is the most common type of thyroid enlargement. It is most often seen at puberty, in pregnancy, or at menopause, but the cause is not usually straightforward. The understood causes include defects in intrinsic thyroid hormone production, ingestion of foods that inhibit thyroid hormone synthesis (goitrogens such as broccoli, cabbage, cassava, and cauliflower, often in countries with ID), and drugs that decrease thyroid hormone synthesis (compounds that contain iodine such as amiodarone, or medications such as lithium).

ENDEMIC GOITER

Endemic goiter is an adaptive disease produced by the persistent stimulation of the thyroid gland due to increased TSH secretion due to ID. Small compensatory elevations in TSH prevent hypothyroidism, but the TSH stimulation causes a goiter to form. Patients may have a history of low iodine intake or over-ingestion of **goitrogens**. The goiter is usually soft, smooth, and symmetric (see **Figure 20.2**). Over time, multiple nodules and cysts can develop.

Epidemiology

Endemic goiter occurs when the prevalence of thyroid enlargement in the population of an area exceeds 10%. The overall prevalence rate of endemic goiter was 50.1%; the prevalence was higher among women (55.1%) than men (47.2%). Prevalence increased with an increase in age. The incidence of goiter is approximately 1,400–1,700 per 100,000 individuals in women and 900 per 100,000 individuals in men worldwide. The prevalence of goiter is about 3,000 per 100,000 individuals worldwide for single thyroid nodules. The frequency of goiter increases in women over 45 years of age. The rate of occurrence of goiter in women is higher than in men by a ratio of 4:1. There is no racial predilection to goiter. Goiter occurs in Asia, the Middle East, Africa, and Europe (see **Figure 20.3**).

Etiology and Risk Factors

The leading cause of endemic goiter is ID, and thyroid growth is presumed to be regulated by TSH. In the United States, where iodized salt is common, goiters are caused by conditions that

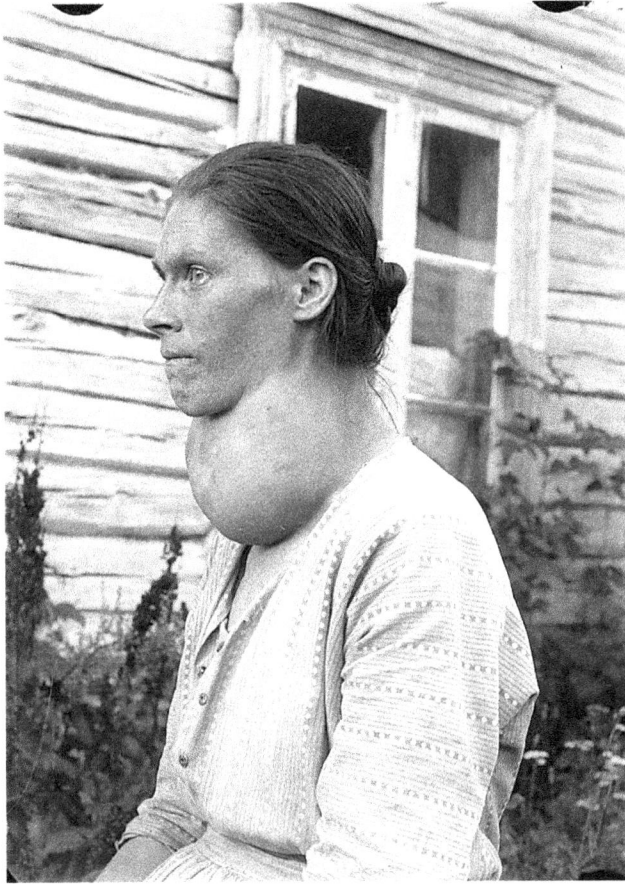

FIGURE 20.2 Endemic goiter.

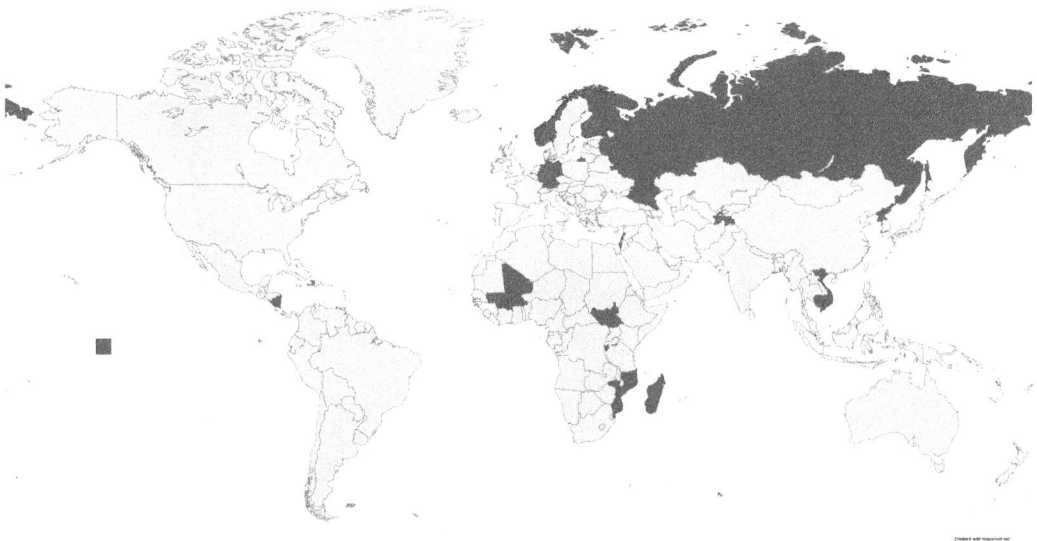

FIGURE 20.3 Global ID.

change thyroid function or factors that affect thyroid growth. Some common risk factors for goiters include a lack of dietary iodine, being female, age, pregnancy, menopause, medications, and radiation exposure.

Clinical Manifestations

Most people with goiters have no signs or symptoms other than swelling at the base of the neck. The goiter is often small enough to be discovered during a routine medical examination or an imaging test for another condition. Symptoms of endemic goiter include enlargement of thyroid glands, a visible goiter, choking, trouble breathing, difficulty swallowing, weight gain, fatigue, thinning hair, dry skin, sensitivity to colds, constipation, **bradycardia**, learning problems, and memory difficulties.

Diagnosis

With endemic goiter, serum TSH may be only elevated slightly, while serum T4 may be low, normal, or somewhat low. The serum T3 is usually normal or slightly higher than usual. Thyroid ultrasonography is performed to determine whether any nodules could suggest cancer. The diagnosis of ID for people of all ages is usually based on thyroid function tests, examination for a goiter, and imaging tests that identify abnormal thyroid function and structure. Every neonate must be screened for hypothyroidism by measuring TSH levels.

Treatment

Treatment depends on the cause of the goiter, symptoms, and complications resulting from the goiter. Small goiters that are not noticeable and do not cause problems usually do not need treatment. Sometimes, suppressing the hypothalamic-pituitary axis with thyroid hormone will block TSH production, stimulating the thyroid. Moderate doses of levothyroxine can be helpful in younger patients to reduce serum TSH to the low-normal range. Based on serum TSH, the average amounts are 100–150 mcg orally, once per day. Levothyroxine should not be used in older patients with non-toxic nodular goiter since this type of goiter usually does not shrink and may have autonomic areas that can result in hyperthyroidism. Large goiters sometimes require surgery or iodine-131 to shrink the thyroid enough to avoid any problems with respiration, swallowing in the neck, or to correct cosmetic abnormalities.

Prevention

Prevention of endemic goiter depends mainly on increasing the iodine intake of people in endemic areas. When iodine intake reaches the estimated adult minimum requirement (100–150 mcg/day), the prevalence of goiter decreases.

YOU SHOULD REMEMBER

Brain development is a complex process that begins in early pregnancy and lasts for the first years of the newborn's life. This is the reason why the most severe consequences of ID are neurological. Thyroid hormones are essential for normal neurological development, myelination, cell differentiation and migration, growth, metabolism, sexual development, and body temperature regulation.

Check Your Knowledge

1. What are the signs and symptoms of endemic goiter?
2. What are the causes of endemic goiter?
3. What are the treatments for endemic goiter?

HYPOTHYROIDISM

Hypothyroidism can occur at any age. However, it may appear more in older adults because it is subtle and complex. It may be primary or secondary. When thyroid hormone levels become extremely low in adults, it is called **myxedema** (see **Figure 20.4**). Primary hypothyroidism results from thyroid disorders, while secondary hypothyroidism is caused by hypothalamus or pituitary gland disease. Primary hypothyroidism occurs from decreased T4 and T3 secretion from the thyroid gland. The serum T4 and T3 levels are low while TSH is increased. It is usually of autoimmune cause and primarily results from Hashimoto thyroiditis. The condition is often related to a firm goiter or, later on, to a shrunken fibrotic thyroid with little or no function. The next most common cause is post-therapeutic hypothyroidism or **iatrogenic** hypothyroidism – usually after radioactive iodine therapy or surgical removal of the thyroid. Hypothyroidism that occurs due to overtreatment with propylthiouracil, methimazole, and iodide will resolve once treatment is stopped.

Epidemiology

Hypothyroidism affects up to 5% of the general population, with a further estimated 5% being undiagnosed. Over 99% of affected patients suffer from primary hypothyroidism.

The prevalence of primary is between 1% and 2%, and it is more common in older women and 10 times more common in women than in men. The frequency of hypothyroidism increases with age.

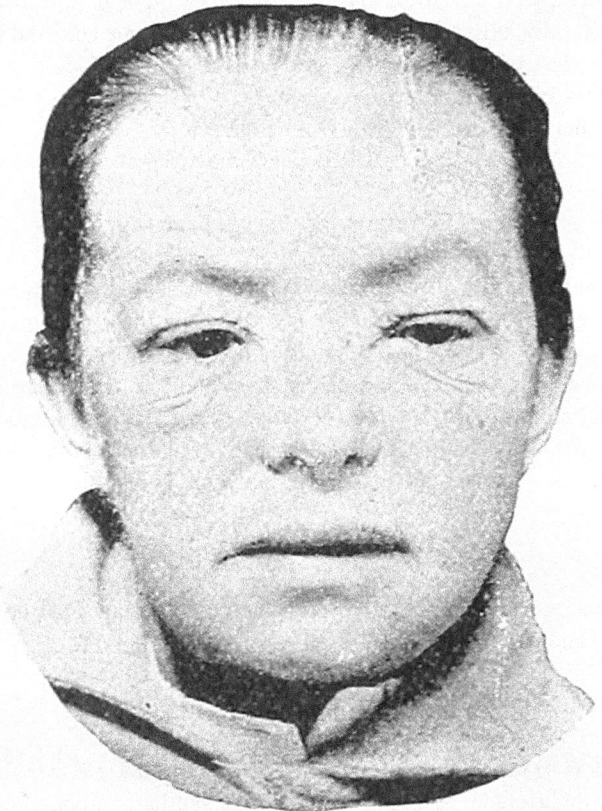

FIGURE 20.4   Myxedema.

ETIOLOGY AND RISK FACTORS

The most common cause of hypothyroidism is an autoimmune disorder. This means the immune system starts to attack itself, making antibodies against the thyroid gland. Another cause may be treatment for an overactive thyroid gland, which may include radioactive iodine therapy or surgery. The risk factors include gender, age, thyroid surgery, family history, genetics, type 1 diabetes, rheumatoid arthritis, and an ID.

CLINICAL MANIFESTATIONS

Hypothyroidism is one of the most common endocrine disorders, with clinical symptoms ranging from mild, such as fatigue, weight gain, cold intolerance, coarse hair, skin, puffy face, thinning hair, memory problems, and depression, to more severe manifestations that may include myxedema and death. Though signs and symptoms of primary hypothyroidism are often slight, the most common images are fluid retention and puffiness of the eyes, cold intolerance, tiredness, and mental fogginess. There are a variety of organ system manifestations, which include the following:

- *Metabolic* – slight weight gain due to fluid retention and decreased metabolism, hypothermia
- *Neurologic* – forgetfulness, hand and foot paresthesias. And it slowed the relaxation phase of the deep tendon reflexes
- *Psychiatric* – depression, personality changes, a dull facial expression, dementia, or frank psychosis known as **myxedema madness**
- *Dermatologic* – hair that is thin, coarse, and dry, skin that is dry, scaly, and thick. Carotenemia (mainly on the palms and soles due to carotene deposits) and **macroglossia**
- *Ocular* – periorbital swelling from infiltration with hyaluronic acid and chondroitin sulfate and drooping of the eyelids due to decreased adrenergic drive
- *Gastrointestinal* – constipation
- *Gynecologic* – menorrhagia or secondary amenorrhea
- *Cardiovascular* – bradycardia, enlarged heart mostly due to pericardial effusion, and rarely, hemodynamic distress
- *Other* – pleural or abdominal effusions, hoarse voice, and slow speech

In older patients, symptoms can differ widely. While secondary hypothyroidism is uncommon, it often affects other endocrine organs that are controlled by the hypothalamic-pituitary axis. In women who have hypothyroidism, signs of secondary hypothyroidism include a history of **amenorrhea** instead of **menorrhagia** and some suggestive physical differences. Secondary hypothyroidism involves the skin and hair being dry but not very coarse, skin depigmentation, macroglossia, atrophic breasts, and hypotension. The heart is smaller than usual, and serous pericardial effusions are not seen. Hypoglycemia is expected due to concomitant adrenal insufficiency or a deficiency of GH.

DIAGNOSIS

Hypothyroidism is diagnosed biochemically, with increased serum TSH concentrations and low triiodothyronine (T3) and thyroxine (T4).

TREATMENT

The goal of treatment is to return the thyroid hormone level to normal. Thyroid hormone preparations can be used for replacement therapy. These include synthetic preparations of T4 (levothyroxine), T3 (liothyronine), combinations, and desiccated animal thyroid extract. The preferred agent is levothyroxine. Maintenance doses are usually 75–150 mcg orally, once per day. This is based on the patient's age, body mass index, and absorption potential. In young or middle-aged patients who are otherwise healthy, the starting dose can be 100 or 1.7 mcg per kg orally, once daily. For patients with heart disease, therapy is started in low doses of 25 mcg once daily. This is adjusted every 6 weeks until a maintenance dose is achieved. This dose may need to be increased for women who are pregnant. It may also need to be increased if drugs that decrease absorption of T4 or that increase its metabolic clearance are also given. The chosen dose should be the lowest, restoring serum TSH to the mid-normal range, but this is not for patients with secondary hypothyroidism. Therefore, the levothyroxine dose in secondary hypothyroidism should achieve a free T4 level in the mid-normal range.

Liothyronine is not used alone for long-term replacement because it has a short half-life and causes prominent peaks in serum T3 levels. Administration of standard replacement amounts quickly increases serum T3 to 300 and 1,000 ng/dL within 4 hours because of its nearly complete absorption. These levels normalize over 24 hours. Also, patients receiving liothyronine are chemically hyperthyroid for several hours (or more) per day. This can increase cardiac risks. When mixtures of T3 and T4 are taken orally, similar serum T3 changes occur, though peak T3 is lower since less T3 is given. Replacement regimens using synthetic T4 show a different serum T3 response. The increases occur slowly, with normal levels being maintained when sufficient doses of T4 are given. Desiccated animal thyroid preparations have varying amounts of T3 and T4. They are only prescribed if the patient takes them and has normal serum TSH. For secondary hypothyroidism, levothyroxine is not given unless there are signs of sufficient cortisol secretion or cortisol therapy is given since levothyroxine could result in an adrenal crisis.

PREVENTION

Hypothyroidism can be prevented from becoming a severe health issue by recognizing the risk factors, understanding the symptoms, and diagnosing them early. The patient can prevent severe complications by starting treatment early. The best way to avoid it is screening. Women aged above 45 should get their thyroid or thyroid hormone levels checked regularly. To avoid developing a severe form of the condition or having the symptoms profoundly impact life, one must watch for signs of hypothyroidism. If you experience any of the symptoms of hypothyroidism, the best thing is to see a healthcare provider.

YOU SHOULD REMEMBER

Infants with hypothyroidism may develop symptoms such as feeding problems, poor growth, poor weight gain, jaundice, dry skin, enlarged tongue, constipation, and umbilical hernia. When hypothyroidism in infants is not treated, even mild cases can lead to severe physical and mental development problems.

Check Your Knowledge

1. What are the signs and symptoms of hypothyroidism?
2. How can it diagnose hypothyroidism?
3. What are the treatments for hypothyroidism?

Clinical Case Studies

CLINICAL CASE STUDY 20.1

A 51-year-old African man presented with a large cervical mass that caused him pain and dyspnea with exertion. Physical examination of the goiter resulted in a diagnosis of a vast, nontoxic, multinodular endemic goiter. A total thyroidectomy was performed. The patient recovered well from the surgery and was given 100 mcg/day of levothyroxine replacement therapy. The patient required no additional treatment.

CRITICAL THINKING QUESTIONS

1. What is an endemic goiter produced by?
2. What is the leading cause of endemic goiter?
3. What does the prevention of endemic goiter require?

CLINICAL CASE STUDY 20.2

A 35-year-old woman who complained of cold intolerance, constipation, and tiredness was diagnosed with ID. Because of familial hypertension, she always avoided salt in her diet and also rarely ate fish or consumed dairy products. The patient had no family history of thyroid disease. She was advised to change her diet to include iodized salt and foods rich in sodium but not excessively. Over 2 months, she improved significantly, with some symptoms lessening.

CRITICAL THINKING QUESTIONS

1. In which global areas do people have a higher risk of ID?
2. If a severe ID causes hypothyroidism, what are the possible outcomes?
3. What methods reverse ID in areas where it is prevalent?

CLINICAL CASE STUDY 20.3

A 27-year-old woman with a previous history of fibromyalgia presented to her physician for a regular checkup. She reported that her mother had just been diagnosed with hypothyroidism and asked for thyroid function tests to be included in her blood work. She had experienced some hair loss over the past 3 months. The test results returned, and her TSH was high, but free T4 was low. A diagnosis of hypothyroidism was confirmed.

CRITICAL THINKING QUESTIONS

1. What are the causes of primary and secondary hypothyroidism?
2. What are the most common signs and symptoms of primary hypothyroidism?
3. What are the signs and symptoms of secondary hypothyroidism in women?

FURTHER READING

1. Agrawal, N.K. (2020). *Goiter: Causes and Treatment*. IntechOpen.
2. Bianco, A.C. (2022). *Rethinking Hypothyroidism: Why Treatment Must Change and What Patients Can Do*. University of Chicago Press.
3. Bonofiglio, D., and Catalano, S. (2020). *Effects of Iodine Intake on Human Health*. Nutrients/MDPI.
4. Brandi, M.L., and Meigs Brown, E. (2015). *Hypoparathyroidism*. Springer.
5. Brito Pateguana, N., and Fung, J. (2020). *The PCOS Plan: Prevent and Reverse Polycystic Ovary Syndrome through Diet and Fasting*. Greystone Books.
6. Burnette, M. (2022). *The Importance of Iodine: Where Iodine Deficiency Is Spread and How People Cope with the Issue*. Burnette.
7. Christianson, A. (2021). *The Thyroid Reset Diet: Reverse Hypothyroidism and Hashimoto's Symptoms with a Proven Iodine-Balancing Plan*. Rodale Books.
8. Cicciarello Andrews, L. (2021). *The Complete Thyroid Cookbook: Easy Recipes and Meal Plans for Hypothyroidism and Hashimoto's Relief*. Rockridge Press.
9. Cohen, L.E. (2016). *Growth Hormone Deficiency: Physiology and Clinical Management*. Springer.
10. Cusano, N.E. (2020). *Hypoparathyroidism: A Clinical Casebook*. Springer.

11. Draznin, B. (2016). *Managing Diabetes and Hyperglycemia in the Hospital Setting: A Clinician's Guide.* American Diabetes Association.
12. Gasparri, G., Camandona, M., and Palestini, N. (2015). *Primary, Secondary, and Tertiary Hyperparathyroidism: Diagnostic and Therapeutic Updates.* Springer.
13. Kellman, R. (2021). *Microbiome Thyroid: Restore Your Gut and Discover the Root Cause of Hidden Thyroid Disease.* Hachette Go.
14. Pappala, A. (2015). *Goiter: Iodine Deficiency Disorder.* Pappala.
15. Pearce, E.N. (2017). *Iodine Deficiency Disorders and Their Elimination.* Springer.
16. Robinson, P. (2018). *The Thyroid Patient's Manual: From Hypothyroidism to Good Health (Recovering from Hypothyroidism).* Elephant in the Room Books.
17. Sussan, B.E. (2020). *Common Iodine Deficiency Symptoms Include Goiter, Bradycardia, Fatigue, Cognitive Problems, Weight Gain, Thin Hair, Dry Skin, Infancy Problems, and Increased Sensitivity to Colds.* Sussan.

21 Copper Deficiency and Toxicity

OVERVIEW

Copper is a crucial micronutrient humans need for proper organ function and metabolic processes such as hemoglobin synthesis, as a neurotransmitter, for iron oxidation, cellular respiration, antioxidant defense peptide amidation, and in the formation of pigments and connective tissue. Multiple hereditary or acquired factors have contributed to the increased clinical copper deficiency over the past decades. Fortunately, severe copper deficiency is relatively rare. It has occurred in premature infants being given milk-based formulas, during recovery from infantile malnutrition, and in those receiving long-term total parenteral nutrition without copper being added. The accumulation of copper in the body may be caused by Wilson disease or chronic copper poisoning. Wilson disease is a genetic disorder that prevents the body from removing extra copper, causing copper to build up in the liver, brain, eyes, and other organs. Without treatment, high copper levels can cause life-threatening organ damage.

COPPER DEFICIENCY

Copper deficiency is rare among healthy people and occurs most commonly among infants with other health problems or inherited genetic abnormalities.

EPIDEMIOLOGY

The classical deficiency diseases have nearly disappeared from the industrialized world and are thought to be found mainly in sub-Saharan Africa and South Asia. More than 80 collected medical articles, mostly from Europe and North America, describe more than 9,000 people with low concentrations of copper in organs or tissues or impaired metabolic pathways dependent on copper. More than a dozen articles reveal improved anatomy, chemistry, or physiology in more than 1,000 patients from copper supplements. The incidence is about 1 in 100,000 to 250,000 live births.

ETIOLOGY AND RISK FACTORS

Because the body mainly absorbs copper in the stomach and the small intestine, problems with either organ often affect a person's ability to absorb copper. Zinc supplementation is also a common cause of copper deficiency. This is because zinc and copper compete for absorption in the stomach, with zinc being the usual winner. As a result, copper isn't absorbed. Many times, copper deficiency is the result of stomach surgery that can affect absorption.

CLINICAL MANIFESTATIONS

Signs and symptoms of copper deficiency include fatigue and weakness due to anemia and depigmentation of hair and skin. Sometimes, there is an increased risk of infection due to decreased white blood cells. Sometimes, osteoporosis develops, or nerves are damaged. Nerve damage can cause tingling and loss of sensation in the feet and hands. Muscles may feel weak. Some people become confused, irritable, mildly depressed, and have impaired coordination.

 DOI: 10.1201/9781003453376-27

DIAGNOSIS

Copper deficiency is usually diagnosed based on symptoms and blood tests that detect low levels of copper and ceruloplasmin. Early diagnosis and treatment of copper deficiency result in a better outcome.

TREATMENT

The treatment of copper deficiency consists of parenteral and oral copper replacement until normal copper levels in the blood are achieved. Copper deficiency anemia is treated with oral or intravenous copper replacement through copper gluconate, copper sulfate, or copper chloride. Hematological manifestations are fully reversible with copper supplementation over a 4—to 12-week period.

PREVENTION

Because the body uses copper frequently and cannot store it in sufficient amounts, the best way to prevent a copper deficiency is to eat foods high in copper, like liver, nuts and seeds, wild-caught fish, beans, certain whole grains, and certain vegetables.

MENKES DISEASE

Menkes disease, also known as Menkes syndrome, is usually inherited, which means it runs in families. The gene is on the X chromosome, so if a mother carries the defective gene, her sons have a 50% (1 in 2) chance of developing the disease, and 50% of her daughters will be carriers of the disease.

EPIDEMIOLOGY

The prevalence at birth is estimated at 1/300,000 and 1/360,000 in Europe and Japan, respectively. In Australia, the birth prevalence is much higher (1/50,000–100,000), likely due to a founder effect. The disorder is X-linked and thus primarily affects males. It is believed to occur in about 1 in 35,000 live male births.

ETIOLOGY AND RISK FACTORS

A mutation of the ATP7A gene causes Menkes disease. This ATP7A gene affects how the body transports copper and maintains copper levels. Menke's disease usually causes low copper levels in blood plasma, the liver, and the brain. The condition also reduces the activity of copper-dependent enzymes in the body.

CLINICAL MANIFESTATIONS

Infants may be born prematurely but appear healthy for 6–8 weeks at birth. Then, symptoms begin. Signs and symptoms of copper deficiency include floppy muscle tone, hypotonia, **pectus excavatum**, seizures, slow physical development, an unstable body temperature, a fair complexion, chubby cheeks, a depressed nasal bridge, and bilaterally large ears. Scalp hairs are sparse, brittle, stubby, and hypopigmented with a steel wire-like feel (see **Figure 21.1**). There is often extensive neurodegeneration in the brain's gray matter—delays in recognition of mother, head control, social smile, or roll-over response. Arteries in the brain may be twisted with frayed and split inner walls. This can lead to rupture or blockage of the arteries.

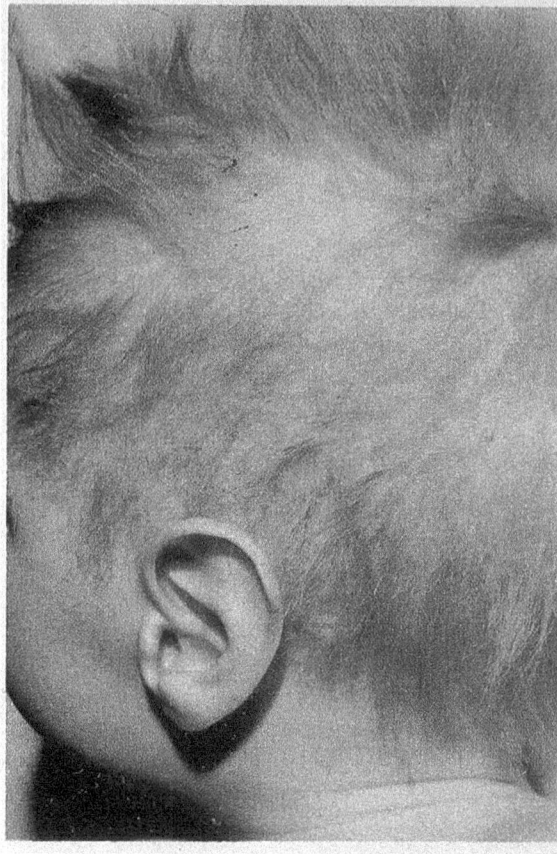

FIGURE 21.1   The characteristics of Menkes disease (wiry and sparse hair, fair complexion, chubby cheeks, irritability).

DIAGNOSIS

The first step in diagnosing Menkes disease includes a physical exam. This can identify some critical signs of Menkes disease, such as thin, kinky hair or poor growth. Blood or genetic tests can confirm the condition and make an accurate diagnosis. For newborns, a diagnostic test known as plasma catecholamine analysis can measure certain natural neurochemicals and help identify the disorder. Genetic testing may also show the ATP7A mutation that causes Menkes disease.

TREATMENT

Because it is a complex, rare disease that affects nearly all areas of the body, treatment of Menkes disease comes with significant challenges. This includes diagnosing Menkes disease and starting treatment as soon as possible, within 28 days of birth. Also, because copper is vital to a developing nervous system, any treatment for Menkes disease must be able to cross the blood-brain barrier. Treatment with daily copper injections may improve the outcome of Menkes disease if it begins within days after birth. Other therapies are symptomatic and supportive. Since newborn screening for this disorder is not available and early detection is infrequent because the clinical signs of Menkes disease are initially subtle, the condition is rarely treated early enough to make a significant difference. The prognosis for babies with Menkes disease is poor.

PREVENTION

It is impossible to prevent Menkes disease. Suppose the patient has a family member or child with the disorder. Pregnant women may choose genetic counseling to undergo genetic testing to see if they have the gene that causes Menke disease.

Check Your Knowledge

1. What is Menkes syndrome?
2. What are the clinical manifestations of Menkes syndrome?
3. How can we prevent Menkes syndrome?

WILSON'S DISEASE (COPPER TOXICITY)

Wilson's disease is a genetic disorder that prevents the body from removing extra copper, causing copper to build up in the liver, brain, eyes, and other organs. Without treatment, high copper levels can cause life-threatening organ damage. The toxic accumulation of copper in the body is known as **hypercupremia**. It can also be acquired, which is sporadic and results in the accumulation of copper in the brain and liver. Inherited hepatic fibrosis develops, which eventually causes cirrhosis.

EPIDEMIOLOGY

Wilson's disease is a rare condition with varying global prevalence rates. Epidemiological surveys have shown that the prevalence of this condition in the United States, Europe, and Asia is 1:30,000–1:50,000, and the prevalence of Wilson's disease in China ranges from 4.93/100,000–6.21/100,000, which can occur at age 2 but is most common between 5 and 35. approximately 40% of patients are primarily young adults. It affects about 1 in every 30,000 people globally. Most people with Wilson's disease are diagnosed between the ages of 5 and 35, but it can affect younger and older people as well.

ETIOLOGY AND RISK FACTORS

Wilson's disease is inherited as an autosomal recessive trait, which means that to develop the disease, you must inherit one copy of the defective gene from each parent. If you receive only one abnormal gene, you won't become ill yourself, but you're a carrier and can pass the gene to your children. The single most significant risk factor for Wilson's disease is a family history of the disease, mainly if first-degree relatives (parents or siblings) exhibit symptoms.

CLINICAL MANIFESTATIONS

Clinical manifestations of Wilson's disease primarily involve liver and brain damage, including liver cirrhosis, jaundice, **dystonia**, tremors, and mental disorders. Copper seriously damages the kidneys. Initial signs and symptoms reflect CNS involvement. Motor deficits are expected, with combinations being dystonia, tremors, **dysarthria**, dysphagia, **chorea**, incoordination, and drooling. The CNS symptoms may be cognitive or psychiatric problems. The clinical manifestations of liver toxicity include abdominal pain, fatigue, jaundice, ascites, and edema. Children most often present with hepatic manifestations, and older patients (teenagers and adults) usually tend to present with neuropsychiatric manifestations.

In some cases, copper may be deposited around the rim of the corneas and edge of the iris, and **Kayser-Fleischer rings** appear. The ring first develops superiorly, then inferiorly, and finally in the lateral and medial areas of the cornea. These occur in approximately 50% of patients with hepatic manifestations and about 95% with neurologic manifestations.

DIAGNOSIS

The diagnosis of Wilson's disease is based on clinical findings as well as biochemical and genetic tests. Patients with Wilson's disease have unexplained liver, neurologic, or psychiatric symptoms, an unexplained chronic elevation of hepatic transaminases, fulminant hepatitis, or a parent, sibling, or cousin with Wilson's disease. A slit-lamp examination for Kayser-Fleischer rings is needed. Serum **ceruloplasmin** levels, complete blood count, and 24-hour urinary copper excretion are assessed. The ceruloplasmin levels are usually sufficient, and the serum copper levels may be measured. Kayser-Fleischer rings plus motor neurologic abnormalities or decreased ceruloplasmin are highly diagnostic.

TREATMENT

Treatment will be lifelong. A low-copper diet is needed, which avoids beef liver, black-eyed peas, cashews, shellfish, vegetable juice, cocoa, and mushrooms. Chelating agents such as d-penicillamine and trientine remain the mainstay of therapy. Zinc is also beneficial, acting synergistically with the chelators, and is often used alone in Wilson's disease with neuropsychiatric manifestations. Drinking water must be checked for its copper content. No vitamin or mineral supplements containing copper should be taken. For patients with Wilson's disease and fulminant hepatic failure or severe hepatic insufficiency for which medications are not effective, liver transplantation may be required.

PREVENTION

There is no way to prevent inherited Wilson's disease. Genetic counseling may determine if current or future children are at risk of developing it. Genetic testing is essential if there is a family or personal history of the condition. The prognosis is usually good unless the disease has advanced before treatment. If untreated, Wilson's disease is usually fatal by age 30.

Check Your Knowledge

1. Which organs are severely damaged by the accumulation of copper?
2. What are Kayser-Fleischer rings?
3. What foods are contained in the copper diet?

YOU SHOULD REMEMBER

Copper plays a crucial role in developing healthy nerves, bones, collagen, and the skin pigment melanin. Usually, copper is absorbed from food, and excess is excreted through a substance produced in bile. But in people with Wilson's disease, copper is not eliminated properly and instead accumulates, possibly to a life-threatening level. When diagnosed early, Wilson's disease is treatable, and many people with the disorder live everyday lives.

YOU SHOULD REMEMBER

Menkes disease and Wilson disease are genetic disorders involving the regulation of copper and ceruloplasmin. These disorders advance the understanding of copper homeostasis's cellular and molecular regulation. Menkes' disease produces copper deficiency, and Wilson's disease leads to copper overload.

CHRONIC COPPER POISONING

Long-term exposure to copper can occur and impair the liver. Therefore, the severe toxicity of copper can cause liver failure and death. In poisonings from a long-term buildup of copper in the body, the outcome depends on how much damage there is to the body's organs. Ingestion of more than 1 g of copper sulfate results in signs and symptoms of toxicity. Copper poisoning is classified as primary when it results from an inherited metabolic defect and secondary from high intake, increased absorption, or reduced excretion due to underlying pathologic processes. Copper toxicity can occur from exposure to excess copper in drinking water or from consuming acidic foods cooked on uncoated copper cookware.

EPIDEMIOLOGY

The incidence of copper poisoning varies mainly by region, but it is uncommon in Western countries. It is more common in South Asian countries and is more prevalent in rural populations. Copper toxicity risks are higher for neonates and infants as they have an immature biliary excretion system and enhanced intestinal absorption. Copper overload is also a feature of Indian childhood cirrhosis, endemic Tyrolean infantile cirrhosis, and idiopathic copper toxicosis.

ETIOLOGY AND RISK FACTORS

Many cases of copper toxicity are often the result of accidental consumption or installation of contaminated water sources, copper salt-containing topical creams for burn treatments, acidic foods cooked in uncoated copper cookware, or suicide attempts (the lethal dose of ingested copper (10–20 g)). Copper sulfate is an easily accessible chemical in many countries and is sold over the counter. It is commonly used in farming as a pesticide, in the leather industry, and in making homemade glue.

CLINICAL MANIFESTATIONS

The clinical signs are caused by the sudden release of a large amount of copper from the liver, which leads to intravascular hemolysis. This leads to anemia, **hemoglobinuria**, jaundice, colic, and depression. There is often an awful odor of diarrhea.

DIAGNOSIS

Diagnosis is typically based on a history of exposure to excess copper in combination with clinical findings of jaundice. Blood, urine tests, and a liver biopsy can diagnose copper poisoning – ceruloplasmin levels in blood or urine are valuable tests. However, a liver biopsy to measure the amount of copper and look for damage in the liver is usually required for diagnosis unless large amounts of copper were consumed.

TREATMENT

The most important treatment is the immediate removal of the source of the excess copper. This will be immediately identifiable in many cases, but in some cases, it may need careful checking of all supplementary feeds. Ideally, all supplementary copper should be removed, as if liver copper concentrations are high, they will remain well above deficient levels for very long periods (1–2 years) even if all copper supplementation is removed.

Feeding sodium thiosulfate and ammonium molybdate may decrease the loss of copper from the liver (by reducing copper uptake). Still, if all supplementary copper can be removed, the impact of this supplementation may be insignificant. Intravenous ammonium tetrathiomolybdate has been used in the past to treat cows that are clinically ill due to copper toxicity.

PREVENTION

Over-supplementation of copper is the leading cause of copper toxicity. In many cases, toxicity has occurred in herds that did not know they were feeding high levels of copper. This is usually because the cattle were being supplemented with copper via various routes–mineral, in-feed, injection, or boluses–and no one had collated them.

YOU SHOULD REMEMBER

Most of the copper in the body is located in the liver, bones, and muscles, but traces of copper occur in all body tissues. The liver excretes excess copper into the bile for elimination from the body. Copper is a component of many enzymes, including ones necessary for forming red blood cells, bone or connective tissues, and energy production.

YOU SHOULD REMEMBER

Although copper is naturally found in water, excessive levels of copper in drinking water are usually caused by leaked copper from old, corroded household pipes and faucets. There is a greater risk if water is stagnant from lack of use or if you use hot tap water (copper more easily dissolves at higher temperatures). In these cases, exposure to excess copper can be decreased by running cold tap water for several minutes before use.

Check Your Knowledge

1. What are the etiology and risk factors for chronic copper poisoning?
2. What are the clinical manifestations of chronic copper poisoning?
3. What are the treatments for chronic copper poisoning?

Clinical Case Studies

CLINICAL CASE STUDY 1

An 8-month-old male infant was referred to a dermatologist because of sparse, hypopigmented, abnormal scalp hair growth since birth. The patient was asymptomatic, born at 32 weeks of gestational age. The child had an abnormally large head at birth, and his birth weight was 1.7 kg). There is a documented history of myoclonic jerks and the gradual onset of hypotonia since 3 months of age. The mother reports delays in attaining developmental milestones such as recognition of the mother, head control, social smile, or roll-over response. The child had two brief hospital admissions in the past 2 months because of recurrent chest infections. The parents have another 6-year-old son who is asymptomatic. Family history is unremarkable. On examination, the child had a characteristic cherubic face with a depressed nasal bridge and bilateral large ears. Scalp hairs were sparse, brittle, stubby, and hypopigmented with a steel wire-like feel. The child failed to make eye contact, and a social smile was absent.

CRITICAL THINKING QUESTIONS

1. What are the causes of Menkes disease?
2. What are the clinical manifestations of Menkes disease?
3. What are the prevention of Menkes disease?

CLINICAL CASE STUDY 2

A 20-year-old man had developed rapid weight loss and increased anxiety, along with suicidal thoughts. A comprehensive series of tests were performed at his local hospital, which revealed abnormal copper levels, resulting in a diagnosis of Wilson's disease. There were Kayser-Fleischer rings in the eyes and low plasma ceruloplasmin. The patient was started on penicillamine, which works by chelation to increase urinary copper excretion.

CRITICAL THINKING QUESTIONS

1. What is the description of Wilson's disease?
2. How does Wilson's disease develop?
3. What do the clinical manifestations of Wilson's disease primarily involve?

FURTHER READING

1. Fischer, R., and Malter, R. (2023). *The Complete Copper Toxicity Handbook: How a Common Copper Imbalance Could Impact Your Health*. Fischer.
2. Lee, Y.J. (2022). *A New Therapeutic Approach to Dystonia: It is Not an Incurable Disease – There is a Cure for It*. Lee.
3. Micheli, F.E., and LeWitt, P.A. (2014). *Chorea: Causes and Management*. Springer.
4. Omine, M., and Kinoshita, T. (2012). *Paroxysmal Nocturnal Hemoglobinuria and Related Disorders: Molecular Aspects of Pathogenesis*. Springer.
5. Purser, D., and Larkin, J. (2019). *Vitamin Deficiency Symptoms and Cures: Modern Deficiency Illness – Using Intracellular Micronutrient Results: Vitamin Deficiencies can Cause Diabetes, Infertility, Anxiety, Fatigue, Depression*. Purser.
6. Qayyum Rana, A., and Hedera, P. (2014). *Differential Diagnosis of Movement Disorders in Clinical Practice*. Springer.
7. Reich, S.G., and Factor, S.A. (2019). *Therapy of Movement Disorders: A Case-Based Approach (Current Clinical Neurology)*. Springer.
8. Schilsky, M.L. (2018). *Management of Wilson Disease: A Pocket Guide (Clinical Gastroenterology)*. Humana Press.
9. Solioz, M. (2018). *Copper and Bacteria: Evolution, Homeostasis and Toxicity (Briefs in Molecular Science)*. Springer.
10. Somsuzen, J. (2023). *Copper Deficiency Symptoms: Understand the Potential Consequences of Copper Deficiency in the Body, Exploring Its Symptoms and Effects on Overall Health*. Somsuzen.
11. Swigert, N.B. (2010). *The Source for Dysarthria*, 2nd Edition. LinguiSystems.

22 Fluoride Deficiency and Toxicity

OVERVIEW

Fluoride is an essential trace element important in dental and bone health. Serum and bone fluoride content generally increases in patients with reduced kidney function. However, there is a lack of evidence linking fluoride accumulation and bone disease in chronic dialysis patients. Fluoride is not considered an essential nutrient but plays a vital role in dental and possibly bone health. A deficiency of fluoride can lead to dental caries and potentially bone problems. Fluoride deficiency is a disease in which a lack of fluoride in the diet can lead to increased tooth decay and osteoporosis. Fluoride salts, especially sodium fluoride, treat and prevent osteoporosis. Symptoms such as hip fractures and brittle and weak bones in older people can be caused by fluoride deficiency in the body. Fluoride stimulates bone formation and increases bone density. However, bone with excessive fluoride content has an abnormal structure, increasing fragility. While low fluoride doses benefit overall teeth integrity, high doses lead to many toxicity phenotypes. Prolonged exposure to high levels of fluoride leads to widespread organelle damage. Over time, fluoride accumulates in soft tissue such as the spleen, kidney, and especially the bone, leading to potential chronic toxicity. Chronic fluoride toxicity is more common than acute toxicity.

FLUORIDE DEFICIENCY

Fluoride is not considered an essential nutrient but plays a vital role in dental and possibly bone health. A lack of fluoride can lead to dental caries and bone problems such as osteoporosis. Most of the fluoride in the body is contained in bones and teeth. Fluoride (the ionic form of fluorine) is widely distributed in nature. The primary source of fluoride is fluoridated drinking water. **Tooth enamel** is constantly undergoing the processes of demineralization and remineralization. Demineralization occurs when tooth enamel loses minerals; regaining those minerals is called remineralization. The saliva in the mouth transports fluoride back into the enamel and helps in remineralization. **Tooth decay** happens when the enamel loses too many minerals (see **Figure 22.1**).

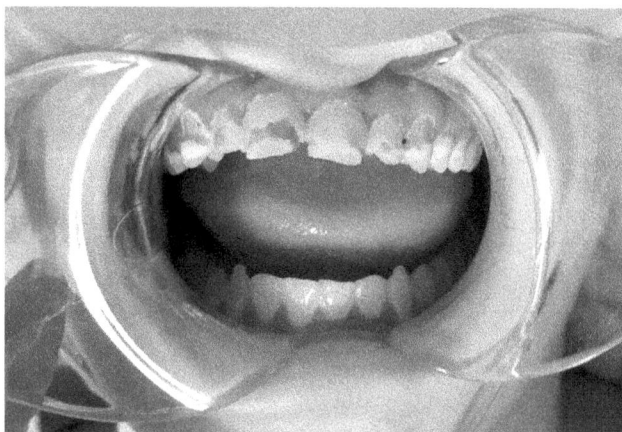

FIGURE 22.1   Tooth decay.

DOI: 10.1201/9781003453376-28

EPIDEMIOLOGY

The prevalence rate of dental fluorosis was highest, 41%, in adolescents and lowest, 8.7%, in those aged 40–49. According to the Centers for Disease Control (CDC), consuming fluoridated water helps reduce the risk of decay by 25% in children and adults. It is estimated that caries of the permanent teeth is the most prevalent of all conditions assessed, with 2.4 billion people globally suffering from caries of permanent teeth and 486 million children from caries of primary teeth.

ETIOLOGY AND RISK FACTORS

Fluoride deficiency is caused by many factors, including bacteria in the mouth, frequent snacking, sipping sugary drinks, and not cleaning teeth well. The risk factors may include diabetes, autoimmune conditions, anorexia, and bulimia. Diabetes has perhaps the most significant cause-and-effect relationship with tooth decay. Autoimmune conditions are a family of diseases that involve the body attacking parts of itself. This can include everything from major organ systems, like the kidneys, to smaller systems, like salivary glands. Many of these diseases have some impact on the mouth, but the one most directly tied to oral health is **Sjogren's syndrome**. Anorexia and bulimia have implications on the teeth because the body is not getting the minerals, vitamins, proteins, and other nutrients that it needs to maintain good oral health and prevent tooth decay from forming.

CLINICAL MANIFESTATIONS

Tooth decay is the primary red flag for fluoride deficiency. Untreated tooth decay can lead to more problems. **Rotting teeth** can be associated with plaque development related to gum disease. As tooth decay advances, it may cause a toothache or tooth sensitivity to sweets, hot or cold. If the tooth becomes infected, an abscess or pocket of pus may form, causing pain, facial swelling, and fever.

DIAGNOSIS

Tooth decay can be found during a regular dental check-up. Signs include white, brown, or black staining on the tooth. If the decay is more advanced, it may form a cavity. The dentist can also check the teeth for soft or sticky areas or take an X-ray, which can show decay.

TREATMENT

If tooth decay is still early, the dentist can apply fluoride to reverse the decline before a cavity forms. A dentist or hygienist can treat patients with fluoride during a routine dental exam or cleaning. They use fluoride gel, foam, or varnish on the teeth. Typically, a fluoride treatment takes less than 5 minutes. Dentists commonly treat cavities by filling them. A dentist will remove the decayed tooth tissue and then restore the tooth by filling it with a filling material.

PREVENTION

To prevent tooth decay, use fluoride, brush with fluoride toothpaste, drink tap water with fluoride, use fluoride mouth rinse, and have a good oral hygiene routine. Make smart food choices that limit sugary drinks and foods high in sugars and starches. Eat nutritious and balanced meals and limit snacking. See a dentist for regular check-ups and professional cleanings. Do not use tobacco products and consider quitting if you use them.

YOU SHOULD REMEMBER

Infants and children between the ages of 6 months and 16 years need an appropriate amount of fluoride. Developing teeth benefit from fluoride just as much as teeth that have already erupted.

YOU SHOULD REMEMBER

Fluoride can be added to infant formula milk or table salt for adults. Fluoride delivery through milk fluoridation could be more efficient than other fluoride delivery methods. This is due to fluoride's tendency to form insoluble complexes with calcium, which makes fluoride absorption difficult. The American Dental Association (ADA) recommends watching the intake of too much fluoride in infants and young children. The ADA recommends avoiding reconstituted formulas, such as liquid concentrate or powdered baby formulas, that require mixing with fluoridated water.

Check Your Knowledge

1. What are the causes and risk factors for fluoride deficiency?
2. What is the primary red flag for fluoride deficiency and its complications?
3. How can we prevent tooth decay?

FLUORIDE TOXICITY

Fluoride can be harmful in large amounts. Acute exposure to dangerous parts of fluoride is rare and usually occurs in small children. **Fluoride toxicity** has been seen in young children after swallowing fluoride solutions or tablets. This rare but acute toxicity can develop quickly and may be life-threatening. Therefore, it is essential to keep children away from fluoridated mouth rinses, supplements, and toothpaste. Chronic intake of excess fluoride during tooth development causes **fluorosis**. This is unrelated to any health risk, but the tooth enamel may become discolored or pitted. Acute fluoride toxicity in humans is rarely reported in adults.

EPIDEMIOLOGY

According to fluoride poisoning data collected by the American Association of Poison Control, toothpaste ingestion remains the primary source of toxicity, followed by fluoride-containing mouthwashes and supplements. The highest proportion (more than 80%) of the cases of fluoride toxicity was reported in children below the age of 6. In India, an estimated 60 million people have been poisoned by healthy water contaminated by excessive fluoride, which is dissolved in the granite rocks. The effects are particularly evident in the bone deformities of children. Similar or more significant problems are anticipated in other countries, including China, Uzbekistan, and Ethiopia.

ETIOLOGY AND RISK FACTORS

A major cause of fluorosis is the inappropriate use of fluoride-containing dental products such as toothpaste and mouth rinses. Sometimes, children enjoy the taste of fluoridated toothpaste so much that they swallow it instead of spitting it out. Ingestion of excess fluoride from drinking water, foods, or industrial pollution also causes chronic toxicity.

CLINICAL MANIFESTATIONS

Severe acute sodium fluoride poisoning occurs after ingesting 120 g of sodium fluoride. Toxic reactions include **tetany**, multiple episodes of **ventricular fibrillation**, and **esophageal stricture**. Other signs and symptoms of a fluoride overdose include headaches, abdominal pain, nausea, vomiting, weakness, cardiac arrest (in severe cases), and abnormal levels of calcium and potassium in the blood. People with fluorosis develop spots on their teeth ranging from light white to dark brown (see **Figure 22.2**). These spots typically occur during tooth development in the early years of life.

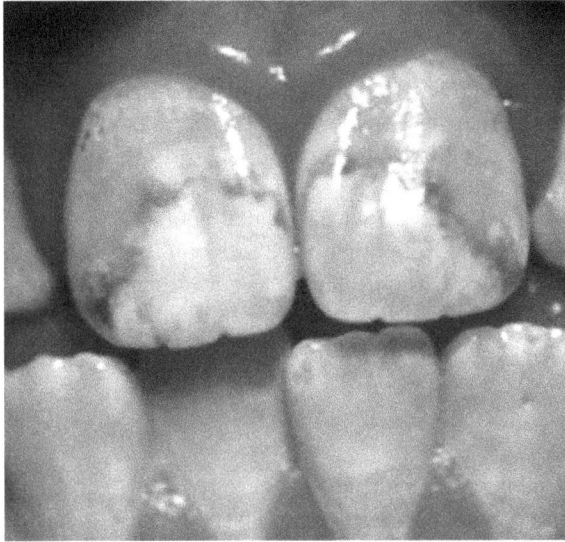

FIGURE 22.2 Fluorosis due to excessive fluoride.

DIAGNOSIS

Diagnosis of fluoride toxicity is based on symptoms. Tests to measure fluoride serum and urine levels are available in most hospitals.

TREATMENT

Treatment of fluoride toxicity involves reducing fluoride intake. Patients should refrain from drinking fluoridated water or taking fluoride supplements in areas with high fluoride water levels. In many cases, fluorosis is so mild that no treatment is needed, and it may only affect the back teeth where it cannot be seen. Treatment involves withdrawing fluoridated water and using foods supplemented with calcium and vitamins C and E.

PREVENTION

To prevent fluoride toxicity, reduce fluoride intake and tell children not to swallow fluoridated toothpaste.

YOU SHOULD REMEMBER

Dental fluorosis is caused by too much fluoride when teeth form under the gums over a long period. Only children aged 8 years and younger are at risk because this is when permanent teeth are developing; children older than eight, adolescents, and adults cannot develop dental fluorosis.

Check Your Knowledge

1. What are the causes of fluorosis?
2. What are the clinical manifestations of fluoride poisoning?
3. What are the treatments for fluoride toxicity?

SKELETAL FLUOROSIS

Skeletal fluorosis is a severe condition resulting from chronic ingesting large amounts of fluoride over many years during bone growth and remodeling. Osteosclerosis and ligament calcifications hallmark the condition and often accompany osteoporosis, osteomalacia, or osteopenia. The most common side effect of fluoride is fluorosis. In skeletal fluorosis, the bones are generally weaker than usual, with stiffness and joint pain being early symptoms. Prolonged, excessive exposure to fluoride can cause a debilitating bone disease known as skeletal fluorosis. The disease develops insidiously and can be difficult to distinguish from other bone and joint disorders. Although skeletal fluorosis used to be considered a non-issue in the United States and other Western countries, recent research suggests that many people – particularly those who consume large amounts of tea and those with kidney damage – may unknowingly be suffering from some form of the disease.

EPIDEMIOLOGY

In the United States, skeletal fluorosis is rare and has been reported to develop via uncommon means of toxicity, including toothpaste ingestion, excessive tea consumption, voriconazole treatment, and inhalant abuse. Industrial fluorosis is on the increase on a global basis. Prevalence of skeletal fluorosis was found to be 29% of grade-I, 51% of grade-II, and 20% of grade-III and was higher in males (63%) compared with females (37%). China and India have the highest prevalence of fluorosis and face the most severe harmful effects of fluorosis in the world. This is because China is located in the fluoride belt.

ETIOLOGY AND RISK FACTORS

Endemic skeletal fluorosis is a chronic metabolic bone and joint disease caused by ingesting large amounts of fluoride either through water or rarely from foods of endemic areas. Fluoride is a cumulative toxin that can alter the accretion and resorption of bone tissue. It also affects the homeostasis of bone mineral metabolism. A combination of varying degrees of osteosclerosis, osteomalacia, osteoporosis, and **exostosis** formation characterizes the bone lesions. The kidney is the primary organ for the excretion of fluorides. Age, sex, calcium intake in the diet, dose, and duration of fluoride intake, as well as renal efficiency in fluoride handling, are the factors that influence the outcome.

CLINICAL MANIFESTATIONS

Individuals with skeletal fluorosis may have deformed bones or bone abnormalities such as bowed legs, knees, or sclerosis. Common symptoms such as joint pain due to skeletal fluorosis are often misdiagnosed as they present similarly to other joint or bone diseases such as arthritis. Skeletal fluorosis is characterized by occasional joint stiffness or pain and some osteosclerosis of the pelvis and vertebra.

The total quantity of ingested fluoride is the most critical factor that determines the clinical course of the disease, which is characterized by the immobilization of joints of the axial skeleton and the major joints of the extremities. In many cases, secondary hyperparathyroidism is observed with associated characteristic bone changes. The osteosclerotic picture is evident when small doses of fluoride are ingested over a long period during which calcium intakes are usual, while osteoporotic forms are common in the pediatric age group and with a higher body load of the element. Alterations in hormones concerned with bone mineral metabolism are seen in skeletal fluorosis.

DIAGNOSIS

Apart from bone ash fluoride measurements, other serum, urine, and imaging tests can be employed to confirm the disease. Elevated serum or 24-hour urine fluoride levels can support the diagnosis. The imaging spectrum to diagnose skeletal fluorosis includes X-rays and CT scans.

TREATMENT

There is no particular treatment for skeletal fluorosis. The longer a person is exposed to fluoride, the more it accumulates and the harder it is to reverse the effects. No effective therapeutic agent can cure skeletal fluorosis. Vitamin E and methionine prevent excessive accumulation of fluoride in the bone by reducing its impact on soft tissues. Acupuncture helps improve **joint motion**, relieves pain, and increases urinary fluoride.

PREVENTION

The most effective way to prevent and treat fluorosis is to improve water quality and reduce water fluoride content. So far, there is no effective clinical treatment for endemic fluorosis, and reducing fluoride exposure levels and reducing fluoride intake are the leading measures most countries adopt. The prevention of endemic fluorosis is related to several factors, including the individual's environment, society, and living habits. Therefore, prevention of skeletal fluorosis may require comprehensive changes. First, providing safe drinking water can protect people against endemic fluorosis. People have recently developed additional techniques to remove fluoride from water. Second, improving people's living standards will help prevent endemic fluorosis. Good living conditions will help people avoid fluoride from water, tea, and coal.

Additionally, education is more critical for the prevention of fluorosis. Knowledge regarding the harmful effects of fluoride and the causes of fluorosis will help people pay more attention to their living habits. Moreover, nutritional supplements can improve human immunity and contribute to treatment approaches. If these preventive measures are taken, people living in areas with a high incidence of fluorosis will show reduced rates of endemic fluorosis and associated morbidities.

YOU SHOULD REMEMBER

According to the WHO, fluorosis has become a significant health problem worldwide, as over 260 million people drink water from sources with high fluoride concentrations. Drinking water is the most critical pathway of fluoride intake, accounting for 75%–90%.

Check Your Knowledge

1. What are the causes of fluorosis?
2. What are the clinical manifestations of fluoride poisoning?
3. What are the treatments for fluoride toxicity?

Clinical Case Studies

CLINICAL CASE STUDY 1

A 3-year-old girl was brought to the emergency department with abdominal pain, diarrhea, headache, and tremors. Her mother was deeply concerned that she may have been poisoned. However, tests revealed that the girl had no actual "poisons" in her bloodstream but that her fluoride levels were extremely high. It was later discovered that the girl had consumed nearly an entire tube of fluoride toothpaste, which she had eaten like candy when no one was supervising her.

CRITICAL THINKING QUESTIONS

1. What is the primary source of fluoride toxicity in younger children?
2. Why may children swallow toothpaste instead of spitting it out?
3. What does the treatment of fluoride toxicity involve?

CLINICAL CASE STUDY 2

A 54-year-old man came to his primary physician and stated that he had 1 year of noninflammatory pain in multiple joints. The pain had begun in both knee joints, followed by low-back ache and neck, wrist, and foot pain. There was no associated fever or swelling of any joint. When questioned, the patient admitted to using fluoridated toothpaste. The patient also lived in a region of India where the fluorosis problem is endemic. On examination, his physician found his teeth had brown strains and were rough and pitted. There was diffuse tenderness at the cervical spine, the lumbosacral spine, the wrist, and the knee joints. There were no neurological findings, and the rest of the physical examination was regular. X-ray scans showed osteosclerosis of the knee, wrist, and vertebral column. 24-hour urinary fluoride levels were elevated. The patient was advised to avoid fluoridated water, toothpaste, and fluoride foods.

CRITICAL THINKING QUESTIONS

1. In which global areas do people have a higher risk for skeletal fluorosis?
2. What are the clinical manifestations of skeletal fluorosis?
3. What are the treatments for skeletal fluorosis?

FURTHER READING

1. Agarwal, A. (2019). *Fluoride Toxicity: Description of History, Mechanism of Fluoride and Perception of Fluoride Toxicity and its Effects: An Overview.* Lap Lambert Academic Publishing.
2. Armstrong, G.P.D. (2020). *How Essential Is Fluoride? What Do the Experts Say?* Armstrong.
3. Birapu, U.K.C., Kovuru, V., and Reddy, J.S. (2023). *Dental Fluorides: A Critical Analysis: Benefits vs. Toxicity.* Lap Lambert Academic Publishing.
4. Connett, P., Beck, J., and Micklem, H.S. (2010). *The Case against Fluoride: How Hazardous Waste Ended Up in Our Drinking Water and the Bad Science and Powerful Politics That Keep It There.* Chelsea Green Publishing.
5. Guan, Z.Z. (2021). *Coal-burning Type of Endemic Fluorosis: Pathophysiology and Clinical Treatments.* Springer.
6. Khandare, A.L. (2021). *Fluoride and Fluorosis Interaction, Symptoms, Prevalence and Mitigation.* Khandare.
7. Meyappan, N., Kumar, A., and Gopal, R. (2022). *Dental Fluorosis.* Lap Lambert Academic Publishing.
8. Nataraj, P. (2023). *Fluorosis: Epidemiological and Histological Perspectives.* Lap Lambert Academic Publishing.
9. Nishu, S., and Ritesh, S. (2015). *Metabolism and Toxicity of Fluorides.* Lap Lambert Academic Publishing.
10. Tandon, V., Tirth, A., and Singh, V. (2015). *Fluoride Toxicity.* Lap Lambert Academic Publishing.

23 Miscellaneous and Rare Mineral Disorders

OVERVIEW

Zinc is essential to human health for average growth, tissue repair, wound healing, intestinal mucosal integrity, formation of testicular hormones, and the immune response. Zinc intake is closely related to protein intake; as a result, zinc deficiency is an essential component of nutritionally related morbidity worldwide. Zinc is relatively nontoxic, especially if taken orally. Manganese (Mn) is a coenzyme that breaks down carbohydrates, proteins, and cholesterol. It also helps enzymes build bones and keep the immune system working. Mn deficiency is rare but can happen, especially with certain medical conditions. Mn toxicity may result in a permanent neurological disorder, with symptoms that include tremors, difficulty walking, and facial muscle spasms. Mg is vital to many bodily reactions that affect cellular function and nerve conduction. The heart, brain, and skeletal muscles use Mg to function correctly. Hypomagnesemia can affect anyone at any age. It can be mild or severe and is treatable. Mg toxicity is frequently caused by the overuse of Mg-containing medication or the under-excretion of Mg by the kidneys. Selenium deficiency may cause various health issues, including neurological symptoms, musculoskeletal abnormalities, impaired immune function, dysfunction of cardiovascular, thyroid dysfunction, and fertility problems. Selenium toxicity can occur with acute or chronic ingestion of excess selenium.

ZINC DEFICIENCY AND TOXICITY

Adequate zinc nutrition is essential for many body functions. It is necessary for average pregnancy outcomes, child growth, immune function, and neurobehavioral development. Nearly all body cells contain zinc and use it for many functions. However, zinc deficiency is a significant problem in areas of the world where the diet is affected by poverty. It occurs after an infant is weaned off of maternal milk and causes impaired intestinal zinc absorption.

Zinc toxicity has been seen when supplements were taken at five or more times the recommended daily allowance (RDA). The upper level of zinc is 40 mg/day. To avoid toxicity and possible mineral-to-mineral interactions, people taking zinc supplements or tablets to relieve cold symptoms should be very cautious and consult with a dietitian.

EPIDEMIOLOGY

An estimated 17.3% of the global population is at risk of inadequate zinc intake. The regional estimated prevalence of inadequate zinc intake ranged from 7.5% in high-income regions to 30% in South Asia. Mild zinc deficiency due to reduced dietary intake is common. Conservative estimates suggest that 25% of the world's population is at risk of zinc deficiency. It is rare in the United States. However, people with a poor diet are more likely to be deficient.

ETIOLOGY AND RISK FACTORS

Zinc deficiency occurs in patients who have nutritional deficiencies, chronic GI diseases, diabetes, liver disease, sickle cell disease, kidney disease, excess alcohol consumption, or HIV infection. Sometimes, newborns experience zinc deficiency if they are premature or very sick or if their

DOI: 10.1201/9781003453376-29

mothers have mild zinc deficiency. Some people are born with zinc deficiency. A rare genetic condition called **acrodermatitis enteropathica** can cause severe zinc deficiency.

CLINICAL MANIFESTATIONS

Signs and symptoms of zinc deficiency include delayed growth and sexual maturation, decreased taste sensitivity, loss of appetite, impaired vitamin A function, immune dysfunction, dermatitis, **alopecia**, poor wound healing, congenital disabilities, severe diarrhea, and higher occurrence of infant mortality. When the body's zinc status is compromised, the integrity of structural proteins that contain zinc is impaired in cell membranes, protein receptors, and **zinc finger proteins**. The proteins become unable to perform normal functions. There are mild zinc deficiencies seen in patients with Crohn's disease, patients undergoing kidney dialysis and **bariatric surgery**, and infants.

Signs and symptoms of toxicity include loss of taste and smell, hair loss, changes in skin and hair, loss of appetite, nausea, vomiting, diarrhea, and intestinal cramps. Toxicities can impair immune function while reducing the absorption of copper and the activity of enzymes that contain copper.

DIAGNOSIS

Detecting zinc deficiencies is complex because methods to assess changes in zinc status need to be revised. Measurement of zinc in blood, neutrophils, lymphocytes, and hair may be the best tool for diagnosing zinc deficiency.

TREATMENT

Clinical zinc deficiency in adults should be treated with zinc supplements at two to five times the recommended dietary allowance. Zinc, in combination with vitamins C and E and beta-carotene, may slow the progression of intermediate and advanced age-related macular degeneration.

PREVENTION

Most people can avoid zinc deficiency by eating zinc-rich foods, especially dairy foods, poultry, meat, and seafood. Zinc can also be found in cereals, legumes, nuts, and seeds.

YOU SHOULD REMEMBER

In populations at risk of zinc deficiency, preventive zinc supplementation reduces the incidence of premature delivery, decreases morbidity from childhood diarrhea and acute lower respiratory infections, lowers all-cause mortality, and increases linear growth and weight gain among infants and young children.

YOU SHOULD REMEMBER

Zinc is crucial for the normal development and function of cells that mediate nonspecific immunity, including neutrophils and natural killer cells. Therefore, zinc is currently used in clinical trials against coronavirus disease 2019 (COVID-19). Some studies have shown that zinc can reduce their duration when administered at the onset of symptoms.

YOU SHOULD REMEMBER

Today, zinc oxide is still a popular over-the-counter treatment skin treatment. It can defend against sunburns by reflecting and scattering ultraviolet rays so they do not penetrate the skin. It also treats inflamed skin conditions like burns, eczema, **bedsores**, and diaper rash. The compound forms a protective barrier on the skin's surface, repelling away moisture and allowing the skin to heal. It may also aid enzymes in breaking down damaged collagen tissue so that new tissue can be formed. No adverse side effects have been reported.

Check Your Knowledge

1. What are the causes and risk factors for fluoride deficiency?
2. What is the primary red flag for fluoride deficiency and its complications?
3. How can we prevent tooth decay?

MANGANESE DEFICIENCY AND TOXICITY

Mn is a trace mineral essential to the body in small amounts. It has been known for a long time, and its effects still need to be understood. It must be obtained from food or supplements. It is a coenzyme that helps several enzymes break down carbohydrates, proteins, and cholesterol. It also assists enzymes in building bones and maintaining the immune and reproductive systems.

Mn is stored mainly in the bone, with smaller amounts in the brain, liver, and pancreas. Its levels are challenging to measure as dietary intake only sometimes correlates with blood levels. Mn is found in various foods, from shellfish to grains to legumes and spices. Drinking water also contains small amounts of Mn.

EPIDEMIOLOGY

Mg deficiency is common in hospitalized patients. Up to 12% of all hospitalized patients and as high as 65% of patients in an intensive care unit have hypomagnesemia. About 57% of the US population must meet the US RDA for dietary Mg intake.

ETIOLOGY AND RISK FACTORS

Inadequate Mn may cause Mn deficiency in the diet. However, according to the Institute of Medicine's review of dietary micronutrients, a clinical deficiency in Mn due to diet has yet to be observed in otherwise healthy people. The risk factors include people with type 2 diabetes, GI diseases, and alcohol use disorder. Older adults are more likely to develop a Mg deficiency than younger people.

Manganism is a well-established result of repeated occupational and nutritional exposures. However, it is relatively uncommon. There are specific populations most at risk for the development of Mn toxicity. This is due to physiological differences between ages and genders, underlying health conditions such as hepatic dysfunction, pre-exposure neurocognitive deficits, and those who are exposed to water sources.

Workers most at risk of being exposed to Mn often perform welding tasks. Welding occurs in the construction, manufacturing, transportation, mining, and agriculture industries and other occupations, such as pipe-fitters or millwrights. Smaller numbers of workers in the metallurgical and other manufacturing industries are also at risk.

CLINICAL MANIFESTATIONS

Signs and symptoms of Mn deficiency include poor growth, nausea, vomiting, reproductive dysfunction, and impaired carbohydrate or lipid metabolism. Toxicity causes extreme neurological impairment and symptoms that resemble those of Parkinson's disease, including muscle stiffness and tremors.

Manganism can result in a permanent neurological disorder, with symptoms that include tremors, difficulty walking, and facial muscle spasms. Other lesser symptoms include irritability, aggressiveness, and hallucinations. The symptoms of Mn toxicity also include muscle spasms, hearing problems, mania, insomnia, depression, loss of appetite, headaches, irritability, weakness, and mood changes. Workers may be harmed from exposure to Mn by breathing Mn fumes or dust. Continued exposure can damage the lungs, liver, and kidneys.

DIAGNOSIS

The diagnosis of hypomagnesemia includes a blood test to measure the level of Mn, calcium, and potassium. A Urine Mn test and EKG are also helpful. If clinical symptoms suggest manganism, blood and urinalysis are initially performed. MRI scans can examine the structure and determine whether manganism has damaged the globus pallidus.

TREATMENT

Treatment for hypomagnesemia depends on its severity and the underlying cause. When it is mild, Mg tablets are taken by mouth. In extreme cases, the patient must be in a hospital and receive fluids and Mg via an IV.

PREVENTION

Workers in steel factories or welding areas should take precautions to prevent inhalation of Mn by wearing an appropriate mask to limit the amount of Mn they breathe.

YOU SHOULD REMEMBER

Mn deficiency results in many medical conditions since Mn is a vital nutrition element in tiny quantities. Poisoning may occur if more significant amounts than 2.3 mg are ingested. Mn is a component of various enzymes and stimulates the development and activity of other enzymes. Several enzymes activated by Mn contribute to carbohydrates, amino acids, and cholesterol metabolism.

Check Your Knowledge

1. What are the causes and risk factors for fluoride deficiency?
2. What is the primary red flag for fluoride deficiency and its complications?
3. How can we prevent tooth decay?

MAGNESIUM DEFICIENCY AND TOXICITY

Mg is naturally found as a silver-white metal in ocean water and soil. It is an essential nutrient for plants and humans and is in many different foods. Mg is a component of **chlorophyll**, so rich sources include broccoli, green leafy vegetables, beans, squash, nuts, seeds, chocolate, and whole grains. Milk and meats supply some Mg but in lower quantities. Hard tap water also contains a lot of Mg. Coffee and tea also provide reasonable amounts of dietary Mg. However, refined foods are usually low in this mineral.

EPIDEMIOLOGY

The prevalence of Mg deficiency in the general population is still being determined because of the uncertainty regarding the Mg intakes needed for optimal health and the lack of an ideal biomarker of Mg status. Mg toxicity occurs in both sexes, and there is a higher rate in the United States than worldwide, likely due to the broader availability of Mg-containing over-the-counter supplements. The prevalence of hypermagnesemia among hospitalized patients in the United States was also 9.3%.

ETIOLOGY AND RISK FACTORS

The causes of hypomagnesemia include inadequate Mg intake and absorption or increased excretion due to hypercalcemia or medications such as furosemide. Risk factors may be anorexia nervosa, starvation, alcohol use disorder, diarrhea, laxative abuse, acute pancreatitis, gastric bypass surgery, and patients receiving total parenteral nutrition. Mg toxicity is frequently caused by the overuse of Mg-containing medication or the under-excretion of Mg due to kidney failure.

CLINICAL MANIFESTATIONS

The signs and symptoms of Mg deficiency include fatigue and weakness, tremors, loss of appetite, nausea and vomiting, and dysrhythmias. Symptoms of Mg toxicity include nausea, weakness, dyspnea, extreme hypotension, malaise, coma, and death. Older patients have a higher risk of Mg toxicity because of declining kidney function. However, if left untreated, Mg toxicity has a high mortality rate due to respiratory paralysis and cardiac arrest.

DIAGNOSIS

Hypermagnesemia is diagnosed when there is a high suspicion index. This can be done by measuring the Mg concentration in the blood. A complete **metabolic panel**, including Mg and phosphorus, will rule out additional electrolyte abnormalities and evaluate the patient's kidney function.

TREATMENT

Hypomagnesemia treatment depends on renal function and the severity of symptoms. Mg sulfate can be given orally or intravenously. The treatment of hypermagnesemia begins with discontinuing Mg-containing supplements and medication. In severe cases, IV calcium gluconate can displace and neutralize the effects of Mg. However, definitive treatment requires reducing Mg levels within the body. In patients with healthy renal function, this is achievable through IV diuretics. For patients with kidney failure, dialysis treatment is required.

PREVENTION

To prevent magnesium deficiency, eat a healthy, balanced diet containing magnesium-rich foods, such as leafy green vegetables. To prevent hypermagnesemia with renal impairment, the patient must avoid medications that contain magnesium, which can help prevent complications. This includes some over-the-counter antacids and laxatives.

YOU SHOULD REMEMBER

Mg deficiency can cause depression, fatigue, numbness, tingling, bone loss, and muscle spasms. Toxicity can lead to diarrhea, nausea, vomiting, hypotension, irregular heartbeat, and cardiac arrest.

Check Your Knowledge

1. What are the causes and risk factors for fluoride deficiency?
2. What is the primary red flag for fluoride deficiency and its complications?
3. How can we prevent tooth decay?

SELENIUM DEFICIENCY AND TOXICITY

Selenium (Se) is crucial in the body's physiological processes and metabolism. This activity investigates the many different roles of selenium, including antioxidant protection, immune system process, and its impact on HIV progression. The presence of selenium in food sources is widely varied based on soil content. The best sources of selenium include cereals, grains, seafood, and other meats. Oysters have the highest content, followed by clams, sardines, egg noodles, and beef.

EPIDEMIOLOGY

Selenium deficiency occurs in approximately 1 billion individuals worldwide due to insufficient dietary intake. However, in the United States, selenium deficiency is thought to be rare. Selenium deficiency was first seen in China, where the soil contained nearly no selenium. Other regions with a lack of soil selenium include Finland and New Zealand. **Keshan disease** can be prevented via selenium supplements. Outbreaks of acute selenium poisoning are periodic in the United States but have been reported.

ETIOLOGY AND RISK FACTORS

Selenium deficiency may result from inadequate dietary intake. Many selenium deficiency illnesses can be associated with concurrent vitamin E deficiency. The risk factors for selenium deficiency include living in low-selenium areas and eating a primarily plant-based diet. Other risks include HIV and kidney failure while undergoing dialysis. Exposure to selenium mainly occurs through food and, in some areas with seleniferous soils, through drinking water. Airborne exposure is rare; however, occupational exposure is possible with the chemical processes to recover selenium, the painting trade, and the metal industries.

CLINICAL MANIFESTATIONS

Selenium deficiency is linked to changes in thyroid hormone metabolism and a higher risk of certain cancers. It is also related to the development of Keshan disease, which is characterized by insufficient cardiac function.

Excessive selenium supplementation can cause toxicity, known as **selenosis**. This has occurred with only 1–3 mg/day taken over many months. Signs and symptoms of selenium toxicity include diarrhea, nausea, vomiting, fatigue, changes in nails, hair loss, and impaired protein and sulfur metabolism. The upper level for daily selenium is 400 μg.

DIAGNOSIS

Determining selenium deficiency and toxicity may be done with laboratory tests, imaging assessments, and other clinical measures. However, it is essential to remember that although some guidelines exist, standardized selenium deficiency evaluation protocols may differ.

TREATMENT

The first-line treatment for selenium deficiency is to try to eat more foods high in selenium. Selenium supplements, generally made from sodium selenite, may be used. Antidotes do not exist or curative treatments for selenosis. Treatment of selenium toxicity includes stopping the exposure and providing supportive care for symptoms.

PREVENTION

Preventing selenium deficiency includes eating foods high in selenium and taking dietary supplements. Preventing selenium toxicity involves stopping the exposure and providing supportive care for symptoms.

YOU SHOULD REMEMBER

Selenium plays a vital role in synthesizing active thyroid hormones, promoting the proper functioning of the immune system, contributing to cognitive well-being, and serving as an antioxidant by protecting cells from oxidative damage.

Clinical Case Studies

CLINICAL CASE STUDY 1

A 63-year-old man had a 1-month history of painful, scaly, edematous palms and soles. The patient had a long history of eczematous dermatitis of the soles, but the palms were affected more recently. Additional skin examination included the body folds and mucosa, which were normal. The patient was first treated with oral prednisone for 2 weeks but did not improve. There were no signs of constitutional symptoms, joint pain, or diarrhea. His weight was stable following the significant weight loss after previous gastric bypass surgery. A punch biopsy revealed significant parakeratosis plus epidermal hyperplasia and spongiosis. Zinc supplementation resulted in near-resolution of the hand dermatitis in 6 days, indicating that a zinc deficiency had been the problem.

CRITICAL THINKING QUESTIONS

1. What are the causes and risk factors for zinc deficiency?
2. What are the clinical manifestations of zinc deficiency?
3. How can zinc deficiency be detected?

CLINICAL CASE STUDY 2

A 57-year-old woman was evaluated for recurring palpitations, supraventricular arrhythmias, and hypomagnesemia. The patient had been taken to the emergency department previously for palpitations and lightheadedness, during which there were abnormal cardiac rhythms and an increased heart rate. On each occasion, the cardiac rhythm quickly converted to sinus rhythm after intravenous administration of adenosine or diltiazem. The patient's Mg levels were deficient, and she was treated with supplementation.

1. What are the causes and risk factors for hypomagnesemia?
2. What are the clinical manifestations of hypomagnesemia?
3. How can we prevent Mg deficiency?

CLINICAL CASE STUDY 3

A 15-month-old boy was found to have a selenium deficiency that caused dilated cardiomyopathy, failure to thrive, prolonged fever, and respiratory distress. Selenium supplementation was administered for 6 months, and the patient's condition improved significantly. Repeated echocardiography was routine after treatment. The patient's selenium levels were measured 3 and 6 months after the supplementation, revealing normalized selenium levels.

CRITICAL THINKING QUESTIONS

1. What are the causes and risk factors for selenium deficiency?
2. What are the clinical manifestations of selenium toxicity?
3. How can we prevent selenium deficiency?

FURTHER READING

1. Bagchi, D., and Swaroop, A. (2016). *Food Toxicology.* CRC Press.
2. Berdanier, C.D. (2021). *Advanced Nutrition: Macronutrients, Micronutrients, and Metabolism,* 3rd Edition. CRC Press.
3. Bever, M. (2015). *Vitamins, Minerals, & More!: Food Sources, Functions of the Body, and Deficiencies (Symptoms).* CreateSpace Independent Publishing Platform.
4. Davies, M. (2021). *Clinical Signs in Humans and Animals Associated with Minerals, Trace Elements, and Rare Earth Elements.* Academic Press.
5. DiNicolantonio, J., and Land, S. (2021). *The Mineral Fix: How to Optimize Your Mineral Intake for Energy, Longevity, Immunity, Sleep, and More.* DiNicolantonio.
6. Gomes, C., and Rautureau, M. (2021). *Minerals latu sensu and Human Health: Benefits, Toxicity, and Pathologies.* Springer.
7. Gualtieri, A.F. (2017). *Mineral Fibres: Crystal Chemistry, Chemical-Physical Properties, Biological Interaction, and Toxicity (EMU Notes in Mineralogy 18).* European Mineralogical Society.
8. Lajusticia Bergasa, A.M. (2021). *Magnesium, Key to Health: The Importance of This Mineral and the Problems Caused by Its Deficiency.* Ennsthaler.
9. Liebermann, S., and Bruning, N. (2007). *The Real Vitamin and Mineral Book: The Definitive Guide to Designing Your Personal Supplement Program,* 4th Edition. Avery.
10. Malavolta, M., and Mocchegiani, E. (2018). *Trace Elements and Minerals in Health and Longevity (Healthy Aging and Longevity Book 8).* Springer.
11. Mozsik, G., and Diaz-Soto, G. (2021). *Mineral Deficiencies: Electrolyte Disturbances, Genes, Diet and Disease Interface.* IntechOpen.
12. Ochsenham, P., and Vormann, J. (2015). *The Magnesium Deficiency Crisis: Is This the World's Number 1 Mineral Deficiency?* MadhouseMEDIA.
13. Rydon, R. (2017). *Profiles of the Nutrients: 2. Minerals and Trace Elements.* Rydon.
14. Tako, E. (2020). *Dietary Trace Minerals (Nutrients).* MDPI AG.
15. Walters, C. (2013). *Minerals for the Genetic Code: An Exposition & Analysis of the Dr. Olree Standard Genetic Periodic Chart & the Physical, Chemical & Biological Connection.* Acres U.S.A.
16. Wartian Smith, P. (2019). *What You Must Know about Vitamins, Minerals, Herbs, and So Much More: Choosing the Nutrients That Are Right for You,* 2nd Edition. Square One.

Part VII

Selective Nutritional Disorders

24 Obesity and Metabolic Syndrome

OVERVIEW

Obesity results from inherited, physiological, and environmental factors combined with diet, physical activity, and exercise choices. Global obesity rates have significantly increased in recent decades. People are becoming obese at younger ages, and morbid obesity is growing, with the complete health implications only beginning to be seen. Usually, as obesity rates rise, there is a related increase in many diseases or conditions. These include type 2 diabetes mellitus, heart disease, stroke, dementia, certain cancers, digestive problems, sleep apnea, osteoarthritis, and even a worsening of COVID-19 symptoms. Other weight-related issues that affect quality of life include depression, disability, shame, guilt, social isolation, and lower work achievement. Therefore, obesity has the potential to shorten life expectancy.

RISK FACTORS FOR OBESITY

There are many risk factors for being overweight or obese. These include knowledge, skills, behaviors, and environmental factors such as school, workplace, and neighborhood. Food industry practices, marketing, social and cultural norms, and values also increase the risks. Not all risk factors can be changed. Lack of physical activity combined with high amounts of television, computer, video game, or other screen time is associated with a high body mass index (BMI). Unhealthy eating behaviors include eating more calories than are burned, consuming too much-saturated fat, and eating foods high in added sugar. Additional risk factors include poor sleep, high stress, **metabolic syndrome**, polycystic ovary syndrome, genetic predisposition, various medications (antidepressants, antipsychotics, beta-blockers, birth control pills, and glucocorticoids), and an environmental lack of areas that promote physical activity.

CARDIOVASCULAR DISORDERS

Obesity is related to an increased risk of developing cardiovascular disorders. It changes the body's composition, affecting **hemodynamics** and altering heart structure. Adipose tissue produces pro-inflammatory cytokines, which can cause cardiac dysfunction and promote the formation of atherosclerotic plaques. When obesity and heart failure or cardiovascular disease coexist, people with class I obesity have a better prognosis compared to those who are average or underweight. This is known as the **obesity paradox**. The cardiovascular disorders that are complications of obesity include dyslipidemia, atherosclerosis, hypertension, myocardial infarction, and stroke, which were discussed in detail before.

DIABETES MELLITUS

Diabetes mellitus is a disease caused by poor control of blood glucose. Its subclassifications include type 1 diabetes, type 2 diabetes, gestational diabetes, neonatal diabetes, and steroid-induced diabetes. Type 2 diabetes involves an imbalance between insulin levels and insulin sensitivity, resulting in a functional insulin deficit. This commonly develops from obesity and aging. Diabetes is a significant cause of death in many countries. Its complications involve nephropathy, retinopathy, neuropathy, dyslipidemia, hypertension, psychological problems, sleep apnea, and osteoarthritis. Approximately 66% of patients with diabetes will die from a myocardial infarction or stroke. Diabetes mellitus was discussed in **Chapter 3**.

DOI: 10.1201/9781003453376-31

OSTEOARTHRITIS

Long-term obesity also affects the musculoskeletal system, mainly the joints, bones, muscles, tendons, and ligaments. **Osteoarthritis**, or degenerative joint disease, is a progressive loss of articular cartilage with related changes at joint margins. It is the most common form of arthritis and usually develops later in life. In most cases, it affects weight-bearing joints, particularly knee joints. Osteoarthritis is the leading cause of disability in many countries, especially those in which the citizens have longer lifespans. Because humans live longer, many more people will probably develop osteoarthritis than ever before. The condition often becomes symptomatic during a person's 40s or 50s. Osteoarthritis was discussed in **Chapter 15**.

SLEEP APNEA

Sleep apnea involves episodes of partial or complete upper airway closure during sleep. Each episode results in breathing cessation. Being overweight or obese is a high-risk factor for sleep apnea, along with other breathing problems during sleep. Alternately, a person who has a sleep-breathing disorder that is not treated can begin to gain weight as a result. In children, excess weight increases the risk of developing lifelong obstructive sleep apnea. The two forms of sleep apnea are *obstructive* and *central*. Obstructive sleep apnea is the most common form, characterized by partial or complete upper airway obstructions. Central sleep apnea is usually less common and is associated with reduced blood oxygen saturation.

EPIDEMIOLOGY

Obstructive sleep apnea syndrome occurs between the ages of 30 and 70. It is currently estimated that up to 4% of children globally suffer from sleep apnea. Many of these children are between the ages of 2 and 8 years. Children are more likely to have other sleep disturbances, including restless leg syndrome, periodic limb movement disorder, narcolepsy, and insomnia.

Overall, sleep apnea affects about five in every 100 people. This is 3%–7% of adult men and 2%–5% of adult women. Prevalence estimates of obstructive sleep apnea from North America, Europe, Australia, and Asia are not very different – it is common everywhere. Obstructive sleep apnea is increasing, affecting more than 25 million adults in the United States alone. Sleep apnea is more common in men than in women in younger adults by a more significant margin, but this reduces with aging. In some elderly groups, obstructive sleep apnea is as high as 90% in men and 78% in women. Incidence averages 4.9% in women but 11.1% in men. It is most common in both women and men in middle age. The prevalence of obstructive sleep apnea is more significant in obese and hypertensive patients. Undiagnosed obstructive sleep apnea is estimated to cost the United States more than $149 billion/year.

ETIOLOGY AND RISK FACTORS

The causes of obstructive sleep apnea are a natural relaxation of throat muscles as sleeping begins. Additional complicating factors may include being overweight or obese, a smaller-than-normal jaw, enlarged tonsils or adenoids that partially block breathing passages, or having a large tongue. In children, who often outgrow the condition, the primary cause is **adenotonsillar hypertrophy**. In adults, those who consume alcohol before sleep or take sleeping pills or tranquilizers experience further relaxation and narrowing of breathing passages. This makes the passages more likely to close. Though many people take sleeping pills or tranquilizers to get better and more continuous sleep, these agents often make things worse.

Endocrine disorders linked to sleep apnea include hypothyroidism, **acromegaly**, and **polycystic ovary syndrome** (since this is related to being overweight or obese). Conditions that interfere with brain signals to the airway and chest muscles may be implicated in sleep apnea. These conditions include stroke, **amyotrophic lateral sclerosis**, Chiari malformations, **myotonic dystrophy**, post-polio syndrome, **dermatomyositis**, and **myasthenia gravis**. Sleep apnea is associated with advanced heart or kidney failure since fluid build-up in the neck may obstruct the upper airway. Genetic syndromes may affect facial or skull structures. These syndromes include cleft lip or palate, **Down syndrome**, and congenital central hypoventilation syndrome. Babies born before 37 weeks of gestation have an increased risk of sleep apnea, but risks usually decrease as the brain matures.

Risk factors for sleep apnea include unhealthy lifestyle habits and environments, age, family history, genetics, race, ethnicity, and gender. Healthy lifestyle changes can decrease risks. With increased age, more fatty tissue builds up in the neck and tongue, raising risks. Studies of twins have revealed that sleep apnea is inheritable. Some genes are associated with obesity and inflammation. Race or ethnicity is a factor, with sleep apnea being more common in African-Americans, Hispanics, and Native Americans than in Caucasians.

CLINICAL MANIFESTATIONS

Sleep quality problems usually manifest slowly over the years, especially with long-term weight increases. Most patients do not recognize the symptoms and rarely remember how often they are awakened at night. Frequently, patients attribute the effects of poor sleep to aging, medications, stress, or an uncomfortable bed. In children, sleep apnea may cause learning and behavioral problems. Apnea-related symptoms include bedwetting, sleepwalking, slow growth, hormone imbalances, worsening of **asthma**, hyperactivity, and failure to thrive. Brain function can be altered, affecting cognition, planning, self-monitoring, organization, and emotions. Signs and symptoms of sleep apnea in children include loud snoring, difficult or labored breathing, and chronic squeaking or gasping when breathing. Snoring during sleep is a sign of sleep apnea. If it is chronic, it can result in hypertension, heart attack, and stroke.

Apnea occurs when the breathing passages become so narrow that no air can pass, and breathing stops. The patient wakes up to breathe, and the cycle starts over. Some patients experience apnea and **hypopnea**, as the throat muscles relax and the breathing passages narrow again. Apnea and hypopnea both drop the blood oxygen levels, causing many other symptoms. Additional signs and symptoms of sleep apnea include mood swings, difficulty concentrating, forgetfulness, irritability, anxiety, falling asleep at inappropriate times, morning headache, unexplained nausea, a frequent need to urinate at night, and chronic darkness of the skin below the eyes. Sleep apnea patients often complain of problems with motor skills and memory, dry mouth, sexual dysfunction, and decreased **libido**. Women more frequently report headaches, fatigue, depression, anxiety, and insomnia than are reported by men.

The impact of untreated sleep apnea on the developing brain and body will lead to changes in metabolism due to systemic stress occurring nightly during sleep. This results in abnormal food cravings, daytime fatigue, low energy levels, behavior problems, and other anomalies that may lead to unhealthy weight gain.

DIAGNOSIS

The diagnosis of sleep apnea is based on symptoms, physical examinations, and tests. The physical examination involves an assessment of the back of the throat, mouth, and nose. The neck and waist circumference may be measured. At the sleep center, your breathing and other body functions are monitored as you sleep. **Polysomnography** monitors the heart, lung, and brain activity and breathing patterns while the patient sleeps (see **Figure 24.1**). The equipment also measures arm and leg movements and blood oxygen levels. The sleep study can also help look for other sleep disorders that cause excessive daytime sleepiness but have different treatments.

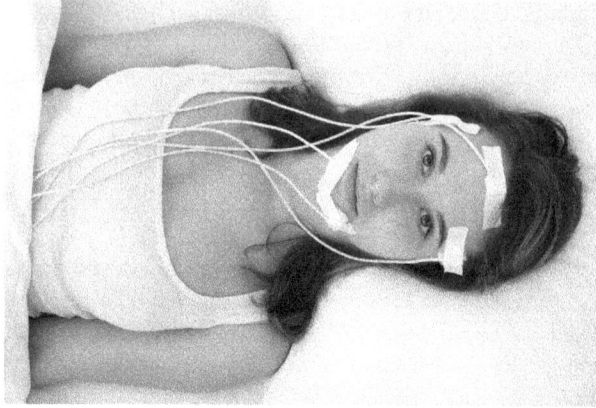

FIGURE 24.1   Polysomnography.

TREATMENT

The most common and reliable treatment method for obstructive sleep apnea is with a continuous positive airway pressure (CPAP) machine (see **Figure 24.2**). This device pushes a steady stream of air
through a mask to keep the airway open, helping the patient to snore less or not at all and to sleep better. Another option is a bi-level positive airway pressure (BiPAP or BPAP) machine. It does not give
the same constant pressure all the time. Since it provides less air while the patient breathes, exhaling is
more manageable than CPAP. Oral appliances, also called mandibular advancement devices (MADs),
are designed to bring the jaw forward to open the airway or hold the tongue in place. Additional treatment options include weight loss, nasal decongestants, breathing strips, implantable upper airway stimulation (UAS) devices, and uvulopalatopharyngoplasty (to remove the tonsils and uvula surgically).

PREVENTION

Sleep apnea can be preventable and even cured in young children if weight management and CPAP
or **tonsillectomy** are undertaken. There are preventive measures against the development or worsening of sleep apnea. It is essential to stop drinking alcohol or sleep medicines because they relax
the muscles in the back of the throat, making it harder to breathe while asleep. Smokers must quit
their habit. Weight loss is an essential method of preventing sleep apnea. Another suggestion is to
sleep on one side instead of the back for most of the night.

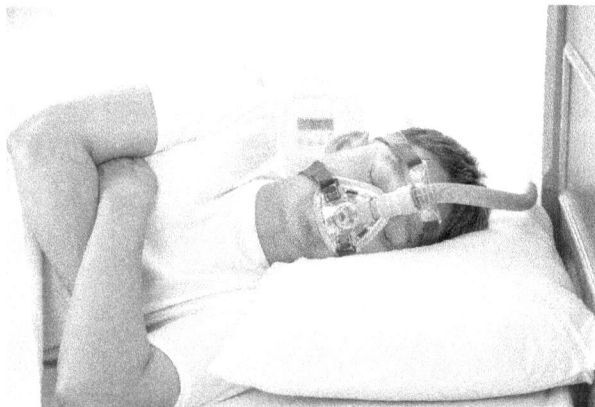

FIGURE 24.2   A CPAP machine.

YOU SHOULD REMEMBER

Untreated sleep apnea is associated with an increased risk of heart disease, hypertension, myocardial infarction, stroke, heart failure, diabetes, asthma, anxiety, depression, and a shortened lifespan.

Check Your Knowledge

1. What are the causes and risk factors for sleep apnea?
2. How does obesity interfere with sleep apnea?
3. What are the treatments for sleep apnea with obesity?

IMPACT OF OBESITY ON PREGNANCY

Obesity during pregnancy puts a woman at risk of severe health problems such as gestational diabetes, **preeclampsia**, **eclampsia**, and sleep apnea. A woman who is short in height and has an increased BMI is more likely to have a difficult labor. Obstetricians counsel patients about all factors related to obesity during pregnancy, including educating them about how obesity reduces the likelihood of actually becoming pregnant and maintaining a healthy and normal pregnancy. Preconception efforts must reduce or prevent fetal exposure to harmful in-utero factors.

EPIDEMIOLOGY

The WHO has estimated that 60% of women between 20 and 40 are overweight or obese. More than 50% of pregnant women in the United States are overweight or obese, with 8% of women in their reproductive years being *extremely* obese. In extremely obese women, 46.3% have chronic or gestational hypertensive diseases or preeclampsia. About 31.8% have progestational or gestational diabetes.

ETIOLOGY AND RISK FACTORS

Obesity increases the risks of other complications, including miscarriage, stillbirth, recurrent miscarriage, and cardiac dysfunction. The baby may be much larger than usual, have excess body fat, and have a higher risk of congenital disabilities.

CLINICAL MANIFESTATIONS

In labor, obese women often have problems that are rare in non-obese women. There may be complications with anesthesia or C-section delivery problems. The infant is at a higher risk of requiring resuscitation and intensive care unit treatment. Complications may continue into the postpartum period, with obese mothers experiencing bleeding, surgical site infections, and abnormal blood clotting. This makes recovery after delivery more prolonged, reducing the mother's ability to care for her infant correctly. Chronic inflammation due to obesity may affect the functioning of the **placenta**, which can influence the fetus's development, growth, and maturity.

DIAGNOSIS

Specialized care for obese mothers includes early testing for gestational diabetes, special accommodations for fetal ultrasound procedures, and screening for obstructive sleep apnea. A glucose challenge test is often recommended at the first prenatal visit for an obese woman and is usually repeated between weeks 24 and 28 of pregnancy. If the results are abnormal, additional tests will be needed. The healthcare provider will advise about blood sugar monitoring and control. Since obesity during pregnancy can interfere with the effectiveness of fetal ultrasound, there may be a need for an experienced sonographer, repeated examinations, or more advanced equipment. If obstructive sleep apnea is suspected, the patient may be referred to a sleep medicine specialist.

TREATMENT

Pregnancy weight control includes dietary control, exercise, and behavior modification. It is essential to avoid excessive gestational weight gain, which is common in obese women. Patients need to work with a nutritionist who can help plan meals for optimum healthy gestational weight gain.

PREVENTION

Pregnant women must be physically active after consulting healthcare providers about safe ways to do this, including walking, swimming, or low-impact aerobics. Pregnant women must avoid smoking, consuming alcohol, or illegal drugs abuse.

YOU SHOULD REMEMBER

Being obese during pregnancy results in many complications. It can cause loss of pregnancy, and obese women have a higher risk of miscarriage compared with women of average weight. Obesity increases the risk of congenital disabilities. Babies born to obese women have an increased risk of heart defects and neural tube defects such as *spina bifida*.

Check Your Knowledge

1. What pregnancy complications are related to obesity?
2. What serious health problems can happen to an obese woman during pregnancy?
3. During labor, what problems can occur concerning obesity?

PSYCHOLOGICAL PROBLEMS

Obesity is a physical, social, and psychological problem. The causative basis of obesity and eating disorders includes combinations of psychosocial, environmental, genetic, and biological attributes. Those with depression and anxiety may have more difficulty in controlling food consumption and in exercising sufficiently. In many obese people, there is a continual cycle of mood disturbances, overeating, and weight gain. A continuous pattern of using food to cope with stress and emotions may appear. Society views obesity with extreme negativity. Obese people are regularly labeled as lacking willpower and being unmotivated to improve their health. They also experience workplace discrimination.

Adults with excess weight have a 55% higher risk of developing depression over their lifetimes compared to people who do not struggle with obesity. Obesity-related anxiety is up to 1.4 times more likely to occur than anxiety occurring in those who are not obese. Individuals are 1.5 times more likely to develop a mood disorder if they are obese. Global statistics on obesity-related depression range between 1.27 and 1.55 times more likely than depression in people who are not obese. Losing weight can significantly impact mental health and well-being, including greater self-esteem and less self-consciousness. One major mental block to weight loss is the desire to lose weight too much and too fast. Weight loss is simply "too slow" for most obese people.

YOU SHOULD REMEMBER

The prevention of social and psychological problems in the obese requires setting realistic goals, staying committed to weight loss, identifying inner motivations, monitoring signals from the body, being accountable, creating meal plans that fit lifestyles, reassessing exercise, and remembering to stay patient.

OBESITY AND CANCER

Excessive body fat contributes to more than 100,500 yearly cases of cancer, as well as 14%–20% of all cancer deaths in the United States. Excess body fat is estimated to be related to more than 33,000 postmenopausal breast cancers, 20,700 endometrial cancers, 13,900 kidney cancers, 13,200 colorectal cancers, 11,900 pancreatic cancers, 5,800 esophageal cancers, and 2,000 gallbladder cancers – annually in the United States. Not all subgroups are equally affected. For example, obese men have a higher risk of colon cancer than obese women. Obesity increases the risks of breast cancer in postmenopausal women but not in those who are not yet menopausal. This may be due to fatty tissue being the primary source of estrogen following menopause.

BREAST CANCER

The breast is mainly comprised of fat and glandular tissues. There are 15–20 distinctive clusters of lobules in each breast, called *breast lobes*. Each breast lobe has 20–40 *lobules*. Breast cancer usually involves the epithelial cells of the ducts or lobules. Patients commonly present with an asymptomatic mass found during examination or mammography. Most breast lumps are benign, do not spread outside the breast, and are not life-threatening. However, some benign breast lumps increase the risk of developing malignant breast cancer.

Epidemiology

Worldwide, breast cancer is the most common invasive cancer in women. It makes up 22.9% of invasive cancers and 16% of all female cancers. The average amount of deaths from breast cancer is over 450,000 annually in the United States. Incidence varies widely around the world. It is lowest in less-developed countries and highest in more-developed countries. The highest incidence is in North America (90 of every 100,000 women), followed by Western Europe (78 of every 100,000). The lowest incidence is in Eastern Asia (18 of every 100,000).

According to the American Cancer Society, in the United States, breast cancer is the second leading cause of cancer death, after lung cancer, in Caucasian, African-American, Asian/Pacific Islander, and American Indian/Alaska Native women. However, in Hispanic women, breast cancer is the leading cause of cancer death – above $3 billion in the United States, over $143 million in Asia, and over $68 million in Africa. Costs per treated patient begin at an average of $24,008.

Etiology and Risk Factors

The actual causes of breast cancer are unclear. The epidemic of obesity is linked to female breast cancer and benign tumors. It is essential to maintain a healthy BMI. In the United States, the cumulative risk of developing breast cancer is about 12%, with much of the risk-focused on those over age 60. However, these data are misleading because they are based on risks up to age 95, and most people do not live that long. The cumulative risk of developing breast cancer in 20 years is much lower. The risk of dying from breast cancer is about 9% within 5 years after diagnosis. Risk factors for breast cancer include age, family history, gene mutations, personal and gynecologic history, breast changes, use of oral contraceptives, radiation therapy, diet, and lifestyle factors.

The most decisive risk factor is age since most breast cancers occur in women older than 50. Having a first-degree relative (mother, sister, or daughter) with breast cancer doubles or triples the risks. However, breast cancer in more distant relatives only increases the risk slightly. If two or more first-degree relatives have breast cancer, the risk may be five to six times higher. Between 5% and 10% of women with breast cancer have a mutated gene. If a relative also carries one of these mutations, there is a 50%–85% lifetime risk of developing breast cancer. For gene mutations, there is also a 20%–40% lifetime risk of developing ovarian cancer. For those without a family history of breast cancer in two or more first-degree relatives, there is a low likelihood of carrying gene mutation.

Risks are increased by early **menarche**, late menopause, or a late first pregnancy. Women with their first pregnancy occurring after age 30 are at higher risk than those who have no children. Diet can contribute to the development or growth of breast cancer, though exactly which diet has not been proven. Obese postmenopausal women have a higher risk, but dietary modification has not been shown to reduce risk. Chances may be decreased in obese women who are menstruating later than is typical. Smoking and alcohol contribute to a higher risk of breast cancer, and women are instructed to stop smoking entirely and limit alcohol consumption.

Clinical Manifestations

The development of breast cancer involves breast pain enlargement or thickening. **Paget's disease** of the nipple causes **erythema**, crusting, scaling, and discharge that usually begin benignly and are often ignored. About half of patients have a palpable mass when first examined. Some patients with breast cancer show signs of metastatic disease, including pathologic fractures or pulmonary dysfunction. Often, physical examination reveals asymmetry or a mass that is very different from surrounding breast tissue. Benign disorders are usually signified by diffuse, fibrotic changes in a breast quadrant (often the upper outer quadrant). A slightly firmer thickening in one breast, but not in the other, may be an indicator of cancer. Advanced breast cancers are characterized by one or more of the following: fixation of the mass to the chest wall or overlying skin, satellite nodules or ulcers of the skin, or exaggeration of common skin markings due to skin edema.

Diagnosis

The diagnosis of breast cancer may include mammograms, MRIs, ultrasound, and biopsy. A diagnostic mammogram is a highly detailed X-ray of the breast or breasts. A breast MRI is a body scan that utilizes computers to create detailed pictures of breast structures. An ultrasound uses sound waves to create sonograms of areas inside the breast. A biopsy can confirm the types of breast cancers. Options include fine-needle aspiration, core biopsy, and open biopsy. If breast cancer is diagnosed, other *staging* tests are done to determine whether cancer cells have spread within the breast or to different areas.

Treatment

Breast cancer treatment is based on the type and degree of the cancer spreading. Often, more than one type of treatment is used. Options include surgery, chemotherapy, hormonal therapy, biological therapy, and radiation therapy.

Prevention

There is no sure way to prevent breast cancer, but there are ways to lower the risks of the disease. These include attaining and maintaining a healthy weight, being physically active, avoiding or limiting alcohol, and choosing to breastfeed infants for at least several months after childbirth. When possible, avoid hormone therapy after menopause. For women at increased risk of breast cancer, options include genetic counseling and testing for breast cancer risks, medications that lower chances, prophylactic surgery, and close observations to monitor for early signs of breast cancer. Genetic counseling is indicated for women with a strong family history of breast cancer or with a family member with a known breast cancer-related gene mutation.

YOU SHOULD REMEMBER

Being obese is linked to a higher risk of getting 13 types of cancer, which make up 40% of all cancers diagnosed annually. These include meningioma, adenocarcinoma of the esophagus, multiple myeloma, kidney, uterine, ovarian, thyroid, breast, liver, gallbladder, upper stomach, pancreatic, and colon cancers.

Check Your Knowledge

1. How much more common are social and psychological problems in obese individuals?
2. What are the statistics between obesity and cancer?
3. What are advanced breast cancers signified by?

COLON CANCER

Colon cancer is also commonly referred to as *colorectal cancer*. It is widespread, with more than 50% of cases affecting the rectum and sigmoid colon. About 95% are adenocarcinomas. Insulin is the primary biochemical mediator between obesity and colon cancer. Hyperinsulinemia is essential for the pathogenesis of colon cancer. Visceral abdominal fat is linked to a higher incidence of colon cancer. Obesity results in a higher risk of colon cancer for men of all ages and for premenopausal women, but not for postmenopausal women.

Epidemiology

Colon cancers are a significant cause of morbidity and mortality throughout the world, accounting for over 9% of all cancers. Colon cancer is the third most common cancer worldwide and the fourth most common cause of death, affecting men and women almost equally. The American Cancer Society's estimate for colon cancer in the United States is approximately 135,000 new cases. Overall lifetime risk is about 1 in 22 men and 1 in 24 women. More than 1 million people are living with this type of cancer in the United States. Countries with the highest incidence include Australia and New Zealand, while countries with the lowest incidence include China and India. Worldwide statistics reveal that colon cancer represents about 9.4% of all cancers in men and approximately 10.1% of all cancers in women.

Colon cancer accounts for more than 50,000 deaths in the United States every year. Incidence increases sharply around the ages of 40 and 50. Costs of colon cancer interventions generally begin at around $14,000 and increase based on the severity of the malignancy.

Etiology and Risk Factors

Colon cancer may occur as a transformation of adenomatous polyps. Approximately 80% of cases are sporadic, with the rest being inherited. The risk factors include chronic ulcerative colitis and Crohn's disease. The diets high in animal protein, fat, and refined carbohydrates with low fiber also account for the risk factors.

Clinical Manifestations

Symptoms of colon cancer include diarrhea, constipation, rectal bleeding, blood in the stool, cramping, fatigue, tiredness, and weight loss.

Diagnosis

The diagnosis of colon cancer includes colonoscopy, biopsy, and blood tests. A colonoscopy can show the entire colon and rectum. Tissue biopsies are often collected during a colonoscopy. Blood tests are used to give clues about overall health, including liver and kidney function, but not actually for the diagnosis of colon cancer. Blood tests can reveal low levels of red blood cells, which may indicate internal bleeding caused by colon cancer. The blood tests can also reveal **carcinoembry-onic antigen** (CEA) over time, indicating whether the tumor responds to treatment. After treatment, CEA blood tests can show if the cancer has recurred.

Treatment

Treatment for colon cancer usually involves surgical removal. A minimally invasive approach can be used if the tumor is microscopic. This may include removing polyps during a colonoscopy, endoscopic mucosal resection, and **laparoscopic surgery**. For more advanced colon cancer, options include partial **colectomy**, surgery to create a port so that feces can leave the body and lymph node removal. If the tumor is highly advanced and metastases, chemotherapy, radiation therapy, targeted therapy, immunotherapy, and palliative care are other options.

Prevention

There is no proven method of preventing colon cancer. However, regular screening is a powerful tool that may help catch the disease early. It allows polyps to be found and removed before they have enough time to become cancerous. Screening can also find colon cancer when it is small and more accessible to treat. Screening should begin at age 45. People with a strong family history of colon polyps or cancer may benefit from genetic counseling to determine whether there is a family cancer syndrome. Risks for colon cancer can be lowered by weight management, physical activity, and diet. Little or no alcohol consumption is beneficial, and smoking should be stopped.

YOU SHOULD REMEMBER

Compared to people of average weight, obese men have about a 50% higher risk of colon cancer. Obese women have almost a 10% higher risk for the disease than nonobese women. Excess risk is also linked to higher abdominal fat, measured by waist circumference or the waist-to-hip ratio, and fat stored in the abdominal cavity.

Check Your Knowledge

1. What is the primary biochemical mediator between obesity and colon cancer?
2. In populations with a high incidence of colon cancer, what do the diets consist of?
3. What is the most common treatment for colon cancer?

GALLBLADDER CANCER

Gallbladder tumors, plus bile duct tumors, can cause extrahepatic biliary obstruction. Nearly all are adenocarcinomas. Papillary adenocarcinoma is a rare type with cells with finger-like projections. Papillary cancers are generally less likely to spread to the liver or lymph nodes and have a better prognosis than most other types of gallbladder adenocarcinomas. Gallbladder tumors may also be adenosquamous carcinomas, squamous cell carcinomas, and carcinosarcomas, but these are rarer. **Cholangiocarcinoma** forms in bile ducts that connect the gallbladder to the liver. They may be described as *intrahepatic, hilar,* or *distal.*

Epidemiology

Cholangiocarcinomas and other bile duct tumors occur in 1 to t2 of every 100,000 individuals but are usually malignant. *Gallbladder carcinoma* occurs in 2.5 of every 100,000 individuals, mainly in American Indians, patients with gallstones larger than 3 cm, and those with signifi-cant gallbladder calcification due to chronic cholecystitis. Between 70% and 90% of patients also have gallstones. Most people who develop cholangiocarcinomas are over age 50, but these tumors can form at any age. Compared to people of average weight, individuals who are overweight have about a 20% higher chance of gallbladder cancer. However, obese people have a 60% increase in this risk, and the risk increase is more significant in women than in men.

Etiology and Risk Factors

The causes of gallbladder cancer are not fully understood, but chronic inflammation and irritation of the gallbladder are believed to influence the development of tumors. Risk factors for cholangio-carcinomas include obesity, old age, primary sclerosing cholangitis, choledochal cysts, and infestation with liver flukes. Other risks include chronic liver disease, bile duct abnormalities that have been present since birth, and smoking.

Gallbladder cancer results from persistent irritation of the gallbladder mucosa over years. This predisposes an individual to malignant transformations or acts as an enhancer for carcinogenic exposure. However, gallbladder cancer is strongly related to gallstone disease, the female gender, and an age above 65 years.

Clinical Manifestations

The primary signs and symptoms of gallbladder cancer include jaundice, **pruritus**, darker urine, and a paler color of the feces. Additional manifestations include loss of appetite or unintended weight loss.

Diagnosis

Blood tests and imaging of the gallbladder are used to diagnose gallbladder cancer. Blood tests to evaluate liver function can help determine the cause of any signs or symptoms. Imaging tests include ultrasound, CT, and MRI. Procedures such as exploratory surgery and examinations of the bile ducts can determine the staging of cancer.

Treatment

Gallbladder cancer has various treatment options based on staging. In stage 1, the tumor is localized in the gallbladder; it can be removed by surgery. Stage 2 (unresectable) cancer cannot be obliterated by surgery. Unfortunately, most patients with gallbladder cancer have unresectable cancer. Recurrent (stage 3) gallbladder cancer may appear in the gallbladder or other parts of the body. Metastatic (stage 4) gallbladder cancer may occur in surrounding tissues, organs, the abdominal cavity, or distant body areas. The treatment of gallbladder cancers includes **cholecystectomy**, radiation therapy, targeted therapy, and immunotherapy.

Prevention

There is no known way to prevent most gallbladder cancers since risk factors such as age, gender, ethnicity, and bile duct defects are beyond our control. Methods of reducing risk factors include attaining and maintaining a healthy weight, keeping physically active, limiting the time spent sitting or lying down, and following a healthy diet with plenty of fruits, vegetables, and whole grains (limiting red and processed meats, sugary drinks, and highly processed foods), plus avoiding alcohol.

Check Your Knowledge

1. What is the most common type of gallbladder cancer?
2. Do obese people have a higher chance of developing gallbladder cancer?
3. What does gallbladder cancer result from?

PANCREATIC CANCER

Most forms of pancreatic cancer involve exocrine tumors, developing from ductal and acinar cells. Adenocarcinomas of the exocrine pancreas develop from duct cells nine times more often than from the acinar cells. They commonly occur in the head of the pancreas. The disease is rare before age 40 and is most common in people older than 70. Approximately 12% of all pancreatic cancers are attributed to being overweight or obese. Obese women carrying most of their excess weight around their waist instead of their hips have a 70% higher chance of developing pancreatic cancer.

Epidemiology

The American Cancer Society's estimates for pancreatic cancer in the United States are nearly 57,000 cases and over 46,000 deaths. Prevalence is estimated to be 1 in 64 people. The highest incidence and mortality rates are in developed countries. Globally, about 338,000 people have pancreatic cancer, making it the 11th most common cancer overall. Trends for incidence and mortality vary widely on a global scale. The 5-year survival rate is about 5% (2% and 9% between developed and developing countries). The highest incidence is in North America and Western Europe, with the lowest rates in Middle Africa and South-Central Asia.

Adenocarcinomas appear at a mean age of 55 years. They occur 1.5–2 times as often in men compared to women. About 1.6% of the population will be diagnosed with pancreatic cancer at some point in life. Overall, pancreatic cancer ranks as the seventh leading cause of cancer death for both genders in the United States.

Etiology and Risk Factors

Pancreatic cancer is fundamentally a disease caused by damage to the DNA. Mutations of DNA can be genetic or by human behaviors. Risk factors include smoking, a history of chronic pancreatitis, gender, obesity, and the African-American race. Alcohol and caffeine consumption are not direct risk factors unless consumption is heavy. A smoker's chance of developing pancreatic cancer decreases after stopping smoking and nearly returns to the risk level for the remainder of the population after 20 years of being tobacco-free. Risks increase with age, and obesity increases relative risks by about 50%. Chronic pancreatitis is believed to triple the risks of pancreatic cancer. Diabetes mellitus is another risk factor since type 2 diabetes, present for more than 10 years, has an almost 50% increased risk.

Clinical Manifestations

The signs and symptoms include abdominal pain and weight loss, but these are nonspecific to the disease until it is later diagnosed because of metastasis. Upon diagnosis, 90% of patients have locally advanced tumors involving retroperitoneal structures, spread to regional lymph nodes, or metastases to the liver or lungs. Severe upper abdominal pain radiation to the back affects most patients, and weight loss is common. When the cancer is in the head of the pancreas, obstructive jaundice leading to **pruritus** occurs in 80%–90% of patients. If the tumor is in the body or tail of the pancreas, there may be splenic vein obstruction, causing splenomegaly, gastric and esophageal varices, and GI bleeding. Between 25% and 50% of patients may develop diabetes, leading to polyuria and polydipsia. The cancers can also lead to pancreatic exocrine insufficiency and malabsorption, resulting in watery, greasy, foul-smelling bloating, gas, and diarrhea. This results in more weight loss and vitamin deficiencies.

Diagnosis

The diagnosis of pancreatic cancers is via computed tomography (CT) or magnetic resonance imaging (MRI)/magnetic resonance cholangiopancreatography (MRCP), followed by endoscopic ultrasonography. Endoscopic ultrasonography with fine-needle aspiration is done for tissue diagnosis and to assess surgical resectability. Routine laboratory tests are also needed to determine the presence of any other conditions.

Treatment

Treatment includes the Whipple procedure, adjuvant chemotherapy, and radiation therapy (see **Figure 24.3**). Medications for pain management include transdermal fentanyl, oxycodone, and oxymorphone. Medication for pruritus includes cholestyramine. It is essential to monitor and maintain a healthy weight for pancreatic cancers. Patients must remain hydrated with at least 64 ounces of fluids per day. Small, frequent meals are indicated. High-protein meals are essential, including baked, grilled, or boiled lean meats, eggs, nut butter, low-fat dairy products, beans, soy products such as tofu, and protein bars. Protein drinks, bone broths, shakes from Greek yogurt or high-protein milk, pureed soups, and smoothies are also suggested. It is essential to choose foods that are easy to digest, such as chopped, soft, or boiled foods. Essential whole grains include oatmeal, whole-grain bread, brown rice, whole-grain pasta, bulgur, corn, farro, and quinoa. Whole fruits and vegetables are highly antioxidants, so at least five servings should be consumed daily. Healthy fats include olive and canola oils, avocados, seeds, nuts, and fatty fish. Sweets and added sugars must be limited. Changes in bowel habits may prompt the addition of dietary alterations or the need for supplemental pancreatic enzymes. Regular exercise helps stimulate appetite.

Prevention

Pancreatic cancer cannot be prevented. However, people can reduce the risk by maintaining a healthy weight, stopping smoking, and limiting alcohol intake. Avoiding workplace exposure to specific chemicals can decrease the risk of pancreatic cancer.

UTERINE CANCER

Endometrial carcinoma is most often an **endometrioid adenocarcinoma**. It is usually signified by vaginal bleeding after menopause has occurred. This cancer is staged via surgical procedures. It begins in the endometrial lining of the uterus and is often detected early since it frequently produces abnormal vaginal bleeding. If discovered early, removal of the uterus is quite usually curative. The upper two-thirds of the uterus, above the internal orifice, is described as the *corpus*. Cancer of the corpus uteri is additionally referred to as endometrial cancer.

Epidemiology

In the United States, endometrial carcinoma is the fourth most common female cancer. It accounts for 6% of all cancers in women and is the most common gynecologic malignancy. About 1 in 40 women will develop endometrial cancer. Approximately 62,000 new cases are diagnosed each year,

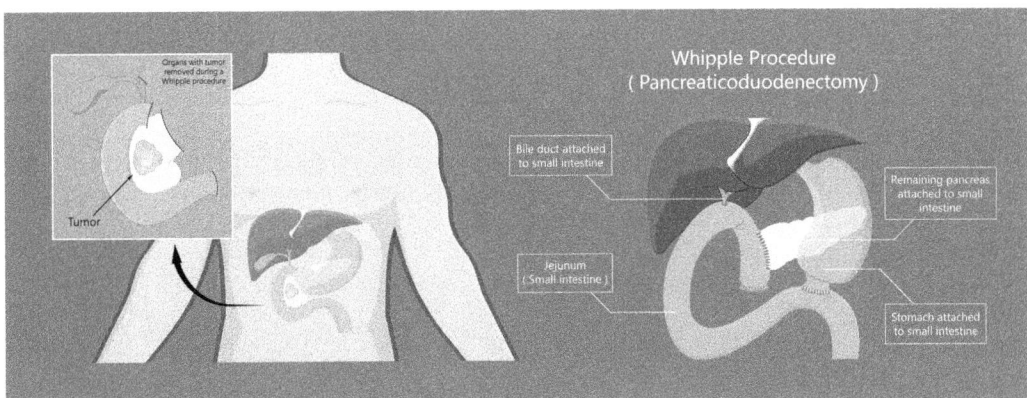

FIGURE 24.3   The Whipple procedure.

and over 12,250 patients are fatal. Caucasian women are affected more than any other racial or ethnic group. Worldwide, more than 287,000 women are diagnosed with endometrial carcinoma annually. As the prevalence of metabolic syndrome increases, this cancer is anticipated to become more common. Incidence has been rising in most countries, which is believed to be linked to increasing rates of obesity, having fewer children, and delaying childbirth until later in life. Endometrial carcinoma is more common in developed countries with diets that are high in fat. This type of cancer is most common in perimenopausal and postmenopausal women. The mean age at diagnosis is 63 years. Most cases are diagnosed between 50% and 60%, and 92% occur in women older than 50. It rarely develops before age 40 (less than 5% of women).

Etiology and Risk Factors

The significant causes of endometrial cancer include age over 50, obesity, and diabetes mellitus. Additional risk factors include the use of tamoxifen for 5 or more years, receiving previous pelvic radiation therapy, personal or family history of breast or ovarian cancer, family history of hereditary nonpolyposis colorectal cancer, and hypertension. Unopposed estrogen involves high circulating estrogen levels, with no progesterone or low levels of progesterone. This may be concerning obesity, nulliparity, polycystic ovary syndrome, estrogen-producing tumors, late menopause, anovulation, and estrogen therapy without progesterone.

Clinical Manifestations

Over 90% of women with endometrial carcinoma have abnormal uterine bleeding, such as postmenopausal bleeding or premenopausal recurrent **metrorrhagia**. About 33% of women with postmenopausal bleeding are found to have endometrial carcinoma. Vaginal discharge may occur weeks or months before postmenopausal bleeding. Additional signs and symptoms include bleeding between periods and pelvic pain.

Diagnosis

The diagnosis of endometrial carcinoma includes pelvic examinations, a transvaginal ultrasound, hysteroscopy, and biopsy. A dilation and curettage may be performed to obtain enough tissue.

Treatment

There are several methods of treatment for uterine cancer, including surgery, radiation, and chemotherapy.

Prevention

There is no way to prevent uterine cancer. Still, methods that can reduce risks include the use of birth control pills, maintaining a healthy weight, being physically active, and, if taking estrogen, adding progesterone.

PREVENTION OF OBESITY

Primary prevention of obesity involves preventing disease before it becomes a problem. Healthy habits that prevent obesity include a good diet, physical activity, healthy weight, stress management, and good sleep quality.

TREATMENTS OF OBESITY

The obesity treatments include initial modest weight loss of 5%–10% of the total body weight by changing eating habits and increasing physical activity. Dietary changes to treat obesity include cutting calories, feeling full on fewer foods, making healthier choices, restricting certain foods, and meal replacements. Behavior changes can be achieved through counseling and support groups.

There is growing interest in the pharmacological treatment of obesity. Before 2012, there were few weight loss medications approved by the FDA. The top medications were phentermine and orlistat (Xenical and Alli). Novo Nordisk is the only US company with FDA-approved semaglutide products, identified under the trade names Wegovy®, Ozempic®, and Rybelsus®.

YOU SHOULD REMEMBER

Endoscopic procedures include sleeve gastroplasty and intragastric balloon placement. Bariatric surgeries include adjustable gastric banding, gastric bypass surgery, and the gastric sleeve procedure, in which part of the stomach is removed.

Check Your Knowledge

1. Is the increased incidence of uterine cancer linked to the increasing rates of obesity?
2. What are the significant risk factors for endometrial cancer?
3. What preventive measures may reduce these risks?

METABOLIC SYNDROME

Metabolic syndrome is related to being overweight, obese, and inactive, plus the condition known as insulin resistance. It is increasing the risks of type 2 diabetes.

Metabolic syndrome involves inflammation, hypercoagulability, and hyperinsulinemia. It is also called *Syndrome X*. Fibrinogen increases in response to high levels of cytokines. It is an acute-phase reactant. Significantly, metabolic syndrome may predispose patients to even more severe complications, such as type 2 diabetes mellitus, heart attack, and stroke.

EPIDEMIOLOGY

Metabolic syndrome is expected in the United States. About one out of every three adults have it.

ETIOLOGY AND RISK FACTORS

The causes of metabolic syndrome include obesity, excessive amounts of fatty tissue, glucose intolerance, hypercholesterolemia, hyperinsulinemia, hypertension, hypertriglyceridemia, and older age. The primary causes of metabolic syndrome are insulin resistance and obesity. Approximately 50% of cases are caused by genetic factors. Because of aging, a genetic predisposition to insulin resistance in voluntary muscle and the liver is worsened by a loss of muscle mass.

CLINICAL MANIFESTATIONS

The signs and symptoms of metabolic syndrome include excess fat around the waist, hyperglycemia, hypercholesterolemia, hypertriglyceridemia, and hypertension. Metabolic syndrome involves having at least three out of five health conditions that increase the risk of cardiovascular disease, stroke, and type 2 diabetes. It can cause other complications as well. It is made worse by abdominal obesity, anxiety, corticosteroids, depression, hypogonadism, infection, lack of aerobic exercise, sleep deprivation, and smoking – fat distribution related to male patterns, mainly the abdomen. In obese women, fat is deposited primarily in the buttocks. Buttock and thigh fat are subcutaneous and are predominantly stored fat with low metabolic activity.

DIAGNOSIS

The criteria for diagnosing metabolic syndrome include having at least three out of five health conditions that increase the risk of cardiovascular disease, stroke, and type 2 diabetes. It can also cause other complications, such as abdominal obesity, BMI above 25, insulin resistance, hypertriglyceridemia, hypercholesterolemia, hypercoagulation, hypertension, and hyperglycemia.

TREATMENT

Management of metabolic syndrome includes controlling BP, lowering LDL cholesterol, increasing HDL cholesterol, and lowering triglycerides. Treatment is also designed to prevent the onset of type 2 diabetes mellitus. Medications can be added when lifestyle changes are entirely practical. These include metformin, statins, and antihypertensives. Allopurinol may also reduce insulin resistance and symptoms of metabolic syndrome. Supplements include alpha lipoic acid, green tea or green tea extract, glycine powder, raspberry ketone, bitter melon extract, potassium, and omega-3 fatty acids.

PREVENTION

Smoking cessation or avoidance means that risks of metabolic syndrome are lowered. Another factor linked to metabolic syndrome is sleep deprivation. Lifestyle modifications include better diets and increased physical activity.

Clinical Case Studies

CLINICAL CASE STUDY 1

An obese 64-year-old man was taken to the local hospital because of chest pain. He had previously experienced exertional chest tightness and mild shortness of breath after minimal physical activity. These symptoms did not occur at rest. The patient has a history of type 2 diabetes and hypertension. He quit smoking 25 years ago. Tests reveal high LDL cholesterol and triglycerides, as well as total cholesterol. An exercise test to evaluate his myocardial perfusion has to be stopped after 8 minutes due to chest pain and leg fatigue. The patient's signs and symptoms are highly indicative of peripheral arterial disease, and most patients with this condition have significant coronary artery disease as well. Treatment for his condition begins immediately.

CRITICAL THINKING QUESTIONS

1. How does obesity lead to cardiovascular disorders?
2. Which cardiovascular disorders are complications of obesity?
3. If this patient eventually requires surgery, how is his obesity potentially linked to postoperative complications?

CLINICAL CASE STUDY 2

An obese 24-year-old man was assessed for symptoms of snoring, orthopnea, and restless sleep patterns. He complained of dyspnea, easy tiredness, extreme exercise intolerance, and poor self-esteem. The man's mother was morbidly obese. Obstructive sleep apnea was suspected in the man. He was prescribed a CPAP machine and discharged. Over 1 year of follow-up, the patient complained of headaches, poor work performance, and progressive weight gain. He was determined to be a good candidate for bariatric surgery, and a laparoscopic sleeve gastrostomy operation was performed successfully. After 1 year, the patient's weight dropped significantly, and the sleep apnea entirely resolved.

1. What is the most common form of sleep apnea, and what is it characterized by?
2. How much do weight increases and decreases affect sleep apnea?
3. What are the causes and complicating factors of obstructive sleep apnea?

CLINICAL CASE STUDY 3

A 69-year-old obese woman found a lump in her left breast. She had a history of hypertension and a 25-year history of smoking one pack of cigarettes per day. Her sister recently had a lumpectomy with radiation therapy, and her mother and aunt died from breast cancer when they were in their 60s. The patient states she has too much stress in her life and cannot quit smoking. A bilateral mammogram and ultrasound are performed, revealing a 4 cm mass in her left breast. A core needle biopsy reveals it to be an infiltrating lobular carcinoma. A lumpectomy and axial lymph node dissection are performed, and six of the nodes are positive for cancer. Further treatment options are then discussed.

CRITICAL THINKING QUESTIONS

1. How common is breast cancer, and what does it usually involve?
2. How fatal is breast cancer?
3. How does having a first-degree relative with breast cancer affect the risks of it developing?

FURTHER READING

1. Angrisani, L., De luca, M., Formisano, G., and Santonicola, A. (2017). *Bariatric and Metabolic Surgery: Indications, Complications, and Revisional Procedures (Updates in Surgery)*. Springer.
2. Banks, D. (2017). *Quadruple Threat: Obesity, Sleep Apnea, Diabetes, and Heart Disease*. Timely Publishing.
3. Crum, C.P., Nucci, M.R., Howitt, B.E., Granter, S.R., Parast, M.M., Boyd, T., Haefner, K.R., and Peters, W.A. (2017). *Diagnostic Gynecologic and Obstetric Pathology*, 3rd Edition. Elsevier.
4. Dannenberg, A.J., and Berger, N.A. (2013). *Obesity, Inflammation and Cancer (Energy Balance and Cancer – 7)*. Springer.
5. Ettinger, S. (2016). *Nutritional Pathophysiology of Obesity and Its Comorbidities: A Case-Study Approach*. Academic Press.
6. Faintuch, J., and Faintuch, S. (2020). *Obesity and Diabetes: Scientific Advances and Best Practice*, 2nd Edition. Springer.
7. Freemark, M.S. (2018). *Pediatric Obesity: Etiology, Pathogenesis, and Treatment (Contemporary Endocrinology)*. Humana Press.
8. Genazzani, A.R., Ibanez, L., Milewicz, A., and Shah, D. (2021). *Impact of Polycystic Ovary, Metabolic Syndrome and Obesity on Women Health: Volume 8: Frontiers in Gynecological Endocrinology (ISGE Series)*. Springer.
9. Govil Bhasker, A., Kantharia, N., Baig, S., Priya, P., Lakdawala, M., and Shah Sancheti, M. (2021). *Management of Nutritional and Metabolic Complications of Bariatric Surgery*. Springer.
10. Kumar, S., and Gupta, S. (2021). *Obesity and Cancer*. Springer.
11. Marini, I., and Stebnicki, M.A. (2017). *The Psychological and Social Impact of Illness and Disability*, 7th Edition. Springer.
12. Martirosyan, D.M. (2009). *Functional Foods for Chronic Diseases, Volume 4: Obesity, Diabetes, Cardiovascular Disorders, and AIDS (Functional Food Science)*. D & A Incorporated.
13. Michaelson, J.A. (2014). *Obesity and Pregnancy: The Dangers and Risks – What You Should Know*. Michaelson.
14. Moini, J., Ahangari, R., Miller, C., and Samsam, M. (2020). *Global Health Complications of Obesity*. Elsevier.
15. Pischon, T., and Niptsch, K. (2016). *Obesity and Cancer (Recent Results in Cancer Research)*. Springer.
16. Ramonde, P.R., and Fochas, E.H. (2009). *Obesity and Cancer Research*. Nova Biomedical.

17. Tappia, P.S., Ramjiawan, B., and Dhalla, N.S. (2020). *Pathophysiology of Obesity-Induced Health Complications (Advances in Biochemistry in Health and Disease).* Springer.
18. Tulasi Latha, A. (2022). *Obesity: Causes, Complications, and Strategies for Weight Loss.* Lap Lambert Academic Publishing.
19. Woodward, B.G. (2006). *A Complete Guide to Obesity Surgery: Everything You Need to Know about Weight Loss Surgery and How to Succeed.* Trafford Publishing.
20. Youness, E.R., and El Toukhy, S.E. (2020). *Obesity: (the) Most Common Metabolic Complication in Prader-Willi Syndrome.* Scholars' Press.

25 Electrolyte and Acid-Base Imbalance

OVERVIEW

The human body's fluids are organized into functional compartments, which must be maintained orderly for everyday health. The composition and distribution of fluids in the internal environment and the roles of various body organs and functions are vital to understanding disorders related to body fluids. Electrolytes dissolved in the body fluids are essential for nearly every life process. As electrolytes move through cell membranes, electrical events occur, influencing nerve conduction, muscle contraction, and metabolic reactions. The body fluids' acidity or alkalinity is maintained within very narrow limits. Nearly all organ systems participate in fluid balance and can be affected by an imbalance. Many diseases alter fluid balance to damage organs or cause them to malfunction. The best treatment results are based on correctly evaluating fluid and electrolyte balances and administering appropriate treatments. Understanding the makeup of body fluids, pathologic changes to standard processes, and how to correct these changes is crucial.

COMPOSITION OF BODY FLUIDS

The **universal solvent** in which many **solutes** are dissolved is water. Solutes are widely classified as *electrolytes* and *nonelectrolytes*. Electrolytes are chemical compounds that dissociate water into *ions*. The ions are charged particles that conduct an electrical current. Electrolytes consist of inorganic salts, inorganic and organic acids and bases, and some proteins. The **nonelectrolytes** have **covalent bonds**, which stop them from dissociating in a solution. Therefore, no electrically charged species are formed as nonelectrolytes dissolve in water. Most nonelectrolytes are organic molecules, including *creatinine*, glucose, lipids, and **urea**.

All dissolved solutes contribute to a fluid's **osmotic** activity, but electrolytes have a much stronger osmotic power than nonelectrolytes since every electrolyte molecule dissociates into two or more ions. For example, a sodium chloride (NaCl) molecule contributes two times as many particles of solute as glucose, which remains undissociated. One molecule of magnesium chloride ($MgCl_2$) contributes three times as many. Water constantly moves according to osmotic gradients, from an area with less **osmolality** to an area with more osmolality. Therefore, electrolytes have the most substantial ability to cause fluid shifts in the body.

The body's fluid separates into two main compartments: intracellular and extracellular. Of the 42 L of water in the body, two-thirds is within the intracellular fluid (ICF) space, equating to 28 L. Each fluid compartment has a unique pattern of electrolytes. The extracellular fluids are similar except for plasma's relatively high protein content. Sodium is their primary **cation**, while chloride is their major **anion**. **Plasma** contains fewer chloride ions than **interstitial fluid** since the non-entering **plasma proteins** are usually anions, and plasma is electrically neutral. However, the **interstitial compartment fluid** (ICF) has only small amounts of sodium and chloride. The most abundant cation is potassium, while the primary anion is hydrogen phosphate. The cells also have large quantities of soluble proteins, about three times higher than the amount in plasma.

The sodium and potassium ion concentrations in the **extra compartment fluid** (ECF) and ICF are practically opposite. These distributions indicate the activity of cellular adenosine triphosphate (ATP)-dependent **sodium-potassium pumps**. These pumps keep intracellular sodium ion concentrations low while potassium ion concentrations remain high. The most abundant solutes in body

DOI: 10.1201/9781003453376-32

fluids determine most chemical and physical reactions, yet they do not make up the majority of dissolved solutes in these fluids. Most comprise large molecules, including proteins and nonelectrolytes, such as cholesterol, phospholipids, and triglycerides. These makeup approximately 97% of the ICF, 90% of the mass of dissolved solutes in plasma, and about 60% of dissolved solutes in the interstitial fluid.

Check Your Knowledge

1. What are the two primary fluid compartments in the human body?
2. What is the difference between each fluid compartment?
3. What is the function of sodium-potassium pumps?

REGULATION OF WATER INTAKE

Water intake is regulated by thirst, which receptors in the hypothalamus trigger. These respond to as little as 2% increased plasma osmolality or decreased body fluid volume. In rare cases, hypothalamic dysfunction reduces thirst capacity. Water excretion by the kidneys is regulated mainly by the **antidiuretic hormone** (ADH), also called vasopressin. ADH increases water reabsorption in the distal nephron. The release of vasopressin is stimulated by increased plasma osmolality, decreased blood volume, and blood pressure. The release of vasopressin can be impaired by substances such as ethanol or phenytoin and posterior pituitary tumors. Water intake decreases plasma osmolality. If the plasma osmolality is low, the secretion of vasopressin is inhibited. This allows the kidneys to produce diluted urine.

REGULATION OF WATER OUTPUT

The kidneys can regulate water levels in the body; they conserve water if a person is dehydrated and make urine more dilute to expel excess water when necessary. Water is lost through the skin through evaporation without overt sweating, and air is expelled from the lungs. Specific amounts of water output cannot be prevented. These obligatory water losses show why humans cannot survive long without drinking fluids. Zero water intake will eventually overcome all of the conservation efforts of the kidneys. Mandatory water loss includes **insensible water** losses, **sensible water** loss of 500 mL/day or more in the urine, and water in undigested food residues in the feces. Obligatory water loss in the urine indicates that the kidneys usually flush 600 mmol of urine solutes daily out of the body water. These solutes, in part, are the end products of metabolism. The maximum concentration of urine is approximately 1,200 mm. Therefore, at least 500 mL of water must be excreted.

Aside from obligatory water loss, the solute concentration and volume of excreted urine are based on fluid intake, diet, and other water loss. A person who sweats heavily on a hot day must pass much less urine than usual to maintain water balance. In normal conditions, the kidneys start eliminating excess water about 30 minutes after it has been taken in. The delay indicates the time needed for the release of ADH to be inhibited.

YOU SHOULD REMEMBER

Diabetes insipidus is a rare, treatable condition in which the body produces too much urine, resulting in polyuria and polydipsia due to a deficiency of ADH. It is mainly caused by an abnormality in the creation and use of ADH. It can be temporary or chronic and mild or severe. Large volumes of urine must be voided daily, and the affected person must drink large amounts of water due to constant thirst.

Check Your Knowledge

1. What are sensible water loss and insensible water loss?
2. What regulates the most water excretion by the kidneys?
3. What do obligatory water losses include?

PATHOLOGY OF WATER BALANCE

Most humans need to understand how vital water is for maintaining the body's peak functions. The primary pathologies of water balance include **dehydration**, hypotonic dehydration, and edema. Fluid imbalance can be related to **hypovolemia**, normovolemia with fluid maldistribution, and hypervolemia.

DEHYDRATION

Dehydration occurs when less fluid is consumed, or more fluid is lost. The body then has insufficient fluids to function normally. Trauma is among the most common causes of hypovolemia, with its often extensive related blood loss. Another common cause is dehydration, which primarily involves a loss of plasma rather than whole blood. Dehydration can be caused by diarrhea, vomiting, sweating, urine abnormalities, fever, an inability to consume enough fluid (such as through unconsciousness), burns, poorly controlled diabetes mellitus, and diabetes insipidus due to a deficiency of ADH. In healthy people, it can occur after heavy exercise, in hot or dry environments, at high altitudes–due to more rapid breathing–or by ignoring thirst.

Usually, the thirst mechanism is controlled by the *hypothalamic thirst center*. This center is activated by **osmoreceptors** that detect extracellular fluid osmolality. The saliva glands then produce less saliva as the osmotic gradient that draws water from the blood into the salivary ducts is reduced – dry mouth results. Next, there is a decrease in blood volume or pressure. If substantial, this also triggers the thirst mechanism. Changes in volume or pressure are signaled by **baroreceptors**, which directly activate the thirst center, and by **angiotensin II**. Baroreceptors in the heart and carotid arteries also affect kidney function by reducing blood pressure and volume. **Table 25.1** summarizes the effects of dehydration based on the extent of water weight lost. With extended physical

TABLE 25.1
The Effects of Dehydration, Based on the Extent of Water Lost

Percentage of Water Weight Lost	Effects
Up to 2%	Thirst
2%–3%	Stronger thirst, slight discomfort and a feeling of oppression, loss of appetite, increased hemoconcentration
4%–5%	Less movement, slow pace, flushed skin, impatience, weariness, sleepiness, apathy, nausea, emotional instability
6%–7%	Tingling, stumbling, headache, faintness, dizziness, fatigue, nausea, increased body temperature, increased pulse, increased respiratory rate, labored breathing, cyanosis
8%–9%	Indistinct speech, increased weakness, mental confusion
10%	Muscle cramps, inability to balance while the eyes are closed, general incapacity, delirium, wakefulness, tongue swelling, circulatory insufficiency, extreme hemoconcentration and decreased blood volume, failing kidney function
11% or higher	Increased risk of death, especially if dehydration is linked to an illness or extreme heat or exercise

activity, 3–8 cups (750–2,000 mL) can be lost per hour. It is essential to plan to have enough water available to maintain hydration.

Mild to moderate dehydration is signified by dry mouth and skin, fatigue, headache, dizziness, confusion, fatigue, dry mouth, chills, decreased urine output, and deep yellow urine. With progressive dehydration, tachycardia, hypotension, and constipation. If the loss of fluid continues, there can be kidney failure, seizures, **delirium**, and coma. Treatment is simply replacing lost fluids. When dehydration is severe, fluid replacement requires medical supervision. Without replenishment, strict progression will lead to death. To avoid exercise-related dehydration, it is essential to consume fluids adequately. This means before, during, and after exercise, as follows:

- *Before exercise*–drink water or sports drinks during the day before the activity begins, even if you are not very thirsty; drink two to three cups (500–750 mL) of fluid 2–3 hours before training, allowing for enough hydration and excretion of excess fluid; drink 250–375 mL of fluid 10–15 minutes before exercising or competing–especially if the event will last a long time
- *During exercise*–drink 1–1.5 cups of fluid every 10–15 minutes; fluid replacement is promoted by flavored juices that are cooler than the temperature of the environment; drink sufficient liquid to maintain body weight during exercise; if the activity lasts for 1 hour or more, fluid replacement beverages must contain 4%–8% carbohydrates to keep blood glucose levels; sodium must be included in the liquid (0.5–0.7 g of sodium per liter) to replace the sodium that is lost in the sweat
- *After exercise*–drink three cups of fluid for each pound lost during exercise; restore body weight before the next period of exercise

YOU SHOULD REMEMBER

Dehydration is the most common fluid and electrolyte problem in older people. The usual causes of water loss are often absent in dehydrated elderly patients. Age-related changes in total body water, thirst perception, renal concentrating ability, and the effectiveness of ADH are probably involved. Dehydration related to infection, high-protein tube feedings, cerebral vascular accidents, and medication-related hypodipsia are especially relevant for elderly patients. Appropriate treatment depends on accurately assessing water deficits and slowly correcting them.

YOU SHOULD REMEMBER

Infants younger than 6 months old should never be given water. Although water intoxication is rare, it can occur in infants whose kidneys are not yet fully developed. Without fully functioning kidneys, giving too much water to an infant can cause the removal of sodium from the body, which is crucial for proper nerve function. Hyponatremia can be deadly to an infant.

Check Your Knowledge

1. What are the causes of dehydration?
2. What happens if more than 10% of body water is lost?
3. What should fluid consumption be while a person is exercising?

HYPOTONIC DEHYDRATION

Hypotonic dehydration refers to a decrease in electrolyte concentration in the extracellular fluid. In hypotonic dehydration, the cells expand as water in the extracellular fluid moves toward the higher sodium concentration inside the cells. Reducing ECF osmolality inhibits ADH release. Less water is reabsorbed. Excess water is flushed quickly out of the body via the urine. If renal insufficiency or vast amounts of water are consumed rapidly, hypotonic dehydration may occur. This is a type of cellular overhydration. Either way, the ECF is diluted. It has an average sodium content, but the excess water results in a low sodium concentration. Therefore, the hallmark sign of hypotonic dehydration is hyponatremia. The low ECF sodium ion concentration promotes net osmosis into the tissue cells. Then, they swell due to being abnormally dehydrated. Various underlying conditions can cause hypotonic dehydration. These conditions result in losing body fluids, usually through the skin, GI tract, or kidneys.

Hypotonic dehydration results in severe metabolic disturbances. Signs and symptoms include nausea, vomiting, dizziness, blurred vision, bradycardia, muscular cramping, **cerebral edema,** and unconsciousness. The neurons can be significantly damaged. If uncorrected, cerebral edema quickly causes disorientation, convulsions, coma, and death. People who have run marathon races have died of overhydration after too much water was consumed too quickly. Sudden, severe hyponatremia is treated with IV hypertonic saline. This reverses the osmotic gradient, pulling water out of the cells. Treatment options include oral fluid replacement if the child is conscious and can drink. Water, fluids, and an oral rehydration solution can be used. In severe cases, intravenous fluids should be used.

EDEMA

Edema is an abnormal accumulation of fluid in the interstitial space that occurs as the capillary filtration exceeds the limits of lymphatic drainage, producing noticeable clinical signs and symptoms. Edema can affect any part of the body. But it is more likely to show up in the legs and feet. The four types of edema include peripheral, pulmonary, cerebral, and macular, which are severe complications of diabetic retinopathy.

Epidemiology

Edema can affect anyone, especially people who are pregnant and adults aged 65 and older. The precise epidemiological data and their impact have not been fully elucidated. Primary lymphedema is rare, affecting 1 in 100,000 individuals. Secondary lymphedema is the most common cause of the disease and affects approximately 1 in 1,000 Americans. Up to 250 million people worldwide have lymphedema, with an estimated 10 million living with lymphedema in the United States, more than HIV. More than 1 million patients are admitted each year with a diagnosis of pulmonary edema secondary to heart failure. African Americans have the highest risk for heart failure as the underlying cause of pulmonary edema, and males are more commonly affected by pulmonary edema than women. Cerebral edema affects all age groups, genders, and ethnic groups. The actual frequency of cerebral edema may be underreported secondary to its sometimes non-specific symptoms.

Etiology and Risk Factors

Medicines and pregnancy can cause edema. It can also be the result of a disease, such as congestive heart failure, kidney disease, venous insufficiency, or cirrhosis of the liver. There are different causes and types of edema. For example, **pulmonary edema** affects the lungs, while **pedal edema** causes swelling in the feet. Pulmonary edema occurs when excess fluid collects in the lungs, making breathing difficult. This can result from congestive heart failure or acute lung injury. It is a severe condition, can be a medical emergency, and may lead to respiratory failure and death. Edema usually starts slowly, but the onset can be sudden. It is a common condition but can also be a sign of a severe illness. Severe lymphedema can affect the ability to move the affected limb, increase the risks of skin infections and sepsis, and lead to skin changes and breakdown.

Cerebral edema occurs in the brain. It can happen for many reasons, many of which are potentially life-threatening. These causes include a sedentary lifestyle, too much dietary sodium, premenstrual signs and symptoms, pregnancy because of certain medications (such as those for hypertension, nonsteroidal anti-inflammatory drugs, steroids, estrogens, and thiazolidinediones), and severe conditions such as congestive heart failure, cirrhosis, kidney disease, weakness or damage to leg veins, an inadequate lymphatic system, and a severe chronic protein deficiency. It most often occurs in the skin, especially in the hands, arms, ankles, legs, and feet. However, it can also affect the muscles, bowels, lungs, eyes, and brain (see **Figure 25.1**).

Clinical Manifestations

Signs and symptoms depend on the underlying cause, but swelling, tightness, and pain are common. The skin may retain a "dimple" after a few seconds of pressure, with visible anomalies. There may be puffiness of the ankles, face, or eyes. Weight gain, weight loss, and decreased urine production also occur. Clinical manifestations of pulmonary edema include dyspnea, anxiety, and wheezing. Cerebral edema can be asymptomatic, merely seen on imaging, or it can cause life-threatening complications. The history can help provide insights into the cerebral edema's etiology. Patients may have an account of trauma, a hypoxic event, cancer, metabolic diseases, or other factors that can help identify the possible etiology of cerebral edema. The physical exam findings of cerebral edema can vary widely depending on the location and extent of the edema. Localized cerebral edema can cause dysfunction of the edematous brain, including weakness, visual disturbances, seizures, sensory changes, diplopia, and other neurologic disorders. For diffuse cerebral edema, the patient may have headaches, nausea, vomiting, lethargy, altered mental status, confusion, coma, seizure, or other manifestations. With diffuse or focal cerebral edema, the patient can develop increased intracranial pressure, which typically presents with headaches, nausea, vomiting, lethargy, cranial neuropathy, altered mental status, coma, and death.

Diagnosis

A physical exam and a medical history might be enough to determine the cause. Sometimes, the diagnosis might require blood tests, ultrasound, vein studies, a chest X-ray, a CT scan, and an echocardiogram.

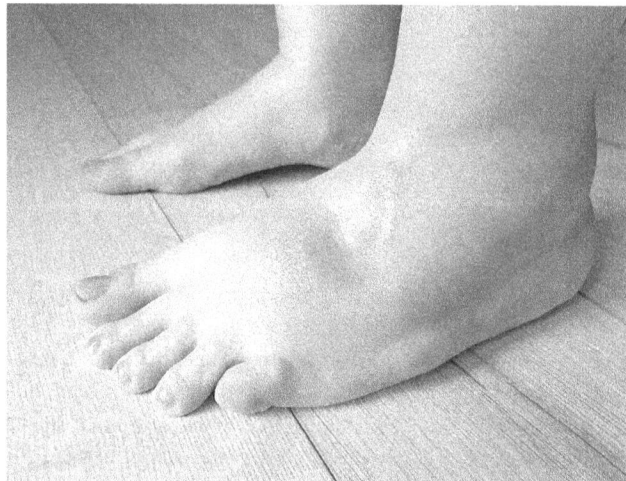

FIGURE 25.1   Edema.

Treatment

Mild edema usually goes away on its own. They wear compression garments, raising the affected arm or leg higher than the heart helps. Treatment depends on the cause of the edema. Wearing compression garments and reducing salt in the diet often relieves edema. When a disease causes edema, the condition needs treatment as well. Diuretics help eliminate excess fluid by increasing the rate of urine production by the kidneys. The first treatment for acute pulmonary edema is oxygen. Narcotic (morphine) may be taken by mouth or given through an IV to relieve dyspnea and anxiety. However, some care providers believe that the risks of morphine may outweigh the benefits. They're more likely to use other drugs. Antihypertension agents are also helpful.

Prevention

Depending on what is causing the edema, the patient may not be able to prevent it from happening. If it is caused by health problems, such as congestive heart failure, liver disease, or kidney disease, the patient will not be able to prevent it but only manage it. If the condition is caused by overeating salt, it can be prevented by reducing salt. Wearing compression stockings, sleeves, or gloves might help if edema affects an arm or leg. These garments keep pressure on the limbs to prevent fluid from building up. Usually worn after the swelling goes down, they help prevent more swelling. Moving and using the muscles in the swollen part of the body, especially the legs, might help move fluid back toward the heart. Hold the swollen part of the body above the level of the heart several times a day. Sometimes, raising the swollen area during sleep can be helpful. Stroking the affected area toward the heart using firm, but not painful, pressure might help move fluid out of that area.

Check Your Knowledge

1. What are the causes of peripheral edema?
2. What are the signs and symptoms of pulmonary edema?
3. What is the diagnosis of cerebral edema?

ELECTROLYTE BALANCE

The body can actively move electrolytes in or out of cells to adjust fluid levels. Thus, having electrolytes in the proper concentrations is essential in maintaining fluid balance among the compartments. The kidneys help maintain electrolyte concentrations. The term electrolyte balance primarily refers to sodium balance in the body. Salts are essential for controlling fluid movements. However, many electrolytes are needed for cellular activity. Regulating sodium, potassium, calcium, and phosphate is most important for electrolyte balance. The flexibility of the kidney's mechanisms that regulate the blood's electrolyte balance is essential. Renal regulation of sodium ions is based on the effects of **aldosterone**.

The kidneys mainly regulate potassium balance. The distal convoluted tubule and collecting ducts achieve potassium balance primarily by changing how much potassium is secreted into the filtrate. **Atrial natriuretic peptide** lowers blood pressure and blood volume by relaxing smooth muscles in the walls of blood vessels.

Estrogens are similar hormones to aldosterone and enhance sodium chloride reabsorption by the renal tubules. Since water follows, many women retain fluid when estrogen levels increase during menstrual cycles. Estrogens are highly responsible for edema, as experienced by many women during pregnancy. Oppositely, **progesterone** has a slight diuretic effect, which is believed to be because it blocks aldosterone receptors. **Glucocorticoids** enhance the tubular reabsorption of sodium ions and promote a higher glomerular filtration rate, which can obscure their effects on the tubules. Another factor is that glucocorticoids have strong aldosterone-like effects when their plasma levels are high, promoting edema. The parathyroid hormone regulates calcium in the extracellular fluid.

ELECTROLYTE IMBALANCE

An electrolyte imbalance occurs when certain mineral levels in the blood get too high or too low. An electrolyte imbalance occurs when a lot of body fluid is lost. The most important electrolytes in body fluids include potassium, sodium, chloride, phosphate, magnesium, and calcium. All of these are important for normal body functions. Burns, medications for chronic kidney disease, insufficient food and fluids, chronic respiratory diseases, and the use of laxatives or steroids may cause electrolyte imbalances. Symptoms of an electrolyte imbalance vary depending on the severity and electrolyte type, including weakness and muscle spasms. Cramps, dizziness, an irregular heartbeat, and mental confusion. Other symptoms include tachycardia, fatigue, **lethargy**, nausea, vomiting, diarrhea, constipation, muscle weakness, irritability, headaches, numbness, and tingling. Conditions caused by electrolyte level imbalances include hyponatremia, hypernatremia, hypochloremia, hypophosphatemia, hyperphosphatemia, hypokalemia, and hyperchloremia. These conditions were discussed in **Chapter 17**.

YOU SHOULD REMEMBER

To prevent electrolyte imbalance, drink plenty of water during physical activity, eat a balanced diet containing electrolyte-rich foods, and avoid strenuous activity outdoors during hot weather. If you are working out inside, do not do it without an air conditioner, especially if you sweat heavily.

ACID-BASE IMBALANCE

Acid-base imbalance results in disorders due to pathologic changes in carbon dioxide partial pressure (PCO_2) or serum bicarbonate (HCO_3^-). They usually produce abnormal arterial pH values. Acidemia exists if the serum pH is below 7.35. Alkalemia exists if it is above 7.45. **Acidosis** causes either the accumulation of acid or the loss of alkali. **Alkalosis** causes either the accumulation of alkali or the loss of acid. Actual pH changes are based on the amount of physiologic compensation and whether multiple processes are present. Primary acid-base disturbances are either metabolic or respiratory, based on whether the main change is in the serum PCO_2 or HCO_3^-.

The pH establishes whether acidosis or alkalosis is the primary process but will move toward the normal range as compensatory efforts occur. Changes in the PCO_2 indicate the respiratory component, while changes in the HCO_3^- indicate the metabolic part. Metabolic and respiratory acidosis and alkalosis are further described here. A *simple acid-base disorder* is an acid-base disturbance with no accompanying compensatory response. A complex acid-base disease consists of two or more primary troubles. Compensated or mild acid-base infections only cause a few signs or symptoms. Severe uncompensated acid-base disorders have many respiratory, cardiovascular, neurologic, and metabolic outcomes. The types of acidosis and alkalosis can be classified as metabolic or respiratory.

METABOLIC ACIDOSIS

The buildup of acid in the body due to kidney disease or kidney failure is called **metabolic acidosis.** There are several types of metabolic acidosis, such as:

- Diabetic acidosis, or diabetic ketoacidosis – develops when ketone bodies build up during uncontrolled diabetes (usually type 1 diabetes)
- Hyperchloremic acidosis – is caused by the loss of too much sodium bicarbonate from the body, which can happen with severe diarrhea.

- Kidney disease (uremia, distal renal tubular acidosis, or proximal renal tubular acidosis)
- Lactic acidosis
- Poisoning by aspirin, ethylene glycol (antifreeze), or methanol
- Severe dehydration

Epidemiology

Metabolic acidosis is a sign of underlying pathology, and while it is not uncommon, especially in acutely ill patients, the overall prevalence in the population is uncertain.

Etiology and Risk Factors

Causes of metabolic acidosis include the accumulation of ketones and lactic acid, renal failure, anemia, heart failure, malnutrition, cancer, **septicemia**, drug or toxin ingestion, unmanageable diarrhea, and renal HCO_3^- loss. Lactic acidosis can be caused by cancer, carbon monoxide poisoning, drinking too much alcohol, exercising vigorously for a very long time, liver failure, medicines such as salicylates and metformin, seizures, and prolonged lack of oxygen from severe anemia, shock, and heart failure.

Clinical Manifestations

Many patients may develop headaches, confusion, nausea and vomiting, long and deep breaths, tachycardia, tachypnea, tiredness, and fatigue. Severe metabolic acidosis can lead to shock or death. In some situations, metabolic acidosis can be mild or chronic.

Diagnosis

Blood tests for metabolic acidosis may include an **anion gap**. A group of blood tests that measure the sodium and potassium levels, kidney function, and other chemicals and functions. Blood and urine ketones, lactic acid test, urine ketones, and urine pH.

Treatment

The management of metabolic acidosis should address the cause of the underlying acid-base derangement. For example, adequate fluid resuscitation and correction of electrolyte abnormalities are necessary for sepsis and diabetic ketoacidosis. Other therapies include antidotes for poisoning, dialysis, antibiotics, and bicarbonate administration in certain situations.

Prevention

Preventing metabolic acidosis includes reducing risk factors, drinking lots of water and other fluids, and managing blood sugar levels if you have diabetes.

YOU SHOULD REMEMBER

The anion gap helps determine the cause of the metabolic acidosis. An elevated anion gap in metabolic acidosis can be caused by salicylate toxicity, diabetic ketoacidosis, and uremia. Non-gap metabolic acidosis is due to GI loss of bicarbonate (diarrhea) or a failure of the kidneys to excrete acid.

METABOLIC ALKALOSIS

Metabolic alkalosis develops from excessive bicarbonate in body fluids due to various conditions. This condition is higher than 28 mEq/L (28 mmol/L). It is caused by acid loss or retention of HCO_3^-. The blood pH increases. Metabolic alkalosis is much less common than metabolic acidosis.

Epidemiology

The mortality rate with metabolic alkalosis is 45% with an arterial blood pH of 7.55%–80% with an arterial blood pH of 7.65.

Etiology and Risk Factors

Common causes include vomiting, gastric suctioning that removes too much of the normal stomach secretions, and the intake of excess bases, such as from too many antacids. Other causes include excessive use of baking soda, diuretics, certain laxatives, or steroids. Medical conditions that can cause metabolic alkalosis include cystic fibrosis, electrolyte imbalances, hyperaldosteronism, hypochloremia, and cyclic vomiting syndrome. People at risk for metabolic alkalosis include those with severe, repeated vomiting, critical illnesses, dehydration, or if gastric suctioning is needed to rid the stomach of abnormal fluid or gas buildup, a poison, or a medication overdose.

Clinical Manifestations

Symptoms include irritability, muscle twitching or cramping, muscle spasms, fatigue, confusion, tremors, tingling, numbness, arrhythmias, seizures, and coma. Healthcare assistance is required once arrhythmias, seizures, or confusion develop.

Diagnosis

The condition is diagnosed via physical examination, blood tests to measure blood gases, acid-base balance, electrolyte levels, an electrocardiogram, and urinalysis.

Treatment

Severe symptoms require immediate treatment. Options include saline infusion, potassium and magnesium replacement, chloride infusion, hydrochloric acid, and stopping causative medications.

Prevention

One prevention method is addressing the underlying cause. This may involve modifying treatments for other medical conditions. Reduce taking water pills and antacids.

RESPIRATORY ACIDOSIS

Respiratory acidosis occurs when the lungs cannot remove carbon dioxide produced by the body, resulting in the blood becoming too acidic. This condition is signified by a PCO_2 higher than 40 mm Hg (**hypercapnia**). It is also called respiratory failure or ventilatory failure. Some people with chronic respiratory acidosis develop the acute form when a critical illness disrupts the acid-base balance. Acute respiratory acidosis develops quickly before the kidneys can rebalance body fluids.

Epidemiology

The epidemiology of respiratory acidosis is quite varied based on the cause. End-stage COPD patients are more likely to develop this acid-base disorder. Also, surgical patients are at a greater risk.

Etiology and Risk Factors

Respiratory acidosis typically occurs due to an underlying disease or condition.

It is caused by hypoventilation. Physiologically, the lungs can eliminate carbon dioxide via **Kussmaul breathing**, a respiratory compensation for metabolic acidosis. Other causes include asthma, chronic obstructive pulmonary disease (COPD), pneumonia, **pulmonary fibrosis, scoliosis**, medications (such as opioids or benzodiazepines, often when combined with alcohol), severe obesity, and obstructive sleep apnea. Respiratory acidosis is a common cause of acid-base imbalances and may be related to pneumonia, cystic fibrosis, or **emphysema**, which all cause carbon dioxide to accumulate in the blood. The blood pH falls while the partial pressure of carbon dioxide rises (see **Figure 25.2**).

Clinical Manifestations

Respiratory acidosis can be acute or chronic; the chronic form is asymptomatic, but the acute or worsening condition causes headache, wheezing, cyanosis, confusion, restlessness, and drowsiness. Signs include tremors, possible seizures, delirium, lethargy, myoclonic jerks, **asterixis**, and coma.

Diagnosis

The diagnosis is clinical and involves arterial blood gas and serum electrolyte measurements. Blood gas measures oxygen and CO_2 in the blood, and electrolyte testing is also required. Lung function tests, such as spirometry, lung volume, gas diffusion, and exercise tests, must also be performed.

Treatment

Treating acute respiratory acidosis usually involves addressing the underlying cause. The patient should receive treatment immediately. The patient may require artificial ventilation through a machine, which assists with breathing and gas transfer without requiring invasive tubing. Medications for treating respiratory acidosis include antibiotics, diuretics, bronchodilators, and corticosteroids.

Prevention

The best way to prevent respiratory acidosis is to avoid the potential causes of the disease.

RESPIRATORY ALKALOSIS

Respiratory alkalosis occurs when high levels of carbon dioxide disrupt the acid-base balance of the blood. This condition is signified by a PCO_2 less than 28 mm Hg (**hypocapnia**). Respiratory alkalosis occurs when carbon dioxide is eliminated faster than it can be produced. The blood, therefore, becomes more alkaline. Respiratory alkalosis and uncontrolled breathing often require immediate medical care in a hospital. The disorder may be prevented by learning methods of coping with stress, anxiety, pain, and anger.

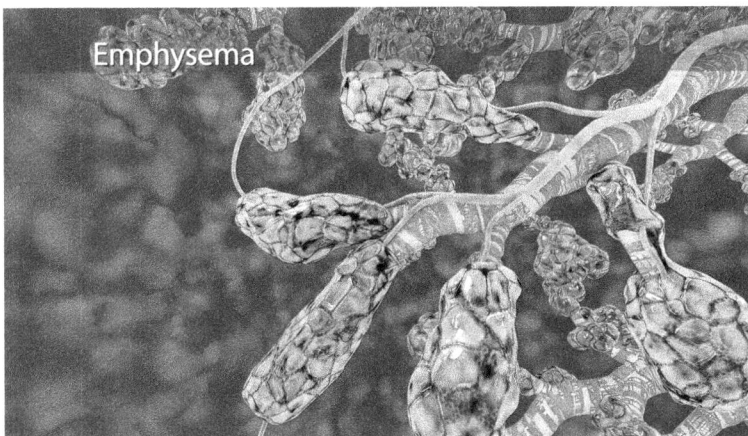

FIGURE 25.2 Damage to the walls of the lung alveoli in emphysema.

Epidemiology

Respiratory alkalosis is the most common acid-base abnormality, and there is no discrimination between genders. The disease's exact frequency and distribution depend on its etiology, morbidity, and mortality rates.

Etiology and Risk Factors

Respiratory alkalosis is caused by increased minute ventilation (hyperventilation). This condition is often related to stress or pain. Other causes of hyperventilation include anxiety, panic, fever, pregnancy, lung cancer, trauma, severe anemia, liver disease, overdose of salicylates or progesterone, pulmonary embolism, asthma, and stroke. People at risk for respiratory alkalosis are those experiencing intense stress, anxiety, panic, or anger. Patients receiving mechanical ventilation are also at risk.

Clinical Manifestations

Symptoms include breathlessness, dizziness, numbness, tingling, irritability, nausea, muscle spasms or twitching, fatigue, lightheadedness, fainting, chest discomfort, shortness of breath, tremors, and confusion.

Diagnosis

With a comprehensive preliminary differential diagnosis list, evaluation should always begin with a thorough history and physical exam to focus on diagnostic considerations. In all cases, arterial blood gas is necessary to diagnose the pH imbalance. Serum electrolytes should be measured with particular attention to sodium, potassium, and calcium levels, as aberrations in these may lead to further complications. Magnesium and phosphate are also essential to measure in hypoxic patients. A chest X-ray is necessary in all patients as it helps discern an anatomical or infectious cause and may rule in/out pulmonary edema. A chest CT can play a vital role in achieving a diagnosis if there is a clinical reason. If there is appropriate clinical suspicion for a neurological insult, a CT or MRI of the head may be right, along with a lumbar puncture for WBC, glucose, and protein analysis.

Treatment

Treatments are based on the underlying cause and focus on increasing blood carbon dioxide levels. Treatment includes supplemental oxygen and therapies to reduce the risk of hyperventilation.

Prevention

Preventive techniques include psychotherapy, relaxation techniques, lifestyle changes, and medications such as antidepressants. It is essential to build a support system of others who can help the patient regain control of rapid breathing before it progresses to hyperventilation.

Clinical Case Studies

CLINICAL CASE STUDY 1

A 62-year-old man was brought to the emergency department because his mental status had changed throughout a single morning. His family reported he had not been eating or drinking as much as usual recently, and he had canceled his weekly social activities, which included playing golf and going to the theater. Past medical history included hypertension, hyperlipidemia, and osteoarthritis. He was also in the early stages of dementia. Upon examination, the patient had signs of wasting, dry mucous membranes, and confusion. He was relatively alert and could follow commands but with some difficulty. Laboratory tests revealed that he had hypernatremia.

CRITICAL THINKING QUESTIONS

1. What are the common causes of hypernatremia?
2. What are the main functions of sodium in the body?
3. Is sodium the central extracellular or intracellular cation, and what are its concentrations in these fluids?

CLINICAL CASE STUDY 2

A 29-year-old woman was brought to the emergency department by relatives after experiencing sudden stiffness and weakness in her arms and legs, plus a lack of sensation and loss of mobility in her left leg. She also felt short of breath, anxious, and sweating heavily. Examination revealed signs of dehydration, and her heart rate was speedy. Laboratory tests revealed hypokalemia, hypochloremia, hypomagnesemia, and alkalemia. She also had a urinary tract infection. Immediate treatment was undertaken, and the patient's electrolytes were normalized within just 1 day of hospitalization.

CRITICAL THINKING QUESTIONS

1. Why is hypokalemia potentially very dangerous?
2. What are the causes of hypomagnesemia?
3. What are the neurologic and respiratory outcomes of alkalemia?

CLINICAL CASE STUDY 3

A 4-year-old boy was taken to the hospital by his parents due to a GI illness and severe dehydration. He had been having diarrhea for a few days, which started as watery and yellow but then turned to a red color with visible clots. The boy also had severe abdominal cramping. Additional symptoms included vomiting and malaise. Examination revealed abdominal tenderness and altered mental status. Vital signs included hypertension and tachycardia. Blood tests showed significant leukocytosis and slight thrombocytopenia. Blood and stool specimens were collected for culture. The patient was started on fluids for rehydration therapy.

CRITICAL THINKING QUESTIONS

1. What can dehydration be caused by?
2. When dehydration is severe, what does fluid replacement require?
3. What is hypotonic dehydration?

FURTHER READING

1. Andersson, D., Mastenbjork, M.D., and Meloni, S. (2018). *Fluids and Electrolytes: A Thorough Guide Covering Fluids, Electrolytes, and Acid-Base Balance of the Human Body.* Anderson/Mastenbjork/Meloni.
2. Connor, G.J. (2021). *Fluids and Electrolytes: A Fast and Easy Way to Understand Acid-Base Balance without Memorization.* Connor.
3. Habibzadeh, F., Yadollahie, M., and Habibzadeh, P. (2021). *Pathophysiologic Basis of Acid-Base Disorders.* Springer.
4. Hale, A., and Hovey, M.J. (2013). *Fluid, Electrolyte, and Acid-Base Imbalances: Content Review plus Practice Questions.* F.A. Davis.
5. Hassan Ketan, S. (2013). *A Guide for Management: Fluids and Electrolytes – Imbalances.* Scholars' Press.
6. Haws, J., and Haws, S. (2015). *A Nursing Guide to Fluids & Electrolytes and Acid-Base Balance.* CreateSpace Independent Publishing Platform.
7. Healy, Z. (2021). *Acid-Base Disturbance Cases (Critical Concept Mastery Series).* McGraw-Hill.

8. Hogan, M.A., Gingrich, M.M., Overby, P., and Ricci, M.J. (2006). *Fluids, Electrolytes, & Acid-Base Balance: Reviews & Rationales*, 2nd Edition. Prentice Hall.

9. Jameson, J.L., and Loscalzo, J. (2016). *Harrison's Nephrology and Acid-Base Disorders*, 3rd Edition. McGraw-Hill/Medical.

10. Johnson, J. (2018). *Fluids and Electrolytes Demystified*, 2nd Edition. McGraw Hill/Medical.

11. Kamel, K.S., and Halperin, M.L. (2016). *Fluid, Electrolyte, and Acid-Base Physiology: A Problem-Based Approach*, 5th Edition. Elsevier.

12. LeFever Kee, J., Paulanka, B.J., and Polek, C. (2009). *Handbook of Fluid, Electrolyte, and Acid-Base Imbalances*, 3rd Edition. Cengage Learning.

13. Mastenbjork, M., Meloni, S., and Andersson, D. (2018). *Fluids and Electrolytes: A Thorough Guide covering Fluids, Electrolytes, and Acid-Base Balance of the Human Body*. Medical Creations.

14. Nurse Academy. (2021). *Fluids and Electrolytes: A Quick and Easy Comprehensive Book to Understand the Acid-Base Balance of the Human Body – Clinical Assessment and Management*. Nurse Academy.

15. Preston, R.A. (2017). *Acid-Base, Fluids, and Electrolytes Made Ridiculously Simple*, 3rd Edition. MedMaster.

16. Reddi, A.S. (2014). *Fluid, Electrolyte and Acid-Base Disorders: Clinical Evaluation and Management*. Springer.

17. Rudiger Kulpmann, W., Stummvoll, H.K., and Lehmann, P. (2006). *Electrolytes, Acid-Base Balance and Blood Gases: Clinical Aspects and Laboratory*, 2nd Edition. Springer.

18. Schrier, R.W. (2017). *Renal and Electrolyte Disorders*, 8th Edition. Lippincott, Williams, & Wilkins.

19. Stephaniak, J. (2016). *The Acid-Alkaline Diet: Balancing the Body Naturally*. Live Healthy Now.

20. Tinawi, M. (2021). *Manual of Fluid, Electrolyte, and Acid-Base Disorders: A Pathophysiologic Approach to Common Clinical Problems*. Tinawi.

26 Malabsorption and Digestive Enzyme Deficiency

OVERVIEW

Malabsorption involves problems with the body's ability to absorb nutrients from food. Many diseases can cause malabsorption. It often involves absorbing certain sugars, fats, proteins, or vitamins. However, it can also cause an overall problem with absorbing food. Problems or damage to the small intestine may lead to problems absorbing essential nutrients. Enzymes produced by the pancreas help absorb fats and other nutrients. Decreased enzymes make it harder to absorb fats and certain nutrients. Cystic fibrosis, celiac disease, Crohn's disease, irritable bowel syndrome, pancreatic cancer, and chronic pancreatitis may cause exocrine pancreatic insufficiency, which can lead to malnutrition. Chronic pancreatitis is the main cause of enzyme deficiency in adults. Digestive enzyme deficiencies can lead to malnutrition and gastrointestinal symptoms.

MALABSORPTION SYNDROMES

Malabsorption is the failure of the intestinal mucosa to absorb the digested nutrients. However, **maldigestion** is often caused by deficiencies of enzymes, such as pancreatic lipase or intestinal lactase, which are necessary for digestion. Inadequate secretion of bile salts and inadequate reabsorption of bile in the ileum also contribute to maldigestion—malabsorption results from mucosal disruption. Gastric or intestinal resection, vascular disorders, or intestinal disease cause it. Various enzymes are involved in the digestion of foods. For example, amylase metabolizes carbohydrates and disaccharides to form monosaccharides. Unabsorbed carbohydrates are fermented by bacteria in the large intestine, forming carbon dioxide, hydrogen, and **methane**. Lipase and colipase from the pancreas split long-chain triglycerides into monoglycerides and fatty acids. Gastric **pepsin** stimulates the release of **cholecystokinin**. The brush border enzyme known as **enterokinase** activates trypsinogen into **trypsin**. This converts many of the pancreatic proteases into their active forms.

EPIDEMIOLOGY

Malabsorption affects millions of people worldwide. Malabsorption syndromes have multiple etiologies, which makes their prevalence and incidence unknown. However, some malabsorption syndromes can be estimated by discussing the epidemiology of subgroups. The prevalence of celiac disease in the United States is 1:13, and it is common in Caucasians of northern European ancestry. The incidence of Crohn's disease appears to be higher in Jews.

ETIOLOGY AND RISK FACTORS

Maldigestion and malabsorption may be caused by insufficient pancreatic enzymes, bile salts, gastric or intestinal resection, vascular disorders, or intestinal disease. Celiac disease is an example of a disorder that impairs the absorption of most nutrients, vitamins, and trace minerals. Fat malabsorption is the most common malabsorption syndrome, arising from fat digestion and absorption defects. Chronic pancreatitis, cystic fibrosis, pancreatic resection, celiac disease, gastric surgery, **Zollinger-Ellison syndrome**, and hepatic cirrhosis impair bile acid synthesis.

DOI: 10.1201/9781003453376-33

CLINICAL MANIFESTATIONS

Unabsorbed substances, especially when there is malabsorption of many nutrients, can cause abdominal bloating, diarrhea, gas, and **steatorrhea**. Additional symptoms are due to nutritional deficiencies. The affected individual eats adequate amounts of food yet loses weight. The most common symptom is chronic diarrhea. The hallmark of malabsorption is steatorrhea, which occurs when more than 7 g of fat per day is excreted. The stool is bulky, greasy, foul-smelling, and pale in color. In advanced malabsorption, there are severe vitamin and mineral deficiencies. Symptoms are based on the specific nutrient deficiency, as follows:

- *Iron*–hypochromic or microcytic anemia
- *Folate and vitamin B12*–macrocytic anemia
- *Vitamins C and K*–bleeding, bruising, and petechiae
- *Calcium and magnesium*–carpopedal spasm
- *Proteins*–edema
- *Vitamins B1, B2, B3, B6, B12, and folate, iron, niacin*–glossitis
- *Vitamin A*–night blindness
- *Calcium, magnesium, potassium, vitamin D*–pain in the limbs and bones; pathologic fractures
- *Vitamins B1, B2, B12*–peripheral neuropathy

Vitamin B12 deficiency can occur in **blind loop syndrome** or following an extensive stomach or distal ileum resection. With mild malabsorption, iron deficiency may be the only present symptom.

DIAGNOSIS

The diagnosis of malabsorption syndromes is based on the patient's history and symptoms. A history of chronic GI disease or surgery may increase the risk of malabsorption.

TREATMENT

Treatment of malabsorption syndromes includes correcting deficiencies, treating the underlying cause, and treating symptoms. For malabsorption syndromes, patients may be put on special supplemental nutrition that is more easily digested and absorbed and given nutritional supplements. Dietary therapy includes a high-protein, high-calorie, low-fat diet, which will help minimize steatorrhea. Adequate treatment requires monitoring serum calcium, magnesium, vitamin D, and parathyroid hormone levels and, ideally, 24-hour urinary collections for calcium. Supplementation of these mineral deficiencies requires continual close observation to prevent hypercalcemia. Foods high in calcium include dairy products, soybeans, dark green leafy vegetables, calcium-fortified foods, salmon, figs, flour tortillas, and baked beans. Foods high in magnesium include many choices: nuts, seeds, whole grains, wheat germ, and wheat and oat bran. Foods high in vitamin D include cod liver oil, swordfish, tuna, fortified orange juice, dairy and plant milk, sardines, and beef liver.

PREVENTION

Malabsorption syndromes can be prevented by changing the diet, eating more fiber, taking digestive enzyme supplements, and chewing food well.

YOU SHOULD REMEMBER

Malabsorption syndromes prevent the body from effectively absorbing foods. Most cases result from damage to the small intestine's mucous lining, where most absorption occurs. Malabsorption syndromes can lead to indigestion and malnutrition.

YOU SHOULD REMEMBER

Zollinger-Ellison syndrome is a rare condition in which one or more tumors grow in the pancreas or the upper part of the small intestine. The tumors are called gastrinomas, which produce a large amount of gastrin hormone.

Check Your Knowledge

1. What are the differences between maldigestion and malabsorption?
2. What are the causes of malabsorption?
3. What is the hallmark sign of malabsorption syndrome?

CELIAC DISEASE

Celiac disease, also known as gluten enteropathy, is an immunologically mediated disease. It occurs in genetically susceptible people who have a gluten intolerance. This results in mucosal inflammation and villous atrophy in the small intestine, causing malabsorption. The actual sensitivity is to the *gliadin* fraction of gluten.

Epidemiology

People of northern European descent are commonly affected. The disorder may affect 1 in every 150 European people (mainly in Ireland and Italy) and as many as 1 in every 250 Americans. However, there are estimated prevalence rates as high as 1 in every 100 people in Northern Africa, Northern India, and Southern Asia. Celiac disease affects 10%–20% of first-degree relatives. Women are affected twice as often as men, with onset usually during childhood, though it can occur later. Risks for celiac disease are higher in people who have **Down syndrome**, lymphocytic colitis, **Hashimoto thyroiditis**, and type 1 diabetes mellitus.

Etiology and Risk Factors

An abnormal immune reaction to eating gluten causes celiac disease. The risk factors include family history, type 1 diabetes, and Down syndrome. A higher number of GI tract infections in infants and young children may also increase the risk factor.

Clinical Manifestations

Signs and symptoms are wide-ranging, with some people being asymptomatic, having signs of a nutritional deficiency, or having extreme GI symptoms. Celiac disease can occur during infancy and childhood once cereals are introduced into the diet. There will be apathy, failure to thrive, anorexia, generalized **hypotonia**, pallor, abdominal distention, and muscle wasting. The stool is bulky, clay-colored, foul-smelling, and soft. Older children may have anemia or slowed growth. Anorexia, **lassitude**, and weakness are the most common signs in adults. The symptoms may be mild, intermittent diarrhea, steatorrhea, and weight loss. The patients often have anemia, angular stomatitis, **aphthous ulcers**, and **glossitis** (see **Figure 26.1**).

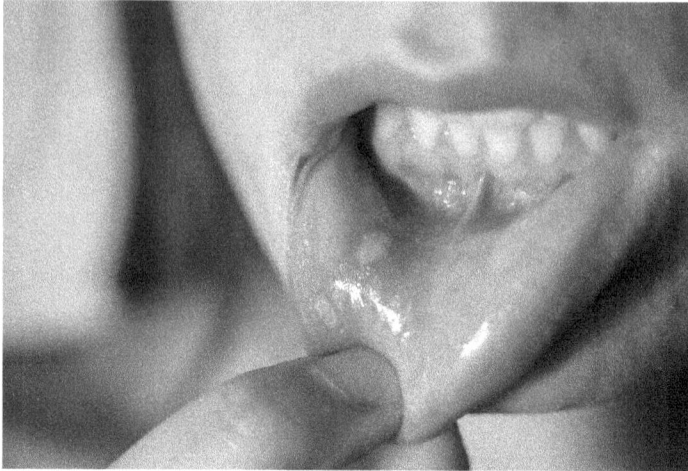

FIGURE 26.1   Aphthous ulcers.

Diagnosis

If the antibody or genetic screening tests are positive, an endoscopic small intestine biopsy must be done. The biopsy can confirm the disease. For children, a biopsy may be avoided when the antibody is positive, and directly starting a gluten-free diet will be recommended.

Treatment

The best treatment for celiac disease is to follow a gluten-free diet for life. This means avoiding gluten-related foods and beverages, like wheat, rye, barley, and triticale.

Prevention

Prevention requires a gluten-free diet to prevent symptoms and damage to the small intestine. All foods containing wheat, rye, or barley must be avoided.

Check Your Knowledge

1. Which group of people is mainly affected by celiac disease?
2. What are the signs and symptoms of celiac disease?
3. What is the likelihood of cancer from celiac disease?

CARBOHYDRATE INTOLERANCE

Carbohydrate malabsorption occurs when the main dietary carbohydrates, sugars, and starches are not absorbed from the small intestine. Sugars include monosaccharides (glucose, galactose, fructose) and disaccharides (lactose, sucrose, maltose). Starches include polysaccharides and consist of glucose sugars linked together. *Carbohydrate intolerance* involves an inability to digest carbohydrates because of a lack of one or several intestinal enzymes. As bacteria ferment carbohydrates, carbon dioxide, hydrogen, and methane gases are produced. There is excessive flatulence, bloating, distension, and abdominal pain.

Epidemiology

The incidence of carbohydrate intolerance is higher in patients with diabetes and Turner syndrome. In the United States, about 36% of people have lactose malabsorption. Worldwide, approximately 65% of adults are affected by lactose malabsorption. Lactose intolerance is also more common in people of West African, Arab, and Jewish descent, while only about 5% of people of northern European descent are lactose intolerant.

Etiology and Risk Factors

Enzyme deficiencies can be congenital or acquired. Congenital deficiencies include rare deficiencies of lactase or sucrase-isomaltase. *Acquired lactase deficiency* (primary adult **hypolactasia**) is the most common carbohydrate intolerance. *Secondary lactase deficiency* is caused by damage to the small intestine mucosa, such as celiac disease, acute intestinal infections, or **tropical sprue**. Congenital enzyme deficiencies are rare and include deficiencies of lactase or sucrase-isomaltase.

Clinical Manifestations

Signs and symptoms of carbohydrate intolerance include diarrhea, bloating, nausea, and abdominal cramps. Diarrhea may be so severe that other nutrients are purged before they can be absorbed. Symptoms mimic those of irritable bowel syndrome. The prognosis is variable since there is no available cure.

Diagnosis

The diagnosis of carbohydrate intolerance is based on clinical symptoms and a hydrogen breath test (also called the lactose breath test). It is the most accurate lactose intolerance test and can inform whether patients are intolerant to sugars such as lactose or fructose. Small intestinal bacterial overgrowth can cause a false positive result test, which is unreliable. An intestinal biopsy must confirm lactase deficiency following the discovery of elevated hydrogen in the hydrogen breath test.

Treatment

Avoiding dietary sugars that cannot be absorbed makes it easy to control carbohydrate intolerance. Many patients can ingest up to 375 mL (18 g of lactose) of milk daily without symptoms. Yogurt and cheese contain lower amounts of lactose than milk and are often tolerated, depending on the amount ingested. Enzyme supplements may be an adjunct to, not a substitute for, dietary restriction. Lactose-intolerant patients must also take calcium supplements.

Prevention

Carbohydrate intolerance cannot be prevented since the causes of enzyme deficiency are unknown. The patients must have a diet restricted to lactose.

YOU SHOULD REMEMBER

Symptoms of lactose intolerance are similar to those in some other digestive disorders, such as irritable bowel syndrome or inflammatory bowel disease. Some people have both lactose intolerance and other disorders of the GI system, like irritable bowel syndrome.

Check Your Knowledge

1. How does carbohydrate intolerance develop?
2. What is the most common type of carbohydrate intolerance?
3. What is secondary lactase deficiency?

CROHN'S DISEASE

Crohn's disease (CD) is a chronic transmural inflammatory bowel disease. It is also known as *regional enteritis*. In most cases, the distal ileum and colon are affected, though effects can occur anywhere in the GI tract. The disease starts with **crypt** inflammation and abscesses that can progress to tiny focal aphthoid ulcers. The mucosal lesions may form deep longitudinal and transverse ulcers and mucosal edema. As the inflammation undergoes transmural spread, lymphedema, the bowel walls, and the mesentery thicken. The mesenteric fat usually extends onto the serosal surface of the intestine. Significant inflammation may cause hypertrophy of the muscularis mucosae, fibrosis, and the formation of strictures – leading to bowel obstruction.

Epidemiology

Approximately 3 million people in the United States have CD. The prevalence of CD has an incidence of 3–20 cases per 100,000. Crohn's disease is more common in the industrialized world, particularly in North America and Western Europe. However, the incidence is rising in Asia and South America. There may be a slightly higher predominance of CD in women, and it is more common in individuals of Ashkenazi Jewish origin than in non-Jews. The disease can occur at any age; it is most prevalent in adolescents and adults between the ages of 15 and 35.

Etiology and Risk Factors

The causes of CD are unknown, but the risk factors for CD development appear to be related to changes in the gut microbiome or disruptions to the intestinal mucosa and genetics.

Clinical Manifestations

The signs and symptoms of Crohn's disease include chronic diarrhea, abdominal pain and tenderness, a sometimes palpable mass, fever, anorexia, and weight loss, except for isolated colonic disease that mimics ulcerative colitis. About one in every three patients has **perianal fistulas** that can be severe. In children, extraintestinal signs and symptoms are often more serious than GI symptoms. Presenting symptoms include arthritis, anemia, fever of an unknown origin, and growth retardation. Abdominal pain and diarrhea are sometimes not present. If there is a severe abscess, the patient may have significant tenderness, rebound, and an overall appearance of toxicity. Stenotic segments may cause bowel obstruction that results in colicky pain, distention, constipation, and vomiting.

While no special diet has been proven to help alleviate the symptoms of Crohn's disease, some foods, such as those high in dietary fiber and fat, dairy products, and carbonated beverages, worsen the condition. Patients should eat small meals every 3–4 hours and stay hydrated by drinking small amounts of water throughout the day. When symptoms are absent, they can consume whole grains, fruits, and vegetables. Starting new foods one at a time, in small amounts, is essential.

Diagnosis

There is no single test to diagnose Crohn's disease. However, a combination of tests, including blood tests, stool studies for occult blood, colonoscopy, CT scan, and MRI, may help to confirm the diagnosis.

Treatment

There is currently no cure for Crohn's disease, and there is no single treatment that works for everyone. One goal of medical treatment is to reduce the inflammation that triggers the signs and symptoms. Another goal is to improve the long-term prognosis by limiting complications. In the best cases, this may lead not only to symptom relief but also to long-term remission.

Prevention

There is no method of prevention, but symptoms and flare-ups can be minimized by stopping smoking and eating a healthy, low-fat diet.

YOU SHOULD REMEMBER

The prognosis for Crohn's disease is varied due to intermittent exacerbations and remissions. If the disease is severe, the pain can be frequent and debilitating. Outcomes are improved with careful choices of medications and surgery. Disease-related deaths are extremely low. The leading cause of excessive disease-related death is GI cancer of the small and large intestines. Often, during active Crohn's colitis, thromboembolic complications can lead to death.

Check Your Knowledge

1. How can bacterial overgrowth occur in the GI system?
2. How can Crohn's disease cause bowel obstruction?
3. What are the causes of Crohn's disease?

SHORT BOWEL SYNDROME

Short bowel syndrome (SBS) is a group of malabsorption conditions resulting from massive resection of the small intestine. Extensive resection may be needed because of Crohn's disease, mesenteric infarction, cancer, congenital anomalies, radiation enteritis, or volvulus. The jejunum is most nutrients' primary digestive and absorptive site so that resection can be significantly reduced.

EPIDEMIOLOGY

SBS is a rare illness with physical and psychosocial morbidity and mortality. The incidence and prevalence of SBS are challenging to determine because of variations in clinical classifications and geographical variations in healthcare provision.

ETIOLOGY AND RISK FACTORS

SBS may be caused by surgically removing half or more of the small intestine. Surgery can be performed to treat Crohn's disease, injury or trauma to the small intestine, or congenital disabilities. SBS is a common cause of chronic intestinal failure with increased morbidity, mortality, and poor quality of life.

CLINICAL MANIFESTATIONS

The symptoms and severity of SBS vary from patient to patient. Diarrhea is common and often severe, and it can cause dehydration, which can even be life-threatening. SBS can lead to malnutrition and weight loss; additional symptoms may be due to losing essential vitamins and minerals. Diarrhea, steatorrhea, cramping, heartburn, dehydration, electrolyte imbalance, and malnutrition are common.

DIAGNOSIS

The diagnosis of SBS includes blood and stool tests to measure nutrient levels. Basic blood tests can determine protein levels, anemia, and electrolytes. Other tests are endoscopy, colonoscopy, a barium X-ray, CT scan, and MRI.

TREATMENT

Treatment options for SBS depend on what parts of the small intestine are affected and whether the colon is intact. Therefore, treatments include nutrition support, fluids, electrolytes, medicines, and surgery. Some patients may receive parenteral nutrition or enteral nutrition. Medications include proton pump inhibitors and antidiarrheals to improve intestinal absorption after surgery. Some patients may have autologous gastrointestinal reconstruction.

YOU SHOULD REMEMBER

Short bowel syndrome is a severe condition because, if left untreated, it can lead to dehydration and malnutrition and can be life-threatening. The extent of the child's problems with SBS usually depends on which sections are affected and how much of the small intestine is affected.

CHRONIC PANCREATITIS

Pancreatitis is either acute or chronic, with *acute pancreatitis* involving inflammation of the pancreas and nearby tissues that resolves. It is usually triggered by alcohol intake and gallstones in 70% or more cases. Severity may be mild, moderately severe, or severe–based on local complications and transient or persistent organ failure. Acute pancreatitis has occurred in susceptible patients after only short periods of high alcohol intake. Low or moderate levels of consumption are related to the progression from acute to chronic pancreatitis. The pancreatic acinar cells metabolize alcohol into toxic metabolites through oxidative and nonoxidative pathways. The cells are predisposed to auto-digestive injury, leading to pancreatic necrosis, inflammation, and cell death. Chronic pancreatitis (CP) is an inflammatory disease characterized by both persistent and irreversible progression of pancreatic lesions that lead to reduced quality of life and a shortened life expectancy. CP is associated with a high incidence of comorbidities, serious complications, and mortality.

EPIDEMIOLOGY

The annual incidence of CP in the United States is 5–8 per 100,000 adults, and the prevalence is 42–73 per 100,000. Globally, the incidence of CP ranges from 5 to 31.7 new cases per 100,000 person-years, and the prevalence of CP ranges from 13.5 to 163 cases per 100,000 individuals. Each year in the United States, more than 80,000 people are diagnosed with CP. Men develop CP at higher rates compared to women. CP is affected more by African Americans than white people.

ETIOLOGY AND RISK FACTORS

The two primary causes of CP are alcohol use and cigarette smoking. The abdominal pain can be continual or wax and wane. The inflammation is progressive and long-lasting. Permanent damage and fibrosis scarring of the pancreas are present. Less common causes of CP include cystic fibrosis, hereditary pancreatitis, and idiopathic or autoimmune pancreatitis. For example, in Nigeria, India, and Indonesia, chronic pancreatitis occurs in children and young adults from unknown causes. This is called **tropical pancreatitis**. CP increases the risk of developing pancreatic cancer. Excessive alcohol intake, obesity, diabetes, cigarette smoking, and family history increase the risks of chronic pancreatitis.

CLINICAL MANIFESTATIONS

The primary symptom of chronic pancreatitis is abdominal pain, which is generally worse after meals and may be reduced by sitting upright or leaning forward. Other symptoms include vomiting, weight loss, fatty stool, chronic diarrhea, and back pain. Chronic pancreatitis may result in pancreatic insufficiency and a decrease in pancreatic enzymes. This can result in malabsorption and steatorrhea. Undigested muscle fibers are sometimes found in the feces. Inadequate absorption leads to undernutrition and vitamin deficiencies. Complications include pancreatic diabetes, pancreatic ascites, pleural effusion, and **pseudocysts**. The pseudocysts can block the bile ducts.

DIAGNOSIS

Chronic pancreatitis can be challenging to diagnose. Family and medical history are essential in diagnosing this illness. Diagnostic tests include laboratory testing, imaging scans, upper endoscopy, endoscopic retrograde cholangiopancreatography (ERCP), and endoscopic ultrasound (EUS).

TREATMENT

Chronic pancreatitis treatment includes analgesics, enzyme replacement, high-protein, high-calorie diets, and surgery such as pancreaticoduodenectomy or total pancreatectomy (see **Figure 24.3**). Drainage and stent placement may manage most complications. Celiac ganglion blockade can decrease pain. Endoscopy is often used to relieve obstruction in the pancreatic duct but only works in 60% of patients.

PREVENTION

Prevention of pancreatitis involves limiting alcohol consumption, eating a heart-healthy diet, exercising regularly to lose excess weight, avoiding crash diets, and quitting smoking.

YOU SHOULD REMEMBER

Tropical chronic pancreatitis (TCP) is a juvenile form of chronic calcific, non-alcoholic pancreatitis. It is seen almost exclusively in the developing countries of the tropical world. The classical triad of TCP consists of abdominal pain, steatorrhea, and diabetes. The prevalence of tropical pancreatitis is about 126 per 100,000 people in southern India. Diets high in cassava (tapioca) predispose individuals to the disease.

Check Your Knowledge

1. What causes short bowel syndrome?
2. How does alcohol intake increase the risk for pancreatitis?
3. What are the two major causes of chronic pancreatitis?

CYSTIC FIBROSIS

Cystic fibrosis (CF) is a progressive genetic disease that affects the lungs, pancreas, and other organs. This condition in the pancreas is also called **mucoviscidosis**. It usually causes death in childhood or young adulthood. Approximately 85% of patients have pancreatic insufficiency. Obstructing the pancreatic ducts with thick mucus blocks the flow of pancreatic enzymes and causes fibrotic changes in the pancreas. Pancreatic damage can eventually affect the beta cells, resulting in diabetes mellitus. Severe problems with maldigestion of proteins, carbohydrates, and fats occur because of insufficient secretion of pancreatic enzymes.

EPIDEMIOLOGY

There are approximately 40,000 people with CF in the United States. An estimated 105,000 people have been diagnosed with CF worldwide. It affects people of every racial and ethnic group. However, it is slightly more common in males. Women have a shortened life expectancy relative to men.

ETIOLOGY AND RISK FACTORS

Cystic fibrosis is an inherited condition in which the lungs and digestive system can become clogged with thick, sticky mucus. It is caused by cystic fibrosis transmembrane conductance regulator (CFTR) gene mutations.

CLINICAL MANIFESTATIONS

Clinical manifestations of cystic fibrosis include **meconium ileus** at birth, which is usually pathognomonic for CF. Poor growth or weight gain in childhood, greasy, bad-smelling stools, and constipation.

DIAGNOSIS

Seventy-two-hour stool fat measurements are used to diagnose pancreatic function. Stools may also be examined for the absence of pancreatic enzymes, particularly fecal elastase, trypsin, and chymotrypsin.

TREATMENT

There is currently no cure for cystic fibrosis, but some treatments are available to help control the symptoms, prevent complications, and make the condition easier to live with. Pancreatic replacement enzymes are administered before or with meals, and high-calorie, high-protein diets with frequent snacks and vitamin supplements are used to treat malnutrition. To combat the worsening problem of growth failure in children with cystic fibrosis, nasogastric or gastrostomy tube feedings are used to supplement oral intake and promote weight gain.

PREVENTION

Since CF is a genetic disease, the only way to prevent or cure it would be with gene therapy at an early age. Amniocentesis and chorionic villus sampling are usually done between 15 and 20 weeks of pregnancy to detect the disease before birth.

YOU SHOULD REMEMBER

All newborns in the United States are screened for CF soon after birth. Finding babies with CF early is essential so that they can start treatment right away, which can help delay or prevent complications of the disorder. Some people with CF show signs of the disorder soon after birth, although in milder cases, signs might not be seen until adulthood.

YOU SHOULD REMEMBER

Today, because of improved medical treatments and care, more than half of people with CF are age 18 or older. Many people with CF can expect to live healthy, fulfilling lives into their 30s, 40s, and beyond.

Clinical Case Studies

CLINICAL CASE STUDY 1

A 17-year-old woman was assessed because of recurrent vomiting, diarrhea, abdominal pain, muscle weakness, fatigue, unintended weight loss, and numbness in her limbs. She had previously been diagnosed with type 1 diabetes mellitus and thyroiditis. After a variety of tests were conducted, the patient was diagnosed with celiac disease.

CRITICAL THINKING QUESTIONS

1. What are the causes and risk factors for celiac disease?
2. What are the signs and symptoms of celiac disease?
3. How can celiac disease be prevented?

CLINICAL CASE STUDY 2

A 24-year-old man was taken to the emergency department because of nausea, vomiting, and abdominal pain. A CT scan revealed ileal thickening and a small bowel obstruction. The patient was hospitalized but developed rectal bleeding. A colonoscopy revealed ulcerations of the ileum and colon, and Crohn's disease was diagnosed. A small bowel study with barium contrast revealed that stenoses and ulcerations extended over the distal 30 cm of the ileum. Treatment was started with medications, which relieved the abdominal pain and bleeding. The diarrhea took longer to correct but was ultimately successfully treated.

CRITICAL THINKING QUESTIONS

1. How does Crohn's disease develop?
2. What are the causes of Crohn's disease?
3. What should patients with Crohn's disease eat when symptoms are not present and when symptoms are present?

CLINICAL CASE STUDY 3

A 48-year-old man was admitted to the hospital complaining of diarrhea, abdominal pain, and general weakness. He had been a heavy drinker for the past 20 years. On examination, he was cachectic, and his abdomen was ascitic. The abdominal CT scan revealed evidence of acute, exacerbated, chronic pancreatitis, including pseudocysts.

CRITICAL THINKING QUESTIONS

1. What are the etiology and risk factors of chronic pancreatitis?
2. How can chronic pancreatitis be diagnosed?
3. What are the treatments for chronic pancreatitis?

FURTHER READING

1. Adams, D.B., Cotton, P.B., Zyromski, N.J., and Windsor, J.A. (2017). *Pancreatitis: Medical and Surgical Management.* Wiley-Blackwell.
2. Caleb, H. (2022). *The Book on Diarrhea Diet: The Best Meal Plan.* Caleb.
3. Corrigan, M.L., Roberts, K., and Steiger, E. (2018). *Adult Short Bowel Syndrome: Nutritional, Medical, and Surgical Management.* Academic Press.
4. DiBiase, J.K., Parrish, C.R., and Thompson, J.S. (2021). *Short Bowel Syndrome.* CRC Press.
5. Gasbarrini, G. (2008). *Malabsorption Syndrome (Digestive Diseases).* S. Karger.
6. Golanna, M. (2022). *Fructose Intolerance Diet: A Beginner's Two-Week Step-by-Step Guide to Managing Fructose Intolerance, with Sample Fructose-Free Recipes and a Meal Plan.* Goanna.
7. Gottschall, E. (2020). *Breaking the Vicious Cycle: Intestinal Health through Diet.* The Kirkton Press.
8. Green, P.H.R., and Jones, R. (2020). *Celiac Disease: A Hidden Epidemic*, 4th Edition. William Morrow Paperbacks.
9. Ishiguro, E., Haskey, N., and Campbell, S. (2018). *Gut Microbiota: Interactive Effects on Nutrition and Health.* Academic Press.
10. Manbacci, M. (2019). *The Comprehensive Guide to Crohn's Disease: All You Need to Know about Crohn's Disease from Diagnosis to Management & Treatment (Autoimmune Disease).* Manbacci.
11. Robillard, N., and Eades, M.R. (2013). *Irritable Bowel Syndrome: Fast Tract Digestion: Diet that Addresses the Root Cause, Small Intestinal Bacterial Overgrowth without Drugs or Antibiotics.* Self-Health Publishing.
12. Strealy, N. (2013). *The Diarrhea Dietitian: Expert Advice, Practical Solutions, and Strategic Nutrition.* Strategic Nutrition Publishing.
13. Sussman, N.L., and Lucey, M.R. (2019). *Alcoholic Liver Disease, An Issue of Clinics in Liver Disease (Clinics Review Articles).* Elsevier.

27 Chronic Liver Disease

OVERVIEW

Chronic liver diseases are progressive impairments of liver functions that last more than 6 months, including detoxifying harmful products of metabolism, production of clotting factors and other proteins, and excretion of bile. These conditions are a continuous process of inflammation, destruction, and regeneration of liver tissues, which can cause fibrosis and cirrhosis. The causes of chronic liver disease include toxins, alcohol abuse for a prolonged time, infection, genetic, autoimmune diseases, and metabolic disorders. Cirrhosis is the final stage of chronic liver disease that disrupts liver architecture, the formation of widespread nodules, vascular reorganization, and deposition of an extracellular matrix. The underlying mechanism of fibrosis and cirrhosis at a cellular level is the recruitment of stellate cells and fibroblasts, resulting in fibrosis, while parenchymal regeneration relies on hepatic stem cells. Chronic liver diseases are a widespread clinical condition.

VIRAL HEPATITIS

Viral hepatitis is a common systemic disease that affects primarily the liver. Different strains of viruses cause other types of hepatitis: hepatitis A virus (HAV), hepatitis B virus (HBV), hepatitis C virus (HCV), hepatitis D virus (HDV), and hepatitis E virus (HEV).

HEPATITIS A VIRUS

HAV is a benign, self-limited disease with an incubation period of 2–6 weeks. HAV does not cause chronic hepatitis or a carrier state and only uncommonly causes acute hepatic failure. The virus can be found in infected individuals' feces, bile, and serum. The usual transmission mode is contaminated food or water, but the transfusion of infected blood can also spread the virus. The disease spreads readily in crowded, unsanitary conditions through contaminated food or water.

The HAV incubation period is 4–6 weeks. It is most contagious during this time. The serum immunoglobulin M (IgM) concentration increases initially. An increase follows in serum immunoglobulin G (IgG), whose levels remain elevated for several years after infection, creating immunity to the disease. The administration of IgG before exposure or early in the incubation period can prevent hepatitis A. HAV vaccine, and the combined HAV and HBV vaccines are available and effective in preventing the disease. Transmission of HAV is prevented by handwashing and using gloves when disposing of fecal matter.

HEPATITIS B VIRUS

Liver disease due to HBV is an enormous global health problem. Approximately 2 billion people have been infected with HBV, and 400 million people have chronic infections. The global prevalence of chronic hepatitis B infection varies widely: it is high in Africa, Asia, and the Western Pacific; intermediate in southern and eastern Europe; and low in Western Europe and North America. HBV is transmitted through blood-blood contact and the sexual route. Immunosuppressed patients who receive hemodialysis and multiple blood transfusions or immunosuppressive drugs; have numerous sex partners; or share needles, syringes, or other drug equipment; or infants born to infected mothers have a greater risk of exposure or less resistance to HBV coinfection with HCV, HDV. HIV is expected because these viruses share the same routes of transmission.

DOI: 10.1201/9781003453376-34

Mother-infant transmission of HBV occurs if the mother becomes infected during the third trimester of pregnancy. Transmission among homosexual men may be by oral or genital contact with bleeding lesions in the rectal mucosa. Up to 400 million people worldwide carry the **hepatitis B surface antigen** (HBsAg) marker for active HBV. HBV is a significant cause of chronic hepatitis, cirrhosis, and hepatocellular carcinoma.

Hepatitis C Virus

HCV (previously known as non-A, non-B hepatitis) is a parenterally transmitted flavivirus with six genotypes. The incubation period for HCV ranges from 4 to 26 weeks, with a mean of 9 weeks. In about 85% of individuals, the clinical course of the acute infection is asymptomatic and typically missed. About 54% of HCV cases involve intravenous drug users, who also have a high incidence of HIV infection. Multiple sex partners, needle stick injuries, and employment in medical or dental offices can lead to infection. Approximately 80% of cases develop chronic liver disease. HCV is diagnosed through the detection of anti-HCV IgG. Persistent infection with recurring acute symptoms and elevated aminotransferase levels indicate the condition. Antiviral drug therapy is available. The progression of disease to cirrhosis or **hepatocellular carcinoma** (HCC) is most significant among individuals with HIV or coexisting liver disease. The variants of HCV make vaccine development difficult, and resistance to drug therapy is common. There is no vaccine for HCV.

Hepatitis D Virus

HDV occurs in individuals with hepatitis B. The delta virus depends on the HBV for its replication because the viral coat consists of HBsAg molecules on the HBV's surface. HDV has been shown to suppress the replication of HBV. Parenteral drug users have a high incidence of HDV infection. Globally, about 15 million people are estimated to have HDV. The prevalence varies in South America, Central Africa, the Middle East, and the Mediterranean. HDV infection is uncommon in Southeast Asia and China. In Western countries, it is restricted mainly to intravenous drug abusers and those who have had multiple blood transfusions. The symptoms can be mild or severe, with progression to severe liver failure. In serum, HDV is diagnosed by antibodies directed against HDAg (anti-HD) and HDV RNA. Treatment for chronic HDV includes pegylated interferon alpha, which is effective in about 25% of individuals.

Hepatitis E Virus

HEV is a water-borne infection, primarily in young to middle-aged adults. HEV is most common in Asian and African countries. It is also found in developed countries and must be differentiated from drug-induced liver injury. It is more prevalent among adults and has the highest mortality in pregnant women. Chronic HEV infection does occur in patients with AIDS and immunosuppressed transplant patients. The average incubation period following exposure is 4–5 weeks. Clinically, it resembles HAV and is diagnosed based on detecting anti-HEV IgM. A vaccine for HEV has been approved in China but not in other countries.

ALCOHOLIC LIVER DISEASE

Abuse of any alcoholic beverage can cause **alcoholic liver disease** (ALD), and the severity of the disease is related to the amount and duration of alcohol consumed and the formation of acetaldehyde. Malnutrition may add to the risk of cirrhosis in alcohol abusers. Many alcoholics are malnourished, and the liver cannot regenerate without adequate nutrition. The spectrum of ALD includes steatosis, alcoholic hepatitis, and alcoholic cirrhosis. ALD is caused by too much alcohol consumption over a long period. Alcohol is absorbed in the digestive tract, and most is metabolized in the liver. During this process, substances are produced that can damage the liver. With increased alcohol consumption, liver damage is increased. The organ can continue functioning for some time because it can sometimes recover from mild injury. It can work commonly even if approximately 80% of the liver is damaged. If the patient continues to drink, liver damage progresses and can be fatal. If an individual quits completely, some damage can be reversed, improving the outlook.

EPIDEMIOLOGY

Approximately 8.5% of adults in the United States alone are estimated to have this disorder. ALD affects an estimated 5.1%–8.6% of the total population globally. About two times as many men abuse alcohol compared to women. Women are more vulnerable to ALD if they drink nearly half as much alcohol as men. Their digestive systems may be less able to process alcohol, increasing the amount of alcohol that reaches the liver. The incidence of alcoholic cirrhosis is most significant in middle-aged men; however, women develop more severe liver injury than men. In the United States, mortality resulting from cirrhosis is highest among Hispanic white males and females; however, the death rates for all groups are declining.

ETIOLOGY AND RISK FACTORS

Genetic factors are likely involved because ALD often runs in families. The family members may have the same genes that make alcohol processing less efficient. Obesity also makes liver damage from alcohol more likely. Accumulation of iron in the liver and viral hepatitis C also increase risks. Iron can accumulate because of **hemochromatosis**, which will be discussed later in this chapter. Over 25% of heavy drinkers also have viral hepatitis C. Heavy drinking plus viral hepatitis C means risks of cirrhosis are significantly increased. Accumulated iron in the liver or the presence of hepatitis C for over 6 months increases risks for **hepatocellular carcinoma**.

CLINICAL MANIFESTATIONS

Initial symptoms of ALD usually appear when a person is in their 30s or 40s, with severe symptoms taking 10 years to appear. ALD is often initially asymptomatic. As alcoholic hepatitis develops, symptoms include fever, hepatomegaly, jaundice, anorexia, nausea, fatigue, edema, insomnia, decreased libido, confusion, and depression. Bands of fibrous tissue in the palms can tighten and **club fingers** (see **Figure 27.1**). The palms may redden, which is known as **palmar erythema**.

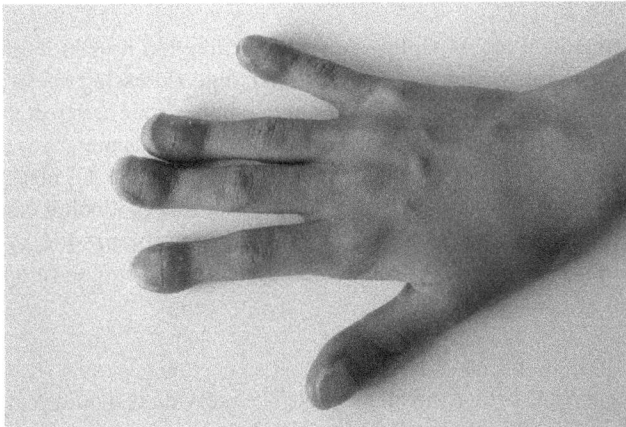

FIGURE 27.1   Clubbed fingers.

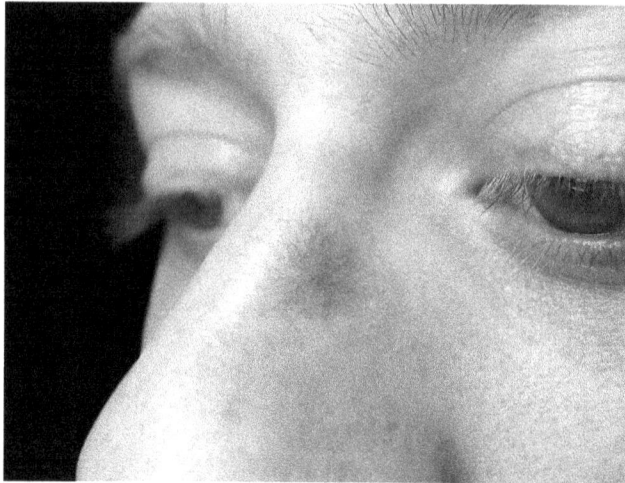

FIGURE 27.2   Spider angiomas.

The skin may develop spider angiomas in the upper body blood vessels resembling spiders (see **Figure 27.2**). The **salivary glands** may enlarge, and there may be muscle wasting. As the peripheral nerves are damaged, sensation and strength are lost. The hands and feet are affected more than the upper arms and legs. Heavy male drinkers may develop female body characteristics such as smooth skin, enlarged breasts, and less body hair. Their testes can also shrink.

DIAGNOSIS

Diagnosis of ALD includes medical history, blood test, ultrasound, CT scan, MRI, and liver biopsy. Liver biopsy is mainly used to clarify atypical cases and to define better the contribution of alcohol in patients with possible non-alcohol-related coexisting conditions, such as hepatitis C and the use of lipid-lowering medications. Many laboratories are researching to evaluate biomarkers or identifier proteins for detecting ongoing alcohol abuse and ALD. Sometimes, diagnosis of ALD can be challenging because patients often minimize or deny alcohol abuse. In addition, there may be no evidence of ALD from the physical exam, and laboratory abnormalities may not expressly point to ALD.

TREATMENT

There is no specific treatment for ALD, but strategies for treating it include lifestyle changes such as reducing alcohol consumption, quitting cigarette smoking, addressing obesity, and implementing nutrition therapy and pharmacological therapy. Many complications are treatable. Perhaps the best treatment for ALD is abstinence from alcohol. However, a nutritious diet, rest, corticosteroids, antioxidants, drugs that slow fibrosis, or managing complications such as GI bleeding, infection, ascites, and encephalopathy can slow disease progression. Cessation of alcohol consumption improves clinical symptoms, slows the progression of liver damage, and prolongs life. A liver transplant is a treatment for liver failure, and artificial liver support systems are being developed.

PREVENTION

The only way to prevent ALD is to avoid all alcohol. The individual should protect against hepatitis C since it infects the liver and leads to cirrhosis. The diet should consist mainly of nutrient-dense foods, including fruits, vegetables, lean proteins, legumes, nuts, seeds, whole grains, heart-healthy fats, water, coffee, tea, herbs, and spices. Foods to avoid include fast food, convenience meals, canned soups, packaged snacks, margarine, vegetable shortening, fried foods, chips, crackers, pretzels, microwave popcorn, hot dogs, sausage, deli meats, bacon, beef jerky, soy sauce, teriyaki sauce, steak sauce, spaghetti sauce, and raw or undercooked foods (meat, poultry, eggs, fish, oysters, or mussels).

YOU SHOULD REMEMBER

ALD can cause three types of liver damage, which usually occurs in the following order: fatty liver, alcoholic hepatitis, and cirrhosis. Almost everyone who drinks too much alcohol develops a fatty liver. Inflammation usually resolves after stopping drinking, but there can still be permanent damage. Once there is scar tissue, it never resolves, even if all alcohol consumption is controlled.

Check Your Knowledge

1. What is cirrhosis of the liver, and what are its complications?
2. What are the clinical manifestations of cirrhosis?
3. What are the treatments for cirrhosis?

FATTY LIVER DISEASE

Fatty liver disease, also called **hepatic steatosis**, occurs when too much fat is accumulated in the liver cells. Fat buildup becomes problematic when it reaches over 5% of the liver's weight. The two types of fatty liver disease include alcohol-related liver disease and metabolic dysfunction-associated fatty liver disease.

EPIDEMIOLOGY

Fatty liver disease occurs in approximately 1 in every 10 people. It occurs in over 90% of people who drink too much alcohol. It is a leading cause of mortality in the United States, with nearly 250,000 deaths attributed to fatty liver disease annually.

ETIOLOGY AND RISK FACTORS

Fatty liver disease can be due to obesity, diabetes, hypertension, hypercholesterolemia, medications, genetic conditions, autoimmune diseases, or drinking too much alcohol. If left untreated, fatty liver disease can progress and cause severe liver problems, including cirrhosis, liver cancer, and liver failure.

CLINICAL MANIFESTATIONS

Fatty infiltration causes no specific symptoms or abnormal liver function test results. The patient has a history of continuous alcohol intake during the previous months. The clinical manifestations of fatty liver can be mild or severe. Nonspecific symptoms include fatigue, weight loss, and anorexia. Manifestations of acute illness include nausea, anorexia, fever, abdominal pain, and jaundice. The toxic effects of alcohol also may cause testicular atrophy, **azoospermia**, reduced libido, **gynecomastia**, and decreased testosterone levels in men. Cirrhosis causes hepatomegaly, splenomegaly, ascites, portal hypertension, **esophageal varices**, GI bleeding, and hepatic encephalopathy. Anemia

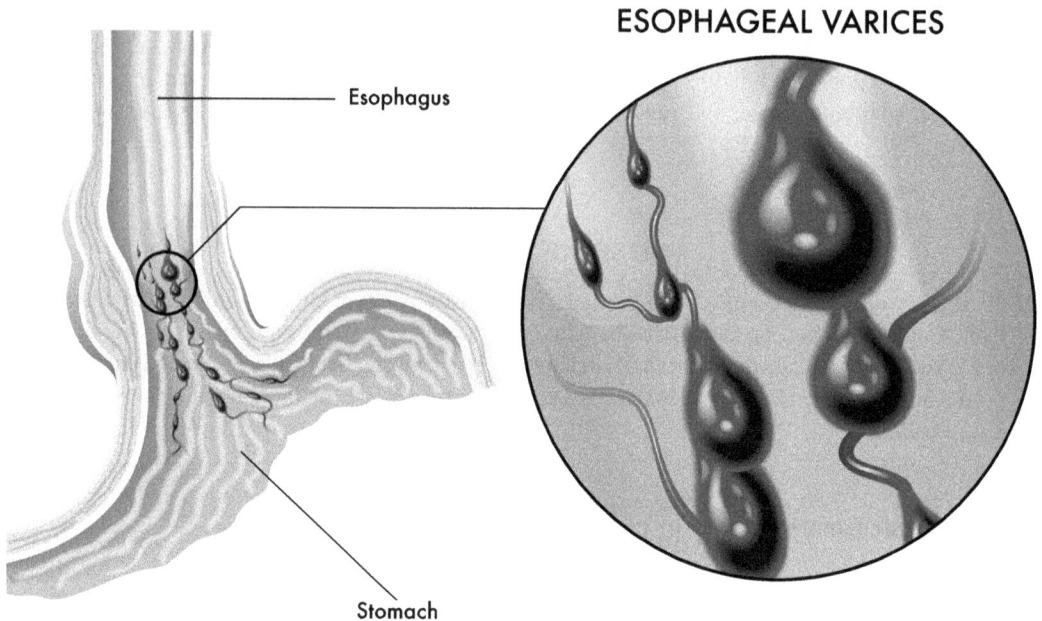

ESOPHAGEAL VARICES

Esophagus

Stomach

FIGURE 27.3   Esophageal varices.

results from blood loss, malnutrition, and hypersplenism. Hepatorenal syndrome is usually a late complication. The infection risk is more significant, partly because of innate immune dysfunction. The presence of numerous and severe manifestations increases the risk of death. The clinical features of alcoholic cirrhosis depend on the duration of the disease and the severity of liver damage (see **Figure 27.3).**

DIAGNOSIS

The diagnosis of fatty liver disease is based on the individual's history and clinical manifestations. The results of liver function tests are abnormal, and serologic studies show elevated levels of serum enzymes and bilirubin and decreased serum albumin levels. Prolonged prothrombin time cannot easily be corrected with vitamin K therapy. Imaging includes an ultrasound, CT scan, or MRI. A liver biopsy can confirm the diagnosis of cirrhosis, but a biopsy is not necessary if clinical manifestations of cirrhosis are evident.

TREATMENT

There is no specific treatment for fatty liver disease, but many of the complications are treatable. Rest, a nutritious diet, weight loss, corticosteroids, antioxidants, drugs that slow fibrosis, and managing complications such as ascites, gastrointestinal bleeding, infection, and encephalopathy can slow disease progression. Cessation of alcohol consumption slows the progression of liver damage, improves clinical symptoms, and prolongs life. Although the liver damage is irreversible, measures that halt the inflammation and destruction of liver cells prolong life. A liver transplant is the treatment for liver failure, and artificial liver support systems are being developed.

PREVENTION

Fatty liver can be reversed if the patient stops drinking and exercises regularly. Fatty liver can be resolved within 6 weeks, but fibrosis and cirrhosis are not reversible.

YOU SHOULD REMEMBER

Liver failure occurs as an acute or chronic condition. It may result from alcohol abuse, a reaction to a medication, high doses of acetaminophen (paracetamol), hepatitis infection, or advanced fatty liver.

Check Your Knowledge

1. What are the causes and the risk factors for fatty liver disease?
2. What are the signs and symptoms of fatty liver disease?
3. What are the treatments for fatty liver disease?

NONALCOHOLIC FATTY LIVER DISEASE

Nonalcoholic fatty liver disease (NAFLD) is the infiltration of hepatocytes with fat, primarily in the form of triglycerides, but it occurs in the absence of alcohol intake. It is associated with obesity, hypercholesterolemia, hypertriglyceridemia, metabolic syndrome, and type 2 diabetes mellitus. It is the most common chronic liver disease in the United States. Some patients with NAFLD will develop nonalcoholic steatohepatitis with liver cell injury, inflammation, and fibrosis. NAFLD is usually asymptomatic and may remain undiagnosed for many years. NAFLD has become the most common form of childhood liver disease in the United States, more than doubling over the past 20 years, partly because of the increase in childhood obesity. NAFLD is a leading cause of liver disease worldwide. The global incidence is 47 cases per 1,000 population and is higher among males than females. The prevalence of NAFLD exceeds 40% in the Americas and Southeast Asia. However, women develop more severe liver injury than men.

CIRRHOSIS

Cirrhosis is an irreversible inflammation, fibrosis, and nodule formation of the liver secondary to chronic injury, leading to alteration of the average lobular organization of the liver. Structural changes result from damage to the liver, such as alcoholism, viruses, chemicals, steatosis, and fibrosis. **Kupffer cells** participate in the process of fibrosis, obstructing biliary channels and blood flow. These changes result in jaundice and portal hypertension. The liver may be larger or smaller than usual and is usually firm or hard when palpated. Cirrhosis develops slowly over the years. Its severity and rate of progression depend on the cause. Cirrhosis develops in about 10%–20% of drinkers; a large amount of normal tissue is permanently replaced with scar tissue. The internal structure is disrupted, and the liver cannot function normally (see **Figure 27.4**).

Epidemiology

The global burden of liver cirrhosis continues to rise. In 2019, cirrhosis was associated with 2.4% of global deaths. With the rising prevalence of obesity, increased alcohol consumption, and improvements in the treatment of hepatitis B virus and hepatitis C virus infections, the incidence and burden of cirrhosis are changing. Although viral hepatitis remains the leading cause of cirrhosis worldwide, the prevalence of NAFLD and alcohol-associated cirrhosis is rising in many parts of the world.

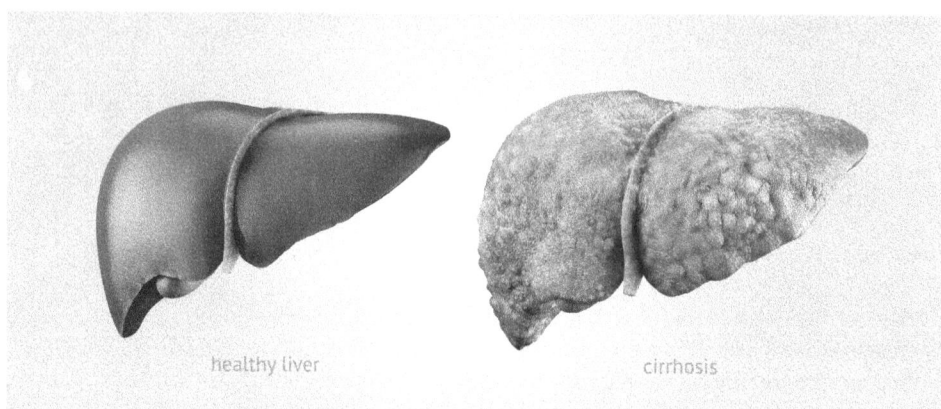

FIGURE 27.4   Cirrhosis of the liver.

ETIOLOGY AND RISK FACTORS

Many disorders can cause cirrhosis of the liver. Among those, alcohol abuse and viral hepatitis are the most common causes. The process of cellular injury depends on the cause of cirrhosis; however, not all causes are clearly understood. Alcoholic cirrhosis is caused by the toxic effects of alcohol metabolism on the liver, immunologic alterations, oxidative stress from lipid peroxidation, and malnutrition. Alcoholic cirrhosis is more severe when associated with HCV. Malnutrition may add to the risk of cirrhosis in alcohol abusers. Many patients are malnourished, and the liver cannot regenerate without adequate nutrition. The spectrum of fatty liver disease includes steatosis, alcoholic hepatitis, and alcoholic cirrhosis.

CLINICAL MANIFESTATIONS

The signs and symptoms of cirrhosis include ascites, hepatic portal hypertension, bleeding in the digestive tract, easy bleeding and bruising, and splenomegaly. Cirrhosis is more likely when large amounts of alcohol are consumed for usually more than 8 years, in the female gender, in the individual with a genetic makeup that increases susceptibility to the disease, and when the individual is obese. One serving of alcohol varies based on the type of drink being consumed.

Other signs and symptoms include gynecomastia, **testicular atrophy**, reduced libido, azoospermia, and decreased testosterone levels in men. Cirrhosis may also cause hepatomegaly, splenomegaly, portal hypertension, ascites, GI bleeding, hepatic encephalopathy, and esophageal varices. Anemia results from blood loss, malnutrition, and hypersplenism.

DIAGNOSIS

The diagnosis of cirrhosis is based on the patient's history and clinical findings. The results of liver function tests are abnormal, and serologic studies show elevated levels of serum enzymes and bilirubin, prolonged prothrombin time, and decreased serum albumin levels. A liver biopsy can confirm the diagnosis of cirrhosis.

TREATMENT

There is no cure for cirrhosis, but some of the complications are treatable. Rest, a nutritious diet, corticosteroids, antioxidants, drugs that slow fibrosis, and managing complications such as GI bleeding, infection, and ascites can slow disease progression. A liver transplant is a treatment for liver failure, and artificial liver support systems have been developed.

PREVENTION

Limiting alcohol intake is the best way of preventing alcohol-related cirrhosis. Avoiding unprotected sex and not sharing needles to inject drugs. Avoid tattooing or body piercing in an unsanitary environment, getting vaccinated against hepatitis B. There is currently no vaccine for hepatitis C.

YOU SHOULD REMEMBER

Biliary cirrhosis differs from alcoholic cirrhosis in that the damage and inflammation leading to cirrhosis begin in bile canaliculi and bile ducts rather than in the hepatocytes. The two types of biliary cirrhosis are primary and secondary. Although both involve bile duct pathology, they differ in cause, risk factors, and mechanisms of obstruction and inflammation.

CHOLELITHIASIS (GALLSTONES)

Gallstones are either cholesterol or pigmented. Cholesterol stones are the most common.

Pigmented stones are black (hard) or brown (soft). They are formed in a sterile environment and consist primarily of calcium bilirubin polymer. They are associated with **hyperbilirubinemia** and hemolytic diseases like **sickle cell anemia**.

EPIDEMIOLOGY

The incidence of gallstones is 10%–15% of the general population. However, many patients with gallstones are asymptomatic, so that the actual incidence may be much higher.

ETIOLOGY AND RISK FACTORS

Risk factors of cholelithiasis include obesity, family history, hypertriglyceridemia, low HDL cholesterol level, middle age, female gender, use of oral contraceptives, and American Indian ancestry.

CLINICAL MANIFESTATIONS

Gallstones may remain in the gallbladder or be ejected, with bile, into the cystic duct. Any gallstones lodged in the cystic duct obstruct bile flow into and out of the gallbladder and cause inflammation (see **Figure 27.5**). Epigastric and upper right abdominal pain and intolerance to fatty foods are the primary clinical manifestations of cholelithiasis. The signs and symptoms include heartburn, flatulence, pruritus, and jaundice. The pain, often called **biliary colic**, is most characteristic and is caused by storing one or more gallstones in the cystic or common duct. The pain can be intermittent or steady. It is usually in the right upper quadrant and radiates to the mid-upper back. Jaundice indicates that the stone is located in the **common bile duct**. Abdominal tenderness and fever indicate **cholecystitis**. Complications can include pancreatitis from the obstruction of the pancreatic duct.

DIAGNOSIS

Diagnosis of cholelithiasis is based on the patient's medical history, physical examination, and imaging evaluation. An oral **cholecystogram** usually outlines the stones. Endoscopic or percutaneous cholangiography and endoscopic or transabdominal ultrasonography are diagnostic options.

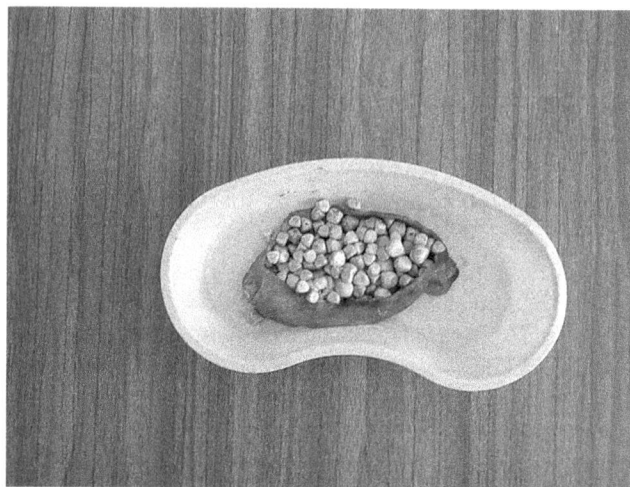

FIGURE 27.5   Gallstones.

TREATMENT

Laparoscopic **cholecystectomy** is the preferred treatment for gallstones that cause obstruction or inflammation. The use of transluminal endoscopic surgery is advancing rapidly. Endoscopic retrograde **cholangiopancreatography** and sphincterotomy with stone retrieval are used for the treatment of bile duct stones. Large stones may be managed with **lithotripsy**. An alternative treatment is the administration of drugs that dissolve smaller stones. For example, bile acid chenodeoxycholic acid can entirely or partially dissolve cholesterol gallstones.

PREVENTION

There is no proven way to prevent gallstones, but eating a well-balanced diet, maintaining an average weight, and exercising regularly (at least 30 minutes a day most days a week) may help reduce the risk. Avoiding fatty foods won't prevent or get rid of gallstones, but it may reduce the frequency of attacks.

YOU SHOULD REMEMBER

Pigmented stones are black (hard) or brown (soft). They are formed in a sterile environment and consist primarily of calcium bilirubin polymer. They are associated with hyperbilirubinemia and hemolytic diseases like sickle cell anemia.

HEMOCHROMATOSIS

Iron overload in adults usually occurs in hemochromatosis (**Figure 27.6**). In this condition, the mucosa of the small intestine protects against excessive iron absorption. In the case of **hepcidin deficiency**, higher amounts of iron are absorbed and transported across the enterocyte to be bound to transferrin and distributed to tissues – eventually, iron deposits in the heart, liver, and other organs. Without treatment, heart failure and liver disease can develop.

Hemochromatosis

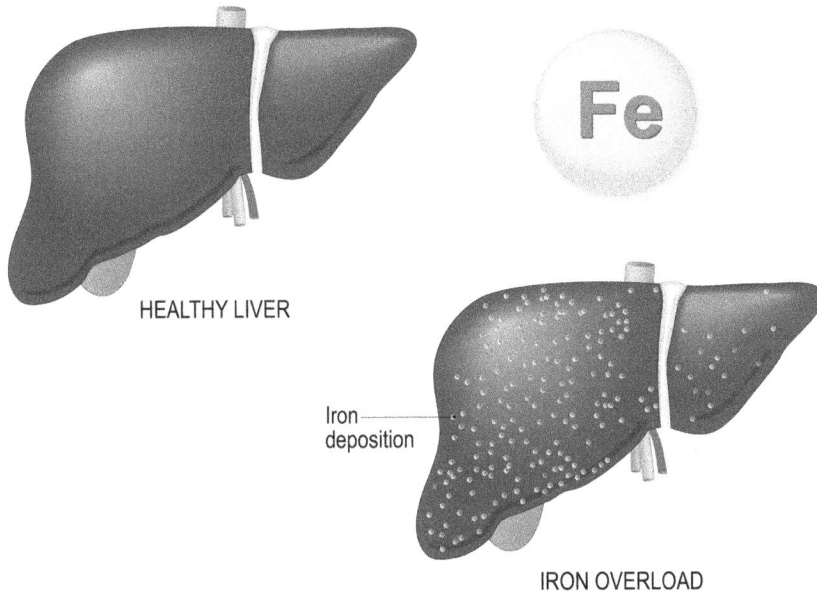

FIGURE 27.6   Hemochromatosis of the liver.

EPIDEMIOLOGY

Hemochromatosis affects about one person of every 200–500. It is one of the most common genetic disorders in the United States.

ETIOLOGY AND RISK FACTORS

The body absorbs and stores too much iron, especially the liver, and can cause severe damage. Without treatment, the disease can cause organs to fail. Excess iron supplementation and regular blood transfusions can cause iron overload in adults.

CLINICAL MANIFESTATIONS

The clinical manifestations of hemochromatosis include fatigue, joint pain (especially in the fingers), abdominal pain, erectile dysfunction, irregular periods, and metallic skin color. With more severe iron overload, patients may develop signs and symptoms of cirrhosis, heart failure, and diabetes mellitus.

DIAGNOSIS

Diagnosing hemochromatosis typically begins with laboratory testing showing elevated serum ferritin and transferrin saturation. Alcohol consumption can elevate ferritin, so serum ferritin has low specificity for primary iron overload syndromes. Transferrin saturation of serum iron-binding capacity is more reliable in diagnosing iron overload and can help determine the need for genetic testing. Other tests to confirm the diagnosis include liver function tests, MRI, genetic tests, and liver biopsy.

Treatment

Treatment of iron toxicity is based on the cause. Iron supplements, if used, should be stopped. With hemochromatosis, treatment requires periodic blood removal, or a chelator drug, which binds the iron and increases excretion, can be administered. The problem with chelator drugs is that they also bind to other trace minerals and can cause secondary deficiencies.

Prevention

The prevention of hemochromatosis is challenging because it primarily inherits the gene mutations link. However, early diagnosis is essential since early treatment with **phlebotomy** can prevent complications of iron overload caused by these gene mutations.

LIVER CANCERS

Liver cancers may be primary or secondary. Primary liver cancer includes *hepatocellular carcinoma, fibrolamellar carcinoma, hepatoblastoma, and angiosarcoma.* HCC usually occurs in patients with cirrhosis and hepatitis B or C virus infections. **Fibrolamellar carcinoma** is a variant of hepatocellular carcinoma with a morphology of malignant hepatocytes enmeshed in lamellar fibrous tissue. It is most common in young adults and has no link to preexisting cirrhosis, HBV, HCV, or other known risk factors. The level of **alpha-fetoprotein** (AFP) is rarely elevated. Fibrolamellar carcinoma has a better prognosis than hepatocellular carcinoma, with many patients surviving for several years after tumor resection. **Hepatoblastoma** is the most common type of childhood liver cancer and usually affects children younger than 3 years of age. **Angiosarcoma** is a rare cancer that develops in the inner lining of blood vessels and lymph vessels. It can occur anywhere in the body but is most often found in the skin, breasts, liver, and spleen.

Liver metastases (secondary liver cancers) are cancerous tumors that have spread to the liver from another part of the body. They can appear shortly after the original tumor develops or even months or years later. They may spread from the GI tract, pancreas, lungs, and breasts. They are more common than primary liver cancers and have similar symptoms.

Epidemiology

HCC is the most common form of *primary liver cancer*, with more than 42,000 new cases and over 30,000 deaths annually in the United States. Approximately 75% of these liver cancers are HCC. Overall, liver cancer is about three times more common in men compared to women. The presence of the hepatitis B virus increases the risk of hepatocellular carcinoma by more than 100 times in HBV carriers. Liver cancer is much more common in countries in sub-Saharan Africa and Southeast Asia than in the United States. In many of these countries, it is the most common type of cancer. More than 800,000 people are diagnosed with this cancer each year throughout the world. Liver cancer is also a leading cause of cancer deaths worldwide, accounting for more than 700,000 deaths each year.

Etiology and Risk Factors

HCC typically develops in people with chronic (long-lasting) liver disease caused by cirrhosis or hepatitis B and C virus infection. Cirrhosis of the liver is the most common cause of HCC. Excessive alcohol consumption, obesity, smoking, and type 2 diabetes are the risk factors.

CLINICAL MANIFESTATIONS

The signs of liver cancer include abdominal pain, a right upper quadrant mass, weight loss, and deterioration from no apparent cause. Some patients develop a fever. Sometimes, the first sign is bloody ascites, **peritonitis**, or shock related to tumor hemorrhage. Some patients have a hepatic **friction rub** or bruit. Systemic metabolic complications may include **erythrocytosis**, hypoglycemia, hypercalcemia, or hyperlipidemia.

DIAGNOSIS

Diagnosis is via AFP measurement. 40% and 65% of diagnosed patients have much higher AFP levels. Initial imaging may be a contrast-enhanced CT scan, MRI, or ultrasonography. A definitive diagnosis is made via liver biopsy guided by CT or ultrasonography.

TREATMENT

Multiple treatment options are available for HCC, including curative resection, liver transplantation, radiofrequency ablation, trans-arterial chemoembolization, radioembolization, and systemic targeted agents like sorafenib. The treatment of HCC depends on the tumor stage, patient performance status, and liver function reserve and requires a multidisciplinary approach. Significant advances in surgical and locoregional therapies have improved in the past few years. Sorafenib is the only approved therapy for patients with advanced disease, but novel systemic molecular targeted agents and their combinations are emerging.

Nutrition can be an essential part of dealing with liver cancers. Eating a well-balanced diet before, during, and after cancer treatment may help patients feel better, maintain strength, and speed up recovery. Strict dieting is not recommended during cancer treatment. Losing weight can lower energy and decrease the ability to fight infection. Frequent small meals will ensure the patient's body gets enough calories, protein, and nutrients to tolerate treatment. Smaller meals may also help to reduce treatment-related side effects such as nausea. Protein helps the body to repair cells and tissues. It also allows the immune system to recover from illness. Fruits and vegetables offer the body antioxidants, which can help fight against cancer. Patients must choose a variety of colorful fruits and vegetables to get the most significant benefits. They should eat at least five servings of whole fruits and vegetables daily. Fresh fruits and vegetables may need to be cooked for patients with a weakened immune system.

PREVENTION

Aside from avoiding, reducing, or quitting the use of alcohol, the incidence of hepatocellular carcinoma may also be reduced by administration of the HBV vaccine, treating chronic HCV, and early detection of hemochromatosis.

Check Your Knowledge

1. What are the classifications of liver cancer?
2. What are the causes of liver cancer?
3. How can we diagnose various liver cancers?

Clinical Case Studies

CLINICAL CASE STUDY 1

A 52-year-old man had a chronic hepatitis C infection, which developed from a much earlier blood transfusion. Previous treatments with pegylated interferon and ribavirin were not helpful. The patient is currently presenting for clearance before evaluation of a kidney transplant. He also has type 2 diabetes mellitus, neuropathy, and nephropathy. The patient had a history of alcohol abuse about 10 years ago, which he was able to stop, but he has been smoking cigarettes for the past 40 years.

CRITICAL THINKING QUESTIONS

1. What is the incubation period for HCV?
2. What are the risk factors for HCV?
3. How is HCV diagnosed?

CLINICAL CASE STUDY 2

A 66-year-old woman with a history of cirrhosis due to alcohol abuse was found to have a lesion in the liver that was consistent with hepatocellular carcinoma. A PET-CT scan indicated there was no extrahepatic disease. The diagnosis was confirmed by a biopsy using ultrasound-guided percutaneous needle puncture. Tests revealed elevated alpha-fetoprotein. The liver cancer was in an early stage. Transcatheter arterial chemoembolization was undertaken, but the alpha-fetoprotein levels continued to increase.

CRITICAL THINKING QUESTIONS

1. What is primary liver cancer usually discovered to be?
2. What are the most common symptoms of liver cancer?
3. What are the options for treatment?

CLINICAL CASE STUDY 3

A 43-year-old woman was evaluated at the emergency department for severe right-sided abdominal pain, nausea, vomiting, and dehydration. The patient was hospitalized, and an ultrasound of her abdomen was performed. Prominent gallbladder wall thickening was present, along with acute cholecystitis. Soon, the patient was scheduled for surgical removal of the gallbladder, which was full of gallstones.

CRITICAL THINKING QUESTIONS

1. What are the risk factors for gallstones?
2. What are the clinical manifestations of gallstones?
3. How can gallstones be prevented?

FURTHER READING

1. About-Alfa, G.K., and DeMatteo, R. (2019). *100 Questions and Answers about Liver Cancer*, 4th Edition. Jones & Bartlett Learning.
2. Anderson, E. (2023). *Liver Disease and Cirrhosis: A Comprehensive Guide to Understanding and Conquering Liver Disease, Fatty Liver, Liver Cancer, Alcohol's Impact, Nutritional Strategies, and a Path to Vibrant Health*. Anderson.
3. Dooley, J.S., Lok, A.S., Garcia-Tsao, G., and Pinzani, M. (2018). *Sherlock's Diseases of the Liver and Biliary System*, 13th Edition. Wiley Blackwell.
4. Friedman, L.S. and Martin, P. (2017). *Handbook of Liver Disease*, 4th Edition. Elsevier.
5. Garrison, C. (2010). *The Iron Disorders Institute Guide to Hemochromatosis: Symptoms, Relief, and Support for Sufferers*. Cumberland House.
6. Mark, Z. (2022). *Cirrhosis of the Liver Treatment Handbook: Everything You Must Know about Cirrhosis of the Liver, Its Treatment, Diagnosis, Causes, Symptoms, Precautions and Prevention*. Mark.
7. McCalvert, J. (2022). *Hemochromatosis: A Comprehensive Strategy for the Management of Hemochromatosis*. McCalvert.
8. Mool, I. (2023). *Gallbladder Wellness: The Ultimate Guide to Eliminating Gallbladder Pain, Managing Gallstones, Inflammation, Biliary Colic Attacks, Cholecystitis and Cholecystectomy Recovery Guide*. Mool.
9. National Comprehensive Cancer Network. (2023). *NCCN Guidelines for Patients' Liver Cancer*. NCCN.
10. Norton, S. (2023). *Alcoholic Liver Disease: An Issue of Clinics in Liver Disease*. American Medical Publishers.
11. Snyder, R. (2016). *What You Must Know About Liver Disease: A Practical Guide to Using Conventional and Complementary Treatments (Understanding and Dealing with Liver Disease and Its Related Problems)*. Square One.
12. Thuluvath, P.J. (2022). *Your Complete Guide to Liver Health: Coping with Fatty Liver, Hepatitis, Cancer, and More*. Johns Hopkins University Press.
13. White, I. (2023). *Non-Alcoholic Fatty Liver Disease: The Ultimate Guide to Diagnosis, Treatment, and Prevention of NAFLD (Things You Must Know)*. White.

28 Nutrition Effects on the Neuro-psychiatric

OVERVIEW

Proper nutrition is essential for the normal functioning of the nervous system. Many deficiencies and toxicities involving vitamins or minerals cause diseases or conditions in the nervous system. Wernicke encephalopathy is a severe, life-threatening illness resulting from vitamin B1 deficiency. If not treated properly, a severe neurologic disorder called Korsakoff psychosis can occur, leading to death. Cognitive dysfunction refers to deficits in attention, verbal and nonverbal learning, short-term and working memory, visual and auditory processing, problem-solving, processing speed, and motor functioning. Cognitive disorders include dementia, amnesia, and delirium, with affected patients no longer fully oriented to time and space. These disorders may be temporary or progressive, based on the cause. While delirium is temporary, dementias such as Alzheimer's disease are generally progressive. Inadequate nutrition can also lead to various types of peripheral neuropathies, which are among the most prevalent of all neurologic conditions. For example, a lack of vitamin B12 damages the protective myelin sheaths, resulting in abnormal functioning of nerves and peripheral neuropathy.

DEMENTIA

Dementia is a loss of memory, language, and problem-solving. It is caused by brain disease or injury. It is classified as Alzheimer's disease (AD), Lewy body dementia, vascular dementia, and frontotemporal dementia (FTD). The affected individual becomes unable to function independently. *Vascular dementia* involves acute or chronic cognitive deterioration. It is usually due to diffuse or focal cerebral infarction from cerebrovascular disease. There are problems with reasoning, planning, judgment, memory, and other thought processes caused by brain damage from impaired blood flow to the brain. Vascular dementia is the second most common cause of dementia in older adults. It may be present concurrently with AD. For more details on AD, see **Chapter 13**.

Lewy body dementia is chronic cognitive deterioration characterized by Lewy body inclusions in the cytoplasm of cortical neurons. Overall, it is the third most common type of dementia. Some patients also have neuritic plaques and neurofibrillary tangles, which also occur in patients with AD. FTD is a group of brain disorders that affects the frontal and temporal lobes. These areas are associated with language, personality, and behavior in FTD, areas of the lobes atrophy. This form is one of the less common types of dementia and may be sporadic or hereditary. One example of FTD is called Pick disease, which includes severe atrophy and loss of neurons. See **Chapter 13** for more details.

Dementia is difficult to prevent since its cause is often unknown. If caused by a stroke, future declines may be preventable by lowering the risk factors. Patients should avoid smoking, control body weight, exercise regularly, eat a healthy diet, manage diabetes, hypertension, or high cholesterol, remain mentally alert and active, engage in regular social activities, and, if recommended by a physician, take aspirin.

DOI: 10.1201/9781003453376-35

COGNITIVE DYSFUNCTION

Cognition is the mental process of acquiring information, knowledge, and understanding through thought, experience, and the senses. It covers various high-level intellectual functions and processes such as attention, memory, learning, decision-making, planning, reasoning, judgment, perception, comprehension, language, and **visuospatial** functions. Cognitive dysfunction describes the impairment of different domains of cognition. Cognitive dysfunction is an impairment in thinking skills such as memory, attention, and processing. It may also impact executive function, the complex thought processes needed for solving problems, making decisions, and reasoning.

Folate deficiency may contribute to cognitive impairment of the brain with continued aging. This may lead to reversible *dementia* and also increase risks for AD and vascular dementia. As confirmed by neuropsychological testing, folate-deficient adults with impaired intellectual function significantly improved after 6–12 months of folic acid supplementation. Chronic folate deficiency can induce **cerebral atrophy**. The highest incidence of folate deficiency is in older adults, and there is a close association with dementia and other cognitive dysfunction. In patients with AD, cognitive decline is significantly related to lower serum folate concentrations. Older people given folate supplements generally improve their cognitive function to a large degree. Folate supplementation can improve **visuomotor** performance, visuospatial memory, associative memory, logical reasoning, and activities of daily living over 4 months.

Epidemiology

The prevalence of cognitive deficits due to various causes is difficult to predict and poorly established. However, increasing age is the most significant factor for cognitive impairment. AD is the most well-known condition associated with cognitive impairment. Approximately 6.9 million people are affected by AD in the United States, and the worldwide prevalence is estimated to be more than 24 million. The prevalence and incidence of AD among African American populations were approximately twice that of those among European Americans. The incidence of dementia is predicted to double every 10 years after age 60.

Etiology and Risk Factors

Cognitive dysfunction may begin from birth or may be caused later by environmental factors such as mental illness, neurological disorders, or brain injury. The cognitive dysfunction is more common in older adults. In early life, cognitive dysfunction may be caused by genetic abnormality, malnutrition, lead poisoning, hypoglycemia, hypoxia, hypothyroidism, prematurity, **kernicterus**, and brain trauma.

In older adults, the causes of cognitive impairment include stroke, brain tumors, delirium, dementia, depression, schizophrenia, chronic alcohol use, substance abuse, vitamin deficiencies, hormonal imbalances, and some chronic diseases. Other causes include AD, Huntington's disease, Parkinson's disease (PD), **prion disease**, and HIV dementia. Cognitive deficits can also be caused by agents such as sedatives, tranquilizers, glucocorticoids, and anticholinergics. Cognitive deficits may develop in children or adolescents due to malnutrition, metabolic conditions, autism, cancer therapy, heavy metal poisoning, and systemic lupus erythematosus.

Clinical Manifestations

The brain, like other parts of the body, changes with age. Many people need to be more mindful as they age. It may take longer to think of a word or to recall a person's name. Mild cognitive impairment is an early stage of memory loss or other cognitive ability loss (such as language or visual/spatial perception) in individuals who can independently perform most activities of daily living.

Cognitive deficits might present with personality or behavioral changes, severe headaches, insomnia, loss of consciousness, imbalance, seizures, vision changes, fatigue, numbness, and paralysis.

DIAGNOSIS

The diagnosis of cognitive deficits includes a detailed medical history from the patient and family members and a clinical assessment of the patient that covers a wide range of information. The neurological exam includes mental status, cranial nerves, motor and sensory functions, reflexes, coordination, balance, and gait. Other tests depend on the signs and symptoms. It may include complete blood count, thyroid tests, vitamin B12 levels, basic metabolic panel, urine analysis, liver function tests, and renal function tests, which may help discover infectious causes and metabolic disorders. Also, brain imaging like CT-scan and MRI may help diagnose brain tumors or stroke.

TREATMENT

The treatment of cognitive deficits depends on the cause. Infections and metabolic syndromes, depression, hypothyroidism, and medication effects are some curable causes of cognitive decline. For mental disorders, a detailed assessment and treatment are needed to improve the quality of life.

There is no pharmacological treatment for mild cognitive impairment. The treatment is focused on promoting functional status. The patients are at risk for recurrent falls – problems with vision and hearing must be corrected. Patients with sleep apnea may need continuous positive airway pressure (CPAP). The use of anticholinergic medications negatively impacts cognitive function in older adults. Treatment with antidepressants, especially those with amitriptyline, nortriptyline, and paroxetine, is contraindicated.

The cause of delirium must be diagnosed first. Drugs such as antipsychotics or benzodiazepines can decrease the symptoms in some patients. Vitamin B supplements are recommended for alcohol abuse or malnourished cases. Ginkgo biloba, a popular herbal supplement, may improve memory and cognition.

Cognitive training, physical activity, exercises, adequate sleep, and relaxation techniques help mental health. The Mediterranean diet may help people with cognitive impairment. Reducing noise around the patient allows the patient to minimize distraction, confusion, and frustration. Psychotherapy and psychosocial support for patients and families have evidence of better outcomes in understanding and proper management of the disorder. Therefore, it is essential to maintain a better quality of life for everyone involved.

PREVENTION

Like the Mediterranean diet, a healthy diet has multiple benefits: improved cognition and decreased risk of dementia in older adults. Exercise offers health benefits. Not only does staying physically active help the brain, but it also helps lower the risk of heart disease, hypertension, type 2 diabetes, breast cancer, and colon cancer.

Check Your Knowledge

1. What are the causes of cognitive deficits?
2. What are the clinical manifestations of cognitive deficits?
3. How can we prevent cognitive deficits?

WERNICKE ENCEPHALOPATHY

Encephalopathy is a disease in which brain function is affected by an agent or a condition, resulting in an altered mental state, confusion, and abnormal actions. **Wernicke encephalopathy** involves an acute onset of confusion, **nystagmus**, ataxia, and partial **ophthalmoplegia** linked to a thiamin deficiency. There may be insufficient intake or absorption of thiamin. Severe alcoholism is often an underlying condition. When alcohol is consumed excessively, it interferes with the absorption of thiamin from the GI tract. Poor nutrition that is related to alcoholism often prevents adequate intake of thiamin. Wernicke encephalopathy may also be caused by recurrent kidney dialysis, hyperemesis, **gastric plication**, starvation, cancer, and AIDS. This condition may develop when a carbohydrate load is given to patients with a thiamin deficiency, such as re-feeding following starvation or administering IV dextrose-containing solutions to patients of high risk.

EPIDEMIOLOGY

Autopsies have identified the typical brainstem lesions of Wernicke encephalopathy, placing the incidence of this condition between 0.8% and 2.8% of the general population. Even so, the incidence can be up to 12.5% in the alcoholic population.

ETIOLOGY AND RISK FACTORS

The prevalence of Wernicke encephalopathy is based on autopsy studies, indicating that it affects 1%–3% of the global population. Incidence is believed to be higher in developing countries because of vitamin deficiencies and malnutrition. The male-to-female ratio is 1.7 to 1, but no studies show any particular racial predisposition to the disease.

CLINICAL MANIFESTATIONS

Central nervous system lesions are usually distributed symmetrically around the ventricles. As Wernicke encephalopathy develops, there are sudden clinical changes. Oculomotor abnormalities include horizontal and vertical nystagmus, partial ophthalmoplegia such as **conjugate gaze palsies**, and **lateral rectus palsy**. The pupils are usually slow-moving or unequal in size. There is commonly vestibular dysfunction but no hearing loss, plus impairment of the **oculovestibular reflex**. Confusion is exemplified by indifference, extreme disorientation, drowsiness, inattention, or stupor. Some patients may have severe autonomic dysfunction with signs of sympathetic hyperactivity such as agitation and tremor. Hypoactivity may be present, signified by hypothermia, postural hypotension, and syncope. **Korsakoff psychosis** is a late complication of persistent Wernicke encephalopathy and can cause memory deficits, confusion, and behavioral changes. This condition occurs in 80% of untreated patients with Wernicke encephalopathy. Without treatment, stupor may progress to coma and death.

DIAGNOSIS

The diagnosis of Wernicke encephalopathy is based on recognizing underlying vitamin B1 (thiamin) deficiencies and poor nutrition. The outlook for Wernicke encephalopathy is based on an early diagnosis and treatment, which can correct all abnormalities.

TREATMENT

The treatment of Wernicke encephalopathy requires immediate thiamin administration. Magnesium is needed as a cofactor for thiamin-dependent metabolism. Supportive treatment involves correcting electrolyte abnormalities, rehydration, and general nutritional therapy, including multivitamins.

When it is advanced, hospitalization is required. The patient must stop drinking alcoholic beverages. This is because the effects of alcohol can lead to permanent damage to the **Wernicke area** of the brain, which is irreversible.

PREVENTION

Wernicke encephalopathy is preventable, so undernourished patients must be given parenteral thiamin, vitamin B12, and folate. Thiamin is advised to be administered before treating a patient with reduced consciousness. Malnourished patients continue to take thiamin on an outpatient basis.

YOU SHOULD REMEMBER

Wernicke encephalopathy is a degenerative brain disorder caused by the lack of vitamin B1. It can result from dietary deficiencies, alcohol abuse, prolonged vomiting, eating disorders, or chemotherapy. The thalamus and hypothalamus are primarily damaged.

Check Your Knowledge

1. What are the signs and symptoms of Wernicke encephalopathy?
2. What is Korsakoff psychosis?
3. What are the treatments for Wernicke encephalopathy?

PERIPHERAL NEUROPATHY

Peripheral neuropathy is a dysfunction of the peripheral nerves, which are the parts of nerves distal to the root and plexus. There are varying degrees of pain, sensory disturbances, diminished deep tendon reflexes, muscle weakness and atrophy, and vasomotor symptoms. All of these can occur singularly or in various combinations. Peripheral neuropathies can be *mononeuropathy* of a single nerve, *multiple mononeuropathy* of two or more discrete nerves in separate areas, or *polyneuropathy*, with many nerves affected simultaneously, suggesting a diffuse disease process. The neuropathy due to thiamin deficiency is known as beriberi (see **Chapter 16**).

EPIDEMIOLOGY

About 2.4% of the population is affected by peripheral neuropathy, which increases to 8% in older populations. The prevalence of peripheral neuropathy is estimated to be between 6% and 51% among adults with diabetes, depending on age and duration of diabetes.

ETIOLOGY AND RISK FACTORS

Peripheral neuropathy may be caused by thiamin deficiency or ingesting megadoses of vitamin B6 (pyridoxine). Such doses are sometimes taken to treat **carpal tunnel syndrome** or **premenstrual syndrome**, even though the effectiveness of these doses has not been proven. The diagnosis of vitamin B6 toxicity is clinical, and treatment is to stop taking vitamin B6 supplements. Recovery, however, is slow, and some patients only partially recover.

CLINICAL MANIFESTATIONS

Peripheral neuropathy may develop with deficits in a **stocking-glove distribution** (see **Figure 28.1**). These include progressive sensory ataxia plus severely impaired position and vibration senses. The senses of pain, temperature, and touch are not affected as much, and the motor system and central

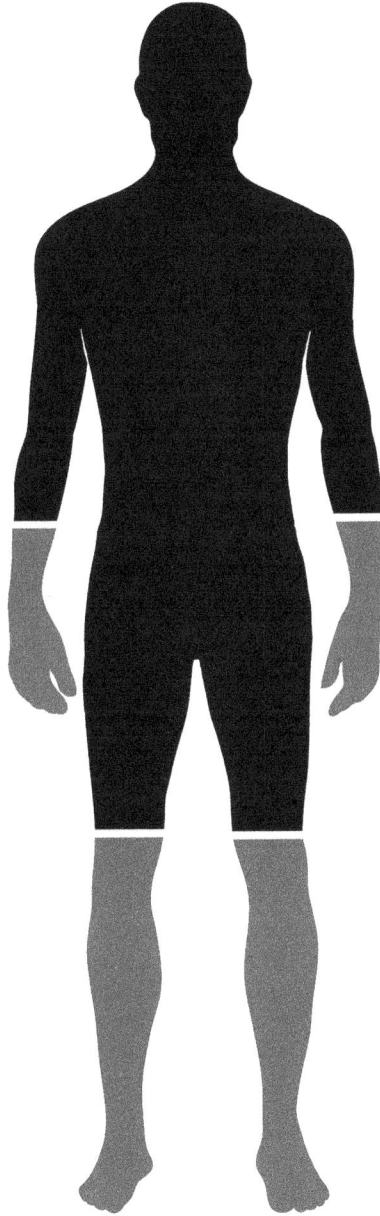

FIGURE 28.1   Stocking-glove distribution of peripheral neuropathy.

nervous system (CNS) are usually standard. There is distal sensory loss, burning pain in the toes and feet, paresthesias, or muscle weakness. The lower legs often ache and cramp. Untreated, the peripheral neuropathy will cause ascending leg weakness, eventually evolving into sensorimotor neuropathy of the hands. The recurrent laryngeal nerve may be affected, causing hoarseness. Cranial nerve involvement is seen as a weakness of the tongue and face.

DIAGNOSIS

The diagnosis of peripheral neuropathy includes a detailed medical history, neurological exam, and blood tests. Imaging tests, such as MRI and CT scans, are helpful. **Electromyography** (EMG) measures and records electrical activity in the muscles to find nerve damage; skin and nerve biopsy must also be done.

TREATMENT

The primary goals of treatment are to manage the condition causing the neuropathy and to improve symptoms. Medicines used to treat peripheral neuropathy include pain relievers, topical application (lidocaine cream), antidepressants, and anti-seizure agents.

Various therapies and procedures might help with the symptoms of peripheral neuropathy. They include **scrambler therapy**, spinal cord stimulation, physical therapy, and surgery for removing tumors.

PREVENTION

The prevention of peripheral neuropathy is based on a nutritious diet, regular exercise, limited alcohol use, avoiding injuries and toxic chemicals, and carefully managing underlying disorders such as diabetes mellitus. Correcting vitamin deficiencies and losing weight also have some preventive effects against peripheral neuropathy.

Check Your Knowledge

1. What are the signs and symptoms of peripheral neuropathy?
2. What are the causes and risk factors of peripheral neuropathies?
3. What are the treatments for peripheral neuropathies?

ATAXIA

Ataxia is a lack of muscle coordination and control. Patients with ataxia have trouble with movement, delicate motor tasks, and maintaining balance. It usually results from damage to the cerebellum, which controls muscle coordination. Some types of ataxia affect children, while others may develop later in adulthood. Depending on the ataxia type, the symptoms may stay the same, progressively worsen, or slowly improve. Various types of ataxia include Friedreich's ataxia, spinocerebellar ataxias, episodic ataxia, ataxia with vitamin E deficiency, and acquired ataxia.

Friedreich's ataxia is the most common form of inheritable ataxia. Ataxia-telangiectasia is a rarer type of hereditary ataxia. **Spinocerebellar ataxias** (SCAs) are a group of hereditary ataxias that often occur in adulthood, affecting people aged 25–80. Episodic ataxia is a rare and unusual type of hereditary ataxia in which someone experiences episodes of ataxia. Episodic ataxia is a rare and unusual type of hereditary ataxia where someone experiences episodes of ataxia, but the rest of the time, they have no or only mild symptoms.

EPIDEMIOLOGY

Friedreich's ataxia affects around 1 in 50,000 people in the United States, and its global prevalence is 1 in 40,000. There is no gender difference in the prevalence of this neurodegenerative disorder. However, other ataxias affect males, and females are equally affected. The disorder occurs in less than 1 in every 1 million people.

ETIOLOGY AND RISK FACTORS

Many conditions may cause ataxia, including genetics, alcohol misuse, brain degeneration, severe head injury, stroke, bacterial meningitis, multiple sclerosis, viral infection (chickenpox and measles), hypothyroidism, mercury poisoning, and vitamin E deficiency. Ataxia with vitamin E deficiency results from gene mutations on chromosome 8.

CLINICAL MANIFESTATIONS

Ataxia is progressive and can affect many different body systems. Some patients may develop tremors or head shaking and poor coordination of hands, arms, and legs: wide-based gait, difficulty with writing, and slow eye movements. However, emotions and intellect are not usually affected. Fatty deposits known as **xanthomas** may affect the **Achilles tendon**. In spinocerebellar ataxia, there is a loss of deep tendon reflexes, truncal and limb ataxia, loss of sensation of vibration and position, muscle weakness, **ptosis**, and ophthalmoplegia (see **Figure 28.2**). Some patients have cardiomyopathy and **scoliosis** (see **Figure 28.3**).

DIAGNOSIS

The diagnosis of ataxia includes medical history, family history, a complete neurological and physical exam, blood and urine studies, spinal tap MRI, and genetic testing. Vitamin E deficiency is diagnosed based on low levels of vitamin E, normal levels of lipoproteins and lipids, and no evidence of fat malabsorption. Vitamin E supplements are given, often stopping the disorder's progression and sometimes improving neurological symptoms.

TREATMENT

Ataxia treatment depends on the cause. If ataxia is caused by a condition such as vitamin deficiency or celiac disease, treating the condition may help improve symptoms. If ataxia results from chickenpox or other viral infections, it will likely resolve independently. Patients with Friedreich ataxia can be treated with an oral medicine called omaveloxolone (Skyclarys). This medication requires regular blood tests because omaveloxolone can affect liver enzymes and cholesterol levels. Physical therapy, occupational therapy, and speech therapy might be helpful. For spinocerebellar ataxia, therapies include medications such as riluzole and valproic acid, botulinum toxin, and physical as well as occupational therapy. Speech therapy is also essential, as dysphagia can lead to aspiration.

PREVENTION

Most forms of ataxia are not preventable since they may be inherited. Genetic counseling and screening are recommended to determine the chance of offspring having the disease or carrying the gene without any symptoms. Prevention of ataxia in some cases requires only drinking alcohol

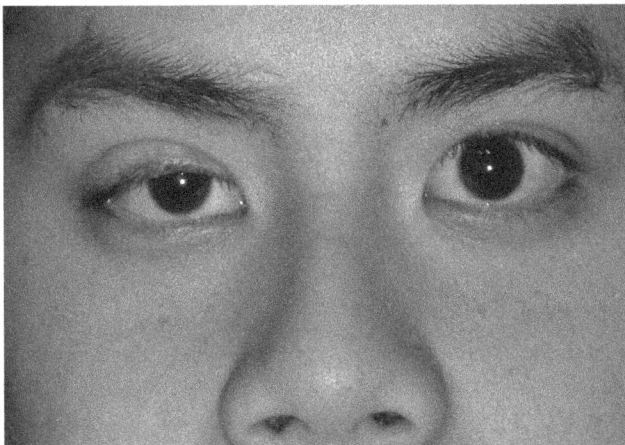

FIGURE 28.2   Ptosis.

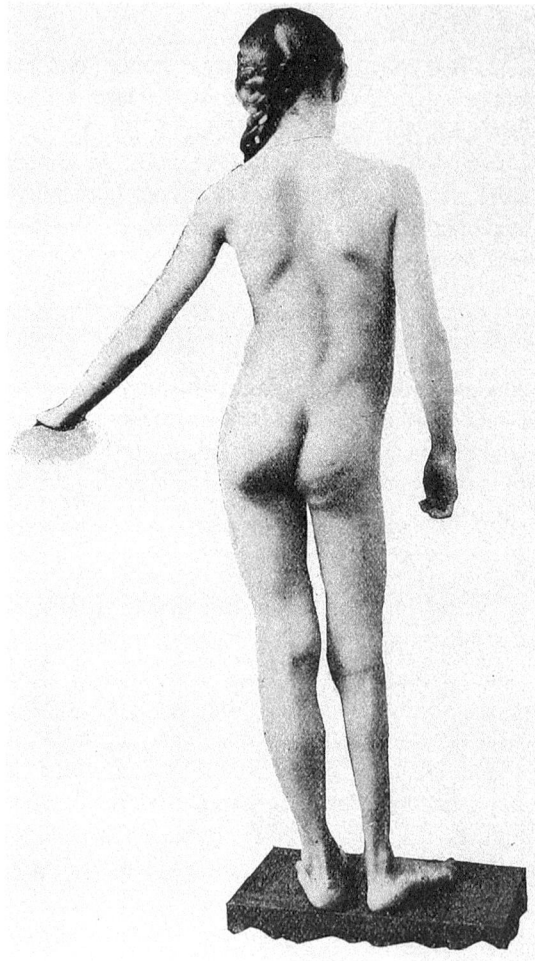

FIGURE 28.3   Scoliosis.

in moderation or not at all, preventing traumatic brain injuries, avoiding recreational drugs, managing fatigue and stress, avoiding exposure to inhalants, preventing or treating infections, controlling body weight, avoiding exposure to chemicals, metals, or toxic substances, and managing vitamin deficiencies or nutritional problems.

Check Your Knowledge

1. What area of the brain damage may cause ataxia?
2. What nutrient deficiency may cause ataxia?
3. What are xanthomas?

WILSON'S DISEASE

Wilson's disease results in the accumulation of copper in the brain and liver. This inherited disease is more common in homozygous patients because of a mutant recessive gene located on chromosome 13. Copper diffuses from the liver into the bloodstream and accumulates in the brain, damaging the brain, liver, and kidneys. **Chapter 21** discussed Wilson's disease in detail.

Clinical Case Studies

CLINICAL CASE STUDY 1

A 54-year-old man was evaluated for possible Wernicke encephalopathy. He had a history of alcoholism and presented with extreme confusion, an upward gaze palsy of the left eye, and gait ataxia over the past week. An MRI of his brain revealed scattered non-enhanced low signal intensity lesions on T1-weighted imaging and high signal intensity lesions on T2-weighted imaging. The bilateral basal ganglia, thalami, midbrain, pons, and periventricular regions were involved. There was evidence of atrophic changes and mammillary bodies. The patient was treated with IV thiamin, 100 mg/day. The left upward gaze palsy was resolved within 1 week, and the other symptoms gradually improved.

CRITICAL THINKING QUESTIONS

1. What does Wernicke encephalopathy involve?
2. What signs and symptoms manifest when autonomic dysfunction is present as part of Wernicke encephalopathy?
3. With Wernicke encephalopathy, in regards to alcohol consumption, what *must* occur?

CLINICAL CASE STUDY 2

A 20-year-old woman presented to her physician with progressive burning sensations on her upper trunk, paresthesias, and numbness of the arms and legs. She also had mild weakness in her hands and feet, insomnia, irritability, and constipation. Extensive testing was undertaken, and eventually, the patient was diagnosed with vitamin B12 deficiency-related peripheral neuropathy. She was treated with sublingual vitamin B12 for 3 months, during which she experienced extreme improvements in her neurological symptoms.

CRITICAL THINKING QUESTIONS

1. What is peripheral neuropathy?
2. How does vitamin B12 deficiency lead to peripheral neuropathy?
3. How does dietary vitamin B12 deficiency usually occur, and what are the later manifestations?

CLINICAL CASE STUDY 3

A 26-year-old woman presented with bilateral cerebellar signs and a history that suggested an autosomal dominant pattern of inheritance. Genetic testing revealed that she had spinocerebellar ataxia. The patient had developed an imbalance while walking over the past 2 years and incoordination of the hands that interfered with her daily activities.

CRITICAL THINKING QUESTIONS

1. What usually causes ataxia?
2. What are the signs and symptoms of spinocerebellar ataxia?
3. What therapies are available for spinocerebellar ataxia?

FURTHER READING

1. Beller, J./Beller Health Research Institute. (2022). *Dementia Overview: 49 Dementia Types, Symptoms, & Risk Factors.* Beller Health Research Institute.
2. Burgess, E.N., and Thornton, L.A. (2013). *Cognitive Dysfunctions: Biological Basis, Management of Symptoms and Long-Term Neurological Implications – Neuroscience Research Progress.* Nova Biomedical.
3. Burlison, L. (2016). *Understanding Alcoholism as a Brain Disease: Book 2 of the "A Prescription for Alcoholics: Medications for Alcoholism" Book Series (Rethinking Drinking).* Addiction Publishing.
4. Campbell, N. (2022). *Cognitive Dysfunction in Aging Adults: A Handbook on Techniques, Therapies, and Simple Hacks to Reversing Memory Loss in Your Old Age.* Campbell.
5. Colajuta, J., and Chapel, J. (2021). *The Gut-Brain Connection: How a Healthy Diet Improves Memory and Cognition through the Relationship of the Immune System, Nervous System, and Hormones.* Nappi.
6. Dave, R. (2022). *Vitamin B12: Truth behind Deficiency.* Dave.
7. Gonzalez, N.J. (2017). *Nutrition and the Autonomic Nervous System: The Scientific Foundations of the Gonzalez Protocol.* New Spring Press.
8. Heinz Weiss, K., and Schilsky, M. (2019). *Wilson Disease: Pathogenesis, Molecular Mechanisms, Diagnosis, Treatment, and Monitoring.* Academic Press.
9. Mayor, J. (2021). *Peripheral Neuropathy Diet: Nerve Repair.* Mayor.
10. McCandless, D.W. (2009). *Metabolic Encephalopathy.* Springer.
11. Mohajeri, H.M. (2020). *Nutrition and Central Nervous System.* Mdpi AG.
12. Pimentel, M., and Rezaie, A. (2022). *The Microbiome Connection: Your Guide to IBS, SIBO, and Low-Fermentation Eating.* Agate Surrey.
13. Quattina, C. (2021). *Wilson's Disease Symptoms: Increased Bleeding, Fatigue, Jaundice, Depression, Aggression, Anxiety, Abdomen Pain and Swelling, Difficulty Speaking and Swallowing, Difficulty Balancing, Tremors.* Quattinla.
14. Schilsky, M.L. (2018). *Management of Wilson Disease: A Pocket Guide (Clinical Gastroenterology).* Humana Press.
15. Stephen, J. (2022). *Peripheral Neuropathy: A Patient's Guide to Self-Management.* Stephen.
16. Veselak, M. (2017). *A Complete Guide to Understanding, Managing, & Improving Your Peripheral Neuropathy.* Veselak.
17. Vink, R., and Nechifor, M. (2011). *Magnesium in the Central Nervous System.* University of Adelaide Press.
18. Warren, S. (2019). *The Pain Relief Secret: How to Retrain Your Nervous System, Heal Your Body, and Overcome Chronic Pain.* TCK Publishing.
19. Weiss, K.H., and Schilsky, M. (2019). *Wilson Disease: Pathogenesis, Molecular Mechanisms, Diagnosis, Treatment, and Monitoring.* Academic Press.
20. Wiesman, J.F. (2016). *Peripheral Neuropathy: What It Is and What You Can Do to Feel Better.* Johns Hopkins Press.

29 Eating Disorders

OVERVIEW

Eating disorders are changes in eating patterns in response to illness, stress, or a need to change the diet for health or personal reasons. These disorders result in altered body weight and nutritional problems. Dieting, skipping meals, eating at incorrect times of day, and having hectic lives all contribute to eating disorders. Obesity is the most common eating disorder, but other significant conditions include anorexia nervosa, bulimia nervosa, and binge-eating disorder. All eating disorders result in some form of malnutrition on a global scale. Dieting, skipping meals, eating at irregular times, or having hectic lives may press individuals with disordered eating to develop actual eating disorders. In the United States, about 20 million women and 10 million men have an eating disorder. Approximately 500,000 adolescents have either disordered eating or an eating disorder.

ANOREXIA NERVOSA

Anorexia nervosa involves extreme weight loss, distortions of body image, and an irrational fear of weight gain and obesity. The affected person often denies their appetite and hates looking in a mirror. People with anorexia believe they are fat no matter what the truth is and what others tell them. Some people focus on body areas, such as the stomach, thighs, and buttocks, which they believe to be excessively fat. The severity of anorexia nervosa is determined by discrepancies between actual and perceived body shape. In part, they blame themselves for the weight gain during puberty. This self-blame is less common in adult women or African-American women of all ages. Men make up only about 10% of all cases since their ideal image is considered normal when they are larger and more muscular. Anorexia nervosa in males occurs more often in homosexuals and athletes participating in sports with weight classes – such as boxers, jockeys, and wrestlers. Eating disorders in men may be encouraged by activities such as cycling, dancing, modeling, and swimming.

Anorexia nervosa is more psychological than related to food. Family conflict is a common underlying factor. If a family's expectations are very high, including expectations about body weight, frustration results in arguments. Anorexic individuals often feel hopeless about human relationships and become socially isolated due to family dysfunction. The two primary forms of anorexia nervosa are as follows:

- *Restricting* – dieting, fasting, and excessive exercising
- *Binge eating/purging* – binge eating, then **purging** in response to severe food restriction

People with anorexia have very low body weights and fear gaining any amount of weight. They have a distorted view of their weight, and their self-worth is nearly entirely based on it. There are continual thoughts about controlling food, eating, and weight while human relationships are reduced. Health professionals can evaluate people with anorexia and make the correct diagnosis. It is essential to seek help sooner rather than later because chances of recovery are much higher when treatment is received as early as possible.

EPIDEMIOLOGY

Although the overall incidence rate of anorexia nervosa has been considerably stable over the past decades, the incidence among younger persons (aged less than 15 years) has increased. Anorexia

DOI: 10.1201/9781003453376-36

nervosa is the third most common chronic condition in adolescent children nationwide. It is unclear whether this reflects earlier detection or earlier age of onset. Nevertheless, it has implications for future research into risk factors and prevention programs. The lifetime prevalence rates of anorexia nervosa might be up to 4% among females and 0.3% among males. While epidemiological studies in the past mainly focused on young females from Western countries, anorexia nervosa is reported worldwide among males and females of all ages.

ETIOLOGY AND RISK FACTORS

A person with anorexia is more likely to come from a family with a history of specific health problems. These include weight problems, physical illness, and mental health problems. Mental health problems may include depression and substance use disorder.

CLINICAL MANIFESTATIONS

Anorexia can cause a variety of symptoms. They may be related to food or weight. They may be physical or emotional. Food- or weight-related symptoms can include low body weight, extreme fear of becoming fat, denial of hunger, excessive physical activity, unusual eating behaviors, and altered body image (see **Figure 29.1**). Loss of interest in sex, irritability, depression, and withdrawal from social situations can occur. There is also a lowered body temperature, cold intolerance, fatigue, fainting, and a greater need for sleep. Some people lose heart tissue to some degree or develop heart rhythm irregularities. The skin becomes rough, dry, scaly, and cold. Bruising can occur because of less protective fat. After eating anything, abnormal fullness or bloating may last for hours. Hair loss is common. **Lanugo hair** may appear, which helps trap air and reduce heat loss caused by reduced fatty tissue. Semistarvation and laxative abuse may cause constipation. Loss of menstrual periods and related hormonal changes cause reduced bone mass and an increased risk of osteoporosis (see **Figure 29.2**). Neurotransmitter function in the brain is altered, leading to depression.

DIAGNOSIS

The two criteria for anorexia nervosa under the *DSM-5* include restriction of calorie consumption leading to weight loss or a failure to gain weight resulting in a significantly low body weight based on that person's age, sex, height, and stage of growth. Intense fear of gaining weight or becoming "fat."

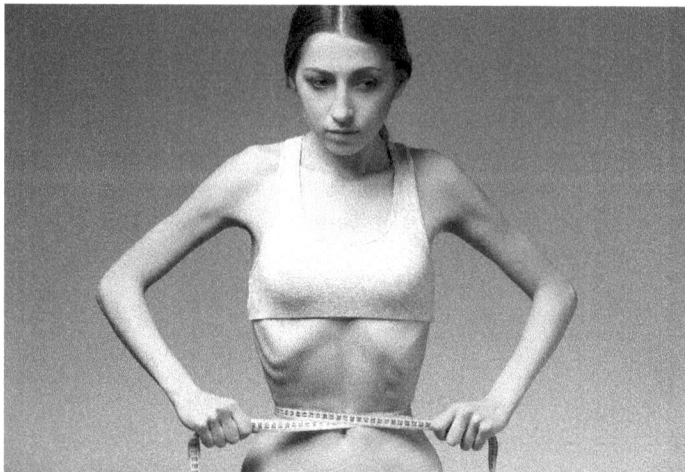

FIGURE 29.1   A patient with anorexia.

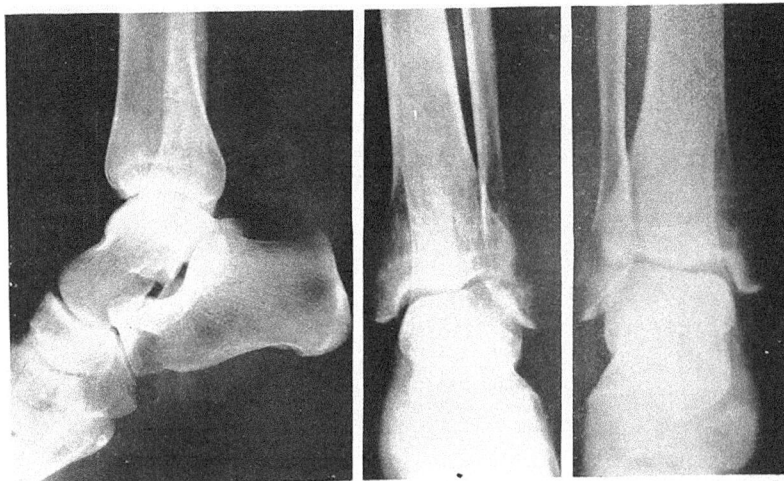

FIGURE 29.2   Decreased bone density, which leads to osteoporosis.

TREATMENT

Treatment of anorexia nervosa requires experienced physicians, registered dietitians, psychologists, and additional health professionals. Eating disorder clinics are often preferred, and treatment may require outpatient therapy, day hospitalization for up to 12 hours, or total hospitalization, which is necessary if the patient is below 75% of expected weight, has acute medical conditions, or has severe psychological problems (suicidal). Efforts sometimes fail regardless of the treatment team, so disease prevention is essential. Many people with anorexia try to hide their weight loss in various ways. It usually takes a person with anorexia about 7 years to recover fully, but many insurers only cover a small amount of the costs of treatment.

Nutrition therapy begins by gaining the patient's cooperation and trust to increase the intake of foods. Weight gain is best if it is sufficient to increase the metabolic rate to average and reverse many physical signs. An early goal is to minimize or stop additional weight loss. Appropriate food habits are slowly restored. Then, slow weight gain of 2–3 pounds/week is attempted. If immediate renourishment is needed, some patients require tube feeding, total parenteral nutrition, or both – but these efforts often cause the patient to distrust the treatment team. Calories are slowly increased, and a multivitamin and mineral supplement is added. Enough calcium is added to increase intake to about 1500 mg/day. Dietitians provide nutritional information, promote healthy food attitudes, and teach patients to eat when hungry and stop when complete. Reassurance is considerable because of uncomfortable bloating and increased body heat and fat. The medical team must assure the patient they will not be abandoned once they regain their average weight.

After this, the underlying emotional problems are addressed. The patient learns to reject a feeling of accomplishment they previously associated with emaciation and starts to accept the healthy body weight. Recovery is based on solid relationships with therapists and other support personnel. Patients are taught to regain control of their lives and cope with adverse situations. Once eating becomes normalized, the patient can return to activities they stopped enjoying while anorexic. Family therapy is essential for younger patients still living at home. Medications are sometimes required for anorexic patients, but these are primarily focused on preventing relapses after treatment when psychiatric disorders are still present. These disorders include depression, anxiety, and obsessive-compulsive disorder.

PREVENTION

Anorexia nervosa can result from various contributing factors, often the perfect storm of biological, psychological, and social triggers. Eradicating anorexia nervosa might not be realistic, but reducing its prevalence is possible by changing the way we talk about food and body image.

YOU SHOULD REMEMBER

Weight loss caused by anorexia nervosa is generally less than 85% of what is expected for the individual's age or a body mass index (BMI) of 17.5 or less. Many people with anorexia find a sense of security in the rigid control of their weight. Even a small weight gain makes them panic. Strict discipline and self-denial provide feelings of purity, power, and superiority. However, they often feel helpless in the presence of food. Anorexic women usually lack menstrual periods after the average age of puberty.

Check Your Knowledge

1. In which age groups do eating disorders usually begin?
2. What are the two primary forms of anorexia nervosa?
3. What are the effects of anorexia nervosa on the heart and brain?

BULIMIA NERVOSA

Bulimia nervosa involves episodes of binge eating that are followed by attempts to purge via vomiting or excessive use of laxatives, diuretics, or enemas. Another way some people with bulimia try to burn off excess energy after binge eating is to exercise excessively. People with bulimia use food to cope with extreme situations. They understand that their behaviors are abnormal, while people with anorexia do not. Often, there is very low self-esteem and depression underlying bulimia. Many people are not diagnosed due to a lack of apparent symptoms. Also, many of them hide their abnormal eating habits.

Epidemiology

For bulimia nervosa, there has been a decline in the overall incidence rate over time.

Regarding bulimia nervosa, up to 3% of females and more than 1% of males worldwide suffer from this disorder during their lifetime. In the United States, the estimated lifetime prevalence of bulimia nervosa is 0.3%; in females, it is 0.5%, and in males, it is 0.08%.

Etiology and Risk Factors

The exact cause of the bulimia is unknown. Several factors may have a role to play in the development of the condition, such as serotonin, dopamine, genetics, childhood trauma, neglect or abuse, and anxiety experienced in childhood. The risk factors include age, gender, and biological makeup.

Clinical Manifestations

Common characteristics of bulimia include erosion of teeth due to excessive vomiting. Many affected individuals have elaborate rules about food, often avoiding all types of sweets. People with bulimia are under a severe misconception that purging soon after binging will prevent excess energy absorption and the gaining of weight. The other option – excessive exercise – is often done at odd times of day, or it continues even though injuries or medical complications occur. They have low self-esteem and feelings of hopelessness. They become distant from other people, spending more time alone and focusing on their bulimia.

Repeated vomiting causes the majority of adverse health outcomes. The teeth become demineralized, making them painful and sensitive to temperatures and acids. Eventually, severe tooth decay occurs, with erosion from fillings, and the teeth fall out over time. Blood potassium may be deficient because of vomiting or certain diuretics, which can disturb heart rhythm and lead to sudden death. Infections and irritation from vomiting may cause inflammation of the salivary glands. In some people, there are esophageal tears and stomach ulcers. Frequent laxative use may lead to constipation. Ipecac syrup, if used to induce vomiting, is toxic to the heart, liver, and kidneys. Repeated doses may result in accidental poisoning. The complications of bulimia nervosa include loneliness, boredom, stress, depression, and death.

Diagnosis

The body weight and BMI can be helpful indicators in the diagnostic process. Most individuals with bulimia nervosa are of normal weight or slightly overweight, in contrast to patients with anorexia nervosa, who are usually underweight. A physical exam and blood and urine tests are performed to ensure another condition is not causing the patient's symptoms.

Treatment

Treatment of bulimia nervosa requires an experienced team. For severe weight loss, treatment begins with measures to gain back the needed weight, followed by psychological therapy and nutritional counseling. For extreme laxative abuse, chronic vomiting, substance abuse, and depression, hospitalization is often required. The initial treatment goal is to reduce how much food is consumed during binging. The patient is instructed about their condition and its likely consequences. They are taught that the disorder is severe, with potentially deadly complications.

Psychological therapy is required due to high rates of depression and suicide. The patient learns self-acceptance and becomes less concerned about their weight. All-or-none thinking is reversed. Group therapy helps supply solid social support. Antidepressants can be used, but they must accompany other therapies. Therapy for bulimia nervosa is long-term due to high relapse potential. Approximately 50% of patients recover complexly. Others battle the disorder in different amounts throughout life. Therefore, the need for prevention of bulimia nervosa is essential.

Prevention

Understanding the risk factors or variables that predict the development of the disorder is vital for prevention efforts. Through recent actions, we have begun to identify risk factors and examine how they increase the probability that an eating disorder will develop.

YOU SHOULD REMEMBER

Bulimia nervosa is an eating disorder that is also classified as a mental disorder. It is among the most fatal mental conditions of all because of related long-term health problems and even suicide. Many patients with bulimia also have depression. Affected individuals often feel shame and guilt about their inability to control their compulsive behaviors, worsening any preexisting depression.

Check Your Knowledge

1. What is the difference between anorexia nervosa and bulimia nervosa, related to how affected individuals perceive their conditions?
2. What often triggers binging?
3. What are the outcomes of bulimia nervosa?

BINGE-EATING DISORDER

Binge-eating disorder (BED) is less severe than bulimia nervosa, yet large amounts of food are still frequently consumed. While binging, food is consumed much more quickly than usual, and eating continues until the individual feels uncomfortable. Other behaviors in the disorder include eating large amounts of food even when not feeling hungry, eating alone due to embarrassment about the condition, and experiencing distress, depression, and guilt after overeating. Food is consumed with no thought about biological needs. It recurs in "ritualistic" behaviors. Some affected individuals eat food continually over long periods, while others have episodes of normal eating broken up by periods of binging.

Obesity and binge eating are not always related since many obese people do not binge eat. Even so, BED is most prevalent in the severely obese and those with chronic restrictive dieting, though many binge-eaters are not obese.

Epidemiology

BED is currently estimated to affect 1.5% of women and 0.3% of men worldwide; a lifetime diagnosis of BED is reported by 0.6%–1.8% of women and 0.3%–0.7% of men. In adolescence, BED is even more prevalent but often transient.

About 40% of binge-eaters are males and feel hungry more often than is typical. Nearly half of severe binge-eaters have clinical depression and isolate themselves.

Etiology and Risk Factors

Triggers for binge eating include stress, depression, and anxiety. Self-permission to eat "forbidden" foods may trigger a binge. Additional triggers include loneliness, fear, anger, alienation, rage, and frustration. Binge eating helps some people feel better or become numb to their emotions, often to avoid emotional pain and anxiety. Some stressed-out or frustrated people eat continually until they go to bed in an attempt to forget about their jobs or other stressors. Some people binge eat only when emotional setbacks happen. Often, affected individuals have dysfunctional families that poorly cope with emotions, so turning to substance use or abuse or binge eating becomes an option.

Clinical Manifestations

People with BED exhibit and experience several of the following symptoms weekly for periods lasting at least 3 months: rapid eating until uncomfortably full, eating large amounts of food without being physically hungry, feelings of guilt after overeating, weight fluctuation, loss of sexual desire, and feelings of low self-esteem.

Diagnosis

About 30%–50% of people in weight-control programs have been diagnosed with BED, though only 1%–2% of people in North America are affected. There are less severe forms of the disease in the general population that lack the criteria for a diagnosis of BED. Cases of the illness are much more numerous than cases of anorexia nervosa or bulimia nervosa. The condition may be preceded by frequent dieting, starting in childhood or adolescence. When little food is eaten, the individual becomes extremely hungry and needs to eat compulsively, without control.

Treatment

The individual often overcomes BED without professional help. If nutrition therapy is needed, it is similar to what is used for bulimia nervosa. Psychological treatment focuses on identifying emotional needs and expressing emotions. Communication issues must be assessed. The individual often requires help to recognize hidden emotions in situations that produce anxiety. They learn simple yet appropriate phrases that help remind them to stop binging when the desire to do so is strong. Treatment tries to create environments of encouragement and accountability. Antidepressants sometimes help to reduce binge eating since depressive triggers are reduced.

Prevention

The chronic nature of BED and its associated comorbidities underscore the significance of prevention. Early intervention and education can allow individuals to adopt healthier eating habits, develop coping mechanisms, and foster a positive relationship with food.

NIGHT EATING SYNDROME

Some individuals only eat or purge large amounts of food at night. This is known as **night eating syndrome**. Most people with eating disorders are in this category. It is classified as an Unspecified feeding or eating disorder because this disorder does not meet the criteria for anorexia nervosa, bulimia nervosa, or binge-eating disorder. In night eating disorder, food is consumed in larger quantities late in the evening, or eating occurs after being awakened during the night in an attempt to fall asleep again. Night eating contributes to weight gain, so treatment should be obtained.

FEMALE ATHLETE TRIAD

The **female athlete triad** is a potentially severe condition affecting many young women. It is a combination of disordered eating, amenorrhea, and osteoporosis. It is often not recognized, but bone mineral density loss can be severe for female athletes. Early osteoporotic fractures can occur, and the lost bone mineral density may never return. The triad requires early recognition by family physicians via assessing risk factors and offering specific screening questions. A good diet and controlled exercise frequency may achieve the natural return of menstruation. To prevent loss of bone density, hormone replacement therapy may be needed. Treatment may require interactive efforts between athletic trainers, coaches, parents, physicians, and athletes. Possibly life-threatening illnesses can be prevented by increased education of everyone involved.

Disordered eating may involve food restriction, binging, and purging to lose weight and remain thin. **Amenorrhea** related to athletic training and weight fluctuations is due to changes in the hypothalamus, which decreases estrogen levels. The amenorrhea may be primary or secondary. With **primary amenorrhea**, there is no spontaneous uterine bleeding by the age of 14 with no development of secondary sexual characteristics or no spontaneous uterine bleeding by age 16 with otherwise normal development. Secondary amenorrhea is the 6-month lack of menstrual bleeding in a female with primary regular **menses** or a 12-month lack with previous **oligomenorrhea**.

Epidemiology

The exact prevalence of the female athlete triad is generally unknown. Disordered eating occurs in 15%–62% of female college athletes. Amenorrhea occurs in 3.4%–66%, which is much higher than the rates of 2%–5% in the general female population.

Etiology and Risk Factors

Premature osteoporosis increases the risks of stress fractures along with severe hip or vertebral column fractures. Morbidity is high, and lost bone density may be permanent. Pathogenic weight-control behaviors may be due to frequent **weigh-ins**, disciplinary actions because of weight gain, increased pressure to always win in competitions, excessive control by coaches or parents, and social isolation because of obsessive focus on athletic activities. The female athlete triad is highest in females who engage in figure skating, gymnastics, swimming, diving, and long-distance running. Prevention requires education for all parties involved. Coaches must never overemphasize weight control. For example, 75% of female college gymnasts use pathogenic behaviors for weight control after being told by coaches that they are overweight.

Clinical Manifestations

Screening for the female athlete triad is best done during physical examinations before competitions. Screening can also be done during acute visits for fractures, disordered eating, weight changes, amenorrhea, arrhythmia, bradycardia, and depression, and during visits for routine Pap smears. A history of amenorrhea is an easy way to detect the triad in the early stages. The condition is abnormal in female athletes and must be reported when it develops. Past eating behaviors should be discussed since this is less threatening to the female athlete than focusing on any current eating disorders. Histories of menstruation, diet, and exercise should be taken as follows:

- *Menstruation* – age at menarche, menstrual cycle frequency and duration, most extended period without any menstruation, last menstrual period, signs of ovulation, any previous or current hormonal therapy
- *Diet* – diet in the last 24 hours, lists of any "forbidden" foods, highest and lowest weight since menarche, happiness with current weight, the patient's "ideal weight," binging or purging, and use of **laxatives**, diuretics, or diet pills
- *Exercise* – patterns and training intensity of exercise (hours/day and days/week), additional activity that is outside of required training, histories of previous fractures or overuse injuries

Common signs and symptoms of disordered eating include anorexia nervosa, bradycardia, cachexia, hypotension, hypothermia, lanugo, cold intolerance, dry hair and skin, hypercarotenemia, alopecia, pruritus, bulimia nervosa, abdominal pain, fatigue, chest pain, sore throat or esophagitis, swollen parotid glands, erosion of tooth enamel, constipation, knuckle scars or calluses, and bloodshot eyes.

Diagnosis

Diagnosis of the female athlete triad includes individual history, physical activity, diet, eating behaviors, past injuries, and menstrual history; blood tests for assessing nutrient and hormone levels; dual-energy X-ray absorptiometry (DXA) test to measure bone density.

Treatment

Early treatment can help prevent further bone compromise and return the child to good health. Common treatments for the female athlete triad include a new diet and nutrition to increase calorie consumption, a change in exercise routine, and hormone and vitamin supplements. It is essential to restore regular menstrual cycling and enhance bone mineral density (BMD). Modifying the diet and exercise regimens to increase overall energy availability is needed. To resume menses, athletes may need to improve their energy availability to at least 30 kcal/kg of fat-free mass daily.

Prevention

To prevent the female athlete triad, eat a nutrient-rich, well-balanced diet, exercise moderately, and get plenty of rest.

YOU SHOULD REMEMBER

Some female athletes who focus on being thinner eat too little or exercise too much, causing long-term damage to health and even death. Abnormal eating habits or excessive exercise prevents the body from getting sufficient nutrition. Often, hormonal changes result, leading to irregular menses or amenorrhea. This disrupts bone-building processes, weakening the skeleton and increasing the likelihood of fractures. In severe cases, young female athletes have even developed early-onset osteoporosis.

Check Your Knowledge

1. In which individuals is the BED most prevalent?
2. What are the three features of the female athlete triad?
3. In which types of athletes is the female athlete triad most common?

Clinical Case Studies

CLINICAL CASE STUDY 1

A 20-year-old woman, previously diagnosed with anorexia nervosa, was admitted to a mental health center. She weighed only 84 pounds (which was about 50 pounds underweight for her height), and tests revealed that she had kidney, liver, and pancreatic damage. The patient remained in the facility for 8 weeks and underwent significant psychiatric and physical treatments. It was found that her anorexia nervosa was based on feelings of "needing to get revenge" on her parents because of feeling emotionally distanced from them. At discharge, the patient gained 23 pounds and agreed to return to the facility if her weight dropped below 100 pounds. She continued to undergo regular weight management regimens and utilized support groups for her condition to prevent any recurrence of her negative behaviors.

CRITICAL THINKING QUESTIONS

1. How is anorexia nervosa described?
2. What is a common underlying factor of anorexia nervosa?
3. What do people with anorexia fear, and how do they perceive themselves?

CLINICAL CASE STUDY 2

A 22-year-old woman had become overly concerned about her weight. Soon, she became obsessed with counting calories and often avoided eating as long as possible. She then started buying sweet foods such as cakes and candy, which she usually ate in large quantities as one meal. She would then force herself to vomit up the food. Her binges began to occur more frequently, and her mood was seriously affected as she became more upset with herself and her uncontrollable behaviors.

CRITICAL THINKING QUESTIONS

1. How common is bulimia nervosa?
2. What can the repeated vomiting of bulimia nervosa cause?
3. Why is psychological therapy necessary for bulimia nervosa?

CLINICAL CASE STUDY 3

A 29-year-old woman has lost control of her eating patterns and often consumes food until she is uncomfortably full, falling asleep afterward. She feels depressed because of her situation. Binge eating occurs at least once per week. The condition even resulted in her husband divorcing her because of her significant weight gain and lack of self-control. The patient tried a variety of substances in an attempt to control her binge eating but has never gone to psychotherapy.

CRITICAL THINKING QUESTIONS

1. In which group of individuals is BED most prevalent?
2. How common is BED?
3. What are the triggers for BED?

FURTHER READING

1. Chukwuemeka, N., Spinn, B., and Treasure, J. (2024). *Eating Disorders Don't Discriminate: Stories of Illness, Hope and Recovery from Diverse Voices.* Jessica Kingsley Publishers.
2. Costin, C., Schubert Grabb, G., and Rothschild, B. (2011). *8 Keys to Recovery from an Eating Disorder: Effective Strategies from Therapeutic Practice and Personal Experience (8 Keys to Mental Health).* W.W. Norton and Company.
3. Crosbie, C., and Sterline, W. (2023). *How to Nourish Yourself through an Eating Disorder: Recovery for Adults with the Plate-by-Plate Approach.* The Experiment.
4. Farrell, N.R., Black Becker, C., and Waller, G. (2024). *Eat without Fear: Harnessing Science to Confront and Overcome Your Eating Disorder.* Oxford University Press.
5. Gaudiani, J.L. (2018). *Sick Enough: A Guide to the Medical Complications of Eating Disorders.* Routledge.
6. Grilo, C.M., and Mitchell, J.E. (2011). *The Treatment of Eating Disorders: A Clinical Handbook.* The Guilford Press.
7. Kalata, A.H., and Thebner Miller, E. (2024). *DBT Principles and Strategies in the Multidisciplinary Treatment of Eating Disorders.* Routledge.
8. Kim, I.M. (2023). *Effective Strategies for Treating and Managing Eating Disorders: Proven Techniques for Overcoming and Controlling Eating Disorders – Transform Your Life Today!* Kim.
9. McClain, D. (2020). *Mindful Eating: An Essential Guide to Eating Based on Mindfulness and Ending Overeating, Binge Eating, Food Addiction and Emotional Eating.* McClain.
10. Mehler, P.S., and Andersen, A.E. (2022). *Eating Disorders: A Comprehensive Guide to Medical Care and Complications*, 4th Edition. Johns Hopkins University Press.
11. Pershing, A., and Turner, C. (2018). *Binge Eating Disorder: The Journey to Recovery and Beyond.* Routledge.
12. Savelle-Rocklin, N. (2019). *The Binge Cure: 7 Steps to Outsmart Emotional Eating.* Adler Press.
13. Seubert, A., and Virdi, P. (2023). *Trauma-Informed Approaches to Eating Disorders.* Springer.
14. Siegel, M., Brisman, J., and Weinshel, M. (2021). *I Survived an Eating Disorder: Strategies for Family and Friends*, 4th Edition. Harper Perennial.
15. Yandel Grabowski, A. (2017). *An Internal Family Systems Guide to Recovery from Eating Disorders: Healing Part by Part.* Routledge.

30 Nutritional Effects on Cancer

OVERVIEW

The development of cancer leads to organ destruction and impaired function, culminating in cachexia and death. In cachexia, there are many metabolic and physiologic alterations, including weakness, anorexia, weight loss, compromised immune function, and depletion and translocation of typical body components, resulting in a condition that resembles malnutrition. To combat the effects of cancer on the body, an extremely healthy diet is required. Nutritional interventions must be implemented as soon as cancer is diagnosed and must be individualized to the needs of each patient. The effects of lifestyle choices, such as alcohol and dietary components like red meat, sodium chloride, and fat, need to be closely assessed since they have a clear impact on certain types of cancers. Also, patients should be educated that cancer can result in changes in appetite, such as early fullness and alterations of taste and smell, which also affect proper nutrition.

DIET AND CANCER

No food can prevent cancer; excluding specific foods does not eliminate the risk. However, eating a diet based on plant foods like vegetables, whole grains, beans, and fruits can help to reduce the risk of cancer and several other chronic diseases.

The risk of developing cancer is linked to the consumption of certain food substances. Diets high in fat are linked to an increased risk of breast, stomach, colon, liver, and prostate cancers. Overweight or obese individuals have higher risks of cancers of the breast, colon, endometrium, esophagus, and kidneys. Alcoholics have a much higher risk of developing cancer of the esophagus. Diets high in smoked or pickled foods or high in meats cooked at high temperatures increase the risks of stomach cancer.

Consuming a diet high in fruits, vegetables, and whole grains can reduce overall cancer risks. Sugary drinks should be avoided, and calorie-dense foods should be limited. Beef, pork, lamb, and processed meats should be limited. Alcoholic beverages should be limited. Salty foods and foods processed with table salt must be specified. Supplements should not be used to protect against cancer because their proven benefits are minimal. Cancer survivors must always follow dietary recommendations after they have been treated.

BREAST CANCER

There are known links between dietary fat and certain cancers, such as breast cancer. However, the percentage of calories consumed from total fat is not significantly linked to higher cancer risks for adults. Animal fat intake is correlated to higher breast cancer risks. Premenopausal women who consume foods high in animal fat have a 40%–50% higher risk of breast cancer compared to women who eat less animal fat. The findings suggest that red meat and high-fat dairy products may contain factors such as hormones, which increase risks for breast cancer. Lower breast cancer risks are related to a high intake of monounsaturated fats (primarily olive oil). Eating fruits and vegetables may also be linked to a decreased risk of breast cancer. Drinking alcohol is related to an increased risk of breast cancer.

Breast cancer invades locally, spreading through regional lymph nodes, the bloodstream, or both. It metastasizes primarily to the lungs, liver, bones, brain, and skin. Some tumors recur earlier, and tumor markers are often able to predict recurrence.

DOI: 10.1201/9781003453376-37

EPIDEMIOLOGY

In the United States, breast cancer is the second leading cause of cancer among women in most racial or ethnic groups, except for Hispanic-American women, in which it is the leading cause of cancer death. There are nearly 282,000 new annual cases of invasive breast cancer, almost 50,000 new cases of in situ breast cancer, and almost 44,000 deaths from the disease. Male breast cancer only makes up about 1% of all cases of the disease, with over 2,600 new cases and over 500 deaths. While the manifestations, diagnosis, and treatment methods are the same, men usually develop breast cancer at a later stage of life.

For American women, there is approximately a 12% lifetime risk of developing breast cancer, mainly after age 60, with the risk of death being about 10% within 5 years of diagnosis.

Lobular carcinoma in situ is often multifocal and bilateral and may be classic or pleomorphic. Invasive carcinoma is usually an adenocarcinoma, with 80% being the infiltrating ductal type. *Inflammatory breast cancer* is a form that proliferates, is highly aggressive, and is often fatal. **Paget disease** is a type of ductal carcinoma in situ (DCIS) that extends into the skin over the nipple and **areola**.

ETIOLOGY AND RISK FACTORS

Breast cancer develops due to DNA damage and genetic mutations that can be influenced by exposure to estrogen. Sometimes, DNA defects or pro-cancerous genes will be inherited. Thus, the family history of ovarian or breast cancer increases the risk of breast cancer development. Factors that may increase risks include age, personal or gynecologic history, breast changes, use of oral contraceptives, hormone therapy, radiation therapy, smoking, and alcohol use.

CLINICAL MANIFESTATIONS

Signs and symptoms of breast cancer include a palpable mass, breast enlargement or thickening, breast pain, skin changes, **erythema**, an "orange peel" appearance of the breast, nipple discharge, abdominal pain, jaundice, dyspnea, breast asymmetry, fixation of a mass to the chest wall or overlying skin, and satellite nodules or ulcers of the skin.

DIAGNOSIS

Diagnosis of breast cancer involves screening by mammography, ultrasonography, and biopsy that analyzes the presence of estrogen receptors and progesterone receptors. After diagnosis, a multidisciplinary evaluation is usually done to plan treatment. There may be a need for bone scanning and abdominal and chest CT (Computerized tomography). Grading is based on histologic examination of biopsied tissues. Staging follows the tumor, nodes, and metastases (TNM) classification. Breast cancer patients should avoid becoming pregnant once treatments begin. The long-term prognosis of breast cancer is based on staging. The 5-year survival rate is as follows for the various breast cancer stages:

- *Localized (primary site only)* – 99%
- *Regional (in regional lymph nodes only)* – 85.8%
- *Unknown* – 57.8%
- *Distant (metastasized)* – 29%

A worsened prognosis is based on younger patient age, non-Hispanic African-American racial or ethnic group, larger primary tumors, high-grade tumors, lack of estrogen and progesterone receptors, presence of the human epidermal growth factor receptor 2 (HER2) protein, and presence of BReast CAncer gene (BRCA) gene mutations.

TREATMENT

Treatments for breast cancer include surgery, radiation therapy (in most cases), and systemic therapy with endocrine therapy, chemotherapy, or both. Mastectomy is the removal of the entire breast and may be described as skin-sparing, nipple-sparing, simple, modified radical, and *radical*. The extreme form is rarely done unless the cancer has invaded the pectoral muscles. Breast-conserving surgery is based on tumor size and the required margins and may be described as **lumpectomy**, wide excision, or **quadrantectomy**. During mastectomy and breast-conserving surgery, the axillary lymph nodes are usually evaluated via *axillary lymph node dissection.*

Reconstructive procedures include *prosthetic* and *autologous* reconstruction. In **prosthetic reconstruction**, a silicone or saline implant is introduced, sometimes after using a tissue expander. With **autologous rebuilding**, there is a muscle flap or muscle-free flap transfer. A contralateral prophylactic mastectomy is an option for breast cancer patients if there is a genetic mutation that results in a high risk of cancer reoccurring in the other breast.

After breast-conserving surgery, radiation therapy significantly reduces local recurrences and can improve overall survival for most patients. Chemotherapy or endocrine treatment can delay or prevent recurrence in nearly all patients and can prolong survival for some. Postmenopausal patients with estrogen receptor-negative tumors have the most benefits from adjuvant chemotherapy. For estrogen receptor-positive tumors, combination chemotherapy or endocrine therapy alone will be indicated.

Generally, combination chemotherapies are more effective than single drugs. Options include doxorubicin, cyclophosphamide, paclitaxel, filgrastim, pegfilgrastim, trastuzumab, pertuzumab, and endocrine therapies such as tamoxifen or aromatase inhibitors. Metastases require immediate evaluation, with treatments based on the hormone-receptor status of the tumor, length of disease-free interval from remission to manifestations of metastases, the number of metastatic sites and organs affected, and the patient's menopausal status. Endocrine therapies, tyrosine kinase inhibitors, radiation therapy, palliative mastectomy, and intravenous bisphosphonates are all options.

PREVENTION

Women should begin monthly self-breast examinations at age 20. They should also be screened for breast cancer via three-dimensional mammography, clinical breast examination, and Magnetic Resonance Imaging (MRI) for high-risk patients. Screening mammography usually starts at ages 40–50, repeated every 2 years until age 75.

YOU SHOULD REMEMBER

Increased consumption of total and saturated fats is positively associated with the development of breast cancer. Although some fat is necessary in the diet, too much can lead to cancers as well as heart disease, obesity, and other health problems. An important consideration is that women with breast cancer who continue to have high *trans fat* intake have an increased risk of all-cause mortality, which is between 45% and 78%.

Check Your Knowledge

1. What is the impact of animal fats in the diet on premenopausal women with breast cancer?
2. What types of foods may decrease the risk of breast cancer?
3. What are the diagnostic procedures for breast cancer?

STOMACH CANCER

A definite link exists between high-salt foods, including meat, fish, and vegetables preserved by salting, and stomach cancer. Many traditional foods in countries such as Japan and Korea are preserved by salting and fermentation instead of the refrigeration methods preferred by many Western countries. Large amounts of salt infuse the foods in the preservation process, resulting in damage to the stomach lining and the development of lesions that may lead to stomach cancer.

Infection with the **Helicobacter pylori** (H. pylori) bacteria also damages the stomach lining, which may be worsened by excessive salt. Much dietary salt is "hidden" in foods, so people may be unaware of how much they consume. With the global population eating out more often and cooking less at home, the proportion of dietary salt is increasing. The limit for dietary salt in the United States is less than 2.3 g daily. Understanding the table salt levels in everyday foods generally not considered "salty," such as bread and soups, is essential. The top 10 foods that contain the highest average amounts of salt are as follows:

- *Pizza* – 640 mg
- *Soups* – 600–700 mg
- *Sandwiches* – 600 mg
- *Burritos and tacos* – 274–985 mg
- *Cold cuts and cured meats* – 214–590 mg
- *Cheese* – 174 mg
- *Savory snacks (chips, popcorn, pretzels, snack mixes, crackers)* – 120–418 mg
- *Breads and rolls* – 117 mg
- *Fried chicken* – 100 mg
- *Eggs and omelets (based on how they are prepared)* – 62–95 mg

EPIDEMIOLOGY

Gastric cancer is among the five most common cancers worldwide, accounting for more than 750,000 deaths in 2020. Most new cases occur in areas with lower socio-economic indices, with approximately half of the newly diagnosed cases in East Asia. Incidence rates are twice as high in men than in women and are increasing with age for both sexes. Approximately 90% of gastric cancers are adenocarcinomas. The global rates of gastric non-cardia cancer are declining, which can be attributed to a lower prevalence of H. pylori infection, a well-established risk factor. In the United States, there are about 27,000 cases and 11,000 deaths from stomach cancer, making it the seventh most common cause of cancer death. It is most common in Africans, Hispanics, and Native Americans. Incidence increases with age since more than 75% of patients are 50 or older. Gastric adenocarcinoma makes up 95% of malignant stomach tumors, with less common forms, including localized gastric lymphomas and **leiomyosarcomas**.

ETIOLOGY AND RISK FACTORS

H. pylori infection has been demonstrated to be a significant risk factor for the development of gastric cancer. Unhealthy diet and lifestyle, including high-salt food, smoking, and drinking, can induce genotypic and phenotypic transformation of gastric epithelial cells.

CLINICAL MANIFESTATIONS

Symptoms of stomach cancer include **dyspepsia**, early satiety, **dysphagia**, weight loss, reduced strength, massive **hematemesis**, **melena**, secondary anemia from occult blood loss, jaundice, ascites, heme-positive stools, epigastric masses, lymph node enlargement, and **hepatomegaly**. There may be pulmonary, central nervous system, or bone metastasis.

DIAGNOSIS

Diagnosis includes upper endoscopy with biopsy, CT scan, and endoscopic ultrasonography. Barium swallow with a series of stomach X-rays and biomarker tests are helpful. Prognosis is usually poor, with a 5-year survival of only 5%–15% since most patients present once the disease is already advanced. However, when the stomach cancer is only within the mucosa or submucosa, 5-year survival may be up to 80%. If the local lymph nodes are involved, survival is 20%–40%. If more widespread, it is usually fatal within 1 year.

TREATMENT

Treatment is with surgical resection, sometimes accompanied by chemotherapy, radiation, or both. Treatment is heavily based on staging. Most or all of the stomach and adjacent lymph nodes are usually removed. Resection of locally advanced regional disease provides a 10-month median survival compared to only 3–4 months without resection. For metastasis or extensive nodal involvement, palliative treatments are usually done.

PREVENTION

Although there is no guarantee that lifestyle changes can entirely prevent stomach cancer, several can reduce the risk of developing the disease. Maintaining a healthy body weight and eating more fruits and vegetables is essential.

Check Your Knowledge

1. How is dietary table salt linked to stomach cancer?
2. In which countries does stomach cancer occur the most?
3. What are the symptoms of stomach cancer?

COLON CANCER

A high consumption of red meat is linked to an increased risk of colon cancer. Individuals who consume at least five ounces of red meat per day are about 33% more likely to develop colon cancer than those who eat less than one ounce per day. White meat, such as chicken, does not increase the risk of colon cancer, and high fish consumption reduces risks by about 33%. High consumption of red meat, as well as processed meats, is linked to a substantial increase in the risk of cancer of the lower colon and rectum. Long-term consumption of large amounts of fish and poultry appears to be protective.

There are several theories as to why red meat is linked to higher rates of colon cancer. The first states that **heterocyclic amines**, produced during high-temperature red meat cooking, are to blame. Another theory states that preservatives such as *nitrates* are causative because the body converts them to a carcinogenic form known as *nitrosamines*. However, fresh red meat is also linked to colon cancer, so preservatives may not be entirely causative. A third theory states that diets high in red meat result in high levels of *N-nitroso compounds*, which are potentially cancer-causing chemicals. These compounds may induce DNA changes that lead to cancer.

Large amounts of red meat can produce genetic damage to the colon cells over just a few weeks. If the body's DNA repair mechanisms fail, cells can experience malignant transformation. Prevention of colon cancer is based on reduced caloric intake, regular exercise, avoiding tobacco products, limiting alcohol intake, reasonable amounts of calcium from dairy products, vitamin D, fruits, vegetables, whole grains, fish, low-dose aspirin, and regular colon cancer screening tests based on age, family history, and risk factors. Red meat should always be considered a "side dish" for meals and not the main focus. Just two 4-ounce portions per week are suggested, and the meat should be lean, with excess fat trimmed away, and not charred on a grill. Processed, cured, and salted meats must be limited as much as possible. The primary protein sources should be fish, chicken, and turkey (without the skin), accompanied by protein sources such as beans.

EPIDEMIOLOGY

There are nearly 148,000 cases of colon cancer in the United States annually and over 53,000 deaths – mostly in people between 40 and 50 years of age. In older adults, the incidence of colon cancer is increased. Over 50% of cases occur in the rectum and **sigmoid colon**, with 95% being **adenocarcinomas**. Colon cancer is slightly more common in men. About 5% of patients have more than one cancer at the same time. Most cases result when **adenomatous polyps** transform, with 80% of cases being sporadic and 20% inherited. Predisposing factors include chronic **ulcerative colitis** and Crohn's disease. Carcinogens are produced mainly by bacterial action upon dietary substances or secretions from the biliary tract or intestines. Colon cancer spreads via direct extension through the colon wall, **hematogenous** metastasis, and regional lymph node metastasis.

ETIOLOGY AND RISK FACTORS

Colon cancer typically affects older adults, though it can happen at any age. It usually begins as small polyps that form inside the colon. Polyps generally are not cancerous, but some can turn into colon cancers over time. The risk factors include a family history of colon cancer, aging, race (African-American), having a history of colon polyps, ulcerative colitis, Crohn's disease, a diet low in fiber and high in fat and calories, diabetes, and radiation therapy.

CLINICAL MANIFESTATIONS

Colon adenocarcinomas grow slowly, with symptoms occurring much later that are based on tumor location, type, size, and any complications. Obstruction of the right colon occurs later in the disease course, with occult bleeding. Some patients only experience fatigue and weakness from severe anemia. Some tumors can be palpated through the abdominal wall before other signs and symptoms occur. The left colon is more often obstructed by tumors, resulting in colicky abdominal pain or complete obstruction, bloody stool, focal pain and tenderness, or, in rare cases, diffuse peritonitis. If the cancer is only in the rectum, there is usually bleeding with defecation. Apparent hemorrhoids, known diverticular disease, or coexisting cancers must be ruled out. There may be tenesmus or a feeling of incomplete evacuation. If there is perirectal involvement, pain is joint. Sometimes, initial signs and symptoms include ascites, hepatomegaly, or supraclavicular lymph node enlargement.

DIAGNOSIS

Diagnosis of colon cancer is based on **colonoscopy**, fecal occult blood testing, and, less often, flexible sigmoidoscopy, fecal DNA testing, and CT colonography. Patients with a family history of a first-degree relative with colon cancer before age 60 should have a colonoscopy every 5 years, starting at age 40 or 10 years before the age at which the relative was diagnosed (whichever is first). Diagnostic tests include colonoscopic biopsy, CT scans to evaluate tumor growth and spread, and genetic testing.

TREATMENT

The treatment of colon cancer is surgical resection, sometimes combined with chemotherapy, radiation, or both. A surgical cure is attempted in 70% of patients who present without metastatic disease. For rectal cancer, the sphincter can be saved via surgical resection if there is a distal margin of 1 cm or more instead of the usual 5 cm length, with no significant risk of local recurrence or decreased long-term survival. If there is liver metastasis, resection of 1–3 of the metastatic lesions is recommended for certain non-debilitated patients as a follow-up procedure. Chemotherapy improves survival by 10%–30% if positive lymph nodes exist. A surveillance colonoscopy is done 1 year after any surgery or after a clearing preoperative colonoscopy. Another colonoscopy is done 3 years later if no polyps or tumors have been found. After that, a surveillance colonoscopy is done every 5 years. If curative surgery is not possible or there are dangerous surgical risks, limited palliative surgery may be done, but the median survival is 7 months. Medications include capecitabine, irinotecan, oxaliplatin, bevacizumab, cetuximab, panitumumab, or floxuridine, sometimes in combination.

PREVENTION

Prevention of colon cancer includes eating a variety of fruits, vegetables, and whole grains, drinking alcohol in moderation, stopping smoking, and maintaining a healthy weight. Screening for colon cancer with colonoscopy is essential around age 45. However, people with an increased risk should think about starting screening sooner.

YOU SHOULD REMEMBER

For average-risk patients, screening for colon cancer should begin at age 45 and continue until age 75. For those over 75, screening choices are individualized based on overall health and previous screening history. Screening may involve colonoscopy (every 10 years) and annual fecal occult blood testing. Flexible sigmoidoscopy should be done every 5 years (or every 10 years if done with fecal immunochemical tests), CT colonography every 5 years, or fecal DNA testing with fecal immunochemical tests every 3 years.

Check Your Knowledge

1. What amount of red meat consumption increases the risk of colon cancer?
2. How prevalent is colon cancer?
3. What are the statistics on colon cancer-related deaths?

LIVER CANCER

Hepatocellular carcinoma (HCC) is the fifth most common form of cancer worldwide and the third most common cause of cancer-related deaths. In the United States and other Western countries, alcohol consumption is relatively high. Approximately 8.5% of U.S. adults have an alcohol use disorder over any 1 year. HCC may develop in patients with **cirrhosis**, primarily if there is coexisting iron accumulation. Liver cancers were discussed in **Chapter 27**.

PROSTATE CANCER

Prostate cancer is the second leading cause of cancer death in American men, after lung cancer. Dietary fat may play a significant role in developing this cancer. Diets high in animal fat are linked to prostate cancer since they may boost testosterone levels. There is also a link between saturated fat and a higher chance of advanced prostate cancer and related death, yet there is no connection to early-stage prostate cancer. In one large study, the primary sources of saturated fat included beef, margarine, and dairy products such as butter and whole milk. Some people may have higher amounts of the insulin-like growth factor 1 hormone, which is implicated in cancer growth. Ongoing studies are focusing on how inflammation, hormone imbalances, and a buildup of lipids from a high-fat diet contribute to prostate cancer.

EPIDEMIOLOGY

Adenocarcinoma of the prostate gland is the most common cancer in men aged 50 or older. However, only 1 in 350 men under the age of 50 years will be diagnosed with prostate cancer. In the United States, there are nearly 288,300 cases and over 34,000 deaths/year. Incidence increases with each decade of age, and autopsies reveal this cancer to be present in 15%–60% of men between 60 and 90 years of age. The incidence rate increases to 1 in every 52 men aged 50–59. The incidence rate is nearly 60% in men over the age of 65 years. The median age at diagnosis is 72, with more than 75% occurring in men over 65. There is an African-American predominance. About one in eight men will be diagnosed with prostate cancer during his lifetime. Prostate cancer is more likely to develop in older men. About 6 cases in 10 are diagnosed in men who are 65 or older, and it is rare in men under 40.

ETIOLOGY AND RISK FACTORS

The exact causes of prostate cancer in an individual patient may not be clear. However, understanding the risk factors may help men take preventive measures to reduce the likelihood of developing prostate cancer. Prostate cancer risk factors include some that cannot be changed, such as having a family history of the disease and a genetic predisposition to developing cancer. However, other risk factors may be adjusted to help lower the likelihood of developing prostate cancer. Diets high in animal fat are linked to prostate cancer since they may boost testosterone levels.

CLINICAL MANIFESTATIONS

Prostate cancer is usually of slow progression, often without symptoms until it has advanced. At that point, symptoms include **hematuria**, straining, hesitancy, weak or intermittent urine stream, incomplete emptying, terminal dribbling, renal colic, flank pain, renal dysfunction, polyuria, and nocturia.

DIAGNOSIS

Prostate cancer is diagnosed by screening via digital rectal examination, **prostate-specific antigen** (PSA) test, and needle biopsy. Sometimes, a prostate-specific membrane is antigen-based. Screening is usually done annually for men aged 50 or older but may be started earlier for high-risk men. Once a prostate cancer diagnosis has been made, determining the stage of the cancer must be done. If cancer spreads beyond the prostate, the following imaging tests are recommended:

- Bone scan
- Ultrasound
- CT scan
- MRI
- Positron emission tomography (PET) scan

TREATMENT

Surgery, radiation therapy, or active surveillance is done for localized cancer. For cancer outside of the prostate, treatments include palliation with hormonal therapy, radiation therapy, or chemotherapy. For some men with low-risk cancers, active surveillance without treatment is done. PSA levels, grade and stage of the tumor, patient age, coexisting disorders, life expectancy, and patient preferences guide treatments. **Radical prostatectomy** is considered best for patients less than 75 years of age with a tumor that is only within the prostate. Other treatments include **cryotherapy**, standard external beam radiation therapy, **hypofractionation**, and **brachytherapy**. For metastatic prostate cancer, hormonal therapy is effective for a limited amount of time; for complications due to bone metastases, denosumab or zoledronic acid can be used.

PREVENTION

There is no proven prostate cancer prevention strategy. However, men may reduce the risk of prostate cancer by making healthy choices, such as exercising and eating a healthy diet. Foods containing fats, including meats, nuts, oils, and dairy products like milk and cheese, should be avoided.

YOU SHOULD REMEMBER

Monounsaturated omega-9 fatty acids and polyunsaturated omega-3 fatty acids are the fats recommended to be included in men's diets to prevent prostate cancer. The omega-9 fatty acids come from avocados, almonds, hazelnuts, pecans, pistachios, extra-virgin olive oil, almond oil, canola oil, and macadamia nut oil. The omega-3 fatty acids come from cold-water fish (salmon, sardines, black cod, trout, herring) and seeds (flaxseed, chia seeds, hemp seeds, and pumpkin seeds).

Check Your Knowledge

1. What are the links between dietary fat and prostate cancer?
2. What are the "good fats" that may help prevent prostate cancer?
3. How is increased age-related to prostate cancer?

Clinical Case Studies

CLINICAL CASE STUDY 1

A 58-year-old woman had been diagnosed with colon cancer that had metastasized to her liver. She presented for management of weight loss since she had lost 22% of her body weight over the past 6 months. Her most significant symptoms were loss of appetite, drowsiness, and shortness of breath. The patient was treated for a vitamin D deficiency, started on a home exercise program to improve her overall strength, and received nutritional counseling. Radiation therapy was given for her abdominal metastases. Slowly, her weight increased, and all other symptoms improved.

CRITICAL THINKING QUESTIONS

1. What is the prevention of colon cancer based on?
2. Which age groups are affected mainly by colon cancer?
3. What are the 5-year survival rates for colon cancer?

CLINICAL CASE STUDY 2

A 62-year-old man had experienced sharp stomach pains and feelings of fullness over about 6 months. He believed it to be from a stomach ulcer and tried his best to self-medicate to reduce the symptoms. However, the pain eventually became severe enough that it affected his ability to work. His appetite diminished, and he began losing weight, finally prompting him to see his physician. He had lost 16 pounds very quickly. Blood tests and an endoscopy with biopsy were done, revealing stomach cancer. A surgical procedure to remove the tumor was scheduled. After surgery, the patient received chemotherapy and radiation therapy. He could not tolerate enteral feeding, so his physician ordered total parenteral nutrition to be administered.

CRITICAL THINKING QUESTIONS

1. How does large amounts of dietary salt lead to stomach cancer?
2. What is the most common type of malignant stomach tumor?
3. What are the symptoms of stomach cancer?

CLINICAL CASE STUDY 3

An obese 69-year-old man had developed all of the symptoms of an aging prostate gland. His diet mainly consisted of fatty foods, which he thoroughly enjoyed, with tiny fruits, vegetables, or whole grains. He was an African-American man whose father had developed prostate cancer but survived, later dying of a pulmonary condition. His mother had died of breast cancer. A thorough review of the patient's diet showed that he always used whole milk and regular dairy products. Testing revealed that his PSA was highly elevated. An ultrasound revealed enlargement of the prostate gland, and a biopsy was ordered, which confirmed that prostate cancer had developed. Fortunately, the cancer had not spread, so the patient was scheduled for surgical resection.

CRITICAL THINKING QUESTIONS

1. How common is adenocarcinoma of the prostate gland?
2. When symptoms of prostate cancer appear, what do they include?
3. What are the treatment options for prostate cancer?

FURTHER READING

1. American Cancer Society, Besser, J., and Grant, B. (2018). *What to Eat During Cancer Treatment*, 2nd Edition. American Cancer Society.
2. Bishoy, S. (2022). *Red Meat Increases the Risk of Colon Cancer*. Bishoy.
3. Dodson, S., Baracos, V.E., Jatoi, A., Evans, W.J., Cella, D., Dalton, J.T., and Stiner, M.S. (2012). *Muscle Wasting in Cancer Cachexia: Clinical Implications, Diagnosis, and Emerging Treatment Strategies*. Annual Reviews of Medicine.
4. Doris, M. (2020). *Managing Cancer with Alkaline Diet: Scientifically Proven Ways to Prevent and Reverse Cancer*. Doris.
5. Gabbert, H., Beach, K., and Lee, C.M. (2014). *Battling Breast Cancer with Nutrition*. Provenir Publishing.
6. Heber, D., Li, Z., and Liang, V. (2021). *Nutritional Oncology*. CRC Press.
7. Jeffrey, D. (2022). *Stomach Cancer: The Complete Guide on How to Cure Stomach Cancer – Everything from Diagnosis to Recovery*. Jeffrey.
8. Kafta, S. (2022). *The Complete Cancer Diet and Nutrition Therapy: Nutritious Anti-cancer Diet Recipes Cookbook for the Newly Diagnosed*. Kafta.
9. Karon, Y. (2021). *Signs of Stomach Cancer Include appetite Loss, Weight Loss, Heartburn, Abdominal Pain, Feeling Full Easily, Anemia, Fatigue, Abdominal Swelling, Regular Vomiting, and Blood in Stools*. Karon.
10. Katzin, C. (2021). *The Cancer Nutrition Handbook*, 7th Edition. Foundation Resources, Inc.

11. Kushi, M., and Jack, A. (2009). *The Cancer Prevention Diet: The Macrobiotic Approach to Preventing and Relieving Cancer*, Revised and Updated 25th Anniversary Edition. St. Martin's Griffin.

12. Lipsky, S.A. (2017). *Beyond Cancer: The Powerful Effect of Plant-Based Eating – How to Adopt a Plant-Based Diet to Optimize Cancer Survival and Long-Term Health*. Wellness Ink Publishing.

13. MB Foundation. (2019). *Outsmart Cancer: Defeat Cancer with Vitamin B17, Healthy Nutrition, and Alternative Medicine*. MB Foundation.

14. McLelland, J. (2018). *How to Starve Cancer: Without Starving Yourself*. Agenor Publishing.

15. Oncology Nutrition Dietetic Practice Group. (2019). *Oncology Nutrition for Clinical Practice*. ONDPG.

16. Rayman, M., Dilley, K., and Gibbons, K. (2020). *Healthy Eating for Prostate Care*. Kyle Books.

17. Rothenberg, T. (2022). *Cancer Diet for the Newly Diagnosed: An Integrative Guide and Cookbook for Treatment and Recovery*. Rockridge Press.

18. Sammut, J. (2015). *Eat Your Way Out of Cancer: The Alternative to Healing the Human Body Using Anti-cancerous Plant Foods*. Blurb.

19. Sears, W., Sears, M., and Van Etten, R. (2022). *Help Heal Yourself from Cancer: Partner Smarter with Your Doctor, Personalize Your Treatment Plan and Take Charge of Your Recovery*. BenBella Books.

20. Werner Gray, L., and Hyman, M. (2019). *Cancer-free with Food: A Step-by-Step Plan with 100+ Recipes to Fight Disease, Nourish Your Body, and Restore Your Health*. Hay House Inc.

31 Environmental Pollutants and Nutrition

OVERVIEW

Environmental contamination from various industrial and agricultural chemicals can compromise our nutritional status and health. This may occur directly or through changes in the diet. Examples of contaminants include heavy metals, organochlorines, and radionucleotides. Environmental factors such as weather, time of day, locations, and advertisements influence food choices. Soil and water quality and temperature significantly affect food systems by impacting production, storage, and transportation. Unfortunately, exposure to environmental chemicals is increasing globally, and nutritional status may modify human susceptibility to chemical exposures. There are many different toxicants, and malnutrition can take many forms. Other environmental impacts on food production include using resources, the production methods required to process foods and food waste.

TOXICITY OF CHEMICAL AND PHYSICAL AGENTS

Chemical and physical agents can be highly toxic to humans, causing various health and biological hazards. Health hazards include carcinogenicity, irritation, and sensitization, while physical hazards include corrosion, explosibility, and flammability. Understanding chemical toxicity requires knowledge of chemicals present as part of manufacturing processes or as related impurities and environmental effects. The outcomes of the metabolism of drugs and chemicals after ingestion are significant. Regarding the skin, percutaneous absorption can be defined as the translocation of surface-applied agents through the various skin layers to where they can enter the systemic circulation through the dermal microvasculature and lymphatics or remain in the deeper layers. The rate-limiting barrier to skin absorption is generally believed to be the outermost, nonviable **stratum corneum**.

Exposure to potentially toxic agents occurs when humans have contact with a chemical or physical agent, either directly or via another substance that has become contaminated or has contacted the poisonous agent. The place where an agent originates is called the *source*. Chemicals can move through air, soil, and water, be present in plants or animals, and find their way into our food sources. The methods by which humans can contact hazardous agents are called *exposure pathways*. These include inhalation, ingestion, and skin contact. Factors that play roles in the outcomes of toxic exposure include the type of chemical or agent, the amount or level an individual was exposed to, the length of the exposure direction, and how many times the exposure occurred. Young and middle-aged adults generally have fewer adverse health effects after exposure than fetuses, children, adolescents, and older adults.

The **potency** and toxicity of a chemical can be affected by its breakdown within the body. Its chemical structure may be changed or metabolized to a more or less toxic substance. The amount of a chemical in its **exposure medium** is its concentration, usually reported in parts per million, milligrams per liter, or milligrams per cubic meter. Acute exposure is short-term exposure to a toxic agent over a few seconds to a few hours. Chronic exposure is continuous or repeated contact over months or years. Chemicals leaking from landfills can enter our groundwater, contaminate wells, or find their way into basements. This can result in chronic exposure. Toxic agents can affect each body system. Delayed health effects can be reversible or permanent, including lung disease and cancer.

DOI: 10.1201/9781003453376-38

Food poisoning occurs when people eat contaminated food. Some microorganisms, such as bacteria or fungi, release a toxin. Sometimes, the toxic byproducts of these organisms cause food poisoning. Therefore, the body reacts to purge the toxins. Most people recover on their own, but some can become gravely ill. Pregnant women, young children, and older adults are more at risk. Food can become contaminated at any production stage, from harvesting to storage to cooking or preparation. Contamination occurs when food is not:

- Fresh
- Washed well
- Handled in a sanitary way
- Cooked to a safe internal temperature
- Held at proper temperatures
- Refrigerated or frozen promptly

Bacteria, viruses, parasites, funguses, toxins, and some chemicals may contaminate food and water. There are more than 250 specific types of food poisoning. Some of the most common microbial causes include:

- *Salmonella* – Raw eggs and undercooked poultry are familiar sources of salmonella poisoning. It can also occur in beef, pork, vegetables, and processed foods containing these items. Salmonella is the most common bacterial cause of food poisoning in the United States. and is responsible for the highest number of hospitalizations and deaths from food poisoning.
- *E. coli (Escherichia coli)* –Normally live in the intestines of healthy people, and most types of *E. coli* are harmless. However, a few strains can cause severe abdominal cramps, bloody diarrhea, and vomiting. Usually found in undercooked meat and raw vegetables, *E. coli* produces a toxin that irritates the small intestine. The **Shiga toxin** is what causes foodborne illness. Most healthy adults recover from an *E. coli* illness within a week. Some people, particularly young children, and older adults may develop a life-threatening form of kidney failure called hemolytic uremic syndrome (HUS), which destroys red blood cells, leading to kidney failure. HUS occurs as a complication of a diarrheal infection (usually *E. coli* O157:H7 infection).
- *Listeria* –Bacteria in soft cheeses, deli meats, hot dogs, and raw sprouts can cause listeriosis, which is especially dangerous for pregnant women.
- *Norovirus* –You can get norovirus by eating undercooked shellfish, leafy greens, and fresh fruits or by consuming food that a sick person prepares. This virus is most commonly associated with the stomach flu.
- *Hepatitis A* – Viral hepatitis A can spread through shellfish, fresh produce, water, and ice contaminated by stool. It is not a chronic infection like other hepatitis viruses, but it can affect your liver.
- *Staphylococcus aureus (staph)* – A staph infection occurs when people transfer the bacteria from their hands to food. Foods often implicated are meats, poultry, milk and dairy products, salads, cream-filled baked goods, and sandwich fillings. The bacteria can affect many parts of your body.
- *Campylobacter* –This common bacterial infection produces severe GI upset and can linger for weeks. Usually, culprits are undercooked poultry, meat or eggs, poorly processed meats, contaminated vegetables, and raw (unprocessed) milk or water sources. It's also spread by cross-contamination. The condition is generally self-limited, causes bloody diarrhea, and is rarely fatal.

- *Shigella (shigellosis) –Shigella* bacteria are typically found in uncooked vegetables, shell-fish, and cream or mayonnaise-based salads (tuna, potato, macaroni, chicken). It can cause blood or mucus in your diarrhea, so the infection is sometimes called bacillary dysentery.

Cyanogenic glycosides are phytotoxins (toxic chemicals produced by plants) that occur in at least 2,000 plant species, of which several species are used as food in some areas of the world. Cassava, sorghum, stone fruits, bamboo roots, and almonds are essential foods containing cyanogenic glyco-sides. The potential toxicity of a cyanogenic plant depends primarily on the potential that its con-sumption will produce a concentration of cyanide that is toxic to exposed humans. In humans, the clinical signs and symptoms of acute cyanide intoxication can include **tachypnea**, hypotension, dizziness, headache, stomach pains, vomiting, diarrhea, mental confusion, cyanosis with twitching, and convulsions, followed by a terminal coma. Death due to cyanide poisoning can occur when the cyanide level exceeds the limit at which an individual can detoxify.

YOU SHOULD REMEMBER

Cyanide is a fast-acting lethal poison. It prevents the body's cells from using oxygen, and the cells die. Cyanide harms the heart and brain more because these organs require more oxygen. The poison may be a colorless gas or a crystal form. Cyanide is released from natural sub-stances in some foods. Signs and symptoms occur within minutes and result in respiratory failure.

Check Your Knowledge

1. How can potentially harmful chemicals reach the food supply?
2. How does food contamination occur?
3. What are the most common microbial causes of food poisoning?

FOOD POLLUTION

Food pollution is the presence of toxic chemicals and biological contaminants in food that are not naturally present. Though these agents' low "background" levels may be present, food pollution occurs when the levels increase. Outcomes of food pollution include mild to severe illnesses, serious hormonal or metabolic problems, and cancer. Sometimes, severe food poisoning and death occur. Over 70 million foodborne illnesses in the United States result in about 5,000 deaths. Any pollutant that comes into contact with food can pollute it. Vegetables from irrigation water, groundwater, or soil can be contaminated with toxic bacteria. Processed, polluted food at very high temperatures may only destroy these bacteria. Harmful chemicals can also get into food sources via the following:

- Growing crops in polluted soils, by using solid wastes as fertilizer, or in areas that have polluted groundwater
- Irrigation of crops with polluted water
- Growing crops in areas with polluted air
- Agricultural treatments such as pesticides, insecticides, or **herbicides**
- Agricultural application of sewage sludge or polluted fertilizers that contain ash from power plants
- Consumption of contaminated water or food by fish or other **creatures**
- Poor food processing, packaging, and handling procedures
- Propagation and concentration of pollutants throughout the food chain

Plants can become contaminated with pollutants when they extract them through their roots, water, and nutrients. Air pollutants may become deposited on the ground with rainwater, entering plants through their roots. Many sources of food pollution include chemicals and microorganisms that contact food while it is grown, processed, or packaged. Risks for food pollution are based on many different factors, which include:

- *The type of pollutant*—persistent and bioaccumulative—has higher risks for food pollution since it can accumulate in food over time, resulting in very high concentrations. Hormones in foods can also pose serious risks that are not fully understood; it is wise to avoid any food source containing hormones.
- *The type of food*—fish are more exposed to a wider variety of contaminants; also, certain compounds can accumulate and become concentrated in fish. Birds or other animals that eat polluted fish can then become contaminated and transmit the pollution further throughout the food chain.
- *The health of individuals* – people most affected by food pollution include children, older adults, pregnant women, and people with chronic food diseases or illnesses.

Water pollution usually first affects fish eaten by other animals, which humans may consume later. When this pollution reaches humans, it may significantly increase compared to its original concentrations. Therefore, human intoxication cases may be severe.

For example, certain fish species are more often contaminated by mercury, which has three forms (organic, inorganic, and metallic), of which the organic form, especially *methylmercury*, is the most dangerous. Contamination mostly comes from mercury in organic sediment, which microorganisms transform into methylmercury. The tissues of **fish gills** absorb this form as they swim and through their digestive tracts as they feed. Fish that contain higher levels of mercury include shark, ray, swordfish, barramundi, gemfish, orange roughy, ling, king mackerel, tilefish, and Southern bluefin tuna. Areas of the world where the waters contain the highest levels of mercury include those near eastern Asia (especially around India and China), Europe, the Mediterranean Sea, and South America.

Another potentially serious problem exists when oil spills into shallow or confined waters. Many species of shellfish are relatively immobile, and because they are filter-feeders, they may be unable to avoid oil exposure. They also do not have the same enzymes needed to break down contaminants as fish with fins have, which detoxify many oil compounds. Oil spills can destroy fish eggs in shallow water. Other areas of concern are lakes, lagoons, and some shallow-water nearshore areas, where spilled oil naturally concentrates—the type of oil and the timing of its release influence the severity of its effects on fish. Light oils and petroleum products may cause acute toxicity, usually resolved relatively quickly. Heavier oils do not affect fish significantly but can kill them in the larval or spawning stages. Only when testing shows that fish are no longer contaminated should they be sold for human consumption.

For example 1989, an oil tanker called the *Exxon Valdez* ran aground in Prince William Sound, Alaska (see **Figure 31.1**). It spilled 11 million gallons of oil into an ecologically sensitive location. The spill affected over 1,300 miles of coastline, killing seabirds, otters, seals, eagles, whales, and billions of salmon and herring eggs. Even today, species not proven to have recovered from the spill include killer whales and birds known as murrelets and pigeon guillemots. Massive protection projects have been created since the spill to help restore the region's species. In 2004, the bulk cargo ship called the *Selendang Ayu* ran aground off of Unalaska Island in western Alaska's Aleutian Islands. The ship broke into two pieces, resulting in a large oil spill. Though not as large as the Exxon Valdez spill, thousands of birds and a smaller number of otters were killed.

Microplastics can move through wastewater into the oceans, where fish and other creatures may consume them (see **Figure 31.2**). This can cause them to accumulate in their bodies, harming humans if they consume the contaminated animals. Microplastics are less than 5 mm in length.

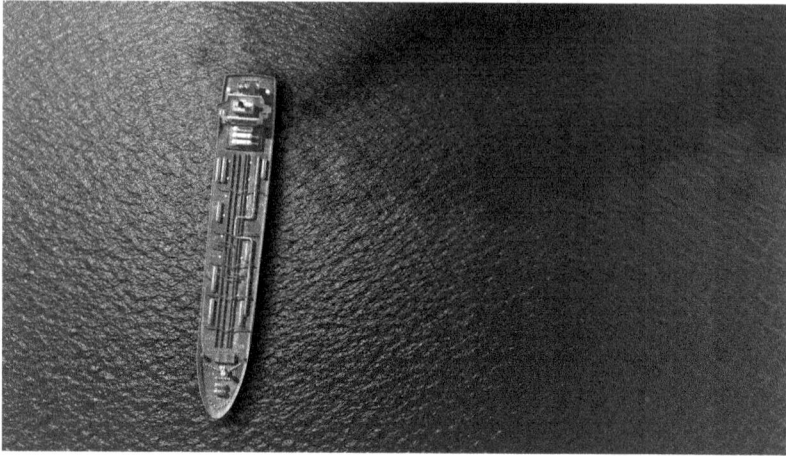

FIGURE 31.1   The Exxon Valdez oil spill.

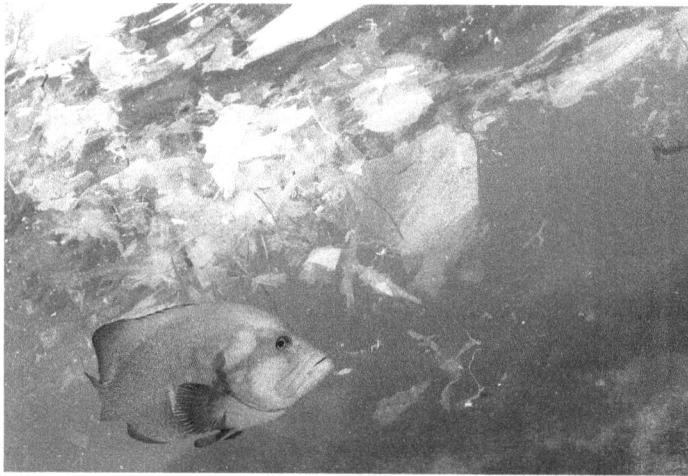

FIGURE 31.2   A fish swimming underneath many microplastics in the ocean.

Larger pieces of plastic can become microplastics as they break down and move through the oceans. Some manufacturers use microplastics, such as in exfoliating products and toothpaste. Any product that lists the word **microbeads** on the label contains microplastics. The closer to the top of the food chain a creature is, the more likely it is to consume significant amounts of microplastics. Smaller animals eat the microplastics, which are consumed by larger creatures, which are consumed by still more giant creatures. This allows for microplastic levels to accumulate, finally reaching humans. There is no way to eliminate microplastics from a creature once they are present. No source of wild seafood is guaranteed to be completely free of microplastics. Potential but not fully proven effects of eating microplastic-contaminated seafood include oxidative stress, neurotoxic effects, endocrine disruption, thyroid damage, and cancer. Additional pollutants that can contaminate the food supply include fertilizer (from water runoff) and other toxic chemicals dumped into waters that reach the oceans.

Microplastics have been detected in bottled and tap drinking water. Hazards include physical particles, chemicals, and microbial pathogens as part of **biofilms**. Fragments and fibers are the main particle shapes in drinking water, and polyethylene terephthalate and polypropylene are the most detected polymers. Plastics and microplastics can contain unbound **monomers** and additives. Biofilms can include pathogens such as *Pseudomonas aeruginosa, Legionella* species, non-tuberculosis *Mycobacterium* species, and *Naegleria fowleri*. However, wastewater and drinking-water treatment systems effectively remove particles of similar sizes and characteristics as microplastics. Water suppliers and regulators must continue to **prioritize** the removal of microorganisms and chemicals from drinking water.

Since, on average, less than 10% of plastics are recycled annually, the problem of plastic contamination in the food supply is ongoing. About 93% of all bottled water contains traces of microplastics. The most commonly used plastic is *polyethylene terephthalate (PET)*, which may disrupt the human endocrine system and its hormones. Another type, called *plastic number 7,* contains **bisphenol A**, which is linked to fertility issues, altered brain development, cancer, and heart complications. While tap water must be tested to show contaminant levels, bottled water does not need to receive the same testing. Therefore, while bottled water costs much more than tap water, it may also be significantly more dangerous. Initiatives to develop more clean water bills and legislation to regulate bottled water quality globally are being debated.

YOU SHOULD REMEMBER

Experts have proposed that growing vegetables in factories in the future could eliminate the effects of environmental pollution. The process could be computerized to control various factors that affect growth. It is estimated that planting crops and growing them in factories could reduce food pollution by more than 33%.

Check Your Knowledge

1. How can toxic chemicals get into food sources?
2. What factors are the risks of food pollution based on?
3. How can mercury, oil, and plastic harm fish and, eventually, humans?

IMPACT OF NUTRITION ON POLLUTANT TOXICITY

Nutrition can positively and negatively modulate toxicity from exposure to pollution. A diet high in pro-inflammatory fats like linoleic acid can increase pollutant toxicity. Diets rich in anti-inflammatory and bioactive components, such as omega-3 fatty acids and **polyphenols**, can reduce toxicant-related inflammation. Nutrition can modulate *epigenetic markers* linked to increased disease risks or protection against diseases. Overnutrition and undernutrition affect prenatal **epigenetic tags**, which may increase the risk of developing the disease later in life. Exposure to pollutants alters epigenetic markers, possibly contributing to inflammation and infection. Through epigenetic modulations, pollutants can increase body factors related to inflammation, cardiac injury, and oxidative damage. Some nutritional components can protect against pollutant-induced inflammation through epigenetic regulation. Overall, exposure to environmental pollutants may increase the risk of developing chronic inflammatory diseases, including cardiovascular disease, diabetes mellitus, and metabolic syndrome. Pollutant exposure inhibits adverse combined effects with less-than-optimal nutrition since pollutants and nutritional components can target identical molecular pathways.

The impact of environmental pollution, primarily chronic low exposures to heavy metals, affects the nutritional status and health of livestock and humans. Malnutrition inhibits the enzyme system, changes **neurotransmitter** levels, degenerates **myelin** and glial and neural elements, lowers **intelligence quotient** (IQ) scores, and impairs fine and gross motor coordination. The additive impact of undernutrition and the adverse effects of heavy metal exposure are becoming a serious threat to health in developing countries. Results are seen in the **hemopoietic**, renal, and nervous systems of neonates, children, postpartum women, and those experiencing occupational exposure to pollution. There are three main ways in which pollutants and nutrition are interconnected. They include the following:

- Food sources may be vehicles for delivering toxicants and can increase exposure and the burden of the toxicants on the body.
- An absorbed toxicant may interact with the nutritional status to determine the amount of the toxicant that is retained and bioavailable so that it can be harmful.
- Once absorbed, nutrients and their metabolism may also interact with the toxicant to determine a specific health outcome; gender and age need to be considered since they affect nutritional status and toxicant exposure.

The impacts of environmental pollution discussed in this chapter include lead, mercury, arsenic, and cadmium toxicities.

Lead Toxicity

Lead is often used in residential installations and metal alloys or chemicals. It is present in pipes, paints, putties, and pesticides. It is one of the heavy metals that can most easily contaminate humans and is extremely harmful to health. Lead is one of the heavy metals that has caused the most harm to the population. Tobacco smoke is another pollutant with a high concentration of this metal. Lead poisoning is known as **plumbism**.

Epidemiology

Lead toxicity is a worldwide pediatric problem. Although data demonstrate a decline in the prevalence of elevated blood lead levels in children in the industrialized world, lead remains a common, preventable environmental health threat. Sequelae of lead intoxication include mental retardation and growth failure. At least 4 million households in the United States have children living in them exposed to high levels of lead. Approximately half a million children ages 1–5 have blood lead levels above 5 μg/dL, the reference level at which the CDC recommends initiating public health actions. Children who belong to minority populations or low-income families or who live in older homes are particularly at risk.

Etiology and Risk Factors

Contamination causes include ingestion, inhalation, prenatal exposure, and dermal exposure, but the most common are ingestion and inhalation. Ingestion is more common in children, while inhalation is more frequent in occupationally-exposed adults. Deteriorating lead paint in pre-1979 housing remains the most common source of lead exposure in children, accounting for up to 70% of elevated levels. Other familiar sources of lead exposure include batteries, putty, cement, imported canned food, cosmetics, jewelry, leaded glass artwork, farm equipment, and illicit intravenous drugs.

Clinical Manifestations

Symptoms of lead poisoning may include abdominal cramping, constipation, mood changes, and tremors. Exposure to high lead levels may cause anemia, weakness, and kidney and brain damage. Very high lead exposure can cause death. Lead can cross the placental barrier, which means pregnant women exposed to lead also expose their unborn child. In children, acute lead poisoning may cause decreased attentiveness and irritability, with **cerebral edema** developing over 1–5 days. The cerebral edema may cause an **ataxic gait**, forceful and persistent vomiting, hair loss, altered consciousness, seizures, and a coma. The **encephalopathy** may follow several weeks of decreased play activity. Chronic lead poisoning may cause intellectual disability, aggressive behavior disorders,

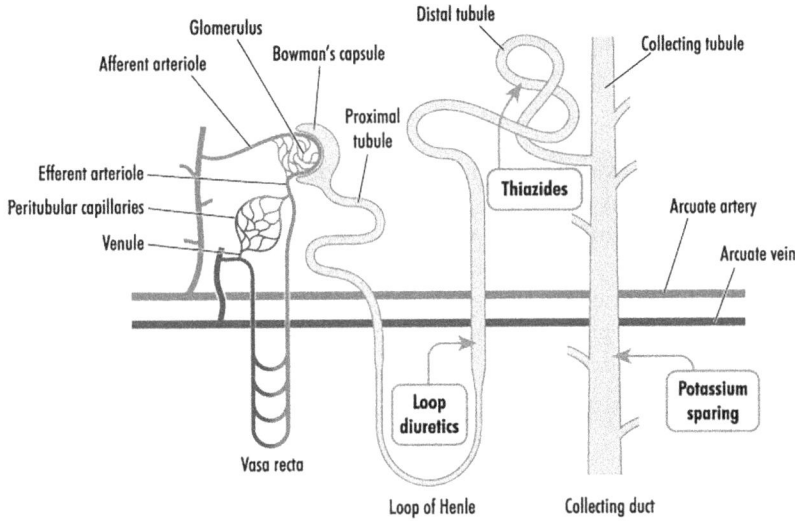

FIGURE 31.3   The structure of a nephron, including the proximal tubule.

seizure disorders, chronic abdominal pain, anemia, and developmental regression. Adults exposed to lead at their jobs may develop headaches, personality changes, abdominal pain, and **neuropathy** over several weeks or more. There may also be impaired libido, infertility, and, in males, erectile dysfunction.

As lead accumulates in the proximal tubular cells, chronic **tubulointerstitial nephritis** results. Short-term lead exposure causes proximal tubular dysfunction (see **Figure 31.3**). This includes decreased urate secretion and hyperuricemia since urate is the substrate for saturnine gout, amino-aciduria, and renal glucosuria. People at the highest risk are children exposed to lead paint chips or dust, battery workers, drinkers of high-proof distilled alcohol (moonshine), and welders.

Diagnosis

Diagnosis is based on lead levels in blood, abdominal X-rays, and sometimes, X-rays of the long bones of children with suspected chronic exposure. **Burton's line** is a blue-purplish line on the gums caused by lead poisoning. It is due to a reaction between circulating lead and sulfur ions released by oral bacterial activity, which deposits lead sulfite at the junction of the teeth and gums. Treatment is based on eliminating the lead source, such as whole-bowel irrigation and chelation (for adults with symptoms plus a high whole blood lead level and children with encephalopathy or a high whole blood level). Chelating agents include **succimer**, calcium disodium ethylenediaminetetraace-tic acid, and dimercaprol. Measures that reduce the risk of household lead poisoning include regular hand washing, regular washing of pacifiers and toys, and regular cleaning of household surfaces.

Treatment

Treatment of lead toxicity involves preventing further lead exposure, decontamination, chelation, and supportive therapy. Any child with blood lead levels (BLLs) of more than 5 µg/dL (0.24 µmol/L) must receive treatment, follow-up testing, serial monitoring, and assessment for vitamin deficiency and overall nutritional status. Outpatient treatment seems to be a good option for asymptomatic children with blood lead levels in the 45–69 µg/dL range. However, be sure that the environment in which the child is placed is safe and lead-free. If this is impossible to ensure, inpatient treatment is needed until the environmental situation is investigated in collaboration with social services and the local health department.

When children have lead encephalopathy, the best approach is to transfer them to a children's hospital where pediatric intensivists and other resources are available. All children being treated for lead poisoning need close follow-up care. Monitoring their BLLs is essential. Closely monitor cardiovascular and mental status in patients with lead poisoning, maintain an adequate urine output, and assess renal and hepatic functions.

Prevention

The key to preventing lead toxicity in children is identifying and eliminating the significant sources of lead exposure. Pediatricians and family practitioners play a fundamental role by providing anticipatory guidance about potential sources of lead exposure and its hazards for the development of children. A successful primary prevention plan should focus on the two main exposure sources for children in the United States: one is lead in housing, and the second is nonessential uses of lead in certain products, such as imported and domestically manufactured toys, eating and drinking utensils, cosmetics, and traditional medicines.

YOU SHOULD REMEMBER

A human-made public health crisis from April 2014 to June 2016) involved Flint, Michigan's municipal water supply system. Tens of thousands of Flint residents were exposed to dangerous levels of lead. Outbreaks of Legionnaire disease killed at least 12 people and sickened dozens more.

YOU SHOULD REMEMBER

Iron deficiency increases the absorption of lead from the stomach and intestines. Prevent iron deficiency by consuming iron-fortified cereals, green leafy vegetables, pureed meats or lean red meats, fish, raisins, dates, prunes, dried beans and peas, skinless poultry, and nuts or sunflower seeds.

Check Your Knowledge

1. What are the three main ways in which pollutants and nutrition are interconnected?
2. Which individuals are at the highest risk for lead poisoning?
3. Which foods help protect children from lead poisoning?

MERCURY TOXICITY

Mercury is a naturally occurring element in air, water, and soil. Even small amounts of mercury exposure may cause severe health problems and threaten a child's development in utero and early in life. People are mainly exposed to methylmercury, an organic compound when they eat fish and shellfish that contain the compound.

Mercury exists in various forms: elemental (metallic), inorganic (to which people may be exposed through their occupation), and organic (methylmercury, to which people may be exposed through their diet). These mercury forms differ in toxicity and effects on the nervous, digestive, and immune systems, as well as the lungs, kidneys, skin, and eyes. Mercury is highly volatile. When it is in the air, we can breathe it through the lungs or absorb it through the skin. The most dangerous form of exposure is inhaled mercury since it enters the body, accumulates, and remains for a long time. The effects of mercury compounds on the body are often extreme. Total blood mercury is usually composed chiefly of methylmercury. Methylmercury levels below 5.8 µg/L are considered safe.

Epidemiology

Mercury poisoning is rare in the United States. Still, it can be more common in other countries, especially among mining communities or near seaside towns where food could become contaminated with mercury. Two major toxic incidents occurred in Minamata Bay, Japan, and Iraq. Mercury was dumped into Minamata Bay, and people developed toxicity from consuming the fish containing methylmercury. In Iraq, more than 6,000 people developed toxicity from eating bread baked with grain that was treated with methylmercury-based fungicide.

Etiology and Risk Factors

People may be exposed to mercury in any form under different circumstances. However, exposure mainly occurs through consuming fish and shellfish contaminated with methylmercury and workers inhaling elemental mercury vapors during industrial processes. Cooking does not eliminate mercury.

Clinical Manifestations

Acute mercury poisoning causes a burning sensation in the mouth, salivation, severe gastroenteritis, abdominal pain, colitis, vomiting, anuria, **nephrosis**, and **uremia**. With the alkyl and phenyl mercurials, there are skin burns. Chronic mercury poisoning may result in mental disturbances, neurologic deficits, and **gingivitis** (see **Figure 31.4**). Mercury may have toxic effects on the immune systems, lungs, kidneys, skin, and eyes. For ingestion of the liquid form, there may be no symptoms. If it is injected intravenously, **pulmonary emboli** may develop. Severe **pneumonitis** occurs because of mercury vapor inhalation.

Mercury poisoning is a neurotoxin and is manifested by tremors, insomnia, memory loss, insomnia, and neuromuscular effects. It can also contribute to cardiovascular disease, metabolic syndrome, chronic fatigue, **fibromyalgia**, autoimmune thyroiditis, hypothyroidism, thyroid cancer, **adrenal fatigue syndrome**, digestive disorders, and allergies.

Diagnosis

Mercury poisoning is diagnosed by testing the blood and urine for mercury levels. Urine might be collected over 24 hours. Assess the history of the possible exposure and also monitor the vital signs. Hair testing may be helpful to detect methylmercury exposures that occurred several months previously, but this type of testing is relatively complex and used infrequently. Other general laboratory tests may be used to help evaluate the health of various organ systems in someone who has been exposed to or is thought to be exposed to toxic levels of mercury. Some examples include a complete blood count (CBC) and a comprehensive metabolic panel.

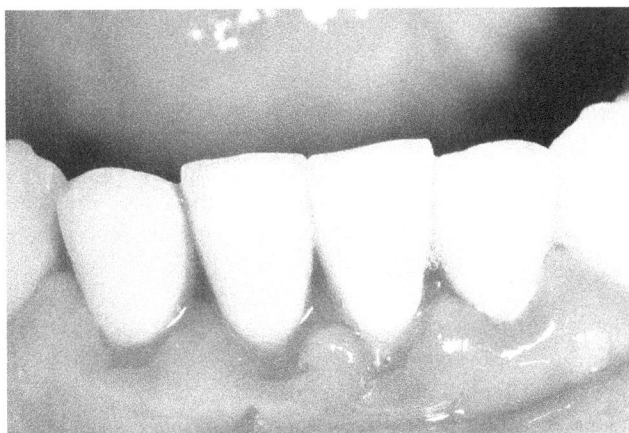

FIGURE 31.4   Gingivitis.

Treatment

For ingestion, **gastric lavage**, activated charcoal, and penicillamine or succimer must be considered. Fluid and electrolyte balance must be maintained, hemodialysis for renal failure must be performed, and observation for GI perforation must be performed.

Prevention

Several ways to prevent adverse health effects include promoting clean energy, stopping mercury in gold mining, eliminating mercury mining, and phasing out non-essential mercury-containing products.

YOU SHOULD REMEMBER

People may be exposed to mercury in any form under different circumstances. However, exposure mainly occurs through consuming fish and shellfish contaminated with methylmercury and worker inhalation of elemental mercury vapors during industrial processes. Cooking does not eliminate mercury.

YOU SHOULD REMEMBER

Burning coal for power and heat is a significant source of mercury. Coal contains mercury and other hazardous air pollutants emitted when the coal is burned in coal-fired power plants, industrial boilers, and household stoves.

YOU SHOULD REMEMBER

Mercury, such as thiomersal (ethylmercury), is used in tiny amounts as a preservative in some vaccines and pharmaceuticals. Compared to methylmercury, ethylmercury is very different. Ethylmercury is broken down by the body quickly and does not accumulate. Therefore, there is no evidence that the amount of thiomersal used in vaccines causes a health risk.

ARSENIC TOXICITY

Arsenic is the most common cause of acute heavy metal poisoning in adults. It is released into the environment by the industrial processing of chemicals and glass and reaches water supplies worldwide, resulting in exposure to marine life. Arsenic poisoning, or **arsenicosis**, occurs after ingesting or inhaling high levels of arsenic. Arsenic is highly poisonous to humans. Arsenic is especially dangerous because it has no taste or odor so that exposure can occur without the affected person's knowledge. Arsenic is a naturally occurring element that combines inorganic or organic substances to form various compounds.

Inorganic arsenic compounds are present in soil, sediment, and groundwater. These compounds occur naturally or may result from mining. Organic arsenic compounds are primarily found in fish and shellfish. People are usually exposed to inorganic arsenic through drinking water. In some locations, water sources have higher natural inorganic levels than other areas. Other sources of inorganic arsenic include contaminated soil or wood previously preserved with arsenic. There is a wide variation in susceptibility to arsenic toxicity, likely related to variations in arsenic metabolism, nutrition status, the body's defense mechanisms, and genetic predisposition. Arsenic induces oxidative stress, compounded by the arsenic-induced inhibition of several antioxidant systems. There is a link between a low degree of arsenic metabolism and the risk of various toxic effects. Arsenic is metabolized in the liver.

Epidemiology

Exposure to arsenic through drinking water is a significant public health problem affecting many countries, but it is most severe in low-income countries. Arsenic poisoning affects at least 140 million people worldwide. This is due to contaminated drinking water. People in 50 countries are exposed to water containing potentially dangerous arsenic levels. The highest mortality rate was recorded between 2016 and 2020. Poisson regressions revealed a positive and significant association between arsenic concentration and mortality due to cancers, particularly liver, breast, stomach, meningeal, brain, and leukemia.

Etiology and Risk Factors

Contaminated water used for drinking, food preparation, and irrigation of food crops poses the greatest threat to public health from arsenic. Long-term exposure to arsenic from drinking water and food can cause cancer and skin lesions. It has also been associated with cardiovascular disease and diabetes.

Clinical Manifestations

Signs and symptoms of arsenic poisoning include dysphagia, throat constriction, burning GI pain, diarrhea, vomiting, dehydration, GI bleeding, pulmonary edema, renal failure, liver failure, and shock. Long-term exposure to arsenic from drinking water and food can cause cancer, skin lesions, muscle cramps, and tingling of fingers and toes. Arsenic is also associated with cardiovascular disease and diabetes mellitus. Exposure in utero and early childhood is linked to poor cognitive development and increased deaths in young adults. Long-term exposure to arsenic can cause more severe symptoms such as darkened skin, a constant sore throat, and persistent digestive issues.

Diagnosis

Various tests are available to diagnose poisoning by measuring arsenic in the blood, urine, hair, and fingernails. A urine test is the most reliable for arsenic exposure over the previous few days. To analyze an acute exposure accurately, urine testing must be done within 24–48 hours.

Treatment

The initial management of acute arsenic intoxication includes gut decontamination and hemodynamic stabilization. Patients with suspected acute arsenic poisoning generally require rapid stabilization with fluid and electrolyte replacement in an intensive care setting, and the following may be necessary:

- *Aggressive intravenous fluid replacement therapy* – this may be life-saving in severe cases.
- *Gastric lavage* – may be helpful soon after an acute ingestion to prevent further absorption.
- *Activated charcoal* – though its efficacy is controversial, administration along with a cathartic (such as sorbitol) is frequently recommended.
- If profuse diarrhea is present, cathartics should be withheld.
- Hemodialysis may be beneficial if there is concomitant renal failure.

Chelating agents administered within hours of arsenic absorption may successfully prevent the full effects of toxicity. The patient's nutritional status may play a role in preventing severe health effects. For example, arsenic and selenium may be mutually antagonistic. Recent reports have shown that a diet rich in selenium and other antioxidants, such as vitamin E, helps promote the methylation of arsenic, which leads to increased excretion. Methyl donors such as folate may also help in arsenic metabolism and excretion. Arsenic-related disease has been shown to increase in individuals who are malnourished, possibly due to decreased arsenic methylation.

Prevention

The most crucial action in affected communities is to prevent exposure to arsenic by providing a safe water supply for drinking, food preparation, and irrigation of food crops. Education and community engagement are critical factors for ensuring successful interventions. People need to understand the risks of high arsenic exposure and the sources of arsenic exposure, including the intake of arsenic by rice from irrigation water and the intake of arsenic into food from cooking water. High-risk populations should also be monitored for early signs of arsenic poisoning–usually skin problems.

YOU SHOULD REMEMBER

In addition to skin cancer, long-term exposure to arsenic may also cause cancers of the bladder and lungs. The International Agency for Research on Cancer has classified arsenic and arsenic compounds as carcinogenic to humans and has also stated that arsenic in drinking water is carcinogenic to humans.

Check Your Knowledge

1. Which foods help to combat mercury poisoning?
2. How can inorganic arsenic affect humans?
3. After a patient with suspected acute arsenic poisoning is stabilized, what else can be done regarding treatment?

CADMIUM TOXICITY

Cadmium is a metal that is soft, malleable, and bluish-white in its elemental form. While it is a relatively widespread element but rarely found as a pure metal. More often, it forms complex compounds in zinc ores. Cadmium is mainly produced through smelting, mining, and refining zinc, lead, and copper. While initially used as a dye for creating shades of yellow, orange, and red, it is most widely used today in nickel-cadmium rechargeable batteries. Cadmium is also found in the following:

- Plating on iron and steel products
- Plastic stabilizers
- Alloy elements for lead, copper, and tin
- Cigarette smoke
- Silver Jewelry

As an industrial byproduct, cadmium is a natural component of the earth's crust and can quickly enter the atmosphere, water, and soil. This may happen through volcanic activity, the weathering of sediment, or the burning of fossil fuels. It can lead to cadmium in drinking water sources and food, including vegetables, fish, and animals. The foods potentially most susceptible to cadmium contamination are mushrooms, shellfish, freshwater fish, dried algae, and potable water.

Epidemiology

Cadmium is a relatively rare heavy metal that occurs naturally when combined with zinc. Over the past century, environmental contamination and consequent human exposure to cadmium have dramatically increased. Cadmium has major industrial applications in galvanizing pigments, alloys, and nickel-cadmium batteries. Over 1 million individuals globally are exposed to cadmium occupationally.

Etiology and Risk Factors

Cadmium toxicity occurs when high levels of cadmium are inhaled from the air or contaminated food or water is consumed. In the general population, exposure to cadmium occurs primarily by eating foods grown in contaminated soil. Cigarette smoke is one of the highest sources of cadmium exposure. High levels of cadmium in the soil can cause some crops to uptake the heavy metal. The rate of cadmium absorption depends on a whole host of factors, like the crop species, the quality of the soil (pH and salinity), and the presence of other elements. Proximity to certain industrial plants, particularly those involving construction and manufacturing, can also affect soil and water sources for crops. Smokers may ingest twice the daily amount of cadmium as non-smokers. People breathing in secondhand smoke also take in more cadmium, as this is a form of environmental exposure. Ingested cadmium is usually stored in the liver, kidneys, and bones. Eliminating cadmium is a naturally slow process that can remain in the human body for decades.

Exposure to cadmium through contaminated workplaces, food, water, or tobacco products causes respiratory diseases, kidney damage, and bone diseases. Cadmium toxicity can affect significant aspects of health, though more studies are necessary to assess the potential risk to humans and the environment thoroughly. Many studies associate chronic occupational inhalation of cadmium dust and cadmium fumes with an increased risk of respiratory problems, such as **emphysema**, bronchitis, chronic rhinitis, damage to the olfactory epithelium, and COPD (see **Figure 31.5**).

Cadmium is also classified as a probable carcinogenic agent when inhaled. This suggests that chronic cadmium exposure through inhalation may contribute to lung cancer. The kidneys receive the most damage from chronic cadmium exposure via ingestion and inhalation. This is because the kidneys act as a filtration system, removing waste and excess fluid from the body. It can take up to 10 years of regular and consistent exposure for cadmium levels to build up enough to cause kidney damage. Most commonly, chronic cadmium exposure has been linked to progressive renal tubular dysfunction.

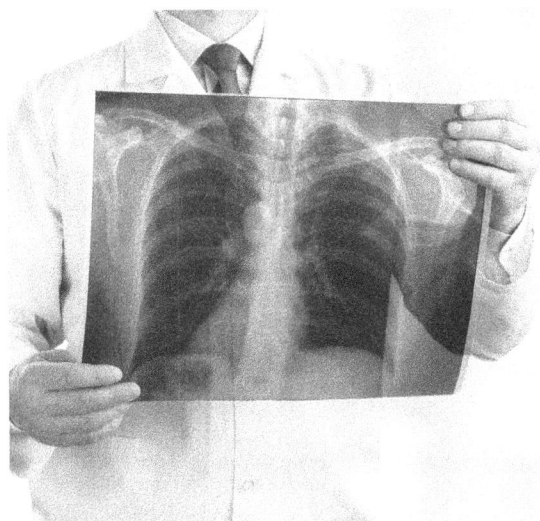

FIGURE 31.5 Chronic obstructive pulmonary disease.

Clinical Manifestations

The general symptoms of acute cadmium poisoning include nausea and vomiting, diarrhea, abdominal pain, and flu-like symptoms. When inhaled consistently over time, cadmium may affect the lungs and breathing.

Diagnosis

The diagnosis is based on the history of occupational exposure to cadmium. Cadmium levels can be measured in blood, urine, hair, nails, and saliva samples. During a radioimmunoassay, increased urinary beta2-microglobulin levels of 7 μg/g creatinine or higher may be found, as well as increased urinary cadmium levels.

Chronic cadmium poisoning may cause renal failure at high concentrations, with increased serum creatinine and urea. There is also fractional excretion of uric acid and elevated phosphate as a urine protein-to-creatinine ratio and a urine albumin-to-creatinine ratio. Kidney stones are also more common in populations experiencing excessive cadmium exposure. Cadmium-related bone diseases and skeletal health issues are often side effects of renal issues since any damage to the kidneys may cause changes in how calcium and vitamin D are metabolized and absorbed. In later stages, severe chronic cadmium poisoning can contribute to bone lesions, including decreased bone density. This can eventually lead to osteoporosis and **osteomalacia**, contributing to certain fractures and other effects;

Treatment

Patients with cadmium toxicity require GI irrigation, supportive care, and chemical decontamination via traditional chelation therapy, using appropriate newer chelating agents and nanoparticle-based antidotes. Treatment focuses on eliminating further exposure. Immediate considerations include evaluation of the airways, breathing, and circulation. Acute or chronic ingestion of cadmium salts is rare but may lead to death. The lowest lethal dose of cadmium is 5 g for a person who weighs 154 pounds (70 kg). If emesis has not occurred, gastric lavage will be performed soon. Activated charcoal cannot effectively absorb cadmium. Therefore, supportive therapy is the best choice.

Prevention

It has also been recommended that the level of food contamination and suspicious exposure areas be determined. Public education and awareness programs for exposed individuals should be considered to prevent additional cadmium poisoning.

YOU SHOULD REMEMBER

Vitamin C, B1, and B6 deficiencies enhance sensitivity to cadmium toxicity. Vitamin C attenuates oxidative damage and histopathological changes in the lungs and brain and protects the kidneys and testes. Vitamin E also protects against cadmium in the blood, liver, and brain. Vegetables, fruits, and other edible plants are important dietary sources of these vitamins. Potentially protective plants include soybeans, garlic, ginger, and onion.

Check Your Knowledge

1. How does cadmium toxicity occur?
2. What are the general signs and symptoms of acute cadmium poisoning?
3. What treatment options exist for cadmium poisoning?

Clinical Case Studies

CLINICAL CASE STUDY 1

A 65-year-old grandmother took her grandchildren to a local taco restaurant. The next day, they awoke with abdominal cramping, which led to the development of diarrhea. The grandmother was the worst affected. Her symptoms also included a fever, fatigue, bruising, and decreased urine output. While the grandchildren recovered, she had to be taken to the local emergency department due to the symptoms. Tests revealed her serum creatinine concentration was high, and her platelet count was low. A blood smear revealed many red blood cell fragments without platelet clumping. The patient was hospitalized and started on hemodialysis. A stool culture was positive for *E. coli*. She was treated but remained hospitalized for 2 weeks. After discussing the restaurant's location with authorities, it was soon discovered that the beef they used in their tacos was contaminated with *E. coli*.

CRITICAL THINKING QUESTIONS

1. Where is *E. coli* bacteria usually found?
2. What toxin is produced by *E. coli* bacteria?
3. What is the life-threatening disease that may be caused by *E. coli*, particularly in young children and older adults?

CLINICAL CASE STUDY 2

A 6-year-old boy was assessed by his pediatrician because of pain in his legs, neck, and abdomen. His appetite had been poor for the last 2 months, and he had lost about eight pounds. The boy was also exhausted. He described pain sensations when his arms, hands, legs, and feet were palpated. Blood tests revealed a high level of mercury. He was given D-penicillamine. Over 2 months, his abdominal pain was reduced, and the pain in his extremities was also lessened. At this time, his mercury levels were assessed again, and they had nearly returned to normal. Over 8 months of follow-up and continued administrations of D-penicillamine, no other symptoms were present.

CRITICAL THINKING QUESTIONS

1. What does acute mercury compound poisoning cause?
2. How can elemental mercury poisoning occur?
3. What symptoms signify mercury poisoning?

CLINICAL CASE STUDY 3

A 42-year-old man presented with increasing skeletal pain. X-rays of his lumbosacral spine and hip revealed reduced bone density and prominent trabecular markings. He also had impaired renal function with high serum creatinine and urea. The patient's fractional excretion of uric acid and phosphate was elevated, as were his urine protein-to-creatinine ratio and urine albumin-to-creatinine ratio. When questioned about his work history, the patient described having been in the silver jewelry industry for several decades. Tests confirmed that he had tubular proteinuria, indicating the likelihood of heavy metal toxicity. Since cadmium is a significant component of working with silver, his blood levels were assessed and found to be extremely high. The diagnosis was severe cadmium toxicity. This was believed to be due to the cadmium fumes released as silver is mixed with cadmium when making silver jewelry.

1. What is cadmium?
2. Where is cadmium most widely used, and where is it also found?
3. When does cadmium toxicity occur?

FURTHER READING

1. Bala Dhull, S., Singh, A., and Kumar, P. (2022). *Food Processing Waste and Utilization: Tackling Pollution and Enhancing Product Recovery*. CRC Press.
2. Birch, C.S., and Bonwick, G.A. (2019). *Mitigating Contamination from Food Processing (Food Chemistry, Function, and Analysis)*. Royal Society of Chemistry.
3. Chatoui, H., Merzouki, M., Moummou, H., Tilaoui, M., Saadaoui, N., and Brhich, A. (2022). *Nutrition and Human Health: Effects and Environmental Impacts*. Springer.
4. Food and Agriculture Organization. (2021). *Global Assessment of Soil Pollution: Summary for Policymakers*. Food and Agriculture Organization.
5. Galal, T., Hassan, L., and Elawa, O. (2019). *Impact Assessment of Environment Pollution on Economic Food Crops*. Lap Lambert Academic Publishing.
6. Gubbels, J.S. (2020). *Environmental Influences on Dietary Intake of Children and Adolescents*. Mdpi AG.
7. Hassan Sabry, A.K. (2019). *Pesticides and Food Contamination*. Lap Lambert Academic Publishing.
8. Institut National de Recherche Chimique Applique. (2014). *Pollution by the Food Processing Industries in the EEC*. Springer.
9. Jones, M.D. (2021). *Toxin Nation: The Poisoning of Our Air, Water, Food, and Bodies*. Visible Ink Press.
10. Li, X., and Liu, P. (2020). *Gut Remediation of Environmental Pollutants: Potential Roles of Probiotics and Gut Microbiota*. Springer.
11. Lichtfouse, E., Schwarzbauer, J., and Robert, Didier. (2014). *Pollutant Diseases, Remediation, and Recycling: Environmental Chemistry for a Sustainable World*. Springer.
12. Mihai Grumezescu, A., and Holban, A.M. (2017). *Microbial Contamination and Food Degradation (Handbook of Food Bioengineering 10)*. Academic Press.
13. Otuu, C.F., Aloh, O., Shu, E. (2018). *Environmental Pollution and Food Quality: Impact of Lead-Zinc Mining on the Quality of Four Dominant Staple Foods*. Lap Lambert Academic Publishing.
14. Pizzorno, J. (2018). *The Toxin Solution: How Hidden Poisons in the Air, Water, Food, and Products We Use Are Destroying Our Health: and What We Can Do to Fix it*. HarperOne.
15. Rakesh, S.S., Ramasamy, M., and Veerasawmy, D. (2021). *Microplastics and Food Contamination: Microplastics on Environment*. Lap Lambert Academic Publishing.
16. Rodriguez Bernalde de Quiros, A., Lestido Cardama, A., Sendon, R., and Garcia Ibarra, V. (2019). *Food Contamination by Packaging: Migration of Chemicals from Food Contact Materials*. De Gruyter.

32 Nutritional Therapy

OVERVIEW

Medical nutritional therapy can range in complexity, from designing a reduced-calorie diet for weight loss to prescribing a high-protein diet to promote wound healing for patients with severe burns. A registered dietitian nutritionist can recommend tube or intravenous feeding to prevent malnutrition in extreme cases, such as for people with cancer. Nutritional therapy is an evidence-based and individualized nutrition process designed to help treat various medical conditions. It can be performed for inpatients and outpatients. Treatment methods include IV therapy (total parenteral nutrition (TPN)), medical foods, tube feeding (enteral nutrition), and oral supplements. Nutritional therapists assist patients with specific health problems through assessment and counseling about their diets. Nutritional therapy is commonly used for those with anorexia nervosa, for patients receiving chemotherapy or radiotherapy, and for dying patients. Nutrition goals during cancer therapy are based on a person's cancer type, stage, and other medical conditions.

ORAL NUTRITIONAL SUPPLEMENTS

Oral nutritional supplements are powerful tools against malnutrition. They provide a concentrated energy source and high levels of nutrition. Though whole foods are usually preferred as much as possible, oral nutritional supplements are an excellent choice to bring in needed calories when eating enough is unrealistic or likely. Diseases and conditions that compromise adequate consumption of whole foods include inflammatory bowel disease, severe malabsorption, oral cancer, **short bowel syndrome**, anorexia, dementia, and severe and unintentional weight loss. Even a 10% decrease in caloric intake can weaken the immune system. Almost 50% of all hospitalized people have some amount of malnourishment, so using oral nutrition supplements can be very helpful.

Oral nutritional supplements provide calories, protein, vitamins, and minerals and can replace meals. Some contain additional fiber, omega-3 fatty acids, prebiotics, and *probiotics*. These supplements are widely available at grocery stores, drug stores, and online. Many oral nutritional supplements provide 100% of the daily recommended intakes (DRIs) for vitamins and minerals within a volume of 1–1.5 L daily. It is important to remember that DRIs are meant for healthy people, so more vitamins and minerals may be required for specific health conditions than these supplements provide.

Generally, calories range from 1 to 2 per mL, mostly from carbohydrates. These carbohydrates often come from corn syrup solids and are very sweet – sometimes too sweet. Many of these supplements can be warmed up before drinking but should never be boiled because it reduces their nutritious capacities. The protein sources in oral nutritional supplements come from **daisy**, soybean, or pea protein (see **Figure 32.1**). Nearly all supplements are lactose-free, gluten-free, or both and may or may not be plant-based. Fat sources may come from corn, sunflower, soy, safflower, coconut, palm, fish, or **medium-chain triglyceride** (MCT) oil. MCT oil-containing supplements may be preferred for people who have problems digesting fat to enhance absorption and optimize tolerance.

Fiber and probiotics are essential for gut health and a healthy microbiome, yet not all oral nutritional supplements contain them. Most oral nutritional supplements, including those with added fiber, are still considered "low fiber" and below the recommended amount of 25–38 g daily. While taking oral nutritional supplements, it is still essential to get additional fiber from vegetables, fruits, legumes, nuts, seeds, whole grains, 100% ground **psyllium husk**, flaxseeds, or **chia seeds** (see **Figure 32.2**). The fiber sources in oral nutritional supplements may come from soy fiber, **guar gum**,

DOI: 10.1201/9781003453376-39

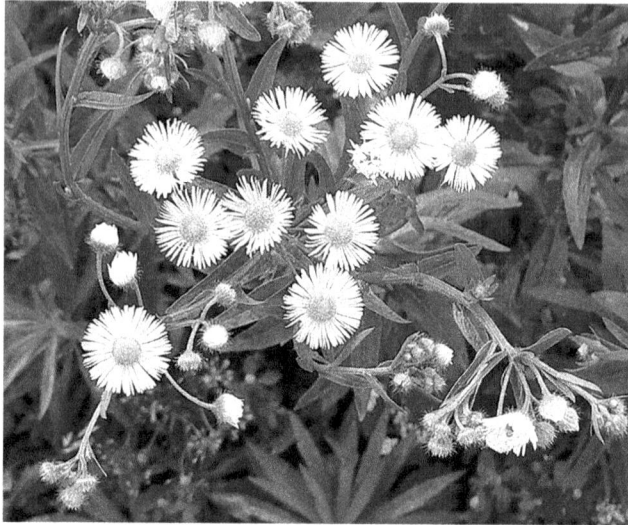

FIGURE 32.1 Daisy flowers.

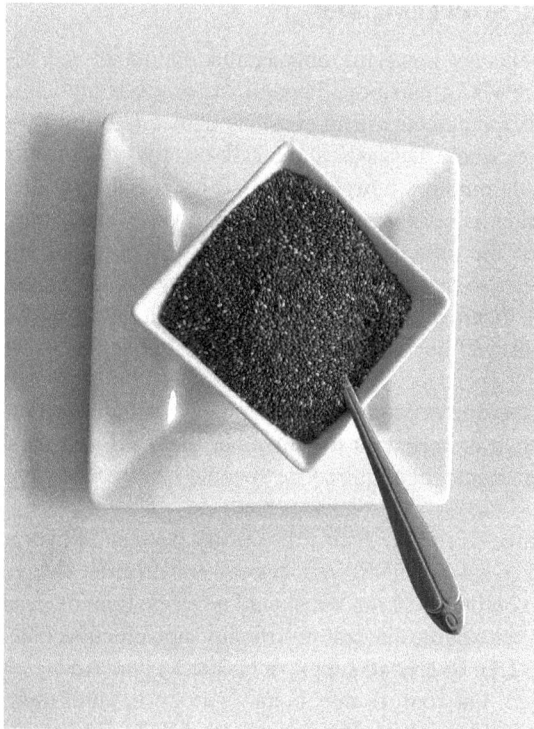

FIGURE 32.2 Chia seeds.

or **inulin**. Discussing oral dietary supplements, with or without fiber, with a physician or dietitian is essential. Sweeteners used in oral nutritional supplements include maple syrup, brown rice syrup, corn syrup, corn maltodextrin, glucose syrup, natural sugar, stevia leaf extract, cane sugar, tapioca dextrin, sucralose, fructose, **acesulfame K**, and rice starch. Therefore, it is essential to check which sweeteners are present, just like all ingredients, in case of allergies to any of them.

Oral nutritional supplements are generally sterile liquids but may also be semi-solids or powders. Some are specifically indicated for certain conditions, including dysphagia, short bowel syndrome, intractable malabsorption, inflammatory bowel disease, preoperative preparation of malnourished patients, bowel fistulae, total gastrectomy, and disease-related malnutrition. These supplements may be prescribed for acute illnesses or long-term chronic conditions. There are also prescription oral nutritional supplements and individual dietetic assessments that consider dietary needs, plus taste and texture preferences, so the prescribed product will be the best the patient can tolerate or enjoy. The most common types of oral nutritional supplements available include the following:

- *Milkshake type* – volume 125–200 mL, energy density 1–2.4 kcal/mL, also available with added fiber
- *Juice type* – volume 200–220 mL, energy density 1.25–1.5 kcal/mL; these products are fat-free
- *High-energy powders* – volume from approximately 125–350 mL, ideally made up of whole milk to provide an energy density of 1.5–2.5 kcal/mL
- *Soup type* – volume 200–300 mL; some are ready-mixed while others are powdered and are made up of water or milk to provide an energy density of 1–1.5 kcal/mL
- *Semi-solid/dysphagia types* – may be thickened liquids (for stage 1 and 2 **dysphagia**) to smooth pudding styles (for stage 3 dysphagia), with an energy density of approximately 1.4–2.5 kcal/mL
- *High protein* – may be jellies, shots, or milkshake types with 11–20 g of protein in volumes of 30–200 mL
- *Low volume high, concentration shots* – fat- and protein-based products, taken in small quantities as "shots," usually 30–40 mL, taken 3–4 times daily

Mixing up the various available flavors is essential to avoid taste fatigue. An emerging group of oral nutritional supplements is designed for people over age 65 who may be at risk of vitamin D deficiency. Others may be good for patients with medical conditions where fluid and electrolyte balance is essential. Patients with short bowel syndrome may not be able to tolerate **hyperosmolar** oral nutritional supplements since they can cause the patency of a stoma to be reduced.

Oral nutritional supplements should only be prescribed and monitored to ensure that they remain appropriate and are being used as prescribed. They may be stopped when dietary intake is sufficient to meet nutritional requirements, the target weight has been reached, the body mass index is within a healthy range, an underlying medical condition has improved sufficiently, or the patient can no longer tolerate them due to taste fatigue.

Check Your Knowledge

1. How can oral nutritional supplements be used to supplement the diet?
2. When taking oral dietary supplements, how can additional fiber be increased?
3. Why do oral nutritional supplements require regular monitoring?

YOU SHOULD REMEMBER

Soybeans are one of the few vegetarian sources of total protein containing all the essential amino acids required in the human diet. Soy protein is the primary protein in soy products, including tofu, tempeh, soy milk, and other soy-based dairy and meat alternatives. It is also found in soy protein powder, which can supplement a workout routine or add more protein to the diet.

ENTERAL TUBE NUTRITION

Enteral tube nutrition (ETN) delivers nutrition directly to the stomach or small intestine. ETN is called tube feeding or *enteral nutrition*. It is used for patients who cannot ingest enough nutrients by mouth due to being unable or unwilling to. Enteral nutrition is better than parenteral nutrition because it offers better preservation of GI structure and function, is less expensive, and, in most cases, involves fewer complications such as infections. ETN is specifically indicated for the following conditions:

- Critical illnesses such as burns, which cause metabolic stress
- Inability to take oral feedings because of head or neck trauma
- Liver failure
- Prolonged anorexia
- Severe protein-energy undernutrition
- Coma or **depressed sensorium**

Additional indications include bowel preparation for surgery in a seriously ill or malnourished patient, enterocutaneous fistula closure, slight intestine adaptation after an extensive intestinal resection, or disorders causing malabsorption, such as Crohn's disease.

If tube feeding is required for 4–6 weeks, the selected tube is usually of a small internal diameter (caliber) and soft, made of silicone or polyurethane. The tube can be a nasogastric or nasoenteric tube. When the patient has a nasal deformity or injury, and nasal placement is complex, an **orogastric** or other oroenteric tube can be put into place. Tube feeding for more than 4–6 six weeks usually utilizes a gastrostomy or jejunostomy tube (see **Figure 32.3**). This is put into place endoscopically, radiologically, or surgically. It is chosen based on the physician's capabilities and the patient's preference.

Jejunostomy tubes are used if the patient has contraindications to gastrostomy, including bowel obstruction proximal to the jejunum or gastrectomy. These tubes do not offer any lower risk of tracheobronchial aspiration than gastrostomy tubes; however, even though many practitioners do not widely believe this. Jejunostomy tubes can be easily dislodged and are mainly used for inpatients. If endoscopic or radiologic placement is unavailable, impossible, or unsafe, feeding tubes are placed via surgery. Open or laparoscopic techniques can be used for order (see **Figure 32.4**).

Liquid formulas used for enteral tube feeding include feeding modules and **polymeric formulas**. A feeding formula is a commercially available product. It contains just one nutrient: protein, fat, or carbohydrate. Feeding modules can be used individually to treat a deficiency or combined with other formulas to satisfy nutritional requirements. Polymeric formulas include blenderized food and commercially available milk-based or lactose-free formulas. These formulas usually provide a complete and balanced diet; tube or oral feedings are generally preferred over feeding modules. In hospitalized patients, lactose-free formulas are the most commonly used type of polymeric formulas. Even so, milk-based formulas usually have a better taste than lactose-free formulas. A patient with lactose intolerance may tolerate milk-based formulas if given slowly by continuous infusion.

Specialized formulas are used for patients who have problems digesting complex proteins. They include **hydrolyzed protein** and amino acid formulas. These formulas are expensive and usually not required. If given enzymes, most pancreatic insufficiency and malabsorption patients can digest complex proteins. Calorie-dense and protein-dense formulas (for patients with fluid restriction) and fiber-enriched recipes (for constipated patients) may be successful for therapy.

For tube feeding, the patient should sit upright at a 30°–45° angle and remain in the same position for 1–2 hours after feeding. This minimizes the likelihood of **nosocomial** aspiration pneumonia as gravity aids in propelling the food downward. Tube feedings are administered in **boluses**, several times daily, or via continuous infusion. Bolus feeding is better physiologically and may be preferred if the patient has diabetes mellitus. Continuous infusion is required if boluses cause the patient to

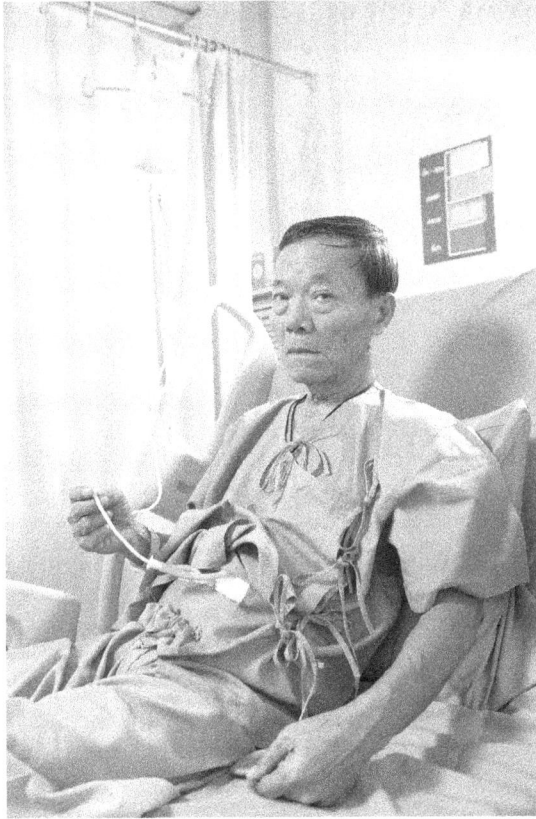

FIGURE 32.3   Gastrostomy tube feeding.

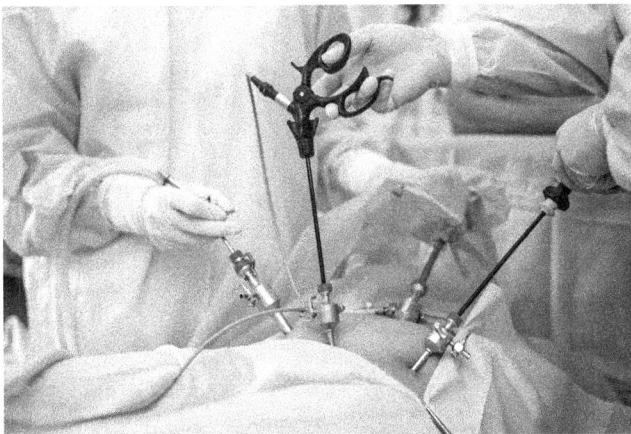

FIGURE 32.4   Laparoscopy.

be nauseous. For bolus feeding, the total daily volume is separated into four to six feedings, injected through the tube with a syringe, or infused via gravity from an elevated bag. The tube is flushed with water after feedings to prevent clogging.

Initially, nasogastric, gastrostomy or nasoduodenal tube feeding often causes diarrhea. Therefore, feedings usually begin with small amounts of diluted preparations and then increase as tolerated. Usually, formulas contain 0.5, 1, or 2 kcal/mL. Formulas with a higher caloric concentration, meaning less water per calorie, may result in decreased gastric emptying and, therefore, higher gastric residuals compared to more dilute formulas with the same number of calories. At the start, a 1-kcal/mL commercially prepared solution may be administered undiluted at 50 mL/hour. If the patient has not been fed for a while, it may be administered at 25 mL/hour. These solutions do not usually supply enough water – significantly if vomiting, diarrhea, sweating, or fever has increased water loss. Therefore, extra water is administered in boluses through the feeding tube or IV. Once a few days pass, the rate or concentration can be increased to meet caloric and hydration needs.

Jejunostomy tube feeding requires more dilution and smaller volumes. Feeding usually starts with a concentration of up to 0.5 kcal/mL at a rate of 25 mL/hour. After a few days pass, the concentrations and volumes can be gradually increased, eventually meeting the patient's caloric and hydration needs. In most cases, the maximum that can be tolerated is 0.8 kcal/mL at 125 mL/hour, which provides 2,400 kcal/day.

Complications of enteral tube feeding are unfortunately common and sometimes severe. They include the following problems, effects, and descriptions:

- *Tube-related complications:*
  - *Presence of the tube* – damage to the esophagus, nose, pharynx, or sinusitis. If the tube is large, it is more likely to irritate tissues and cause them to erode. With sinusitis, the sinus ostia can become blocked.
  - *Blockage of the tube lumen* – inadequate feeding. Thick feedings or pills sometimes block the lumen (mostly of small tubes). Blockages are sometimes dissolved by instilling a solution of pancreatic enzymes or other commercially available products.
  - *Misplacement of a nasogastric tube intracranially* – brain trauma or an infection. A tube can be misplaced intracranially if the cribriform plate is disrupted by severe facial trauma.
  - *Misplacement of a nasogastric or orogastric tube in the tracheobronchial tree* – pneumonia. A responsive patient will immediately cough and gag. An obtunded patient will have few immediate symptoms. If the misplacement is not discovered, feedings can enter the lungs (and cause pneumonia).
  - *Dislodgement of a gastrostomy or jejunostomy tube* – peritonitis. Once dislodged, a tube can be replaced into the peritoneal cavity. If a tube was initially placed with an invasive technique, replacement is more difficult to achieve and more likely to cause complications.
- *Formula-related complications:*
  - *Intolerance of one of the leading nutrient components of the formula* – diarrhea, GI discomfort, nausea, vomiting, and occasional mesenteric ischemia. Intolerance occurs in about one of every five patients and half of all critically ill patients. It is more common with bolus feedings. GI discomfort may have other causes, which include reduced stomach compliance because of shrinkage caused by lack of feeding, distention due to volume of feedings, and decreased gastric emptying because of pyloric dysfunction.
  - *Osmotic diarrhea* – stools that are loose and frequent. Sorbitol, often a component of liquid drug preparations administered through feeding tubes, can worsen diarrhea.
  - *Nutrient imbalances* – electrolyte disturbances, hyperglycemia, volume overload, hyperosmolarity. The patient's body weight and blood levels of electrolytes, glucose, magnesium, and phosphate must be monitored frequently. During the first week, this is done daily.
- *Other complications:*
  - *Reflux of tube feedings or difficulty with oropharyngeal secretions* – aspiration, which may occur even if rigid tubes are correctly placed, and the head of the bed is elevated if the patient has either of these problems.

Check Your Knowledge

1. What are the reasons that enteral nutrition is better than parenteral nutrition?
2. When is a jejunostomy tube indicated?
3. How does tube feeding occur?

YOU SHOULD REMEMBER

Enteral nutrition is generally preferred to parenteral nutrition as it is more physiological, straightforward, cheaper, and less complicated. However, even nasogastric feeding requires care, and the more complex types of enteral nutrition, such as gastrostomy and jejunostomy, need great care due to the possibility of becoming dislodged or skin irritation at the insertion site.

TOTAL PARENTERAL NUTRITION

Total parenteral nutrition (TPN) is administered intravenously and supplies a patient's daily nutritional requirements. It can be used in hospitals or at home since TPN solutions are concentrated and can cause peripheral venous **thrombosis**; a central venous catheter is usually required. This type of nutrition is not for routine use in a patient with an intact GI tract. Compared with enteral nutrition, TPN causes more complications, does not preserve the structure and function of the GI tract as well, and is more expensive. Another form, *partial parenteral nutrition*, supplies only part of the daily nutritional requirements and is used to supplement oral intake. Many hospitalized patients receive dextrose or amino acid solutions via this method. TPN is sometimes the only realistic option if a patient does not have a functional GI tract or has disorders requiring entire intestine rest. These include bowel obstruction, short bowel syndrome (because of surgery), some stages of ulcerative colitis, and conditions such as congenital GI abnormalities and prolonged diarrhea (regardless of its cause) in children. TPN requires the following components:

- *Water* – 30–40 mL/kg of body weight/day
- *Energy* – 30–35 kcal/kg of body weight/day based on energy expenditure (up to 45 kcal/kg/day for a critically ill patient) – medical patients usually need 30–35 kcal/kg/day; postoperative patients need 30–45 kcal/kg/day; and hypercatabolic patients need 45 kcal/kg/day – note that requirements for energy increase by 12% for every 1°C of fever
- *Amino acids* – 1–2 g/kg of body weight/day based on degree of catabolism – medical patients usually need 1 g/kg/day; postoperative patients need 2 g/kg/day; hypercatabolic patients may require 3 g/kg/day
- *Essential fatty acids* – commercially available lipid emulsions are often added to supply these crucial fatty acids as well as triglycerides; 20%–30% of total calories are usually provided as lipids; however, withholding lipids as well as their calories may help an obese patient mobilize endogenous fat stores, which increases insulin sensitivity
- *Vitamins* – ascorbic acid (100 mg), biotin (60 μg), cobalamin (5 μg), folate (folic acid, 400 μg), niacin (40 mg), pantothenic acid (15 mg), pyridoxine (4 mg), riboflavin (3.6 mg), thiamin (3 mg), vitamin A (4,000 International units), vitamin D (10 μg, or 400 units), vitamin E (15 mg), vitamin K (200 μg)
- *Minerals* – acetate/gluconate (90 mEq), calcium (15 mEq), chloride (130 mEq), chromium (15 μg), copper (1.5 mg), iodine (120 μg), magnesium (20 mEq), manganese (2 mg), phosphorus (300 mg), potassium (100 mEq), selenium (100 μg), sodium (100 mEq), zinc (5 mg)

Children who require TPN may have different fluid requirements and need more energy and amino acids. They may require up to 120 kcal/kg/day of energy and 2.5 or 3.5 g/kg/day of amino acids.

Essential TPN solutions require sterile techniques for their preparation, which is often done in liter batch sizes based on standard formulas. Usually, 2 L/day of the standard TPN solution is required. Solutions are modified based on laboratory test results, underlying conditions, hypermetabolism, and other factors. Most calories are supplied as carbohydrates. Usually, 4–5 mg/kg/minute of dextrose is administered. Standard solutions contain as much as 25% dextrose. However, the amount and concentration are based on the patient's metabolic needs and the proportion of caloric requirements supplied by lipids.

Many TPN solutions are commonly used. Electrolytes can be added based on the patient's requirements. TPN solutions are adjusted based on other present disorders and the patient's age. For a patient with renal insufficiency who is not being treated with dialysis or if a patient has liver failure, the TPN solution contains reduced protein content and has a high percentage of essential amino acids. For a patient with heart or kidney failure, there is a limited volume of liquid intake. For a patient with respiratory failure, a lipid emulsion will provide most non-protein calories to reduce carbon dioxide production via carbohydrate metabolism. Dextrose is present in lower concentrations for neonates, 17%–18%.

A strict sterile technique is required during insertion and maintenance of the TPN line since the central venous catheter will remain in place for a long time. The TPN line is not to be used for any other purpose. External tubing must be changed every 24 hours, with the first bag of the day. In-line filters do not decrease complications. Dressings must be kept sterile. They are usually changed every 48 hours, with strict sterile techniques followed. If TPN is administered outside of a hospital, the patient must be taught to recognize infection symptoms. Qualified home nursing must be provided. The solution starts slowly at 50% of the calculated needs, using 5% dextrose to balance fluid requirements. Energy and nitrogen are given simultaneously. The patient's plasma glucose level determines the amount of regular insulin given, which is added directly to the TPN solution. If the glucose level is average and the final solution contains 25% dextrose, the usual starting dose will be 5–10 units of regular insulin per liter of TPN fluid.

The patient's progress with the TPN line is followed on a flowchart. An interdisciplinary nutrition team should be involved in monitoring. A complete blood count should be obtained, and the patient's weight, electrolytes, and blood urea nitrogen (BUN) should regularly be monitored. This may be done daily for inpatients. The plasma glucose level should be monitored every 6 hours until the patient and the glucose level have stabilized. Continuous monitoring of fluid intake and output must be performed. When the patient is stable, blood tests can be done less regularly. Liver tests are required, with twice weekly measurements of **plasma proteins**, plasma, **prothrombin time**, urine osmolality, calcium, magnesium, and phosphate. The plasma proteins monitored include serum albumin and sometimes **transthyretin**. When possible, blood tests should not be performed during glucose infusion. A complete nutritional assessment will be repeated every 2 weeks, including body mass index calculation and anthropometric measurements.

Between 5% and 10% of patients with a TPN line experience complications related to central venous access. Catheter-related sepsis rates have occurred less often since the introduction of guidelines emphasizing sterile techniques for catheter insertion and skin care in the area surrounding the insertion site. Infections have been reduced because dedicated healthcare terms specializing in specific procedures, including catheter insertion, are standard in today's healthcare systems.

It is important to note that hyperglycemia, hypoglycemia, or liver dysfunction affects more than 90% of patients on TPN. Hyperglycemia can be avoided by monitoring plasma glucose often, adjusting the insulin dose in the TPN solution, and giving subcutaneous insulin when required. Hypoglycemia can be avoided by suddenly stopping constant concentrated infusions of dextrose. Treatment is based on the degree of hypoglycemia. Short-term hypoglycemia can be reversed with an IV of 50% dextrose. Extended hypoglycemia may require an infusion of 5% or 10% dextrose for 24 hours before TPN via the central venous catheter can be resumed.

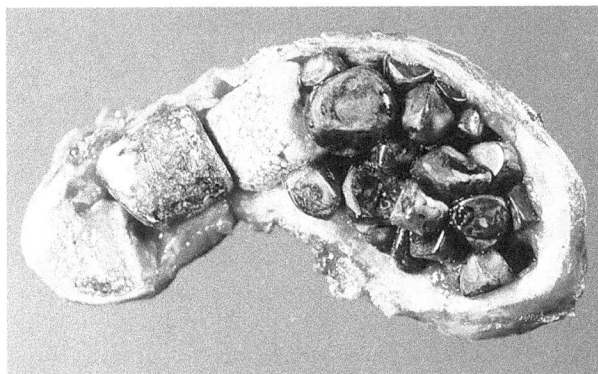

FIGURE 32.5   Resected gallbladder with cholelithiasis (gallstones).

Liver complications include dysfunction, painful hepatomegaly, and hyperammonemia. These can occur at any age but are usually seen in infants – especially those delivered prematurely. Liver dysfunction can be transient, indicated by increased transaminases, bilirubin, and alkaline phosphatase. It usually occurs when TPN is started. Any delayed or persistent elevations may be due to excess amino acids. The pathogenesis is unknown, but **cholestasis** and inflammation may be involved. Sometimes, progressive fibrosis develops, so reducing the delivery of proteins may be helpful. Painful hepatomegaly suggests an accumulation of fat, so carbohydrate delivery should be reduced. In infants, **hyperammonemia** can develop, resulting in lethargy, twitching, and generalized seizures. The arginine supplementation can correct this at 0.5–1 mmol/kg/day. If any liver complication develops in an infant, the amino acids may need to be limited to 1 g/kg/day.

Abnormalities of serum electrolytes and minerals can be corrected by modifying the additional infusions or, if correction must occur quickly, by starting appropriate infusions into the peripheral veins. When TPN solutions are correctly administered, vitamin and mineral deficiencies are rare. Elevated BUN may indicate dehydration, which can be corrected by administering free water as 5% dextrose into a peripheral vein. Any volume overload, suggested by more than 1 kg/day of weight gain, can occur if the patient has high daily energy requirements and requires large fluid volumes.

Osteoporosis or osteomalacia sometimes develops in patients on TPN for over 3 months and is not fully understood. Advanced disease may cause severe pain that can be periarticular, leg, or back pain. Adverse reactions to lipid emulsions are not common but can occur early, especially if the lipids are given as more than 1 kcal/kg/h. The reactions may include cutaneous allergic reactions, dyspnea, headache, back pain, nausea, sweating, and dizziness. Temporary hyperlipidemia can occur, especially in kidney or liver failure patients, but treatment is usually unnecessary. Delayed adverse reactions to lipid emulsions include hepatomegaly, slight elevation of liver enzymes, splenomegaly, leukopenia, thrombocytopenia, and (mostly in premature infants with respiratory distress syndrome) pulmonary function abnormalities. These adverse reactions can be prevented or reduced by temporarily or permanently slowing or stopping the infusion of lipid emulsions.

Gallbladder complications may include **cholelithiasis**, **cholecystitis**, and gallbladder sludge (see **Figure 32.5**). The complications can be caused or exacerbated by chronic gallbladder stasis. Stimulating gallbladder contraction by providing 20%–30% of calories as fat and stopping glucose infusion for several hours per day is helpful, as is oral or enteral intake. Metronidazole, ursodeoxycholic acid, phenobarbital, or cholecystokinin are helpful for some patients with cholestasis.

Check Your Knowledge

1. When is TPN the only realistic option for feeding a patient?
2. What components are present in TPN?
3. What conditions affect most patients who are on TPN?

NUTRITIONAL THERAPY FOR ANOREXIA NERVOSA

For patients with **anorexia nervosa**, nutritional supplementation is often used along with behavioral therapy. Supplementation begins by providing 30–40 kcal /kg/day and can result in weight gains of up to 1.5 kg/week in inpatient care and 0.5 kg/week in outpatient care. Oral feedings with solid foods are preferred, but many weight restoration plans include liquid supplements. Resistant undernourished patients may require nasogastric tube feedings. Elemental calcium at 1,200–1,500 mg/day and vitamin D at 600–800 International units per day are often prescribed for bone loss. Long-term treatment begins only after nutritional, fluid, and electrolyte status are stabilized, with psychotherapy being essential. Treatments continue for 1 year after weight has been restored. For adolescents, family members are taught correct feeding techniques with supervised family meals. Nutritionists can provide specific meal plans or information about calories to restore weight to an average level. Some patients also require medications such as olanzapine to aid weight gain.

For a person with anorexia nervosa, long periods of starvation may have caused biochemical abnormalities, including deficiencies in proteins, micronutrients, and fatty acids. Therefore, unique dietary plans must be created so that additional problems are not generated as the imbalances are corrected. Weight should not be gained until deficiencies are corrected. Aggressive attempts to boost weight gain in the early stages of treatment may be very hazardous. The patient may find nutritional therapy challenging and upsetting because of their altered connection with food. If weight loss symptoms are severe and health is critical, the patient is admitted to a particular recovery unit in a hospital. Forced nutritional therapy is only done if the patient is likely to die without medical help. For patients discharged from inpatient treatment who still require support and monitoring, daycare treatment is beneficial. It is usually recommended if an outpatient suffers a slight relapse.

For recovery, patients should start by eating tiny amounts of food, gradually increasing intake. It is essential to develop a routine, eating food regularly at specific times each day, consisting of three well-balanced meals. A target weight should be set, providing a goal for the patient. A weight gain of just 0.5–1 kg/week is widely recommended, achieved by eating 3,500–7,000 extra calories per week. Daily intake of foods containing high biological value protein, such as whey, casein, and egg white, with a high concentration of essential amino acids per gram and calorie density, is recommended. Consuming these foods and foods the patient perceives to be less "challenging" – usually vegetables – helps restore nutrient status quicker, even when the body is still underweight. Various protein sources, including fleshy fish and poultry, should be encouraged. Recommended daily allowances for vitamins and minerals are varied by age and gender. They can be met by use of multivitamin and multimineral tablets or liquids. Emphasizing nutrient intake instead of caloric intake can help reduce anxiety and resistance to refeeding.

Check Your Knowledge

1. What type of agreement should be drawn up regarding nutritional therapy for a dying patient?
2. What biochemical abnormalities does anorexia nervosa cause?
3. For recovery, what food regimen is used for a patient with anorexia nervosa?

NUTRITIONAL THERAPY FOR CHEMOTHERAPY AND RADIOTHERAPY

The effects of chemotherapy and radiotherapy on cancer patients have been well-documented for many years. Chemotherapy agents can be single or combined, based on the type of cancer and the patient's overall health status. There are several functional categories of chemotherapy agents, which are systemic treatments that affect the whole body. More potential adverse effects may occur in chemotherapy than in radiotherapy. Common nutrition-related adverse effects include anorexia, early satiety, taste changes, nausea, vomiting, diarrhea, mucositis or esophagitis, and constipation.

Since cancer and the adverse effects of chemotherapy can significantly impact nutrition, healthcare providers must anticipate possible problems and design a plan with the patient to prevent malnutrition and weight loss. Malnutrition and weight loss can affect a patient's ability to regain normal health and acceptable blood counts between cycles of chemotherapy. This can directly affect the ability to follow the treatment schedule, which is essential for achieving a positive outcome.

Radiation therapy can cause nutrition-related adverse effects such as changes in taste or the ability to swallow, nausea, vomiting, and diarrhea. Effects of radiation therapy are based on the irradiated area, total dose, **fractionation**, duration, and volume. Most acute effects begin around the 2nd or 3rd week of treatment. They usually reduce by about 2 or 3 weeks after the completion of radiation therapy. Some effects are chronic, continuing, or occurring after treatment is done. Nutrition support during radiation therapy is essential since changes in normal physiologic function can diminish the nutrition status via interference with ingestion, digestion, or absorption of nutrients. Aside from the effects of radiation therapy on areas within the head and neck, it may cause dysphagia, **odynophagia**, esophagitis, nausea, vomiting, loss of appetite, esophageal stenosis, fibrosis or necrosis, diarrhea, chronic enteritis or colitis, and intestinal stricture or obstruction. The adverse effects of chemotherapy and nutritional therapies that may combat them are described as follows:

- *Constipation* – gradually increase intake of foods higher in dietary fiber by including them in meals and snacks, drink plenty of water
- *Nausea without vomiting* – eating the right foods at the correct times may help (small, more frequent meals, foods containing ginger, cool and light foods instead of greasy and high-fat foods)
- *Diarrhea* – eat small and frequent meals, eat easy-to-digest foods that are lower in fiber, slowly sip non-caffeinated fluids throughout the day, limit beverages and foods with sugar alcohols
- *Sore or dry mouth and throat* – prescribed medications may be required; tips to reduce irritation include soft and liquid foods, softening foods with milk, broth, sauces, or gravy, regular sipping of water, frozen fruits, avoiding acidic, crunchy, dry, or hot food sources, alcohol, and foods with tiny seeds
- *Lack of appetite* – eating smaller and more frequent meals, keeping healthy snacks nearby, eating favored foods any time of the day, discussing fiber intake with a dietitian since higher fiber foods can promote fullness, drinking fat-free or low-fat milk, 100% fruit juice, or smoothies
- *Weight gain or increased appetite* – choose healthy snacks, ask for help managing anxiety and stress, and avoid fatigue with light to moderate physical activity such as walking

Radiation therapy often causes cancer patients to lose weight, so maintaining proper nutrition can increase chances for successful outcomes and improve quality of life. Getting the right amount of protein during radiation therapy is very important, so every meal or snack should have some source of protein. This helps to spare lean muscle mass while repairing damage from the radiation. Protein-rich foods include eggs, nuts and nut butter, seeds, soy and tofu, dairy products, meats, poultry, and fish. Meal replacement drinks containing protein may be good if there is difficulty eating solid foods. Hydration helps make the adverse effects of radiation therapy less severe and reduces the chances of missing or delaying cancer treatments. Avoiding dehydration during treatment protects body organs from long-term damage. All non-alcoholic beverages count toward keeping the body hydrated. Flavored waters or waters infused with fruits or vegetables can replace regular water. For radiation therapy patients, 8–12 cups are recommended per day. Caffeinated drinks such as tea or coffee should be reduced to no more than 1–2 glasses per day since they worsen dry mouth, a common adverse effect of treatment. Alcoholic beverages are best to avoid during radiation therapy – this should be discussed with a physician. Antioxidant supplements must be avoided during radiation therapy since they can protect the cancer cells – consult all supplements with a physician or dietitian/nutritionist.

YOU SHOULD REMEMBER

Radiotherapy may be used in the early stages of cancer or after its spread. It can be used to try to cure the cancer completely (curative radiotherapy) or to make other treatments more effective. For example, it can be combined with chemotherapy or used before surgery.

Check Your Knowledge

1. What are the functional categories of chemotherapy agents?
2. If chemotherapy causes a lack of appetite, what can be done?
3. During radiation therapy, why must dehydration be prevented?

NUTRITIONAL THERAPY FOR DYING PATIENTS

A terminally ill patient eventually loses all appetite, and tube feeding or IV feeding methods may be required – this is often a concern for family members. Even so, for a dying patient, nutritional support does not seem to have any benefit since it does not prolong or improve the quality of life. Many healthcare professionals believe that in the days before death, the patient may made less comfortable if given nutritional support or made to eat more than they want. Dying patients are usually not distressed by hunger and are more comfortable eating and drinking as they wish. As the body starts to shut down, the person may lose all desire to eat or drink. When death is not expected within hours or days, nutritional support may be attempted for a limited time to see if the patient's comfort, energy, or mental clarity improves. There should be an explicit agreement between the patient, family members, and the healthcare team about when to try nutritional support and stop it. An *advance directive* is used for this purpose.

Regardless, family members and caregivers may slowly offer food to the dying patient in small portions. The patient's favorite, intensely flavored, or easy-to-swallow foods are suggested. Even a tiny amount of a preferred alcoholic drink can be offered 30 minutes before meals. Allowing the dying patient to choose all food or drink is most important. Sometimes, appetite stimulants or antidepressants such as megestrol or dronabinol are helpful. Comforting care to the dying patient may include brushing the teeth, moistening the mouth with wet cloths as needed, giving the patient ice chips, or applying lip balm. Hospice care personnel are trained to provide these types of support (see **Figure 32.6**). Sometimes, family members need counseling to understand the use or stoppage of nutritional support.

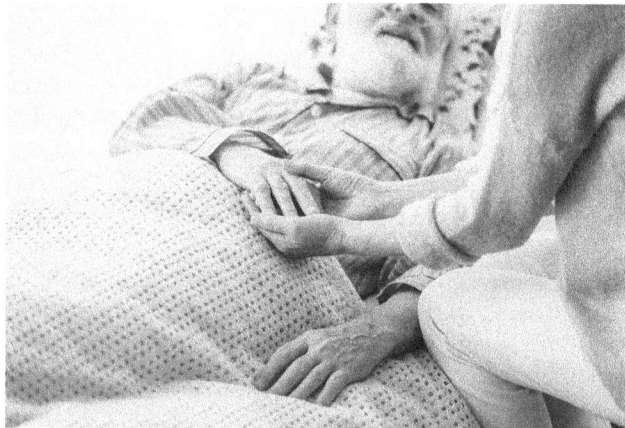

FIGURE 32.6   A patient in hospice care.

Clinical Case Studies

CLINICAL CASE STUDY 1

A 60-year-old woman had a past medical history of alcohol abuse and depression. She was hospitalized after being found unconscious at home and suffered from tachycardia, hypotension, and an inability to follow commands. She had GI bleeding that resulted in significant blood volume loss. The patient was intubated and placed on broad-spectrum antibiotics but also required cardiac support with vasopressors. A CT scan revealed hepatic steatosis. The patient was started on pantoprazole and octreotide infusions. An upper endoscopy revealed esophageal necrosis. After a few days, the patient was placed on TPN. Eventually, she was discharged to home care, and the TPN continued there until she could transition to a soft diet.

Critical Thinking Questions

1. How is TPN used?
2. What steps of the sterile technique are required for TPN?
3. What complications affect more than 90% of patients receiving TPN?

CLINICAL CASE STUDY 2

A 17-year-old girl was hospitalized because of anorexia nervosa. Though she stood 5¢2² tall, her weight was only 89 pounds. Her continued attempts to lose weight resulted in damage to her heart, resulting in bradycardia, hypotension, and the development of heart failure. The girl's family worked relentlessly to get her help, and fortunately, they found a family-based therapy program that was highly successful. Four years later, the now 21-year-old girl is a healthy, happy woman whose weight is well within normal ranges for her height.

Critical Thinking Questions

1. How does nutritional supplementation for anorexia nervosa begin?
2. How do long periods of starvation affect treatments for anorexia?
3. For recovery from anorexia, what incremental food changes are suggested?

CLINICAL CASE STUDY 3

A 67-year-old woman had been diagnosed with ovarian cancer. Her symptoms included pelvic discomfort, reduced appetite, weight loss, abdominal distension, reflux, and worsening shortness of breath. Though ambulatory and capable of self-care, she could no longer work at her job. Imaging revealed a large pelvic mass, which a biopsy confirmed as ovarian cancer. Chemotherapy was initiated. Upon meeting her dietitian, the patient's diet consisted of soups, clear fluids, and milk. She was given oral nutritional supplements, which she tolerated well, and encouraged to add small amounts of semi-solid foods, which she did. Over time, the patient improved and could add some solid foods to her diet. She underwent a total abdominal hysterectomy, bilateral salpingo-oophorectomy, total omentectomy, and excision of bulky paracaval nodes. The patient had additional chemotherapy and remains cancer-free and well-nourished over several months of follow-up due to the combined types of treatments.

Critical Thinking Questions

1. What are the common nutrition-related adverse effects of chemotherapy?
2. What considerations are required for cancer patients receiving chemotherapy?
3. How important is it to prevent cancer patients' chemotherapy-related malnutrition and weight loss?

FURTHER READING

1. Aadhaar O'Gormon, E. (2012). *Complete Tubefeeding: Everything You Need to Know about Tubefeeding, Tube Nutrition, and Blended Diets*. CreateSpace Independent Publishing Platform.
2. American Cancer Society, Besser, J., and Grant, B. (2018). *What to Eat During Cancer Treatment*, 2nd Edition. American Cancer Society.
3. Balch, P.A. (2010). *Prescription for Nutritional Healing: A-to-Z Guide to Supplements*. Avery.
4. Creagan, E.T., and Wendel, S. (2018). *Farewell: Vial End-of-Life Questions with Candid Answers from a Leading Palliative and Hospice Physician*. Write On Ink Publishing.
5. Douglas, D. (2022). *Pancreatitis Diet for Beginnings: Comprehensive Guide on Control, Management, and Treatment with Healthy Recipes, Food List, and Meal Plan for Healthier Lifestyle*. Douglas.
6. Jeejeebhoy, K.N. (2018). *Total Parenteral Nutrition in the Hospital and at Home*. CRC Press/Taylor & Francis Group.
7. Kalamian, M., and Seyfried, T.N. (2017). *Keto for Cancer: Ketogenic Metabolic Therapy as a Targeted Nutritional Therapy*. Chelsea Green Publishing.
8. Kane, K., and Prelack, K. (2018). *Advanced Medical Nutrition Therapy*. Jones & Bartlett Learning.
9. Lazarides, L. (2011). *Principles of Nutritional Therapy*. Nature study.
10. Leigh, I. (2022). *A Guidebook to Nutrition: A Comprehensive Guide to Essential Vitamins, Minerals, and Omega Oils*. Inara Leigh.
11. Lock, J., and Le Grange, D. (2015). *Treatment Manual for Anorexia Nervosa: A Family-Based Approach*. The Guilford Press.
12. McKay, J., and Schacher, T. (2009). *The Chemotherapy Survival Guide: Everything You Need to Know to Get Through Treatment*, 3rd Edition. New Harbinger Publications.
13. Nelms, M., and Sucher, K.P. (2019). *Nutrition Therapy and Pathophysiology*, 4th Edition. Cengage Learning.
14. Nelms, M., and Roberts, K. (2021). *Medical Nutrition Therapy: A Case Study Approach*, 6th Edition. Cengage Learning.
15. Ouren, M. (2022). *Cancer Treatments: Good Nutrition for Cancer Patients*. Ouren.
16. Plaskett, L. (2018). *The Nutritional Therapy of Cancer*. Lulu.com,
17. Schlenker, E., and Gilbert, J.A. (2018). *Williams' Essentials of Nutrition and Diet Therapy*. Elsevier.
18. Stephen, N. (2022). *Nutritional Therapy on High Fiber Diet: A Complete Guide with Benefit, Delicious and Healthy Recipes for the Diet*. Stephen.
19. Viola, S., and Evans, N. (2021). *When Waves Rise: Navigating Difficult Moments Associated with Dementia*. SV Grace LLC.

Appendix A
Answer Key to Clinical Case Studies

CHAPTER 1: HEALTHY NUTRITION

CLINICAL CASE STUDY 1.1

1. Health education teaches about various health conditions to improve preventive methods and early treatments. It is often focused on target populations such as poorer neighborhoods that lack sufficient ways to learn about nutrition, physical activities, and conditions such as type 2 diabetes mellitus.
2. A triglyceride is an **ester** formed from **glycerol** and three fatty acid groups. Triglycerides are the main constituents of natural **fats** and oils, and high concentrations in the blood indicate an elevated risk of stroke.
3. Carbohydrates provide energy for the brain, muscles, heart, and lungs. Lipids provide energy, help manufacture the coverings around nerves, and produce some hormones. Proteins also provide power and help build and repair cells and tissues.

CLINICAL CASE STUDY 1.2

1. Health promotion includes concentrating on quitting smoking, increasing access to healthy foods, increasing physical activity, preventing excessive alcohol use, promoting lifestyle changes and disease management, promoting reproductive health, promoting clinical preventive services, and promoting community water fluoridation.
2. The primary dietary guidelines required for good nutrition include a variety of vegetables – including dark green, orange, and red, as well as legumes and starchy vegetables; fat-free or low-fat dairy products – milk, yogurt, cheese, and fortified soy products; fruits – especially whole fruits; grains – especially whole grains; healthy oils; and protein foods – lean meats, poultry, seafood, legumes, nuts, seeds, and soy products.
3. Simple carbohydrates are found in fruits, milk, and sweeteners such as sugar, honey, and high-fructose corn syrup. Complex carbohydrates are found in cereals, fruits, grains, pasta, and vegetables.

CLINICAL CASE STUDY 1.3

1. Fiber is a complex carbohydrate that helps the body feel full, making overeating less likely. It can also help lower cholesterol and blood glucose. Fiber is found in many plant foods, including beans, fruits, nuts, seeds, vegetables, and whole grains.
2. The healthiest sources of carbohydrates are unprocessed or slightly processed beans, fruits, vegetables, and whole grains. They promote good health by delivering fiber, phytonutrients, minerals, and vitamins.
3. Several cholesterol types are based on various lipoproteins: VLDLs, LDLs, and HDLs.

CHAPTER 2: DIGESTION, ABSORPTION, AND METABOLISM

CLINICAL CASE STUDY 2.1

1. Hydrochloric acid causes the stomach contents to be highly acidic, with a pH between 1.5 and 3.5 – this is required for activation and for the highest activity of pepsin, which digests proteins.
2. Therefore, pancreatic fluid has a high pH that helps neutralize acidic chyme that enters the duodenum, providing the best environment for intestinal and pancreatic enzymes.
3. Gastric secretion is inhibited when the gastric contents are highly acidic, with a pH below 2. This often occurs between meals.

CLINICAL CASE STUDY 2.2

1. Absorption is the process of moving nutrients from the intestines into the bloodstream. Most nutrients are absorbed through the small intestine's lining, but water-soluble nutrients are absorbed differently than fats or fat-soluble compounds.
2. Concerning absorption, carbohydrates are absorbed in the duodenum, while proteins are found in the jejunum. The jejunum also functions to absorb most fats.
3. The plicae circulares, villi, and microvilli increase the absorptive surface area of the small intestine.

CLINICAL CASE STUDY 2.3

1. Problems with metabolism can result in illness, and one of the most common metabolic diseases is diabetes mellitus. It occurs when the body cannot process glucose and other sugars properly.
2. *Stage 1* – digestion and absorption, with absorbed nutrients transported in the bloodstream to tissue cells; *Stage 2* – in tissue cells' cytoplasm, newly arriving nutrients are built into lipids, proteins, and glycogen, an essential metabolic intermediate; *Stage 3* – in the mitochondria, oxygen is used to complete the breakdown of remaining products; most are converted to *acetyl CoA*, producing carbon dioxide and water, requiring large amounts of ATP.
3. The three processes regulating blood glucose are glycogenesis, glycogenolysis, and gluconeogenesis. Glycogenesis is the formation of glycogen from glucose. Glycogenolysis involves glycogen breaking down into glucose-1-phosphate and glucose. Gluconeogenesis is the formation of glucose from non-hexose precursors (glycerol, lactate, pyruvate, and glucogenic amino acids). Gluconeogenesis is the reversal of glycolysis.

CHAPTER 3: DIABETES MELLITUS

CLINICAL CASE STUDY 3.1

1. Hypoglycemia is generally signified by a fasting blood sugar of 70 mg/dL or 3.9 mmol/L.
2. Patients with type 1 diabetes have an increased frequency of symptomatic hypoglycemia, with about one severe episode per year. The proportion of patients with diabetes mellitus with an observed extreme hypoglycemia event in insulin-treated type 2 diabetes is approximately 30% of the rate seen with type 1 diabetes. The event rate for severe hypoglycemia ranges from 40% to 100% of patients with type 1 diabetes.
3. The mainstay of therapy for hypoglycemia is glucose. Pure glucose is available in tablets, gels, and other forms. Commonly, four glucose tablets (usually available OTC) can be

taken, or one serving of *glucose gel*, five to six pieces of hard candy or jelly beans, four ounces of fruit juice or regular (not diet) soda, or one tablespoon of sugar, corn syrup, or honey. Generally, food or drinks with 15–20 g of carbohydrates can return blood glucose levels to the safe range.

CLINICAL CASE STUDY 3.2

1. Type 2 diabetes is more common in males than females and usually occurs after the age of 40 years. However, when diagnosed before age 40, the average reduction in lifespan is 12 years in men but 19 years in women.

2. Since 1940, type 2 diabetes has been increasing in the United States. It has doubled in all adult age-groups in just the past 25 years. Type 2 diabetes varies between ethnic groups but is most common in African-American women. It affects 34% of people between the ages of 65 and 74.

3. According to the American Diabetes Association, hypertension plus type 2 diabetes is much more likely to be fatal because it dramatically increases the risks of heart attack or stroke. Chronic hypertension can also cause faster development of Alzheimer's disease and dementia.

CHAPTER 4: HEREDITARY CARBOHYDRATE DISORDERS

CLINICAL CASE STUDY 4.1

1. All types of glycogen storage disorders are caused by deficiencies in enzymes involved in glycogen synthesis or breakdown. The defects may occur in the liver or muscles, causing hypoglycemia or deposition of abnormal types of glycogen or its intermediate metabolites in tissues.

2. The signs and symptoms of glycogen storage disorders include jaundice, malaise, weight loss, chronic abdominal pain, inability to concentrate, and bruises. In some cases, hypoglycemia, hepatomegaly, exercise intolerance, muscle cramps, weakness, cirrhosis with dysplastic nodules, and splenomegaly are present. These disorders sometimes affect the myocardial tissue, leading to cardiomyopathy and cardiac conduction defects.

3. Treatments vary by the type of glycogen storage disorder present but usually include dietary supplementation with cornstarch. This provides a sustained source of glucose for the hepatic subtypes, while exercise avoidance is needed for the muscle subtypes.

CLINICAL CASE STUDY 4.2

1. Fructose is a monosaccharide present in significant concentrations in fruit and honey. It is a constituent of sucrose and sorbitol.

2. Infants are healthy until they ingest fructose. Then, fructose 1-phosphate accumulates. This causes hypoglycemia, nausea, vomiting, abdominal pain, sweating, confusion, excessive sleepiness, tremors, lethargy, failure to thrive, mental deterioration, and coma. Repeated ingestion of fructose-containing foods can lead to liver and kidney damage. Liver damage can result in jaundice, hepatomegaly, and cirrhosis. Continued exposure to fructose may result in seizures, coma, and, ultimately, death from liver and kidney failure.

3. Only the primary manifestations of hereditary fructose intolerance can be prevented with dietary restrictions of fructose, sucrose, sucralose, and sorbitol.

CLINICAL CASE STUDY 4.3

1. The two examples of these disorders are pyruvate dehydrogenase deficiency and carboxylase deficiency.
2. Pyruvate carboxylase is an enzyme needed for gluconeogenesis from pyruvate and alanine generated in muscles.
3. Pyruvate carboxylase deficiency is suspected in patients with non-specific clinical signs. Diagnosis requires identifying test abnormalities in amino acid, organic acid, glucose, and ammonia serum concentrations. A pyruvate carboxylase enzyme activity assay that shows a deficiency of the enzyme in fibroblasts is also diagnostic, along with mutations in the PC gene via molecular genetic testing.

CHAPTER 5: DISORDERS OF LIPID METABOLISM

CLINICAL CASE STUDY 5.1

1. Xanthomas are yellowish fatty nodules under the skin, especially around the eyes, knees, and elbows.
2. Complications include increased mortality, coronary artery disease, peripheral artery disease, cancer, infection, adrenal failure, mental disorders, and suicide.
3. Since secondary hypercholesterolemia is acquired, lifestyle modifications are essential for treatment, along with cholesterol-lowering medications. Most underlying metabolic causes, such as diabetes mellitus and hypothyroidism, are chronic and must be controlled. Other reasons, such as hepatitis C, can be cured, though there can still be resultant damage to the liver, leading to elevated lipid levels even after treatment. Medication-induced hypercholesterolemia can often be stopped by stopping or lowering doses of the causative drug. Patients are advised to reduce their intake of saturated fats to less than 6% of total daily calories. They should be replaced with healthier polyunsaturated or monosaturated fats. Fruits, vegetables, whole grains, low-fat dairy products, and oily fish rich in omega-3 fatty acids should be increased.

CLINICAL CASE STUDY 5.2

1. If an individual inherits the situation from both parents, symptoms usually appear during childhood. This is a rare and more severe subtype, and if untreated, it usually causes death before the age of 20 years.
2. Primary hypercholesterolemia is an autosomal dominant genetic disorder caused by a genetic alteration from one or both parents. Affected individuals are, therefore, born with the condition. It prevents the body from removing LDL, "bad cholesterol," resulting in a buildup in the arteries that leads to heart disease.
3. Adults with primary hypercholesterolemia usually have LDL levels over 190 mg/dL (4.9 mmol/L).

CLINICAL CASE STUDY 5.3

1. Secondary hypercholesterolemia may begin with endocrine disorders, renal disorders, medications, liver disease, storage disease, and other causes. Endocrine disorders include diabetes mellitus and hypothyroidism. Renal disorders include nephrotic syndrome and renal failure.
2. Atherosclerosis or hypertension can cause shortness of breath and fatigue, especially with exertion. Once advanced, more severe complications can develop.

3. Medications used include the drugs used for primary hypercholesterolemia, plus a few more: *statins, ezetimibe, PCSK9 inhibitors, bile acid sequestrants* – they clear bile from the body, forcing the liver to produce more bile and less cholesterol, *adenosine triphosphate-citrate lyase (ACL) inhibitors* – inhibit the biosynthesis of cholesterol in the liver, *fibrates* – mainly used to reduce triglyceride levels and increase HDL levels, and *niacin (nicotinic acid)* – a prescription form of vitamin B3; it may help lower LDL and increase HDL.

CHAPTER 6: DYSLIPIDEMIA AND ATHEROSCLEROSIS

CLINICAL CASE STUDY 6.1

1. Dyslipidemia is divided into primary and secondary types. Primary dyslipidemia is inherited. Secondary dyslipidemia is an acquired condition. That means it develops from other causes, such as obesity or diabetes and genetics – in the majority of cases, autosomal recessive inheritance. It is one of the most prevalent monogenic disorders, identified in approximately 1 of every 500 individuals in the general population.
2. In most patients with newly diagnosed dyslipidemia, and when a component of the lipid profile has worsened, tests for secondary causes should be done. Creatine, fasting glucose, liver enzymes, thyroid-stimulating hormone (TSH), and urinary protein should be measured.
3. Children with risk factors such as diabetes, hypertension, and a family history of severe hyperlipidemia should have a fasting lipid profile once between ages 2 and 8. For children with no risk factors, the lipid profile is done once before puberty – usually between ages 9 and 11 – and again between ages 17 and 21.

CLINICAL CASE STUDY 6.2

1. Atherosclerosis is the most common form of arteriosclerosis and is related to dyslipidemia, diabetes mellitus, cigarette smoking, family history, hypertension, obesity, and a sedentary lifestyle. Once the plaques grow or rupture, blood flow can be reduced or obstructed.
2. Screening for dyslipidemia is done using a fasting lipid profile. Lipid measurement should occur along with assessment for other cardiovascular risk factors, including diabetes mellitus, hypertension, smoking, and family history of coronary artery disease in a male first-degree relative before age 55 or a female first-degree relative before age 65.
3. Regular physical activity reduces the incidence of diabetes mellitus, dyslipidemia, hypertension, CAD, and atherosclerotic-related death. This is true whether there have been any previous ischemic events. It is recommended that patients engage in 30–45 minutes of walking, cycling, swimming, or running for 3–5 days/week. Aerobic exercise helps prevent atherosclerosis while promoting weight loss.

CLINICAL CASE STUDY 6.3

1. When an unstable plaque ruptures and occludes a significant artery and a superimposition of embolism or thrombosis, symptoms may develop, including unstable angina, heart attack, and ischemic stroke.
2. Preventing atherosclerosis involves quitting or avoiding smoking, managing hypertension and high cholesterol, becoming more physically active, eating a heart-healthy diet, and managing diabetes mellitus. Aerobic exercise is very beneficial for reducing atherosclerosis. At-risk patients should see their healthcare providers regularly for check-ups to check their BP and cholesterol levels.

3. Atherosclerosis is a common condition that develops when a sticky substance called plaque builds up inside the artery – the development of plaques collecting in the lumens of routes such as the coronary, carotid, and cerebral arteries.

CHAPTER 7: HYPERTENSION

CLINICAL CASE STUDY 7.1

1. Early signs and symptoms of hypertension include dizziness, facial flushing, early morning headache, epistaxis, vision changes, ear buzzing, and nervousness.
2. The development of primary hypertension is highly complex and multifactorial. The kidneys are the contributing organs and the target organs of hypertension. There is an interaction between multiple organ systems and various mechanisms of independent or interdependent pathways. Factors include genetics, activation of the sympathetic nervous system and renin–angiotensin–aldosterone system, obesity, and high dietary sodium.
3. The generally recommended lifestyle modifications include increased physical exercise; weight loss; a diet rich in fruits, vegetables, whole grains, and low-fat dairy products, with reduced saturated and total fat content; reduced dietary sodium; enhanced dietary potassium intake; moderate or no use of alcohol; and smoking cessation.

CLINICAL CASE STUDY 7.2

1. Uncontrolled hypertension is one of the leading causes of malignant hypertension. Other causes include Conn's syndrome, Cushing's syndrome, pheochromocytoma, a renin-secreting tumor, stroke, traumatic brain injury, medications, and substance and medication withdrawal.
2. The clinical diagnosis of malignant hypertension is based on high blood pressure at or above 180/120 mmHg and evidence of organ damage from a urinalysis, a chest X-ray, a fundoscopic eye exam, and blood tests. Other tests include a CT scan, MRI, an EKG, and an echocardiogram.
3. Antihypertensive medications are administered via an intravenous (IV) line for quick onset of action. IV beta-blockers (labetalol and esmolol) or calcium channel blockers (nicardipine and clevidipine) are administered to reduce systolic blood pressure levels by no more than 25% within the first hour. They will aim to avoid low blood flow to the organs, which may worsen organ damage. Several other parenterals are recommended to treat MHT, such as nitroprusside sodium, hydralazine, nicardipine, fenoldopam, nitroglycerin, and enalaprilat. The most commonly used intravenous drug is nitroprusside. An alternative for patients with renal insufficiency is intravenous fenoldopam. Labetalol is another common alternative, providing an easy transition from intravenous to oral dosing.

CLINICAL CASE STUDY 7.3

1. The pathophysiology of hypertension involves an impairment of renal pressure natriuresis. This is the feedback system in which hypertension causes an increase in sodium and water excretion by the kidney, which leads to a reduction in blood pressure.
2. Common causes of secondary hypertension include primary aldosteronism, parenchymal diseases of the kidneys, renovascular disease, and sleep apnea.
3. The prevention of secondary hypertension requires a healthy lifestyle. A healthy diet with limited sodium and increased potassium is needed. Foods should be lower in fat and include many fruits, vegetables, and whole grains. The *DASH eating plan* helps lower blood pressure. Regular exercise, including aerobic exercise, is essential.

CHAPTER 8: CORONARY ARTERY DISEASE

CLINICAL CASE STUDY 8.1

1. Chest pain or discomfort are the common symptoms of unstable angina. However, these are usually more intense, longer in duration, precipitated by little exertion, or occur while resting.
2. Unstable angina is caused by blood clots that block an artery wholly or partially. They can form, partially dissolve, and reform, with unstable angina occurring each time. The condition is related to coronary heart disease from the buildup of atherosclerotic plaques along arterial walls.
3. Treatment of unstable angina begins with establishing an excellent intravenous route. Oxygen is usually given in 2 L via nasal cannula. Single-lead ECG monitoring is initiated. If the patient is clinically unstable due to continuing symptoms, arrhythmias, or hypotension, urgent angiography with revascularization must occur. Morphine must be used carefully, such as when nitroglycerin is contraindicated, or the patient still has symptoms after nitroglycerin has been administered.

CLINICAL CASE STUDY 8.2

1. Chest pain or discomfort is the common symptoms of unstable angina. However, these are usually more intense, longer in duration, precipitated by little exertion, or occur while resting. Unstable angina is classified by severity and the clinical situation as follows:
   - *Class 1 severity* – the new onset of severe angina or increasing angina, but no angina at rest
   - *Class 2 severity* – there is angina at rest over the previous month but not within the preceding 48 hours; this is designated as subacute angina at rest
   - *Class 3 severity* – there is angina at rest over the preceding 48 hours; this is designated as acute angina at rest; the troponin status as negative or positive is evaluated, which affects the prognosis
   - *Clinical situation A* – the condition develops secondary to an extracardiac condition that worsens the myocardial ischemia, designated as secondary unstable angina
   - *Clinical situation B* – the condition develops without a contributing extracardiac need being present; the troponin status as negative or positive is evaluated, which affects prognosis; designated as primary unstable angina
   - *Clinical situation C* – the condition develops within 2 weeks of an acute MI, designated as post-myocardial infarction unstable angina
     1. Angina symptoms can sometimes include shortness of breath, nausea, or upper abdominal pain. The patient often believes that indigestion is the cause. Ischemic symptoms usually require a minute or longer to resolve, so very brief sensations are generally not from angina. Pain from stable angina lasts an average of 1–15 minutes.
2. A stable angina diagnosis is likely when a patient has chest discomfort caused by exertion and is relieved by rest. It is more accurate when significant risk factors for CAD are present. It is essential to understand that anxiety, panic attacks, costochondritis, GI disorders, and hyperventilation can also cause chest discomfort. A blood cholesterol profile is done. ECG is performed, and stress testing with ECG or myocardial imaging and coronary angiography may be ordered in some cases. Myocardial imaging methods include echocardiography, MRI, and radionuclide imaging.
3. Sublingual nitroglycerin is the most effective drug for relieving symptoms during an acute angina attack. It can also be taken before exertion to prevent an attack. Effective relief

occurs in 1.5–3 minutes in most cases, entirely by 5 minutes, and lasting as long as 30 minutes. Antiplatelet drugs, beta-blockers, long-acting nitrates, and calcium channel blockers prevent ischemia. Antiplatelet drugs inhibit the aggregation of platelets. Aspirin binds to the platelets irreversibly, inhibiting platelet aggregation and cyclooxygenase. Calcium channel blockers are used for persistent symptoms after nitrates are used or if they cannot be tolerated. Sodium channel blockers and sinus node inhibitors can also stabilize angina.

CHAPTER 9: MYOCARDIAL INFARCTION

CLINICAL CASE STUDY 9.1

1. The three types of myocardial infarction include ST-segment elevation myocardial infarction, non-ST-segment elevation myocardial infarction, and silent myocardial infarction.
2. Acute myocardial infarction is caused by narrowing or blockage of the coronary arteries with atherosclerotic plaque. Factors that lead to this include high LDL and excessive saturated fat and trans fats in the diet. Modifiable risk factors represent over 90% of the risks for acute MI. Risk factors include diabetes mellitus, obesity, smoking, hypertension, high cholesterol, high triglycerides, increased age, and family history of heart disease. Additional risk factors include high-stress levels, lack of physical exercise, cigarette smoking, use of amphetamines or cocaine, and a history of preeclampsia.
3. Even if it recurs, prevention of AMI includes a heart-healthy diet with plenty of whole grains, fruits, vegetables, and lean protein. There must be significant reductions in cholesterol, saturated fat, trans fat, and sugar. This is critical for people with diabetes mellitus, high cholesterol, and hypertension. Exercising regularly and following an approved exercise plan created by a physician improves cardiovascular health. Any new exercise plan must only be started by consulting a physician. Quitting smoking significantly lowers risks for acute MI and improves heart and lung health. Secondhand smoke must also be avoided.

CLINICAL CASE STUDY 9.2

1. Dyslipidemia is a significant risk factor for STEMI, along with diabetes mellitus, hypertension, smoking, obesity, and a family history of coronary artery disease. For most patients, STEMI is a type 1 myocardial infarction.
2. Quitting smoking significantly lowers risks for acute MI and improves heart and lung health. Secondhand smoke must also be avoided.
3. Coronavirus disease 2019 (COVID-19) is caused by severe acute respiratory syndrome. The coronavirus likely affects the risk of HF development after MI.

CLINICAL CASE STUDY 9.3

1. The most common causes of heart failure include CAD, AMI, arrhythmia, hypertension, myocarditis, diabetes, obesity, alcohol use, tobacco and recreational drug use, and chemotherapy.
2. The clinical signs and symptoms of heart failure after MI include chest pain, dyspnea, persistent coughing or wheezing, edema, tiredness, fatigue, lack of appetite, nausea, nocturia, confusion, impaired thinking, tachycardia, and weight gain.
3. The primary medicines for heart failure include angiotensin-converting enzyme, angiotensin II receptor blockers, beta-blockers, potassium-sparing diuretics, and digoxin.

CHAPTER 10: STROKE

CLINICAL CASE STUDY 10.1

1. A hemorrhagic stroke usually occurs in the basal ganglia, cerebral lobes, cerebellum, or pons. However, it can also occur in the brainstem or midbrain.
2. Arteriovenous malformations (AVMs) are abnormal tangles of blood vessels that cause abnormalities in the connections between the arteries and veins. They usually occur in the brain and spinal cord.
3. Extensive hemorrhages in the brain hemispheres cause hemiparesis. If they occur in the posterior fossa, cerebellar or brainstem deficits arise. These include conjugate eye deviation, ophthalmoplegia, pinpoint pupils, breathing that resembles snoring, and coma. In about half of patients, extensive hemorrhages are fatal in a few days. Those that survive experience a return to consciousness. Neurologic deficits slowly reduce as extravasated blood is resorbed.

CLINICAL CASE STUDY 10.2

1. An ischemic stroke is caused by a blockage cutting off the blood supply to the brain and is the most common type of stroke. Of the forms of stroke, 80% are ischemic, and 20% are hemorrhagic. The five leading causes of a stroke include hypertension, hypercholesterolemia, smoking, obesity, and diabetes.
2. Stroke occurs suddenly with numbness, weakness, paralysis of the contralateral limbs and face, aphasia, confusion, visual disturbances, headache, dizziness, and loss of balance and coordination.
3. Complications of strokes include aphasia, spasticity, confusion, depression, sleep problems, incontinence, pneumonia, and swallowing dysfunction, which can lead to aspiration, dehydration, or undernutrition.

CLINICAL CASE STUDY 10.3

1. A transient ischemic attack involves symptoms of stroke that usually last for less than 1 hour. It is defined as focal brain ischemia with sudden neurologic deficits. There is no visualization of any acute cerebral infarction when evaluation is done with diffusion-weighted MRI.
2. Most TIAs are caused by emboli, usually from the carotid or vertebral arteries. Rarely, TIAs occur from impaired perfusion caused by severe hypoxemia, a lowered oxygen-carrying capacity of the blood, or increased viscosity – especially in stenotic brain arteries.
3. The cause of a TIA is evaluated the same way as the reasons for ischemic strokes. There are tests for cardiac sources of emboli, carotid stenosis, atrial fibrillation, and hematologic abnormalities. These tests include transesophageal echocardiography, transthoracic echocardiography, cardiac CT angiography, 24-hour Holter monitoring, ultrasonography, magnetic resonance angiography, electrocardiography, event recording (also called event monitoring), implantable loop recorders, and blood tests. Stroke risk factors are screened. Evaluation continues quickly, usually with the patient being hospitalized since the risks of an ischemic stroke are very high and often happen quickly.

CHAPTER 11: HEREDITARY LIPID DISORDERS

CLINICAL CASE STUDY 11.1

1. Niemann–Pick disease (NPD) is a group of autosomal recessive disorders involving splenomegaly, variable neurologic deficits, and the storage of lipids, including sphingomyelin and cholesterol. It is a rare, inherited disease that affects the ability to metabolize lipids within cells, causing them to malfunction and die. Affected individuals have abnormal lipid metabolism that causes a buildup of harmful amounts of lipids in various organs.
2. The accumulation of lipids and cellular dysfunction eventually leads to cell death, causing tissue and organ damage.
3. Mutations in either the NPC1 or NPC2 gene cause Niemann–Pick disease type C. The proteins produced from these genes are involved in the movement of lipids within cells. Mutations in these genes lead to a need for more functional proteins. This prevents the movement of cholesterol and other lipids, leading to their accumulation in cells. Because these lipids are not correctly located in the cells, many normal cell functions that require lipids (such as cell membrane formation) are impaired.

CLINICAL CASE STUDY 11.2

1. Tay-Sachs disease is a rare genetic disorder passed down from parents to their children. It develops from the absence of beta-hexosaminidase A enzyme, which is required to break down GM2 ganglioside. The enzyme helps break down gangliosides, which are fatty substances. When gangliosides build up to toxic levels in the CSN, the function of nerve cells is affected.
2. In the most common and severe form of Tay-Sachs disease, signs and symptoms start at about 3–6 months of age. With disease progression, development slows, and the muscles begin to weaken. Over time, this causes seizures, paralysis, vision and hearing loss, and other significant abnormalities. Children with this form typically live only a few years. Less often, some children have the juvenile form of the disease and may live into their teen years. In rare cases, adults may have a late-onset form of Tay-Sachs disease, which is often less severe.
3. A thorough clinical evaluation and specialized tests confirm the diagnosis of Tay-Sachs disease. These include blood tests to measure the enzyme activity levels of hexosaminidase A. Molecular genetic testing for mutations in the HEXA gene is confirmative.

CLINICAL CASE STUDY 11.3

1. Gaucher disease is a rare, inherited metabolic disorder in which a fat molecule called glucocerebroside accumulates in different organs and tissues in the body. Type 1 is the most common type of disease reported in Western countries. It is a non-neuropathic form of the disease and is usually treatable. It affects bones and multiple organs, but the severity of the symptoms varies. The fatty substances that form due to this disease can build up in bone tissue. This occurrence weakens bones and increases the risk of fractures. It is often mild, affecting children as well as adults.
2. Type 1 is non-neuropathic and usually treatable. Type 2 (acute infantile neuronopathic Gaucher disease) is a severe form that is generally fatal within 2 years of birth. Type 3 (chronic neuronopathic Gaucher disease) is the most common worldwide, especially in India, the Pacific Rim, China, and the Middle East. The onset usually occurs later than type 2 and progresses slowly into adulthood.
3. Splenomegaly and hepatomegaly develop in about 90% of Gaucher disease type 1 patients.

CHAPTER 12: PROTEIN DEFICIENCIES

CLINICAL CASE STUDY 12.1

1. Protein–energy malnutrition is most prevalent in areas of Africa (Ethiopia, Kenya, Somalia, South Sudan, Sudan, Uganda), Southeast Asia (India, China, Bangladesh, Indonesia, Philippines, North Korea), Central America (Guatemala, Honduras, Mexico, El Salvador, Nicaragua), and South America (Peru, Bolivia, Colombia, Paraguay, Venezuela).
2. Hypoproteinemia can be caused by malnutrition or malabsorption due to intestinal disease, excessive loss of plasma protein either into the urine (nephrotic syndrome) or into the gut lumen (protein-losing enteropathy), or hepatic failure, the liver being the site of the synthesis of the plasma protein albumin.
3. Treatment to cure hypoproteinemia includes steroids and immune suppressors to lower intestine inflammation, antibiotics or antiparasitic drugs to counter infections, dialysis or kidney transplant for treatment of kidney disease, and treatment of liver damage with medications or surgery.

CLINICAL CASE STUDY 12.2

1. Marasmus is severe undernutrition – a deficiency in all the macronutrients the body requires to function, including carbohydrates, protein, and fats.
2. The underlying social cause of marasmus in children is poverty. Poverty may occur as a result of low status and insufficient education of mothers, along with natural disasters, war, and civil instability. Poverty directly influences the ability of a household to secure a reliable food source for children, leading to an insufficient calorie supply.
3. The primary treatment of marasmus is to rehydrate, prevent infections, and avoid the complications of the treatment of marasmus, such as refeeding syndrome. The immediate treatment lasts approximately 1 week.

CLINICAL CASE STUDY 12.3

1. Hypoalbuminemia is a common problem among persons with acute and chronic medical conditions. At the time of hospital admission, 20% of patients have hypoalbuminemia. The prevalence of hypoalbuminemia is higher amongst hospitalized, critically ill, and elderly patients.
2. Hypogammaglobulinemia is a disorder caused by low serum immunoglobulin (Ig) or antibody levels.
3. Primary causes of hypogammaglobulinemia are genetic conditions that affect the production of antibodies. In contrast, secondary causes are external factors that affect antibody levels.

CHAPTER 13: PROTEIN MISFOLDING DISEASES

CLINICAL CASE STUDY 13.1

1. In Alzheimer's disease, the processing of the amyloid precursor protein is altered, resulting in the deposition and fibrillar aggregation of beta-amyloid, the primary component of senile plaques. These plaques contain degenerated axonal or dendritic processes, astrocytes, and glial cells surrounding an amyloid core.
2. Alzheimer's disease is more common in women than men, partially because women live longer. Prevalence in industrialized countries will likely increase as the population ages. There is a rapid increase globally in people living with Alzheimer's disease. About

44 million people are now estimated to live with Alzheimer's disease or a related form of dementia.

3. The first sign of Alzheimer's disease is the loss of short-term memory. The affected individual asks questions repeatedly, often misplaces items, and needs to remember meetings or appointments. Additional problems with cognition may involve difficulty with complicated tasks, impaired reasoning, poor judgment, language dysfunction, and an inability to recognize faces or everyday objects. The disease progresses slowly and can plateau occasionally. Common behavioral disorders include agitation, feelings of persecution, wandering, and yelling.

CLINICAL CASE STUDY 13.2

1. Parkinson's disease is caused by the destruction of the nerve cells that make dopamine. Therefore, the risk factors include longstanding nerve cell destruction, increased age, the male gender, presence of visual hallucinations, family history of dementia, and severe motor symptoms.
2. Parkinson's disease is best treated with carbidopa/levodopa. Levodopa is the metabolic precursor of dopamine. Coadministration with carbidopa prevents levodopa from being decarboxylated into dopamine outside the brain. Levodopa is highly effective at relieving bradykinesia and rigidity while significantly reducing tremors.
3. Later in the disease course, postural instability may develop in a stooped position, with the patient having problems initiating walking, turning, and stopping. Short steps are taken, and the walk is described as *shuffling*. The arms are flexed to the waist and swing very little or not at all with each step. Some patients experience accidental quickening of steps, with progressive shortening of the stride length. This is festination, which often precedes freezing of the gait. With no warning, voluntary movements such as walking may suddenly stop. When the center of gravity is displaced, the patient tends to fall forward or backward. Dementia develops in about 33% of patients, usually late in the disease course.

CLINICAL CASE STUDY 13.3

1. *Huntington's disease* affects men and women equally. About 1in every 10,000 people globally has the disease. In the United States, nearly 30,000 people are affected every year. The condition is not prevalent within any particular population.
2. Before or along with the movement abnormalities, dementia or psychiatric disturbances develop. These may include apathy, depression, anhedonia, irritability, antisocial behaviors, and fully developed bipolar or schizophreniform disorder. The patient will likely have suicidal thoughts and attempts more often than the general public.
3. There is no cure for *Huntington's disease*. It is treated supportively to help manage some symptoms. Antipsychotic medications may partially suppress the chorea and agitation. Doses of antipsychotics are increased until symptoms are controlled or unwanted adverse effects such as lethargy or parkinsonism develop. Alternative medications include vesicular monoamine transporter type 2 inhibitors, such as tetrabenazine or deutetrabenazine. They deplete dopamine and help reduce chorea and dyskinesias.

CHAPTER 14: PROTEIN MISFOLDING DISEASES

CLINICAL CASE STUDY 14.1

1. Phenylketonuria causes a clinical syndrome that involves intellectual defects and behavioral and cognitive abnormalities caused by elevated serum phenylalanine.

2. The primary sign of untreated PKU is severe intellectual disability. There is also significant hyperactivity, gait disturbances, microcephaly, seizures, and psychoses. Often, there is a musty odor in the breath, skin, or urine because of too much phenylalanine in the body.
3. The treatment of phenylketonuria is a lifelong restriction of dietary phenylalanine. All-natural protein contains approximately 4% phenylalanine. This means that the diet requires low-protein natural foods such as certain cereals, plus fruits and vegetables, phenylalanine-free elemental amino acid mixtures, and protein hydrolysates that are treated to remove phenylalanine.

CLINICAL CASE STUDY 14.2

1. Patients with severe neonatal MSUD are usually typical for the first 2 or 3 days of life. They then develop lethargy, hypertonia with authoritarian opisthotonic posturing, loss of appetite, poor feeding, vomiting, seizures, respiratory failure, and coma that can lead to death.
2. Classic maple syrup urine disease is the most severe type of MSUD. It is also the most common. Symptoms usually develop within the first 3 days of birth.
3. Treatment of an acutely ill newborn with maple syrup urine disease includes hypercaloric nutritional support (high glucose concentrations, an insulin infusion to avoid hyperglycemia, and a source of leucine, isoleucine, and valine-free protein). Protein catabolism must be suppressed, and an anabolic state must be induced.

CLINICAL CASE STUDY 14.3

1. Lesch–Nyhan syndrome is caused by a deficiency of hypoxanthine-guanine phosphoribosyl transferase. The degree of the deficiency and its resulting manifestations vary between the specific gene mutations that are present.
2. Lesch–Nyhan syndrome causes brain and behavior problems, including severe arthritis, poor muscle control, and mental disability. A key symptom is uncontrollable self-injury. Hyperuricemia predisposes patients to gout and its complications – an orange, sandy precipitate known as xanthine appears in infants' urine.
3. Treatment for Lesch–Nyhan syndrome (LNS) is symptomatic. Gout can be treated with allopurinol to control excessive amounts of uric acid. Kidney stones may be treated with lithotripsy or laser beams. There is no standard treatment for the neurological symptoms of LNS, so management of the disease is supportive. Physical restraints, dental extractions, and drug therapy may be needed for self-mutilation. Hyperuricemia is treated with a low-purine diet, which avoids beans, organ meats, and sardines. The xanthine oxidase inhibitor called allopurinol prevents the conversion of collected hypoxanthine to uric acid. Since hypoxanthine is highly soluble, it is excreted.

CHAPTER 15: FAT-SOLUBLE VITAMINS

CLINICAL CASE STUDY 15.1

1. Vitamin A is a fat-soluble vitamin that is naturally present in many foods. Vitamin A is essential for normal vision, the immune system, reproduction, and growth and development. Vitamin A also helps the heart, lungs, and other organs work properly.
2. Risk factors include celiac disease, cystic fibrosis, chronic diarrhea, bile duct blockage, zinc or iron deficiency, and alcohol use disorder.

3. To prevent vitamin A deficiency, people should eat dark green leafy vegetables, yellow and orange fruits (such as papayas and oranges), carrots, and yellow vegetables (such as squash and pumpkin). Other food sources include milk and cereals fortified with vitamin A, liver, egg yolks, and fish liver oils.

CLINICAL CASE STUDY 15.2

1. Rickets is a metabolic disease of childhood, characterized by softening of the bones as a result of inadequate intake of vitamin D and insufficient exposure to sunlight, also associated with impaired calcium and phosphorus metabolism. It was a common metabolic disease of bone a century ago in North America, Europe, and East Asia (mainly due to vitamin D deficiency).
2. Osteomalacia occurs in adults because of insufficient calcium and phosphorus, making the bones soft and deformed. The diet usually causes low levels of vitamin D, inadequate sunlight, or a problem with how the body uses vitamin D. There is poor calcification of newly synthesized bone. Hence, fractures of the hips or spine are common.
3. Osteoporosis is a medical condition in which the bones become brittle and fragile from tissue loss, typically due to hormonal changes or deficiency of calcium or vitamin D. Around the world, one in three women and one in five men over the age of 50 will suffer a broken bone due to osteoporosis. Throughout life, bone is constantly being renewed, with new bone replacing old bone, which helps keep the skeleton strong. But for people with osteoporosis, more and more bone is lost and not replaced.

CLINICAL CASE STUDY 15.3

1. In the newborn, the typical presentation includes bleeding, which can be spontaneous or associated with surgery. There is often a history of easy bruising, mucosal bleeding, and developmental and skeletal anomalies. In adults, vitamin K deficiency may manifest as bleeding at venipuncture sites or after minor trauma. Patients may also administer antibiotics, anticonvulsants, warfarin, or other prescription medications interfering with vitamin K metabolism. Physical examination often reveals the presence of ecchymoses or petechiae.
2. Laboratory tests can diagnose vitamin K deficiency, including the prothrombin time test, which helps identify the time the plasma takes in the blood to clot. Prothrombin is a component that is involved in the process of blood clotting.
3. Intramuscular vitamin K injection is the recommended prophylactic method for all newborns and infants due to its increased efficacy compared to oral administration. If a newborn vomits or regurgitates an oral dose of vitamin K within 1 hour, another dose is recommended.

CHAPTER 16: WATER-SOLUBLE VITAMINS

CLINICAL CASE STUDY 16.1

1. Vitamin B2 (riboflavin) is essential for energy production, red blood cell generation, enzyme function, and ordinary fatty acid and amino acid synthesis. In addition to producing energy for the body, riboflavin is an antioxidant and necessary for producing glutathione, a free radical scavenger. Additionally, it is essential for normal development, growth, reproduction, lactation, physical performance, and well-being. A small amount is stored in the liver, kidneys, and heart. Excessive amounts are excreted in the urine. If excessive riboflavin supplements are taken, the urine becomes yellow and glows under a black light. Riboflavin is a component of the coenzymes needed.

2. Riboflavin deficiency can be associated with inadequate dietary intake and malabsorption. Pregnant and breastfeeding women may require higher riboflavin intake, and deficiency can occur if dietary intake is insufficient. Chronic alcohol consumption can interfere with the absorption and utilization of vitamin B2. Some medications, particularly those used to treat migraines, may interfere with the absorption or utilization of riboflavin. The risk for riboflavin deficiency also includes alcoholics and people with inferior diets. Certain GI disorders, such as Crohn's disease, celiac disease, and irritable bowel syndrome, can impair the body's ability to absorb nutrients from this vitamin. Long-term use of phenobarbital also affects riboflavin levels since the drug increases its breakdown, along with other nutrients in the liver.

3. The signs and symptoms of riboflavin include fatigue, sore throat, angular stomatitis, cheilosis, anemia, disorders, blurred vision, hair loss, and reproductive problems. Skin cracking around the corners of the mouth and seborrheic dermatitis. Some people have confusion, sensitivity to light, headaches, and poor growth.

CLINICAL CASE STUDY 16.2

1. The primary cause of pellagra is an inadequate diet. Drugs, alcoholism, GI tract diseases, and malignancies are the common causes of secondary pellagra. Excessive and chronic alcohol intake can induce pellagra due to reducing the absorption of niacin. Niacin is primarily absorbed in the small intestine; therefore, malabsorptive disorders such as chronic diarrhea, inflammatory bowel disease, and malignancy can impair niacin absorption. Also, a drug used for tuberculosis, such as isoniazid, may cause an increase in the risk of niacin deficiency.

2. The signs and symptoms of severe niacin deficiency lead to pellagra, a condition that causes chronic diarrhea, sometimes bloody, nausea, vomiting, and loss of appetite. Dermatology symptoms include a thick, scaly, pigmented rash on skin areas exposed to sunlight. Neurological symptoms of severe niacin deficiency include fatigue, headache, apathy, depression, memory loss, and hallucinations.

3. To diagnose pellagra, medical history, and diet are essential. Clinical symptoms may be straightforward when skin and mouth lesions, diarrhea, delirium, and dementia co-occur. More often, the presentation could be more specific. Laboratory testing should be completed to confirm the results, and it should include testing for tryptophan, NAD, NADP, and niacin levels. Urinary excretion of N1-methyl nicotinamide (NMN) of less than 5.8 µmol (0.8 mg/day) may suggest niacin deficiency.

CLINICAL CASE STUDY 16.3

1. Vitamin B12 plays an essential role in RBC formation, cell metabolism, nerve function, and the production of DNA, the molecules inside cells that carry genetic information. Absorption of vitamin 12 requires an intrinsic factor. Free B12 combines with an intrinsic factor, enhancing the absorption of the vitamin in the ileum.

2. Vitamin B12 deficiency has three primary causes: autoimmune (pernicious anemia), malabsorption, and dietary insufficiency. It can also occur because of Chron's disease or certain medications. Deficient intake of animal food products also causes B12 deficiency. Severe deficiency causes megaloblastic anemia.

3. A vitamin B12 deficiency can lead to anemia, fatigue, muscle weakness, intestinal problems, nerve damage, and mood disturbances. There are sensory disturbances in the legs, including burning, prickling, tingling, and numbness of fingertips. Walking and balance become affected. Mental problems include loss of concentration and memory, disorientation, and

dementia. Bowel and bladder control is eventually lost, and visual disturbances are common. Gastrointestinal problems include tongue soreness and constipation.

CHAPTER 17: NATREMIA, CHLOREMIA, AND KALEMIA

CLINICAL CASE STUDY 17.1

1. Hyponatremia can be caused by excessive fluid loss due to sweating or burns, severe vomiting, diarrhea, poor nutrition, alcohol use disorder, overhydration, chronic hypothyroidism, diabetes insipidus, adrenocortical deficiency, use of certain diuretics or seizure medications, antidepressants and pain medication, and liver, congestive heart failure, or kidney failure.
2. Signs and symptoms may include nausea and vomiting, headache, fatigue, hypotension, irritability, lethargy, muscle weakness or muscle cramps, seizures, confusion, and coma.
   Hyponatremia is very dangerous for many organs, but especially for the brain.
3. The treatment of hyponatremia depends on its cause and severity. The mainstay of management is rehydration with sodium chloride (0.9% solution) and discontinuation of diuretic therapy where appropriate. Correction or maintenance of other serum electrolytes is vital. Correction of hypokalemia is significant because low potassium can impair correction of hyponatremia.

CLINICAL CASE STUDY 17.2

1. In general, hypokalemia is associated with diagnoses of cardiac disease, renal failure, malnutrition, and shock. Hypokalemia may be caused by severe vomiting or diarrhea, dehydration, excessive sweating, dehydration, excessive alcohol use, chronic kidney disease, diabetic ketoacidosis, malnutrition, Cushing's syndrome, excessive aldosterone, hypomagnesemia, excessive laxatives, certain diuretics, and corticosteroids. Hypomagnesemia often occurs with and may worsen hypokalemia, especially in the presence of chronic diarrhea, alcoholism, genetic disorders, diuretic use, and chemotherapy. Both promote the development of cardiac dysrhythmias. Psychiatric patients are at risk for hypokalemia due to their drug therapy.
2. Clinical symptoms of hypokalemia become evident once the serum potassium level is less than three mEq/L unless there is a sudden severe fall or the patient has a process that is potentiated by hypokalemia. The severity of symptoms also tends to be proportional to the degree and duration of hypokalemia. Clinical manifestations include muscle cramps, severe muscle weakness (leading to paralysis of GI muscles), hypotension, faintness, polyuria, and polydipsia. Severe hypokalemia can also lead to muscle cramps, rhabdomyolysis, and resultant myoglobinuria. Hypokalemia can result in a variety of cardiac dysrhythmias. Although dysrhythmias are more likely to be associated with moderate-to-severe hypokalemia, there is a high degree of individual variability, and it can occur with even mild decreases in serum levels. Affected muscles can include the muscles of respiration, which can lead to respiratory failure and death.
3. Diagnostic evaluation of hypokalemia involves measuring urinary potassium excretion and assessing acid-base status. Measuring urinary potassium excretion can help distinguish renal losses from other causes of hypokalemia. Measurement of potassium excretion is ideally done via a 24-hour urine collection. After determining the presence or lack of renal potassium wasting, acid-base status should be assessed.

CLINICAL CASE STUDY 17.3

1. Patients with chronic hyperkalemia may be asymptomatic at increased levels, while patients with acute hyperkalemia may develop severe symptoms. Infants have higher baseline levels than children and adults. Signs and symptoms of hyperkalemia include fatigue, lethargy, muscle weakness, loss of appetite, nausea and vomiting, increased thirst, craving for salty foods, depression, irritability, polyuria, and poor concentration. Dangerously high potassium levels affect the heart and cause sudden chest pain, palpitations, dyspnea, paresthesias, and arrhythmia, which are life-threatening problems.

2. To diagnose hyperkalemia, ECG shows changes in the heart rhythm. T wave elevation is the earliest sign of this condition. Laboratory testing includes serum blood urea nitrogen and creatinine to assess renal function and urinalysis to screen for renal disease. In patients with renal disease, the serum calcium level should also be checked because hypocalcemia may exacerbate the cardiac effects of hyperkalemia. A complete blood count to screen for leukocytosis or thrombocytosis may also be helpful. Serum glucose and blood gas analysis should be ordered in diabetics and patients with suspected acidosis. Lactate dehydrogenase should be contained in patients with suspected hemolysis. Creatinine phosphokinases and urine myoglobin should be called in patients with suspected rhabdomyolysis. Uric acid and phosphorus should be ordered in patients with suspected tumor lysis syndrome. Digoxin toxicity may cause hyperkalemia, so serum levels should be checked in patients on digoxin. If no other cause is found, consider cortisol and aldosterone levels to assess for mineralocorticoid deficiency.

3. Treatment of hyperkalemia includes discontinuing sources of potassium intake. Calcium therapy will stabilize the cardiac response to hyperkalemia and should be initiated first in the setting of cardiac toxicity. Calcium does not alter the serum concentration of potassium but is a first-line therapy in hyperkalemia-related arrhythmias and ECG changes. Calcium chloride contains three times more elemental calcium than calcium gluconate. Still, it is more irritating to peripheral vessels and more likely to cause tissue necrosis with extravasation, so it is usually only given through central venous lines or peripherally in cardiac arrest. Thus, calcium gluconate is the usual initial drug of choice in patients with evidence of cardiac toxicity. Beta-2 adrenergic drugs such as albuterol will also shift potassium intracellularly. Loop or thiazide diuretics may help enhance potassium excretion, and hemodialysis should be performed in patients with end-stage renal disease or severe renal impairment.

CHAPTER 18: CALCEMIA AND PHOSPHATEMIA

CLINICAL CASE STUDY 18.1

1. Osteoporosis occurs when too much bone mass is lost, and changes occur in the structure of bone tissue. Many people with osteoporosis have several risk factors, but others who develop osteoporosis may not have any specific risk factors. There are some risk factors that we cannot change and others that we may be able to change. However, understanding these factors may prevent the disease and fractures. The risk factors include age, sex, race, family history, body size, and hormone changes. Examples of modifications to hormones include low estrogen levels in women after menopause, low levels of estrogen from the abnormal absence of menstrual periods in premenopausal women due to hormone disorders, extreme levels of physical activity, and low levels of testosterone in men.

2. Osteoporosis is called a "silent" disease because there are typically no symptoms until a bone is broken. Symptoms of spine fracture include severe back pain, loss of height, or spine malformations such as kyphosis. Bones affected by osteoporosis may become so

fragile that fractures occur spontaneously or result from minor falls, such as a fall from a standing height that would not usually cause a break in a healthy bone. Fractures may occur from everyday stresses such as bending, lifting, or coughing. Osteoporosis-related breaks most commonly occur in the hip, wrist, or spine.

3. The goals for treating osteoporosis are to slow or stop bone loss and to prevent fractures: proper nutrition, lifestyle changes, exercise, and medications. The US FDA has approved bisphosphonates, calcitonin, combined estrogen, progestin therapy, human parathyroid hormone, and calcium with vitamin D.

Clinical Case Study 18.2

1. The risk factors include family or personal history, dehydration, obesity, and certain supplements and medications, such as vitamin C, dietary supplements, laxatives (when used excessively), and calcium-based antacids, which can increase the risk of kidney stones.

2. A kidney stone usually will not cause symptoms until it moves around within the kidney or passes into one of the ureters. The ureters are the tubes that connect the kidneys and bladder. If a kidney stone becomes lodged in the ureters, it may block the flow of urine and cause the kidney to swell and the ureter to spasm, which can be very painful. At that point, the patient may experience sharp pain in the side and back below the ribs. Pain that radiates to the lower abdomen and groin comes in waves and fluctuates in intensity. Other signs and symptoms may include cloudy or foul-smelling urine, hematuria, nausea, vomiting, fever, and chills.

3. If you can pass a kidney stone, it may pass through the urinary tract without treatment. Larger kidney stones or kidney stones that block the urinary tract or cause great pain may need urgent treatment. Therefore, a kidney stone may be treated with shockwave lithotripsy, ureteroscopy, percutaneous nephrolithotomy, or nephrolithotripsy. The procedure involves surgically removing a kidney stone using small telescopes and instruments inserted through a small incision in the back.

Clinical Case Study 18.3

1. Hyperphosphatemia is usually caused by low calcium levels, chronic kidney disease, metabolic or respiratory acidosis, hypoparathyroidism, severe muscle injury, and excessive use of laxatives that contain phosphate. Renal failure is the most common cause of hyperphosphatemia. A glomerular filtration rate of less than 30 mL/min significantly reduces the filtration of inorganic phosphate, increasing its serum level. Other less common causes include a high intake of phosphorus or increased renal reabsorption. High phosphate can result due to excessive use of phosphate-containing laxatives or enemas and vitamin D intoxication.

2. Most patients with hyperphosphatemia are asymptomatic. However, it may cause tetany, muscle cramps, and perioral numbness or tingling. Other symptoms include bone and joint pain, pruritus, and rash. Soft-tissue calcifications are common among patients with chronic kidney disease; they manifest as quickly palpable, hard, subcutaneous nodules, often with overlying scratches.

3. Treatment includes eliminating phosphate intake and administering phosphate-binding antacids like calcium carbonate. The mainstay of therapy in patients with advanced chronic kidney disease is the reduction of phosphate intake, usually accomplished by avoiding foods containing high amounts of phosphate and using phosphate-binding medications taken with meals. Although quite effective, aluminum-containing antacids

should not be used as phosphate-binding agents in patients with end-stage renal disease because of the possibility of aluminum-related dementia and osteomalacia. Saline diuresis can enhance phosphate elimination in cases of acute hyperphosphatemia in patients with intact kidney function. Hemodialysis can lower phosphate levels in cases of severe acute hyperphosphatemia.

CHAPTER 19: IRON DEFICIENCY AND TOXICITY

CLINICAL CASE STUDY 19.1

1. *Iron-deficiency anemia* develops when the body's iron stores drop too low to support average red blood cell production.
2. The three stages of iron-deficiency anemia are as follows: (1) iron requirement exceeds intake – this causes progressive depletion of bone marrow iron stores; (2) as stores decrease – absorption of dietary iron increases to compensate; and (3) later stages – deficiency impairs red blood cell synthesis, and anemia results.
3. Most iron-deficiency symptoms are related to anemia. They include extreme fatigue, loss of stamina, dyspnea, chest pain, tachycardia, headache, dizziness, pale skin, brittle nails, and weakness. Restless legs syndrome is another common symptom, in which there is an urge to move the legs while remaining inactive.

CLINICAL CASE STUDY 19.2

1. Iron tablets may look like candy to children, and prenatal multivitamins are the source of iron in most fatal childhood iron ingestions. The cause and risk factors for pediatric iron poisoning are based on the amount of elemental iron consumed. Ingestion of less than 20 mg/kg of elemental iron is non-toxic. Ingestion of 20–60 mg/kg results in moderate symptoms. Ingestion of more than 60 mg/kg can result in severe toxicity and lead to severe morbidity and mortality.
2. The diagnosis of iron toxicity is based on the history and clinical presentation. Serum iron levels are used to determine a patient's potential for toxicity. The most helpful laboratory test is a serum iron level measured at its peak, 4–6 hours after ingestion. Sustained-release or enteric-coated preparations may have erratic absorption, and therefore, a second level of 6–8 hours post-ingestion should be checked.
3. The steps for treating pediatric iron poisoning include the following: administration of deferoxamine, a chelating agent that can remove iron from tissues and free iron from plasma; IV crystalloid infusion is then administered to correct hypovolemia and hypoperfusion; whole-bowel irrigation with polyethylene glycol solution may then clear the GI tract of iron pills before absorption.

CLINICAL CASE STUDY 19.3

1. Plummer–Vinson syndrome is defined by the classic triad of dysphagia, iron-deficiency anemia, and esophageal webs.
2. Symptoms resulting from anemia, such as weakness, pallor, fatigue, and tachycardia, may dominate the clinical picture. Furthermore, it is characterized by glossitis, angular cheilitis, and koilonychia. Spleen and thyroid enlargement may also be observed.
3. Plummer–Vinson syndrome is related to an increased risk of squamous cell carcinoma of the pharynx and the esophagus.

CHAPTER 20: IODINE DEFICIENCY

CLINICAL CASE STUDY 20.1

1. Endemic goiter is an adaptive disease produced by the persistent stimulation of the thyroid gland due to increased secretion of the thyroid-stimulating hormone (TSH) due to iodine deficiency. Small compensatory elevations in TSH prevent hypothyroidism, but the TSH stimulation causes a goiter to form.
2. Iodine deficiency is the leading cause of endemic goiter, and thyroid growth is presumed to be regulated by TSH.
3. Prevention of endemic goiter depends mainly on increasing the iodine intake of people in endemic areas. When iodine intake reaches the estimated adult minimum requirement (100–150 µg/day), the prevalence of goiter decreases.

CLINICAL CASE STUDY 20.2

1. People living far away from oceans or at higher altitudes are at a higher risk for iodine deficiency. Iodine is present as iodide in seawater. Small amounts enter the atmosphere and then fall back to earth in the rain, entering groundwater and soil near oceans. Iodine deficiency is uncommon in areas where iodized salt is used, yet it is relatively common worldwide.
2. If a severe iodine deficiency causes hypothyroidism, it can decrease fertility and increase risks for stillbirth, spontaneous abortion, and prenatal or infant mortality.
3. In areas of iodine deficiency, methods that reverse the condition include iodine supplementation of salt, oral administration of iodized oil, annual intramuscular administration of iodized oil, and iodination of water, crops, or animal fodder. Any goitrogens that are being eaten should be removed from the diet. Sometimes, suppressing the hypothalamic-pituitary axis with thyroid hormone will block TSH production, stimulating the thyroid.

CLINICAL CASE STUDY 20.3

1. Primary hypothyroidism is caused by thyroid disease, while secondary hypothyroidism is caused by hypothalamus or pituitary gland disease.
2. Though signs and symptoms of primary hypothyroidism are often slight, the most common manifestations are fluid retention and puffiness of the eyes, cold intolerance, tiredness, and mental fogginess. Organ system manifestations may be metabolic, neurologic, psychiatric, dermatologic, ocular, gastrointestinal, gynecologic, cardiovascular, or described as "other" (pleural or abdominal effusions, hoarse voice, and slow speech).
3. In females that have hypothyroidism, signs and symptoms of secondary hypothyroidism include a history of amenorrhea instead of menorrhagia and some suggestive physical differences. Secondary hypothyroidism involves the skin and hair being dry but not very coarse, skin depigmentation, macroglossia, atrophic breasts, and hypotension. The heart is smaller than usual, and serous pericardial effusions are not seen.

CHAPTER 21: COPPER DEFICIENCY AND TOXICITY

CLINICAL CASE STUDY 21.1

1. Menkes disease is a genetic condition that usually causes low copper levels in blood plasma, the liver, and the brain. The condition also reduces the activities of copper-dependent enzymes in the body.

2. The signs and symptoms of Menkes disease include being born prematurely but appearing healthy for 6–8 weeks at birth. Then, floppy muscle tone, hypotonia, seizures, slow physical development, an unstable body temperature, fair complexion, chubby cheeks, depressed nasal bridge, and bilateral large ears. Scalp hairs are sparse, brittle, stubby, hypopigmented with a steel wire-like feel. There is often extensive neurodegeneration in the brain's gray matter – delays in recognition of mother, head control, social smile, or roll-over response. Arteries in the brain may be twisted with frayed and split inner walls.

3. It is impossible to prevent Menkes disease. Suppose the patient has a family member or child with the disorder. Pregnant women may choose genetic counseling to undergo genetic testing to see if they have the gene that causes Menkes disease.

CLINICAL CASE STUDY 21.2

1. Wilson's disease is a genetic disorder that prevents the body from removing extra copper, causing copper to build up in the liver, brain, eyes, and other organs. Without treatment, high copper levels can cause life-threatening organ damage.

2. Wilson's disease is inherited as an autosomal recessive trait, which means that to develop the disease, you must inherit one copy of the defective gene from each parent.

3. Clinical manifestations of Wilson's disease primarily involve liver and brain damage, including liver cirrhosis, jaundice, dystonia, tremors, and mental disorders.

CHAPTER 22: FLUORIDE DEFICIENCY AND TOXICITY

CLINICAL CASE STUDY 22.1

1. According to fluoride poisoning data collected by the American Association of Poison Control, toothpaste ingestion remains the primary source of toxicity, followed by fluoride-containing mouthwashes and supplements. The highest proportion (more than 80%) of the cases of fluoride toxicity was reported in children below the age of 6.

2. Sometimes, children enjoy the taste of fluoridated toothpaste so much that they swallow it instead of spitting it out.

3. Treatment of fluoride toxicity involves reducing fluoride intake. Patients should refrain from drinking fluoridated water or taking fluoride supplements in areas with high fluoride water levels.

CLINICAL CASE STUDY 22.2

1. China and India have the highest prevalence of fluorosis and face the most severe harmful effects of fluorosis in the world. China is in the fluoride belt, and India contains more fluoride.

2. *Skeletal fluorosis* is characterized by occasional joint stiffness or pain and some osteosclerosis of the pelvis and vertebra.

3. There is no particular treatment for skeletal fluorosis. The longer a person is exposed to fluoride, the more it accumulates and the harder it is to reverse the effects. No effective therapeutic agent can cure skeletal fluorosis. Vitamin E and methionine prevent excessive accumulation of fluoride in the bone by reducing its impact on soft tissues. Acupuncture helps improve joint motion, relieves pain, and increases urinary fluoride.

CHAPTER 23: MISCELLANEOUS AND RARE MINERAL DISORDERS

CLINICAL CASE STUDY 23.1

1. Zinc deficiency occurs in patients who have nutritional deficiencies, chronic GI diseases, diabetes, liver disease, sickle cell disease, kidney disease, excess alcohol consumption, or HIV infection. Sometimes, newborns experience zinc deficiency if they are premature or very sick or if their mothers have mild zinc deficiency. Some people are born with zinc deficiency. A rare genetic condition called acrodermatitis enteropathica can cause severe zinc deficiency.

2. The signs and symptoms of zinc deficiency include delayed growth and sexual maturation, decreased taste sensitivity, loss of appetite, impaired vitamin A function, immune dysfunction, dermatitis, alopecia, poor wound healing, congenital disabilities, severe diarrhea, and higher occurrence of infant mortality. When the body's zinc status is compromised, the integrity of structural proteins that contain zinc is impaired in cell membranes, protein receptors, and zinc finger proteins. The proteins become unable to perform normal functions. There are mild zinc deficiencies seen in patients with Crohn's disease, patients undergoing kidney dialysis and bariatric surgery, and infants.

3. Detecting zinc deficiencies is complex because methods to assess changes in zinc status need to be revised. Measurement of zinc in blood, neutrophils, lymphocytes, and hair may be the best tool for diagnosing zinc deficiency.

CLINICAL CASE STUDY 23.2

1. The causes of hypomagnesemia include inadequate magnesium intake and absorption or increased excretion due to hypercalcemia or medications such as furosemide. Risk factors may be anorexia nervosa, starvation, alcohol use disorder, diarrhea, laxative abuse, acute pancreatitis, gastric bypass surgery, and patients receiving total parenteral nutrition.

2. The signs and symptoms of Mg deficiency include fatigue and weakness, tremors, loss of appetite, nausea and vomiting, and dysrhythmias. Symptoms of magnesium toxicity include nausea, weakness, dyspnea, extreme hypotension, malaise, coma, and death. Older patients have a higher risk of Mg toxicity because of declining kidney function. However, if left untreated, *magnesium toxicity* has a high mortality rate due to respiratory paralysis and cardiac arrest.

3. To prevent magnesium deficiency, eat a healthy, balanced diet containing magnesium-rich foods, such as leafy green vegetables. To prevent hypermagnesemia with renal impairment, the patient must avoid medications that contain magnesium, which can help prevent complications. This includes some over-the-counter antacids and laxatives.

CLINICAL CASE STUDY 23.3

1. Selenium deficiency may result from inadequate dietary intake. Many selenium-deficiency illnesses can be associated with concurrent vitamin E deficiency. The risk factors for selenium deficiency include living in low-selenium areas and eating a primarily plant-based diet. Other risks include HIV and kidney failure while undergoing dialysis. Exposure to selenium mainly occurs through food and, in some areas with seleniferous soils, through drinking water. Airborne exposure is rare; however, occupational exposure is possible with the chemical processes to recover selenium, the painting trade, and the metal industries.

2. Symptoms of selenium toxicity include diarrhea, nausea, vomiting, fatigue, changes in nails, hair loss, and impaired protein and sulfur metabolism. The upper daily limit for selenium is 400 µg.
3. Preventing selenium deficiency includes eating foods high in selenium and taking dietary supplements.

CHAPTER 24: OBESITY AND METABOLIC SYNDROME

CLINICAL CASE STUDY 24.1

1. Obesity is related to an increased risk of developing cardiovascular disorders. It changes the body's composition, affecting hemodynamics and altering heart structure. Adipose tissue produces pro-inflammatory cytokines, which can cause cardiac dysfunction and promote the formation of atherosclerotic plaques.
2. The cardiovascular disorders that are complications of obesity include atherosclerosis, dyslipidemia, hypertension, stroke, and pulmonary embolism.
3. Obesity is a risk factor for the development of postoperative complications. Obese patients experience more concomitant diseases, increased risks of wound infection, more intraoperative blood loss, and longer operation times.

CLINICAL CASE STUDY 24.2

1. Obstructive sleep apnea is the most common form, characterized by partial or complete upper airway obstructions. An uncommon condition, obstructive sleep apnea syndrome, occurs between the ages of 30 and 60.
2. Just a 10% increase in body weight was associated with an average 32% increase in the apnea-hypopnea index and a six times higher risk of developing moderate-to-severe obstructive sleep apnea. A 10% decrease in body weight was associated with a 26% decrease in the apnea-hypopnea index.
3. The causes of obstructive sleep apnea are a natural relaxation of throat muscles as sleeping begins. Additional complicating factors may include being overweight or obese, having a smaller-than-normal jaw, enlarged tonsils or adenoids that partially block breathing passages, or having a large tongue.

CLINICAL CASE STUDY 24.3

1. Breast cancer is the second most common cancer in women in the United States, and worldwide, it is the most common invasive cancer in women. Breast cancer usually involves the epithelial cells of the ducts or lobules.
2. Breast cancer is the second leading cause of cancer death in Caucasian, African-American, Asian/Pacific Islander, and American Indian/Alaska Native women. However, in Hispanic women, it is the leading cause of cancer death.
3. Having a first-degree relative (mother, sister, or daughter) with breast cancer doubles or triples the risks. However, breast cancer in more distant relatives only increases the risk slightly. If two or more first-degree relatives have breast cancer, the risk may be five to six times higher.

CHAPTER 25: ELECTROLYTE AND ACID–BASE IMBALANCE

CLINICAL CASE STUDY 25.1

1. Hypernatremia is usually caused by insufficient water consumption, severe dehydration, excessive body fluid loss (from vomiting, diarrhea, sweating, or respiratory illnesses), and corticosteroids.
2. Sodium helps control body fluids and impacts blood pressure. It is also necessary for muscle and nerve function.
3. Sodium is the principal extracellular cation. The extracellular sodium concentration averages 140 mEq/L (140 mmol/L). The intracellular sodium concentration is only at 12 mEq/L (12 mmol/L).

CLINICAL CASE STUDY 25.2

1. The heart is especially sensitive to potassium levels, and hypokalemia (or hyperkalemia) can disrupt its electrical conduction and lead to sudden death.
2. Hypomagnesemia is usually caused by alcohol use disorder, malnutrition, malabsorption, chronic diarrhea, excessive sweating, heart failure, and the use of certain diuretics or antibiotics.
3. The neurologic outcomes of alkalemia include delirium, lethargy, seizures, stupor, and tetany. The respiratory outcomes include compensatory hypoventilation with hypercapnia and hypoxemia.

CLINICAL CASE STUDY 25.3

1. Dehydration can be caused by diarrhea, vomiting, sweating, urine abnormalities, fever, an inability to consume enough fluid (such as through unconsciousness), burns, poorly controlled diabetes mellitus, and diabetes insipidus due to a deficiency of ADH.
2. When dehydration is severe, fluid replacement requires medical supervision. Without replenishment, severe progression will lead to death.
3. Hypotonic dehydration refers to decreased electrolyte concentration in the extracellular fluid. In hypotonic dehydration, the cells expand as water in the extracellular fluid moves toward the higher sodium concentration inside the cells. Reducing ECF osmolality inhibits ADH release. Less water is reabsorbed. Excess water is flushed quickly from the body via the urine – hypotonic dehydration results in severe metabolic disturbances.

CHAPTER 26: MALABSORPTION AND DIGESTIVE ENZYME DEFICIENCY

CLINICAL CASE STUDY 26.1

1. An abnormal immune reaction to eating gluten causes celiac disease. The risk factors include family history, type 1 diabetes, and Down syndrome. A higher number of GI tract infections in infants and young children may also increase the risk factor.
2. Celiac disease may be asymptomatic or symptomatic. An infant may have apathy, failure to thrive, anorexia, generalized hypotonia, pallor, abdominal distention, and muscle wasting. The stool is bulky, clay-colored, foul-smelling, and soft. Older children may have anemia or slowed growth. Anorexia, lassitude, and weakness are the most common signs in adults. The symptoms may be mild, intermittent diarrhea, steatorrhea, and weight loss. The patients often have anemia, angular stomatitis, aphthous ulcer, and glossitis.
3. Prevention requires a gluten-free diet to prevent symptoms and damage to the small intestine. All foods containing wheat, rye, or barley must be avoided.

CLINICAL CASE STUDY 26.2

1. In most cases of Crohn's disease, the distal ileum and colon are affected, though effects can occur anywhere in the GI tract. The disease starts with crypt inflammation and abscesses that can progress to tiny focal aphthoid ulcers. These mucosa lesions may form deep longitudinal and transverse ulcers and mucosal edema. This is followed by a cobblestone appearance of the intestine, spreading inflammation, lymphedema, thickening of the bowel wall and mesentery, hypertrophy, strictures, and obstruction.

2. The causes of Crohn's disease are not yet well understood, but recent research suggests deficiencies in the immune system and hereditary, genetic, and environmental causes must be considered. The disease can occur at any age, most prevalent in adolescents and adults between the ages of 15 and 35.

3. When symptoms of Crohn's disease are absent, patients can eat whole grains, fruits, and vegetables. Starting new foods one at a time, in small amounts, is essential. When symptoms are present, such as diarrhea or abdominal pain, it is necessary to avoid high-fiber foods, raw and gas-producing vegetables, most raw fruits, and beverages that contain caffeine.

CLINICAL CASE STUDY 26.3

1. The two primary causes of cystic fibrosis (CP) are alcohol use and cigarette smoking. The abdominal pain can be continual or wax and wane. The inflammation is progressive and long-lasting. Permanent damage and fibrosis scarring of the pancreas are present. Less common causes of CP include cystic fibrosis, hereditary pancreatitis, idiopathic or autoimmune pancreatitis. For example, in Nigeria, India, and Indonesia, chronic pancreatitis occurs in children and young adults of unknown causes. This is called tropical pancreatitis. CP increases the risk of developing pancreatic cancer. Excessive alcohol intake, obesity, diabetes, cigarette smoking, and family history increase risks for chronic pancreatitis.

2. Chronic pancreatitis can be challenging to diagnose. Family and medical history are essential in diagnosing this illness. Diagnostic tests include laboratory testing, imaging scans, upper endoscopy, endoscopic retrograde cholangiopancreatography, and ultrasound.

3. Chronic pancreatitis treatment includes analgesics, enzyme replacement, high-protein, high-calorie diets, and surgery such as pancreaticoduodenectomy or total pancreatectomy. Management of most complications may be done by drainage and stent placement. Celiac ganglion blockade can be performed to decrease pain. Endoscopy is often used to relieve obstruction in the pancreatic duct but only works in 60% of patients.

CHAPTER 27: CHRONIC LIVER DISEASE

CLINICAL CASE STUDY 27.1

1. The incubation period for HCV hepatitis ranges from 4 to 26 weeks, with a mean of 9 weeks.

2. About 54% of HCV cases involve intravenous drug users, who also have a high incidence of HIV infection. Multiple sex partners, needle stick injuries, and employment in medical or dental offices can lead to infection.

3. HCV is diagnosed through the detection of anti-HCV IgG. Persistent infection with recurring acute symptoms and elevated aminotransferase levels indicate the condition.

CLINICAL CASE STUDY 27.2

1. Primary liver cancer is usually discovered to be hepatocellular carcinoma, with other types being uncommon or rare. They include fibrolamellar carcinoma, cholangiocarcinoma, hepatoblastoma, and angiosarcoma.
2. The most common symptoms of liver cancer include abdominal pain, weight loss, right upper quadrant mass, and unexplainable deterioration.
3. Options for treatment of liver cancer include liver transplantation, surgical resection, ablative therapies, radiofrequency ablation, and medications (sorafenib, levatinib, regorafenib, and nivolumab). Systemic immunotherapies are quickly evolving and include atezolizumab and bevacizumab.

CLINICAL CASE STUDY 27.3

1. Risk factors of gallstones (cholelithiasis) include obesity, family history, hypertriglyceridemia, low HDL cholesterol level, middle age, female gender, use of oral contraceptives, and American Indian ancestry.
2. Epigastric and upper right abdominal pain and intolerance to fatty foods are the primary clinical manifestations of cholelithiasis. The pain can be intermittent or steady. It is usually in the right upper quadrant and radiates to the mid-upper back. Jaundice indicates that the stone is located in the common bile duct. Abdominal tenderness and fever indicate cholecystitis.
3. There is no proven way to prevent gallstones, but eating a well-balanced diet, maintaining an average weight, and exercising regularly (at least 30 minutes a day most days a week). Avoiding fatty foods won't prevent or get rid of gallstones, but it may reduce the frequency of attacks.

CHAPTER 28: NUTRITION EFFECTS ON THE NEURO-PSYCHIATRIC

CLINICAL CASE STUDY 28.1

1. Wernicke encephalopathy involves an acute onset of confusion, nystagmus, ataxia, and partial ophthalmoplegia linked to a thiamin deficiency. There may be insufficient intake or absorption of thiamin. The condition is also linked to continuous ingestion of carbohydrates. Severe alcoholism is often an underlying condition.
2. Many patients with Wernicke encephalopathy have severe autonomic dysfunction with signs of sympathetic hyperactivity, such as agitation and tremor. In some, hypoactivity may be present, signified by hypothermia, postural hypotension, and syncope.
3. For spinocerebellar ataxia, therapies include medications such as riluzole and valproic acid, botulinum toxin, and physical as well as occupational therapy. Speech therapy is also essential, as dysphagia can lead to aspiration.

CLINICAL CASE STUDY 28.2

1. Peripheral neuropathy is dysfunction of the peripheral nerves, which are the parts of the nerves distal to the root and plexus. There are varying degrees of pain, sensory disturbances, diminished deep tendon reflexes, muscle weakness and atrophy, and vasomotor symptoms. All of these can occur singularly or in various combinations.
2. Vitamin B12 deficiency may result in demyelination, damaging the myelin sheath. Nerve conduction is slowed down. Demyelination mainly heavily affects myelinated fibers and causes large-fiber sensory dysfunction.

3. Dietary vitamin B12 deficiency usually occurs from inadequate absorption, but vegans who do not take vitamin supplements can also develop it. Deficiency of vitamin B12 causes damage to the white matter of the CNS, peripheral neuropathy, and megaloblastic anemia. Subacute combined nervous system degeneration may result in demyelinating or axonal peripheral neuropathies. Later, spasticity, extensor plantar responses, increased loss of position, vibratory sensation in the legs, and ataxia will appear. Some patients develop irritability and slight depression.

CLINICAL CASE STUDY 28.3

1. Many conditions may cause ataxia, including genetics, alcohol misuse, brain degeneration, severe head injury, stroke, bacterial meningitis, multiple sclerosis, viral infection (chicken-pox and measles), hypothyroidism, mercury poisoning, and vitamin E deficiency. Ataxia with vitamin E deficiency results from gene mutations on chromosome 8.
2. Ataxia is progressive and can affect many different body systems. Some patients may develop tremors or head shaking and poor coordination of hands, arms, and legs: wide-based gait, difficulty with writing, and slow eye movements. However, emotions and intellect are not usually affected. Fatty deposits known as xanthomas may affect the Achilles tendon. In spinocerebellar ataxia, there is a loss of deep tendon reflexes, truncal and limb ataxia, loss of sensation of vibration and position, muscle weakness, ptosis, and ophthalmoplegia. Some patients have cardiomyopathy and scoliosis.
3. For spinocerebellar ataxia, therapies include medications such as riluzole and valproic acid, botulinum toxin, and physical as well as occupational therapy. Speech therapy is also essential, as dysphagia can lead to aspiration.

CHAPTER 29: EATING DISORDERS

CLINICAL CASE STUDY 29.1

1. Anorexia nervosa involves extreme weight loss, distortions of body image, and an irrational fear of weight gain and obesity. The affected person often denies their appetite and hates looking in a mirror. People with anorexia believe they are fat no matter what the truth is and what others tell them. Some people focus on body areas, such as the stomach, thighs, and buttocks, which they believe to be excessively fat.
2. Family conflict is a common underlying factor of anorexia nervosa. If a family's expectations are very high, including expectations about body weight, frustration results in arguments. Anorexic individuals often feel hopeless about human relationships and become socially isolated by family dysfunction.
3. People with anorexia have very low body weights and fear gaining any amount of weight. They have a distorted view of their weight, and their self-worth is nearly entirely based on it. There are continual thoughts about controlling food, eating, and weight while human relationships are reduced.

CLINICAL CASE STUDY 29.2

1. Regarding bulimia nervosa, up to 3% of females and more than 1% of males worldwide suffer from this disorder during their lifetime. In the United States, the estimated lifetime prevalence of bulimia nervosa is 0.3%; in women, it is 0.5%, and in men, it is 0.08%.
2. Repeated vomiting causes the majority of adverse health outcomes. The teeth become demineralized, making them painful and sensitive to temperatures and acids. Eventually, severe tooth decay occurs, with erosion from fillings, and the teeth fall out over time.

Blood potassium may be deficient because of vomiting or certain diuretics, which can disturb heart rhythm and lead to sudden death. Infections and irritation from vomiting may cause inflammation of the salivary glands. In some people, there are esophageal tears and stomach ulcers.

3. Psychological therapy is required due to high rates of depression and suicide. The patient learns self-acceptance and becomes less concerned about their weight. All-or-none thinking is reversed. Group therapy helps supply solid social support.

CLINICAL CASE STUDY 29.3

1. Binge-eating disorder (BED) is most prevalent in the severely obese and those with chronic restrictive dieting, though many binge-eaters are not obese.
2. Binge-eating disorder is currently estimated to affect 1.5% of women and 0.3% of men worldwide; a lifetime diagnosis of BED is reported by 0.6%–1.8% of women and 0.3%–0.7% of men. In adolescence, BED is even more prevalent but often transient. About 40% of binge-eaters are men and feel hungry more often than is typical. Nearly half of severe binge-eaters have clinical depression and isolate themselves.
3. Triggers for binge eating include stress, depression, and anxiety. Self-permission to eat "forbidden" foods may trigger a binge. Additional triggers include loneliness, fear, anger, alienation, rage, and frustration.

CHAPTER 30: NUTRITIONAL EFFECTS ON CANCER

CLINICAL CASE STUDY 30.1

1. The prevention of colon cancer is based on reduced caloric intake, regular exercise, avoiding tobacco products, limiting alcohol intake, reasonable amounts of calcium from dairy products, vitamin D, fruits, vegetables, whole grains, fish, low-dose aspirin, and regular colon cancer screening tests based on age, family history, and risk factors.
2. There are nearly 148,000 cases of colon cancer in the United States annually and over 53,000 deaths – mostly in people between 40 and 50 years of age. In older adults, the incidence of colon cancer is increased.
3. The 5-year survival rates for colon cancer are nearly 90% (if limited to the mucosa), 70%–80% (if there is an extension through the colon wall), 30%–50% (if there are positive lymph nodes), and less than 20% (if there is metastatic disease).

CLINICAL CASE STUDY 30.2

1. Large amounts of salt infuse foods in the preservation process, resulting in damage to the stomach lining and the development of lesions that may lead to stomach cancer. Also, many dietary salts are hidden in foods, so people may need to know how much they consume.
2. Gastric adenocarcinoma makes up 95% of malignant stomach tumors, with less common forms, including localized gastric lymphomas and leiomyosarcomas.
3. Symptoms of stomach cancer include dyspepsia, early satiety, dysphagia, weight loss, reduced strength, massive hematemesis, melena, secondary anemia from occult blood loss, jaundice, ascites, heme-positive stools, epigastric masses, lymph node enlargement, and hepatomegaly. There may be pulmonary, central nervous system, or bone metastasis.

CLINICAL CASE STUDY 30.3

1. Adenocarcinoma of the prostate gland is the most common cancer in men age 50 and older. In the United States, there are nearly 249,000 cases and over 34,000 deaths per year. Incidence increases with each decade of age, and autopsies reveal this cancer to be present in 15%–60% of men between 60 and 90 years of age. About one in every six men is diagnosed with prostate cancer.
2. Once symptoms of prostate cancer appear, they include hematuria, straining, hesitancy, weak or intermittent urine stream, incomplete emptying, terminal dribbling, renal colic, flank pain, renal dysfunction, bone pain, pathologic fractures, or spinal cord compression.
3. PSA levels, grade and stage of the tumor, patient age, any coexisting disorders, life expectancy, and patient preferences guide treatments for prostate cancer. Radical prostatectomy is considered best for patients less than 75 years of age with a tumor that is only within the prostate. Other treatments include cryotherapy, standard external beam radiation therapy, hypofractionation, and brachytherapy.

CHAPTER 31: ENVIRONMENTAL POLLUTANTS AND NUTRITION

CLINICAL CASE STUDY 31.1

1. *E. coli* is usually found in undercooked meat and raw vegetables.
2. *E. coli* bacteria produce a toxin that irritates your small intestine. The Shiga toxin is what causes foodborne illness.
3. Some people, particularly young children and older adults, may develop a life-threatening form of kidney failure called hemolytic uremic syndrome (HUS), which destroys red blood cells, leading to kidney failure.

CLINICAL CASE STUDY 31.2

1. Acute mercury compound poisoning causes burning mouth pain, salivation, severe gastroenteritis, abdominal pain, colitis, vomiting, anuria, nephrosis, and uremia.
2. Elemental mercury poisoning may occur in liquid form (ingestion or skin contact) or through mercury vapors. Ingestion of the liquid form may cause no symptoms. If it is injected intravenously, pulmonary emboli may develop. Severe pneumonitis occurs from mercury vapor inhalation.
3. Tremors, insomnia, memory loss, neuromuscular effects, headaches, and cognitive and motor dysfunction signify mercury poisoning.

CLINICAL CASE STUDY 31.3

1. Cadmium is a soft, malleable, and bluish-white metal in its elemental form. While it is a relatively widespread element, it is rarely found as a pure metal. Most often, it forms complex compounds in zinc ores.
2. Cadmium is most widely used today in nickel–cadmium rechargeable batteries. It is also found in plating on iron and steel products, plastic stabilizers, alloy elements (for lead, copper, and tin), cigarette smoke, and silver jewelry.
3. Cadmium toxicity occurs when high levels of cadmium are inhaled from the air or when contaminated food or water is consumed. In the general population, exposure to cadmium occurs primarily by eating foods grown in contaminated soil.

CHAPTER 32: NUTRITIONAL THERAPY

CLINICAL CASE STUDY 32.1

1. Total parenteral nutrition (TPN) is administered intravenously and supplies a patient's daily nutritional requirements. It can be used in hospitals or at home since TPN solutions are concentrated and can cause peripheral venous thrombosis; a central venous catheter is usually required. This type of nutrition is not for routine use in a patient with an intact GI tract.

2. A strict sterile technique is required during insertion and maintenance of the TPN line since the central venous catheter will remain in place for a long time. The TPN line is not to be used for any other purpose. External tubing must be changed every 24 hours, with the first bag of the day. In-line filters do not decrease complications. Dressings must be kept sterile. They are usually changed every 48 hours, with strict sterile techniques followed.

3. It is important to note that hyperglycemia, hypoglycemia, or liver dysfunction affects more than 90% of patients on TPN. Hyperglycemia can be avoided by monitoring plasma glucose often, adjusting the insulin dose in the TPN solution, and giving subcutaneous insulin when required. Hypoglycemia can be avoided by suddenly stopping constant concentrated infusions of dextrose. Treatment is based on the degree of hypoglycemia. Short-term hypoglycemia can be reversed with an IV of 50% dextrose. Extended hypoglycemia may require an infusion of 5% or 10% dextrose for 24 hours before TPN via the central venous catheter can be resumed. Liver complications include dysfunction, painful hepatomegaly, and hyperammonemia.

CLINICAL CASE STUDY 32.2

1. Supplementation begins by providing 30–40 kcal/kg/day and can result in weight gains of up to 1.5 kg/week in inpatient care and 0.5 kg/week in outpatient care. Oral feedings with solid foods are preferred, but many weight restoration plans include liquid supplements.

2. Long periods of starvation may have caused biochemical abnormalities in a person with anorexia nervosa, including deficiencies in proteins, micronutrients, and fatty acids. Therefore, unique dietary plans must be created so that additional problems are not generated as the imbalances are corrected. Weight should only be gained once deficiencies are corrected.

3. For recovery, patients should start by eating tiny amounts of food, gradually increasing intake. It is essential to develop a routine, eating food regularly at specific times each day, consisting of three well-balanced meals. A target weight should be set, providing a goal for the patient. A weight gain of just 0.5–1 kg/week is widely recommended, achieved by eating 3,500–7,000 extra calories per week. Daily intake of foods containing high biological value protein, such as whey, casein, and egg white, with a high concentration of essential amino acids per gram and calorie density, is recommended.

CLINICAL CASE STUDY 32.3

1. Common nutrition-related adverse effects of chemotherapy include anorexia, early satiety, taste changes, nausea, vomiting, diarrhea, mucositis or esophagitis, and constipation.

2. Since cancer and the adverse effects of chemotherapy can significantly impact nutrition status, healthcare providers must anticipate possible problems and design a plan along with the patient to prevent malnutrition and weight loss.

3. Malnutrition and weight loss can affect a cancer patient's ability to regain normal health and acceptable blood counts between cycles of chemotherapy. This can directly affect the ability to follow the treatment schedule, essential for achieving a positive outcome.

Index

Note: **Bold** page numbers refer to tables and *italic* page numbers refer to figures.

anemia (*cont.*)
  megaloblastic 219, 256
  microcytic hypochromic 251
  pernicious 257
  sickle cell 389
anencephaly 254, *255*
aneurysms 101, *102*
angina
  atypical 129
  nocturnal 129
  unstable 132–134, 465
  variant 135–136
angina inversa *see* variant angina
angina pectoris 121, 127–129
angiographically-directed intraarterial thrombolysis 162
angiography 100
  coronary 111, 130, 133, 138
angiokeratomas 177
angiomas, spider *384*
angiopathy, cerebral amyloid 158
angioscopy 101
angiotensin-converting enzyme (ACE) inhibitors 104, 105,
    115, 134, 151, 272
angiotensin II 357
angiotensin II receptor blockers (ARBs) 151
angular cheilitis 297, 302
angular stomatitis 247, *247*
anhedonia 205
anion 287, 355
anion gap 363
anisopoikilocytosis 293
anorexia 234, 321
anorexia nervosa 51, 407, 454, 485
  clinical manifestations 408, *408*, *409*
  diagnosis 408
  epidemiology 407–408
  etiology and risk factors 408
  nutritional therapy for 454
  prevention 410
  treatment 409
antibodies 52, 191
antidiuretic hormone (ADH) 265, 356
antigen 27
  carcinoembryonic 346
antihypertensive medications 54, 464
antioxidants 58, 240
antiplatelet drugs 105, 131
anxiety, obesity-related 342
apathy 188, 190, 205
aphthous ulcers 371, *372*
apical murmur 143
apnea 339
  sleep 338–340
apolipoprotein epsilon (apo E) alleles 199
apolipoproteins 89, 90
appetite 40, 62, 190, 455
arachnodactyly 219
ARBs *see* angiotensin II receptor blockers (ARBs)
areola 418
ariboflavinosis 247
arrhythmia 143
arsenicosis 438
arsenic toxicity 438–439
  clinical manifestations 439

diagnosis 439
epidemiology 439
etiology and risk factors 439
prevention 440
treatment 439–440
arteries, middle cerebral 155
arteriosclerosis, Mönckeberg 103
arteriovenous malformations (AVMs) 158, 467
arthralgia 234
arthritis, rheumatoid 278
aspartame (NutraSweet) comprises 58
asterixis 365
asthma 339
ataxia 76, 245, 402, 485
  clinical manifestations 403
  diagnosis 403
  epidemiology 402
  episodic 402
  etiology and risk factors 402
  Friedreich 222–223, 402
  prevention 403
  spinocerebellar ataxia 239, 402, 485
  treatment 403
  truncal 239
ataxic gait 434
atheroma 103
  clinical manifestations 104
  diagnosis 104
  epidemiology 103–104
  etiology and risk factors 104
  prevention 106
  treatment 104–105
atherosclerosis 94, 98, *99*, 99–100, *100*, 240, 462–464
  clinical manifestations 101
  diagnosis 101, *102*
  epidemiology 101
  etiology and risk factors 69
  prevention 103
  treatment 102
athlete triad, female 413–414
atrial natriuretic peptide 361
atrophic gastritis 292
atrophy
  cerebral 397
  testicular 388
atypical angina 129
autism 255
autologous rebuilding 419
autonomic nervous system 23
autosomal recessive enzyme 69
autosomal recessive inheritance 98
azoospermia 385

bacterial microbiota 27
"bad" high-density lipoprotein (HDL)
    cholesterol 56
balanced diet 6–7
bariatric surgery 251, 328
baroreceptors 155, 357
basal ganglia 76
basilary artery 155
BED *see* binge-eating disorder (BED)
bedsores 329
beriberi, infantile 246

For Product Safety Concerns and Information please contact our EU
representative GPSR@taylorandfrancis.com
Taylor & Francis Verlag GmbH, Kaufingerstraße 24, 80331 München, Germany

www.ingramcontent.com/pod-product-compliance
Lightning Source LLC
Chambersburg PA
CBHW060953210326
41598CB00031B/4815